Nervous Control of Cardiovascular Function

Nervous Control of Cardiovascular Function

Edited by

Walter C. Randall, Ph.D.

PROFESSOR OF PHYSIOLOGY
LOYOLA UNIVERSITY STRITCH SCHOOL OF MEDICINE

New York Oxford
OXFORD UNIVERSITY PRESS
1984

Library of Congress Cataloging in Publication Data
Main entry under title:

Nervous control of cardiovascular function.

Bibliography: p.
Includes index.
1. Heart—Innervation. 2. Nervous system,
Vasomotor. 3. Heart—Diseases. I. Randall, Walter C.
[DNLM: 1. Autonomic nervous system—Physiology. 2. Cardiovascular system—Innervation. 3. Heart—Physiology.
4. Heart conduction system. WG 202 N456]
QP113.4.N47 1984 612′.17 83-23619
ISBN 0-19-503390-6

Printed in the United States of America

Printing (last digit): 9 8 7 6 5 4 3 2 1

Preface

Just 20 years ago I was deeply involved in organizing a symposium on The Nervous Control of the Heart to be presented at the annual meeting of the American Physiological Society. A volume carrying the same title [3] and describing the papers presented at the meeting was dedicated to Dr. Carl J. Wiggers who was deeply interested in the topic but could not attend because of serious illness. He died less than two weeks later on April 29, 1963. This volume represents the continuing influence and inspiration of this giant among cardiovascular teachers and investigators.

The impetus for the 1963 symposium was the awakening of interest in central nervous control of the circulation, as discussed in Washington, D.C. in 1959, when the National Academy of Sciences brought together a small group of investigators in either cardiovascular *or* neurophysiological research. At the time, very few considered the circulation from *both* perspectives. Approximately one-hundred interested researchers and specialists were invited to attend the sessions, and discussions were open to the entire group. Relatively few new data were actually revealed at the meeting, but there was recognition of how amazingly little was known about the relationship between the brain and the heart. This recognition encouraged laboratories all over the world to actively pursue research in the field, funding became available, and recent history has seen an almost explosive development of new information and understanding about cardiovascular and neurophysiological control mechanisms. The interrelations between the two systems progressively became dramatically emphasized.

It is important to realize from our present perspective in 1983 that no more than 20% of the knowledge and technical know-how now available to the patient with serious cardiovascular disease was known at the time of the Washington meeting only 20 years ago. Intensive research in virtually every area of cardiovascular physiology has expanded knowledge of the many ways in which the nervous system regulates the heart and circulation.

Levy (2) recently illustrated this deficit in understanding of the circulation in describing the development of insight into clinical abilities to recognize and treat hypertension (in 1948) at the time of the organization of the National Institutes of Health. Very little research was being done, and the main therapeutic alternative was the rice diet. It was not clear whether hypertension was a disease, a symptom of a disease, or a possibly beneficial circulatory adaptation to aging. In fact, a popular theory at the time held that hypertension was essential to maintain critical perfusion pressure in areas like the brain, and there was concern that harm might be done if the blood pressure were lowered. The intervening generation of research has revealed much about the complexities of this disease. The involvement of the central and autonomic nervous systems in control of blood pressure, the role of kallikreins and kinins, prostaglandins, renin and angiotensin, the vessel wall and its intrinsic reactivity, the role of the heart and kidneys, and the importance of nutrition and salt and water balance have all been elaborated. There is penetrating (but still incomplete) insight into the importance of psychological and sociological factors. By selective pharmacological treatment, deaths due to clinically associated cerebrovascular disease, strokes, heart, and renal failure, have been reduced by 30 to 40%. Still, despite all that has been learned about the complexities of hypertension, its cause remains unknown in more than 95% of patients suffering from the disease.

Before 1950, cardiovascular research was confined almost exclusively to experimental animals. Following the genesis of new excitement and insights of both basic and clinical scientists, findings from the experimental laboratory were promptly tested and introduced into the practice of human medicine. Indeed, many of the new observations were made by physicians upon patients admitted to superbly instrumented hospital critical care units. The modern, well-equipped coronary care unit was born during this period and under this research emphasis. Cardiac catheterization was first conceptualized, tested, and applied. New information from "invasive" studies was translated into advanced diagnosis and treatment so soon after the original research that it was sometimes difficult to separate research from clinical application. The NIH sponsored the development and testing of such direct applications of research information to the patient through use of hospital-based concentrations of highly specialized personnel and instrumentation in dramatically new installations such as the myocardial infarction research unit (MIRU). Spectacular improvements in the management of cardiovascular disease resulted in an incredibly short period of time, and deaths from these diseases declined remarkably. Cardiovascular mortality rates in the United States fell 25% in the decade ending in 1979, and the decline continues. However, 30 million Americans still suffer from heart and vessel diseases. The cost of cardiac care was estimated at 28.5 billion dollars in 1978. This is a huge, continuing burden of disability and suffering, as well as a staggering strain upon the American economy. More than 650,000 died of coronary heart disease in 1979. Explanations for the decline in cardiovascular disease mortality include better fundamental knowledge of underlying cardiovascular mechanisms; advances in diagnosis and treatment; improvement in preventive measures; and changes in life-style such as improving one's diet, quitting smoking, and exercising regularly (1). Perhaps even more important, the quality of life that patients can expect has improved, and the productivity of literally thousands of previously doomed individuals has been greatly extended. I do not hesitate to assert that virtually *all* of these dramatically optimistic statistics stem from cardiovascular research. Therefore, it is hard to understand the current curtailment of health-related research emphasis and funding by the responsible government authorities. Given the firm information that cardiovascular diseases kill more people, many in their most productive years, than all other causes of death combined, it is difficult to rationalize decisions to cut back on the very research that has had such spectacular success during the past 20 years. Such research would appear to offer the best bargain available for tax dollar expended.

Perhaps the reader will indulge me in a brief personal expression of appreciation for this research. At the present writing I am recuperating from a recent quadruple aorto-coronary arterial bypass operation. As I sustained the unique experiences of the cardiac catheterization laboratory, a few recollections may be of interest. During the procedure, it occurred to me that I had known Drs. Andre Cournand and Dickinson Richards who initially conceived of and implemented cardiac catheterization in 1941, and that Dr. Mason Sones, who actually applied the technology to the diagnosis of human cardiac disease in the late 1950s, was a colleague and close friend on an NIH Program-project Committee for many years. The cardiologist in charge of my catheterization was among his early trainees at the Cleveland Clinic. Also, as he "cut down" to insert the Schwann-Ganz catheter, I recalled that I had participated in the NIH Site Visit to evaluate and ultimately to fund the original experiments designed to develop and test this instrument. Similarly, when I awakened from the anesthesia of the bypass surgery, I became aware of a pair of tiny lead wires protruding through my chest wall, and realized that the original use of direct pick-up electrodes (also available for direct cardiac pacing) was the product of a close friend's research, and they were first employed clinically only five or six years ago. They were vividly reminiscent of similar leads emerging from the chronic dog models employed in my own current experimental protocols. Thus, procedures now routinely employed in the modern cardiology-thoracic surgery suite, would have been considered "pie-in-the-sky" only a few years ago.

Following the catheterization, I told Dr. Gunnar, my cardiologist, that I thought I had noted evidence on the oscilloscopic monitor of relatively rich collateralization of the ventricles. He informed me that I certainly had, and that I was undoubtedly "dependent upon such collaterals since my conduit arteries were substantially occluded." My commitment to regular exercise (vigorous walking for 2–4 miles per day) for the past twelve years, following an earlier episode of myocardial ischemia, flashed through my mind. It also piqued my interest because we have not successfully demonstrated such collateral development in experimental animals whose anterior descendens are experimentally tied off while they undergo a regimen of treadmill exercise. Thus, it is abundantly clear to me that while dramatic progress has been made through research in my time, much remains to be learned. To quote from one of Dr. Cournand's classic articles, "*Knowledge is proud that it has learned so much, Wisdom is humble that it knows no more.*"

In 1977, a second volume, entitled *Neural Regulation of the Heart* (4), updated the first with information derived from cardiovascular research between 1963 and 1977, the fourteen chapters detailing new approaches and new conclusions. Many chapters in this book still stand as current understanding in their field, and there has been no attempt or intention to detract from their authoritative positions. Thus, it is not our intention to prepare a second edition of that volume. We wish, rather, to approach the research of the past several years differently, and to examine many different areas in which newly discovered facts have bearing on the neural regulation of the cardiovascular system. Examination of the table of contents reveals that the majority of chapters concern topics that were not explored previously, which now appear to represent areas in which real breakthroughs in knowledge have been, or are about to be achieved. We feel also that new insights will offer great challenges to current researchers, and hold even greater potential for direct contributions to understanding cardiovascular disease. All of the authors stand as authorities in their fields, and each has personally participated in experiments at the cutting edge of rapidly expanding cardiovascular research. The resulting chapters in this book represent up-to-the minute statements of new facts and their implications for existing concepts of neurophysiological regulation of the heart and vascular system. Each author also elaborates how, in his judgment, the new data will enhance our understanding and treatment of disease.

I wish to acknowledge the contribution of Dr. David C. Randall who read the page proofs and developed the index. Finally, I wish to thank Mrs. Bette Kalina for her secretarial assistance.

Maywood, Illinois W.C.R.

REFERENCES

1. Kannel, W. B., Meaning of the downward trend in cardiovascular mortality. *JAMA 247:* 877–80, 1982.
2. Levy, R. I., The National Heart, Lung, and Blood Institute Overview, 1980. The Director's Report to the NHLBI Advisory Council, *Circulation 65:* 217–25, 1982.
3. Randall, W.C., ed., *Nervous Control of the Heart,* Williams and Wilkins, Baltimore, Maryland, 1965.
4. Randall, W. C., ed., *Neural Regulation of the Heart,* Oxford University Press, New York, 1977.

Contents

1. Regulation of the Heart in Health and Disease
WILLIAM H. WEHRMACHER and WALTER C. RANDALL 3

2. Anatomy of the Extrinsic Efferent Autonomic Nerves and Ganglia Innervating the Mammalian Heart
J. ANDREW ARMOUR and DAVID A. HOPKINS 21

3. Selective Autonomic Innervation of the Heart
WALTER C. RANDALL 46

4. Parasympathetic Control of the Heart
MATTHEW N. LEVY and PAUL MARTIN 68

5. Adrenergic Receptors in the Heart: Pre- and Postsynaptic Mechanisms
JARL E. S. WIKBERG and ROBERT J. LEFKOWITZ 95

6. Cellular Mechanisms of Muscarinic Regulation of Cardiac Function
AUGUST M. WATANABE 130

7. Neural Modulation of Cardiac Metabolism
STEPHEN B. JONES and JOHN X. THOMAS, JR. 165

8. Neural Modulation of Coronary Blood Flow
JOHN X. THOMAS, JR., CARL E. JONES, and WALTER C. RANDALL 178

9. Subsidiary Atrial Pacemakers and Their Neural Control
WALTER C. RANDALL, STEPHEN B. JONES, STEPHEN L. LIPSIUS, and GEORGE J. ROZANSKI 199

10. Sympathetic Imbalance and Cardiac Arrhythmias
PETER J. SCHWARTZ 225

11. Neural Influences in Myocardial Ischemia: Effects of Neural Ablation
CARL E. JONES and JOHN X. THOMAS, JR. 253

12. Denervation and Reinnervation of the Heart
MICHAEL P. KAYE 278

13. Central Nervous System Regulation of the Heart: An Overview
ROBERT D. WURSTER 307

14. Spinal Cord Control of the Cardiovascular System
SUSAN M. BARMAN 321

15. Brainstem Systems Involved in Cardiovascular Regulation
GERARD L. GEBBER 346

16. Mechanisms of Cardiac Pain: Processing of Cardiac Afferent Information in Ascending Spinal Pathways
ROBERT D. FOREMAN 369

17. Neural Control of the Heart in the Intact Conscious Animal with Implications Concerning the Etiology of Cardiovascular Disease
DAVID C. RANDALL and ORVILLE A. SMITH 391

18. Neural Control of the Heart and the Coronary Circulation During Exercise
STEPHEN F. VATNER 414

19. The Rationale for Therapeutic Cardiac Denervation
WALTER C. RANDALL, JOHN X. THOMAS, JR., and ROLF M. GUNNAR 425

20. Clinical Significance of Neural Control of the Heart
THOMAS N. JAMES 435

Index 465

CONTRIBUTORS

J. ANDREW ARMOUR, M.D., Ph.D., Associate Professor, Physiology and Biophysics, Dalhousie University Faculty of Medicine, Halifax, Nova Scotia, Canada

SUSAN M. BARMAN, Ph.D., Assistant Professor, Pharmacology and Toxicology, Michigan State University, East Lansing, Michigan

ROBERT D. FOREMAN, Ph.D., Associate Professor, Physiology and Biophysics, University of Oklahoma Health Sciences Center, Oklahoma City, Oklahoma

GERARD L. GEBBER, Ph.D., Professor of Pharmacology and Toxicology, Michigan State University, East Lansing, Michigan

ROLF M. GUNNAR, M.D., Professor and Chairman of Internal Medicine and Professor of Cardiology, Loyola University Stritch School of Medicine, Maywood, Illinois

DAVID A. HOPKINS, Ph.D., Professor of Anatomy, Faculty of Medicine, Dalhousie University, Halifax, Nova Scotia, Canada

THOMAS N. JAMES, M.D., Mary Gertrude Waters Professor of Cardiology and Distinguished Professor of Medicine, University of Alabama School of Medicine, Birmingham, Alabama

CARL E. JONES, Ph.D., Professor and Chairman of Physiology, Texas College of Osteopathic Medicine, Fort Worth, Texas

STEPHEN B. JONES, Ph.D., Associate Professor of Physiology, Loyola University Stritch School of Medicine, Maywood, Illinois

MICHAEL P. KAYE, M.S., M.D., Professor and Director, Cardiovascular Research in Surgery, Mayo Clinic Foundation and Mayo Graduate School of Medicine, Rochester, Minnesota

ROBERT J. LEFKOWITZ, M.D., Professor of Medicine, Duke University Medical Center, Durham, North Carolina

MATTHEW N. LEVY, M.D., Chief, Investigative Medicine, Mt. Sinai Hospital, and Professor of Physiology, Case-Western Reserve University School of Medicine, Cleveland, Ohio

STEPHEN L. LIPSIUS, Ph.D., Associate Professor of Physiology, Loyola University Stritch School of Medicine, Maywood, Illinois

PAUL MARTIN, Ph.D., Head, Bioengineering Section, Department of Investigative Medicine, Mt. Sinai Hospital, and Professor of Physiology, Case-Western Reserve University School of Medicine, Cleveland, Ohio

DAVID C. RANDALL, Ph.D., Associate Professor of Physiology, University of Kentucky School of Medicine, Lexington, Kentucky

WALTER C. RANDALL, Ph.D., Professor of Physiology, Loyola University Stritch School of Medicine, Maywood, Illinois

George J. Rozanski, Ph.D., Research Scientist, Masonic Medical Research Laboratory, Utica, New York

Peter J. Schwartz, M.D., Associate Professor of Medicine, Centro per lo Studio della ritmie e Fisiologia Clinica, Istituto di Clinica Medica IV, Universita di Milano, CNR, Ospedale Maggiore, Milan, Italy

Orville A. Smith, Ph.D., Professor of Physiology and Director, Primate Center, University of Washington School of Medicine, Seattle, Washington

John X. Thomas, Jr., Ph.D., Assistant Professor of Physiology, Loyola University Stritch School of Medicine, Maywood, Illinois

Stephen F. Vatner, M.D., Associate Professor of Medicine, Harvard University Medical School and Peter Bent Brigham Hospital, Boston, Massachusetts

August M. Watanabe, M.D., Professor of Medicine and Pharmacology, Indiana University School of Medicine, Indianapolis, Indiana

William H. Wehrmacher, M.D., Adjunct Professor of Physiology and Clinical Professor of Medicine, Loyola University Stritch School of Medicine, Maywood, Illinois

Jarl E.S. Wikberg, M.D., Assistant Professor of Medicine, Duke University Medical Center, Durham, North Carolina

Robert D. Wurster, Ph.D., Professor of Physiology, Loyola University Stritch School of Medicine, Maywood, Illinois

Nervous Control of Cardiovascular Function

1

Regulation of the Heart in Health and Disease

WILLIAM H. WEHRMACHER and WALTER C. RANDALL

Recognition of the complex, interrelated physiological mechanisms responsible for preservation of the "milieu interne," and their dependence on the heart and vascular system requires a constantly renewing perspective for both practicing physician and basic scientist in keeping pace with the ever increasing body of fundamental knowledge. In considering cardiovascular adjustments to changing external and internal stresses, lines of distinction between a wide variety of causes and effects tend to become blurred. Emphases shift from one to the other, particularly in clinical practice where the clinical syndrome becomes the specific target for diagnostic and/or therapeutic attention. The cardiovascular system ordinarily maintains appropriate performance for the circumstances, but the response may have limits beyond which its integrity breaks down or decompensates. Although the heart appears to function independently when isolated from the body, it is actually balanced among powerful neural, humoral, and hydrostatic forces. Disturbance of critical balance impairs functional integrity [20], but appropriate interactions provide for finely tuned cardiac response throughout a lifetime of complex challenges. Those mechanisms that preserve overall integrity, as well as those that may fail and lead to life-threatening decompensations must be fully appreciated. It is a primary objective of this book to assist both the practicing physician and the cardiovascular investigator in comprehending these interrelated mechanisms and to update his understanding of recent research in neural regulation of the cardiovascular system.

The healthy heart pumps 3.5 liters of blood per square meter of body surface at rest, with heart rates varying between 60 and 100 beats per minute. Untrained subjects can increase this volume of ejection to 12 liters, and athletes to about 20 liters during exercise, with heart rates between 160 and 190 beats per minute. Such broad changes in capacity with the common challenge of

The data reported were derived from experiments supported by Grant HL 08682, The James R. DePauw Fund, Chicago Illinois, and the Bane Charitable Trust Fund, Chicago Illinois.

exercise demonstrate the remarkable adaptability of the unique cardiac pump. Adaptations to internal derangements produced by congenital abnormalities, shunts, plugs within branches of the system, injury, inflammation, and neoplastic disease are not only astonishing but absolutely essential for preservation of life. Life expectancy was 49 years in 1900 and now approaches 73 years. It should be expected to extend still further if the spectacularly successful research of this century continues. Special recognition of Federal support of health-related research through such agencies as the National Institutes of Health, National Science Foundation, and the Veterans Administration Hospital System during the period from 1950 to the present should be continued and augmented by properly stimulated private philanthropy.

Adaptation to external forces has extended to nonterrestrial environments within the past twenty years. Consider the incredibly effective adaptations which have been elaborated in the conquest of extremes of heat, cold, wet, dry, wakefulness, fatigue, anxiety, excitement, aggression, fear, frustration, sorrow, aversion, love, and delight—a remarkable range of stresses requiring unique physiologic adjustments for maintenance of the overall system. Most current operational knowledge of the cardiovascular system was totally unknown a score of years ago, and much of this will be summarized and updated by the contributors to this volume.

Looking back over the 19th century for mileposts of progress in understanding cardiovascular adaptive mechanisms, I. P. Pavlov [12] in his M.D. thesis (1883) drew attention to the four functions of the "centrifugal nerves of the heart": (1) those which inhibit (slow) the heart, (2) those which weaken its contraction, both via the vagus, (3) those which accelerate contractions, and (4) those which augment them. In 1929, Cannon [2] published a book on his concept of "fight or flight," emphasizing sympathetic reactions to stress characterized by tachycardia and hypertension. In 1957, Richter [16] extended Cannon's view of the sympathetic mechanism to stress to include a fatal parasympathetic reaction: "A phenomenon of sudden death in man, rats, and other animals, apparently resulting from hopelessness, seems to involve overactivity of the parasympathetic system." His experimental model (dewhiskered swimming wild rats) showed that the animal, hopeless because of loss of sensory clues to guide behavior, simply sank to the bottom of the vessel and died (before drowning) with bradycardia. The heart stopped in diastole—a vagal death—unless atropine was given previously, which substantially increased survival. Sudden death of captured wild animals may represent a similar phenomenon. In 1972, attention was focused on highly localized alterations in cardiac function that can be induced by excitation of small branches of the vagosympathetic nerves [13]. This recognition made the remarkably localized adaptations of the heart clear for the first time, and accounted for essential moment-to-moment adjustments in cardiac functions which could not previously be explained from classical concepts of generalized autonomic regulation.

More recently, parasympathetic reactions to stress have received attention as part of the aversion reaction with vagal components of bradycardia or even of cardiac arrest, hypotension, faintness, and vomiting. It is unlikely that these autonomic reactions occur entirely independently or in pure form, but rather appear in combinations depending on the stressor and the responsiveness of the subject to stress. Either predominant dysautonomia may prove fatal in the extreme case: sympathetic excess terminating in ventricular fibrillation and parasympathetic excess terminating in asystole.

In health, reaction to stress results in an appropriate balance among a variety of cardiocirculatory adjustments, often with overall feelings of invigoration and enthusiasm. People exercise with pleasure, seek excitement, and promote love and affection as they enter into interpersonal activities and competition. Some avoid competition because they experience symptoms of decompensation when they attempt to compete. Are they as healthy? Should one conclude that competition and athletics make one healthy or that one is able to compete because of good health? Can one expect to cure the ill person who avoids competition by forcing him to change his way of life?

The competitive choice may be one way to look at the Type A personality described by Friedman and Rosenman [15], a personality type or behavior pattern sometimes considered to be coronary disease-prone. This is the personality characterized by an intense, chronic struggle to achieve more and more in less and less time, and may be associated with exaggerated hostile reactions to others. Type-B behavior personalities lack these behavioral components. Radically different responses can be expected when stress acts upon these different types of people. Thus it is not only the stressor but also the receptivity of the stressed that must be considered in determining the response. Even those who are healthy may decompensate if stressed beyond their ability to adjust; the unhealthy decompensate with still less stress. The physician must recognize the reserves available, and be prepared to exploit these reserves but not overwhelm the system.

EXERCISE

Energy requirements for physical work are maintained by large volumes of blood flow delivered by the cardiovascular system, adequacy of pulmonary ventilation, and diffusion capacity of the lungs. Physical work increases metabolic rate, initially elevating metabolites, decreasing oxygen tension in the immediate vicinity of the working muscle, and causing local vasodilatation through autoregulation. Local receptors and central activation of autonomic activity improve the adjustments.

At the onset of physical exercise, catabolism of high-energy phosphates (ATP and creatine phosphate) utilizes oxygen stored in the blood and myoglobin, aerobically, to produce the necessary energy. Thereafter, anaerobic glycogenolysis and glycolysis produce energy with the formation of lactic acid. As oxygen is supplied, lactates are metabolized and energy stores are repleted. Cardiac output is increased by increased stroke volume and heart rate; systolic blood pressure is increased to supply the microcirculation with increased perfusion pressure throughout both systemic and pulmonary systems. Regional blood flow increases by recruitment of capillary beds not perfused at rest. Diffusion distances are shortened. Increased hydrostatic pressures and diminished reabsorption contribute to elevated extracellular fluid volume, plasma protein concentration, and colloidal osmotic pressure—a hemoconcentration. This, in turn, results in reabsorption from tissues other than the active muscles, adjustments within the venous system, and contraction of capacitance vessels consequent to sympathetic stimulation. All these combine to improve venous return to the heart and facilitate its performance.

Perhaps the circulatory system is the weakest link in any prolonged demand for aerobic transformation of energy required by vigorous muscular activity. Therefore, it is likely to show the first signs of decompensation if exercise becomes excessive. This furnishes a basis for use of exercise stress testing in noninvasive cardiovascular studies. Unless significant lung disease is present, neither the ventilatory nor diffusion capacity of the lung are likely to be limiting factors except at high altitude or in circumstances which limit oxygen intake. Actually, maximal ventilatory volumes and the transfer coefficients for oxygen transport across alveolar membranes are remarkably similar in sedentary subjects and in olympic athletes. Not so for the circulatory system; the well-trained subject adjusts his cardiac output much more quickly than does the untrained.

HYPERBARIC CONDITIONS (SUBMERSION UNDER WATER)

Barometric pressure increases as one dives beneath the water at sea level, increasing one atmosphere for each 10 meter descent. The most significant effect of the increased pressure is not on oxygen saturation of the blood or on cardiovascular function, but rather on gases trapped within the body, especially in the lung, middle ear, paranasal sinuses, and bowel. Circulatory adjustments come not with increasing compression but rather with release of the compressing force (dysbarsim) as the subject returns to normal atmospheric conditions. Equilibration of gases, and particularly nitrogen, which is only slowly removed as the pressure is reduced, may not occur smoothly and produce small bubbles, particularly in joints, to become painful (bends) or in the pulmonary circulation to disturb function (chokes). If bubbles form in the brain, severe nervous system dysfunction may evolve. Rapid ascent from hyperbaric conditions to increased altitude is particularly hazardous.

HYPOBARIC CONDITIONS (HIGH ALTITUDES)

Barometric pressure decreases approximately exponentially with distance from the earth's surface; at 18,000 ft, it is about half ordinary sea-level pressure of 760 mm Hg. Thus the oxygen pressure of moist imspired air is only 80 mm Hg at 18,000 ft in comparison to 160 mm Hg at sea level (each minus water vapor 47 mm Hg for moist air reaching the lungs). Although newcomers complain of headache, dizziness, dyspnea, palpitation, nausea, and insomnia on arrival at high altitude, this acute mountain sickness is usually dissipated promptly. Some long-term residents fail to maintain tolerance and develop chronic mountain sickness (Monge's disease), complaining of fatigue and reduced exercise tolerance associated with hypoxemia and polycythemia. The acute syndrome probably results from hypocapnia of hyperventilation associated with the hypoxemia incident with lowered atmospheric pressure. Acclimatization results from hyperventilation, polycythemia, and shift to the right in the oxygen dissociation curve. The adjustment is hampered by tendencies to pulmonary vasoconstriction, and may be complicated by high-altitude pulmonary edema, which may become life threatening. Residents at very high altitudes, as in the Peruvian Andes, make remarkable adjustments over a period of time, permitting excellent work capacity and development of astonishing athletic prowess.

STRESS OF AMBIENT TEMPERATURE

Body tempreature is ordinarily well maintained between 98 and 100° F (36.7–37.8° C) in spite of wide shifts in environmental temperature. The nude body in dry, quiet air will tolerate variations between 60 and 130° F (16–54° C) ambient temperature. Normal individuals respond to sensations of cold and heat by altering temperature of the surroundings and air flow or clothing to maintain temperature homeostasis. When compensatory mechanisms are exhausted, severe impairment may result. Heat exchanges are maintained by physical processes of radiation, conduction, convection, and vaporization (sweating). The natural insulators of the body, supplemented by clothing, contribute to heat conservation. Both the integrity and critical responsiveness of the heart and circulatory system are essential for adaptation to excessive heat. Loss of plasma volume through profuse sweating requires extensive adjustments, including altered cardiac output, splanchnic constriction, and response to decreased venous return. Decompensation is heralded by falling cardiac output, decreasing central blood volume, and cessation of sweating. Facial color changes from pink to ashen grey as core temperature rises. With acclimatization, three critical adjustments prevent decompensation: increased maximal cardiac output, decreased peak heart rate, and increased stroke volume. Oxygen delivery to muscle is increased through training; myoglobin content may increase; the density of mitochondria per unit muscle mass also increases. Thus, energy utilization is improved and heat production per unit amount of work is less in trained, acclimatized man.

Facilitating the sweating mechanism requires simultaneous cardiovascular increments in blood flow to the skin and to the exercising muscle. More blood, greatly warmed by metabolic processes, is brought to the body surface to facilitate heat loss. High ambient temperatures alone make strenuous demands upon the circulation. In dry, moderately hot environments, increased cutaneous flow is accomplished by reduction in peripheral vascular resistance. This may be accompanied by falling blood pressure with relatively little augmentation in cardiac output. Greater environmental stress, particularly when the increased temperature is accompanied by high humidity, requires greater increments in cardiac output; central venous pressure rises and the heart may be seriously challenged to maintain compensation. This is an especially challenging stress for patients with damaged cardiac compensatory reserves. The subject may become ashen and cyanotic with falling blood pressure; pulmonary edema may occur. Symptoms of congestive heart failure or angina pectoris may appear. Elderly people tolerate heat stress poorly because they lack cardiovascular reserve.

Although the cardiovascular system is essential to the cooling mechanism of the body, it is tightly coordinated with sweating in the facilitation of heat loss. As acclimatization occurs, more sweat is produced with lower sodium concentration, aldosterone secretion increases, and blood volume and total body water increase, thus facilitating heat loss by vaporization. In hot, moist environments (as in India and African tropics) people customarily facilitate loss of sweat by wearing light clothing and providing spacious areas with liberal ventilation. Contrariwise, the Bedouin in the hot, dry Arabian desert wears long, rather heavy robes to hold sweat close to the body for its continuing cooling effect. Hospitals in such areas must be constructed with recognition of these differing needs.

Fever

Since the beginning of history, fever has been associated with disease. Ancient inscriptions of the sixth century B.C. carried the symbol of a flaming brazier to denote fever and the local warmth accompanying inflammation. The four primary features of inflammation—heat, redness, swelling, and pain—were first annunciated by Celsus (first century), but specific experimental investigations of casual relations between inflammation, disease, and fever were not recognized until late in the nineteenth century. Clinically accurate temperature measurements have been available for only about 100 years. Hippocratic writings (fifth century B.C.) contained descriptions of febrile disease so accurate that it is possible to recognize malaria and bacterial pneumonia or enteric fevers as the disorders observed. However, explanations of fevers were entirely lacking at the time. Claude Bernard determined that the source of heat arose from metabolic processes, and defined the role of the autonomic nervous system in modifying heat loss. Thermoregulation was a primary model for his theory of homestasis. William Welsh, Professor of Pathology at Johns Hopkins, hypothesized that the central nervous system regulated body temperature. He also believed fevers were not necessarily harmful and that they might even be beneficial in controlling infection.

It was not until 1943 that Menkin proposed, and Bennett and Beeson demonstrated, that granulocytes in sterile lesions and exudates contain an agent that produced fever when injected intravenously. Bacterial endotoxins produced fever by activating these and other phagocytic cells to manufacture and release "endogenous pyrogen" (EP), the messenger molecule now thought to mediate all clinical fevers. Subsequent research has shown that monocytes and macrophages are also sources of EP. It now appears that no body cell normally stores transferable fever-producing substances. If, however, phagocytic cells are activated by highly specific stimuli, they may synthesize pyrogenic factors which, in turn, initiate physiological changes resulting in fever. Such a system meets criteria of an endocrine system. EP is thus believed to alter the "set point" of a thermostat-like control mechanism in the anterior hypothalamus, to initiate via neural pathways, cutaneous vasoconstriction, inhibition of sweating, and other heat loss mechanisms [8].

Frostbite

Frostbite is manifested by vasoconstrictor pallor which replaces an initial compensatory vasodilatation produced by exposure to cold. Some cells are probably frozen while others are only impaired, so that partial recovery is possible if the body is warmed and vasodilatation is induced promptly. When ischemia is severe and prolonged, thrombosis occurs in the smaller arteries with ischemic necrosis and gangrene. Both the crystallization of ice within the tissue and deprivation of blood supply contribute to frank gangrene, most commonly in fingers, toes, ears, and nose.

Total Body Hypothermia

When compensatory mechanisms fail and the body is exposed to extreme cold, the central body temperature falls and the subject may die in circulatory arrest. As failure approaches, sleepiness is likely to overcome the subject, preventing active effort to alter the unfavorable course. Metabolic processes deteriorate slowly, internal heat production fails, and the progressive course to death accelerates. Controlled hypothermia is used therapeutically to slow metabolic processes for open heart surgery.

BLOOD LOSS OR SEQUESTRATION OF BLOOD VOLUME ON HYPOTENSIVE HEMORRHAGE

Loss of less than 10% of blood volume, as in normal menstrual bleeding or blood donation, produces no fall in blood pressure because both atrial and arterial baroreceptors induce sufficient cardiac stimulation, venoconstriction, and renal vasoconstriction to completely restore pressure. However, if more than 10% total blood volume is lost, reflex mechanisms may fall short in supporting cardiac output and arterial blood pressure.

ACUTE HYPOTENSION

Clinical shock is the model of acute hypotension most frequently encountered in medical practice. Shock can be caused by hypovolemia, cardiogenic mechanisms, obstruction to blood flow, neuropathy, infection, anaphylaxis, endocrine failure, or anoxia. Hypovolemic shock may be related either to external fluid loss (hemorrhage) or to internal sequestration of fluid (soft tissue injury, ascites, intestinal obstruction, hemothorax, hemoperitoneum). The shock syndrome supervenes when cardiovascular compensation is overwhelmed, resulting in decompensation.

Many subjects normally exhibit arterial blood pressure lower than described in average tables, and systolic pressure between 85 and 110 mm Hg are commonly found; such pressures do not appear to impair life expectancy. Symptoms of tiredness, easy fatigue, or aesthenia in healthy persons with low arterial pressure do not ordinarily improve when blood pressure is artificially raised; only placebo effects have been observed. However low blood pressure caused by an underlying syndrome does respond to treatment of the syndrome. As the subnormal product of cardiac output and peripheral resistance, hypotension can be brought about by malfunction or inadequacy of (1) autoregulatory mechanisms essential for constant perfusion of each vascular bed, (2) neurogenic vasoconstrictors (alpha-adrenergic receptors on vascular smooth muscle), (3) neurogenic vasodilators (muscarinic receptors and beta-2-adrenergic receptors, possibly histaminic and others), (4) circulating and locally released vasoactive substances (prostaglandins, bradykinin, angiotensin II, catecholamines, etc.), (5) chronotropic, and (6) inotropic influences on the heart. Prolonged hypotension may result from cardiac dysfunction, vascular or neurological dysfunction, metabolic and endocrine disturbances, and drug toxicity.

Orthostatic hypotension may arise from primary degenerative disorders imparing the autonomic nervous system through the action of vasoactive drugs, from disorders of central or peripheral nervous systems, from cardiovascular deconditioning, from venous pooling in diseased veins of the lower extremities, from surgical sympathectomy, from pathologic infiltration (amyloidosis) of blood vessel walls, and from the peculiar obstruction of venous return via the inferior vena cava as in the supine hypotensive syndrome of pregnancy. *Chronic idiopathic orthostatic hypotension* (Bradbury-Eggleston syndrome) is characterized by postural hypotension without compensating tachycardia, hypohydrosis, impotence, and disturbed sphincter control. Common complaints include giddiness, presyncope, and visual disturbances on standing. The *Shy-Drager syndrome* manifests somewhat similar symptoms, but also includes degeneration within the central nervous system, particularly the basal ganglia and extrapyramidal system, dorso-motor nucleus of the vagus, pigmented brainstem nuclei, intermediolateral cell columns of the spinal cord, and the sympathetic ganglia. It is recognized as orthostatic hypotension in a patient who has characteristics of Parkinson's syndrome. *Familial Dysautonomia* (Riley Day syndrome) is a progressive, inherited autonomic instability marked by both hypotensive and hypertensive episodes associated with defective reflex control of the circulation. Almost exclusively limited to Ashkenazic Jews, it is inherited as an autosomal recessive trait, manifest shortly after birth, and progressing through life with fever, impaired pain perception, temperature and taste sensibility, impaired lacrimation, diminished deep tendon reflexes, ataxia, and susceptibility to pulmonary infections.

SYSTEMIC HYPERTENSION

As a state of sustained elevated blood pressure that affects approximately 20% of the mature population of the United States, this syndrome is identified with resetting of homeostatic mechanisms for blood pressure regulation at a substantially higher level (by definition, 150/90 mm Hg) than is expected in the healthy population. As this pressure load is carried for years, hypertrophy of the heart, accelerated sclerosis of blood vessels, and target organ damage occurs, particularly in the brain, kidney, and heart. As a result, life span is significantly shortened, but the condition can often be corrected by changes in habits and drug therapy. Systemic hypertension arises from a variety of disturbances in circulation, with either increased cardic output, peripheral resistance, or both. Compensatory mechanisms are retained when hypertension has become fixed, but rather than adjusting pressure within a normal range, it is maintained at higher than normal pressure ranges.

Early in the clinical course of hypertension, blood pressure is often only slightly (borderline) or transiently (labile) elevated. During this period, cardiac output is increased in one-third to two-thirds of the subjects consequential to increased stroke volume, heart rate, or both [17]. Some manifest only increased peripheral resistance with normal stroke volume, heart rate, and plasma volume. Overactivity of the sympathetic nervous system has been recognized frequently in the early history of hypertension, but controversy persists as to its implications. Abnormal parasympathetic response, particularly as related to baroreflexes, has received less attention, but has also been suggested from regression lines relating increased blood pressure to cardiac slowing and specific sensitivity to graded blockade by atropine. Julius et al. [7] demonstrated simultaneous increase in sympathetic and decrease in parasympathetic activity among patients with borderline hypertension. In 1975, both Chalmers [3] and Reid et al. [14] provided strong evidence for autonomic impairment, particularly in central neural connections, which they believed may represent trigger mechanisms for the initiation of hypertension.

Alternatively, one may consider retention of salt and water by the kidney [1], and increased activity of the sympathetic nervous system as the intermediary hypertensive mechanism. Guyton et al. [6] drew attention to the kidney's normal response to increased blood pressure characterized by increased sodium and water excretion, which returns blood pressure towards normal. In the hypertensive patient, a defective resetting of the pressure-natriuresis curve exists so that compensation is incomplete. The increasing renal vascular resistance, relative to renal blood flow, augments glomerular filtration rate. The resulting oncotic pressure in the peritubular capillary bed increases tubular reabsorption of sodium, thereby expanding the plasma volume and setting off a dynamic cascade increasing cardiac output and blood pressure. Such renal effects can result from intermittent, stress-induced, and sympathetically mediated vasoconstriction. This is completely compatible with the autonomic dysfunction concept of the origin of hypertension.

Regardless of the early role of elevated cardiac output in the genesis of hypertension, it ordinarily declines as peripheral resistance rises as the disease progresses. Late in the clinical course, cardiac output generally falls sufficiently to decompensate the circulation and produce a classical picture of congestive heart failure, if the course is not interrupted by such complications as cerebrovascular disease or myocardial infarction. Nonetheless, some patients may sustain high cardiac output for as long as 20 years after the onset of the syndrome.

Multifactorial Etiology

Many pathophysiologic factors act together to initiate and sustain hypertension. A final elevation in peripheral resistance with increased amounts of vascular smooth muscle and mural interstitium of collagen and other materials in the vascular walls is seldom reversed when the elevated pressure is reduced.

While not continuously manifest, hypertension generally begins in youth, has strong familial tendencies (either because of genetic factors or living habits), and is influenced by overlying environmental circumstances: stress, nutrition, salt intake, and perhaps by subclinical bacterial, viral, or immunologic processes. Experimentally, hypertension was induced by Goldblatt et al. in 1934 [5] by renal artery constriction and renal ischemia, now recognized to be associated with renin and angiotensin release. By 1956, induction by increasing amounts of sodium in the diet or the effect potentiated by administration of DOCA became another standard model for experimental hypertension. In 1963, a strain of spontaneously hypertensive rats (SHR) was developed in which the hypertension was related to elevated peripheral resistance [10]. The resistance vessels respond excessively to normal levels of humoral and neuronal stimulation as well as to a variety of artificial stimuli including barium chloride. Whether this hyperreactivity should be considered a primary or secondary cause of hypertension and whether it may be clinically applicable remain controversial.

For each of these experimental models, a human counterpart has been suggested in clinical practice (familial essential vascular hypertension, renal artery stenosis, primary aldosteronism, pheochromocytoma, and the hypertension associated with stress). Regardless of the cause in the experimental model or its human counterpart, the resulting hypertension tends to persist even after correction of the precipitating cause. Yet, modern therapy directed to the hemodynamics of hypertension which resulted from a great variety of primary causes, substantially reverses the serious injury which would otherwise occur [21].

CONGESTIVE HEART FAILURE

The healthy heart is remarkably adaptable to demands for pumping from one-third to five times the normal resting cardiac output. As the product of cardiac rate and stroke volume, about 3.5 liters/minute/sq. meter of body surface are pumped by the heart.

One speaks of the heart's *preload* as the volume of blood within the ventricle just before systole. For the normal heart, increased filling volume (and pressure) induces more vigorous contraction of the ventricle (Frank-Starling relation). Sarnoff termed this relationship heterometric autoregulation. With increased myocardial fiber stretch to optimal (approximately 2.0 microns), cardiac output increases but with further stretch as in the dilated heart, cardiac efficiency decreases.

One also speaks of the heart's *afterload* as the resistance against which the ventricle must pump, a load determined by the impedance of the aorta, resistance of the arterial tree, and viscosity of the blood. The normal heart continues to eject even more blood against existing afterloads despite greater resistance (homeometric autoregulation or the Anrep Phenomenon). The failing myocardium is unable to do so, as observed in congestive heart failure regardless of its cause.

Finally, one speaks of *contractility* or inotropic state of the heart. As inotropic influences increase (catecholamine or digitalis stimulation), augmented cardiac contractility results in greater stroke volume in the presence of a given preload or afterload; on the otherhand, impaired contractility reduces cardiac ejection capacity.

Supplementing autoregulation, several additional neuroregulators may function in congestive heart failure. Abboud and Schmid [1] suggest three separate phases: Phase I is characterized by increased plasma renin activity and aldosterone levels, associated with avid sodium retention and thirst, resulting in substantial expansion of total fluid content of the body. In this stage, increased humoral and neural drives result from reductions in arterial and intracardiac pressures (stretch receptors). Phase II also occurs early, usually within the first two weeks of developing decompensation, and is characterized by return of renin and aldosterone levels toward normal as the blood volume increases and sodium excretion is restored. This hypervolemic stage is associated with supressed neurohumoral drive, partly related to cardiac distension and activation of cardiac sensory endings. After this transiet Phase II, Phase III appears with established heart failure, and is characterized by loss of activity of cardiac sensory endings. Renin, angiotensin, aldosterone, and increased sympathoadrenal drive all increase. Vasoconstriction and antidiuretic hormone (ADH) secretion result in substantial expansion of extravascular fluid volume with impairment of overall blood flow through the constricted vascular system. It is this third phase which has received the most clinical attention, often considered teleologically as beneficial by redirecting the major blood flow to essential organs (brain and heart) and away from skin, kidneys, splanchnic organs, and skeletal muscle. Increased venous tone contributes to elevated venous pressures above normal levels to return blood to the heart. The Abboud-Schmid classification will help organize otherwise confusing data, but probably cannot be pursued as a certain chronological table of the entire process, which still requires considerable investigation.

Afferent nerves reduce neurohumoral drive to the circulation by a negative feedback mechanism. Receptors are distributed in the atria, ventricles, and pulmonary veins, as well as in well recognized sites in the carotid sinus, aortic arch, and left coronary artery. They are sensitive to stretch, but some may respond to chemicals (veratridine, nicotine, bradykinin, prostacyclin, digitalis). Receptors respond to stretch in congestive failure. Their impulses are carried in both myelinated and nonmyelinated afferents accompanying both sympathetic and parasympathetic pathways en route to the central nervous system. Here they may influence the vasomotor centers and modulate efferent sympathetic discharges that would otherwise elicit tachycardia, renin and ADH release, and vasoconstriction. These may sum to elevate arterial pressure with reflex activation of the vagi and bradycardia. These integrated functional mechanisms are all consequential to the three stages of heart failure according to the Abboud-Schmid schema [1]. Normally integrated function is not restored until congestive failure is brought under control, but normal function may be restored by different routes: correction of the cardiac overload or ischemia, upright posture in acute pulmonary edema, salt and water management, diuretics, and digitalis. The latter may produce part of its beneficial effect by restoring sensitivity to the cardiac sensory receptors. Interventions which increase vascular resistance and release renin, norepinephrine, and angiotensin may elicit opposite effects and contribute to further decompensation. The paradoxical effects of reflex mechanisms in heart failure may be considered to result from shifts in the myocardial response to a different position on its ventricular compliance curve and consequent resetting of the entire neuroregulatory system.

Thus, while the normal heart is able to compensate for tremendous differences in cardiac demand, the abnormal heart may be unable to eject even a normal resting blood volume. Valvular disease, myocardial ischemia, inflammation, tissue degeneration, excessive afterloads as in sustained hypertension, or excessive preloads resulting from shunts may all contribute to congestion and impairment in circulatory function.

SHUNTS

Abnormal communications between chambers of the heart, or between arteries and veins bypassing the capillary networks, greatly alter cardiac pumping demands, resistance to outflow, and preload upon the heart. The magnitude of these alterations is determined by (1) length and diameter of the shunt, (2) pressure differences accross the shunt, (3) compliance of the chambers and vessels, (4) resistance of the circulatory beds on either side of the shunt, and (5) cardiac pumping performance. The shunts will produce cyanosis if they direct nonoxygenated blood into the systemic circulation (tetrology of Fallot), where as a result of pulmonary hypertension, blood from the right side of the heart is misdirected into the aorta which overrides the ventricular septal defect. Shunts do not produce cyanosis when blood is directed in the opposite direction as in ordinary atrial or ventricular septal defects in the absence of outflow obstructions, but produce overloads of the heart and circulatory beds. Arteriovenous connections may be congenital but are often acquired from injuries that interrupt both artery and veins. When near the surface, such fistulae produce a pulsatile mass over which a thrill can be felt and a bruit heard. Obliteration of the fistula by compression (Branham's bradycardiac sign) is followed by prompt decrease in pulse rate, indicating prompt responsiveness of the circulatory control system.

Restoration of tachycardia following compression indicates the effectiveness of the chronotropic stimulation in compensation for the increased blood flow through the shunt.

Plugs

Emboli, thrombosis, atheromatous narrowing, and stenosis can plug many vessels in the body. As these vessels are narrowed, there is ordinarily available collateral circulation to compensate for the impairment and bypass the occluded area to again provide flow to the dependent organ. When this fails, ischemia or frank necrosis is responsible for grave consequences.

SUDDEN CARDIAC DEATH

Of the 650,000 Americans who die of ischemic heart disease, 400,000 die suddenly. Although concern about sudden cardiac death dates back at least to Lancisi (1707), modern upsurge in experimental studies date from the emphases of Pantridge and Geddes (1967) upon mobile intensive care units demonstrating effective resuscitation of patients who suddenly undergo cardiac crisis [11]. Ventricular fibrillation is generally conceded to be the common mechanism of sudden cardiac death, although asystole may be involved in many instances. Those with prolonged asystole are rarely resuscitated. After return to the community, survivors face formidable mortality statistic of 20% during the first year and 28% by the end of the second year for those who sustained infarction. Those who did not have infarction faced even worse statistics of 32% within the first year and 47% by the end of the second year. These statistics, while certainly formidable, are seen by physicians in the perspective of a situation previously acknowledged as uniformly fatal. Training of civilians in cardiopulmonary resuscitation qualifies them to support many (60–70%) potential sudden cardiac death victims until they get to a hospital. Beta-adrenrgic blocking drugs, and specifically Timolol, have been shown to reduce the incidence of sudden death following myocardial infarction [9].

Recurrence of ventricular fibrillation marks some 15% of survivors at a median interval of 17 weeks. Survival from the recurrences have also been reported (29% in a second episode; rarely from a third).

Sudden cardiac death represents a disintegration of cardioregulatory mechanisms rather than simple death of heart muscle, although most victims also have ischemic heart disease, or some form of cardiomyopathy. The Sudden Infant Death syndrome (cot death or SIDS) is the most frequent mechanism of death beginning after the neonatal period and continuing through the second year of life. It lacks demonstrable structural abnormality and is presumably a functional derangement whose mechanism remains obscure. Possible implications of autonomic nervous system dysfunction, cardiac rhythm disturbance, prolonged Q–T interval (disturbed myocardial repolarization), and idiopathic apnea have been examined. Some authorities relate sudden deaths to direct psychogenic origins as in "voodoo deaths," Bangungut among Filipino men, and

Pokurri deaths among apparently healthy Japanese soldiers during World War II. Only recently has linkage been established between sudden cardiac death and psychologic or physical stress and scientific evidence. This book presents much information relating neuroanatomical pathways and mechanisms relating to that linkage, but many fundamental questions must be resolved and research areas investigated before the chain of events is securely understood.

Sudden Death and Stress

Engle gathered 170 instances of sudden death during psychological stress from reports in the daily press and added that "people are described as dying suddenly while in the throes of fear, rage, grief, humiliation, joy . . . as far back as written records exist . . . intense emotional distress may induce sudden death"[4]. While these reports stand dramatically on their own merit, they are not suitable for statistical or epidemiological evaluation. Studies of 45,000 workers at Eastman Kodak Company highlighted the cause of death in 22 who had died suddenly, and whose background revealed they had been depressed for varying periods. Death had occurred in "a setting of acute arousal endangered by increased work activity or circumstances precipitating reactions of anxiety or anger." It was suggested that "the combination of depressive and arousal psychological states, or abrupt transition from one such state to another, may produce disharmonious responses in hormonal and autonomic systems as well as in centrally mediated behavior which are conducive to sudden death." Unfortunately, well-controlled studies are lacking.

Type A individuals, as mentioned earlier, have been considered to have "coronary disease-prone personality profiles," manifested by aggressiveness, ambitiousness, competitiveness, and time urgency [15]. A prospective study of risk factors showed that "the enhanced prognostic risk associated with hypertension and abnormal lipoprotein pattern became significant only when either or both findings occurred in a subject with type A behavior." In 1981, a Task Force at a working conference on Circulation, Neurobiology and Behavioral Medicine of the NHLBI [22] concluded that " . . . sufficient evidence exists to establish that biological factors powerfully influence cardiac vulnerability . . . This means that pursuit of neural mechanisms by which psycho-social stressors regulate cardiac vulnerability will have a scientific payoff quite independent of results obtained from research on ischemic heart disease."

Truly applicable animal models of the sudden death syndrome do not exist, but are being planned to incorporate the following characteristics: (1) ability to develop atherosclerotic plaques similar to those in man, (2) develop chronic ventricular arrhythmias, (3) spontaneously develop ventricular fibrillation, (4) possess large enough heart to permit localized electrical recordings, (5) coronary artery anatomy and ventricular conduction system similar to those in the human heart. Extensive studies on animals in the Philadelphia zoo tend to link psychological stress and coronary disease. However, even though extensive research using animal models has been proposed, essential ingredients are missing, and conclusive protocols have not yet been designed.

EMOTIONAL BEHAVIOR

Violence

An outstanding form of Cannon's "Bodily Changes in Pain, Hunger, Fear and Rage" is found in twentieth century violence. Within our lifetime the world has been almost continuously at war. In World War I, 65 million men from 29 nations fought for 4 years, leaving 8½ million dead. World War II, beginning less than a generation later, was unlike anything before: execution of more than 6 million people and 16 million known dead from combat, 100 million men under arms from 27 nations, and continuing violence for 6 years and a day, ending in uneasy peace that continues to erupt periodically throughout the world. There is an ever-present threat to engulf the entire planet and likely destroy every living thing. This is organized violence.

Unorganized violence threatens the peace and security of everyone in society. There is unbridled aggression facing almost every individual at every turn. The prison system, supposedly designed to contain violence, seems rather to incubate it, increasing the destructiveness and hazard both within and without the prison.

Charles Darwin saw aggressive emotion "as proof of the exciting nature of anger, that a man when excessively jaded will sometimes invent imaginary offences to put himself into a passion for the sake of invigorating himself." Cannon saw these reactions as adrenergic responses. With the increasing recognition of the cerebral pentopeptides, one may logically see the aggressive individual as seeking Darwin's reaction, like addiction, compatible with the known addictive properties of enkephalins that simulate the action of morphine and other opiates.

Seeking Excitement or Challenge

Common experience identifies large numbers in society who deliberately seek challenge with financial and personal risk, seek adventure with variable risk, or put themselves in peril for their lives in hazardous sport. Taggart and others report studies of race car drivers during competition, with radioelectrocardiographic monitoring to demonstrate tachycardias of 190–205 beats per minute during the racing event [19]. In later studies they found increased catecholamine and lipemia after the race, incident to endogenous triglyceride production associated with the stress of racing. Parachutists and mountain climbers show similar changes although their behavior lacks the aggressive element. Even driving a conventional motor car in busy traffic elicits elevated sympathetic activity, sometimes accompanied by repolarization phonemena mimicking those expected in coronary insufficiency. Taggert et al. (1978) demonstrated tachycardia (150–180), repolarization changes simulating those seen in coronary insufficiency, and elevated catecholamines in public speakers, including experienced lecturers and television performers. These sympathetic-like effects were ameliorated by preliminary use of beta-adrenergic blocking drugs.

Aversion

Cannon described preponderant parasympathetic activity in individuals with the emotion of aversion. Common experience includes the observation, if not the actual sensation, of faintness when viewing a particularly revolting sight: an automobile accident with people severely injured, a first experience in the cadaver dissection laboratory, the visible trauma of violence on the street, etc. Associated fainting or vasovagal collapse is manifest by pallor, bradycardia, hypotension, and sometimes nausea and vomiting [19]. All of these phenomena involve autonomic mechanisms of cardiovascular regulation.

Sexual Intercourse

In the four phases of sexual intercourse, (1) excitement-erotic sexual arousal, (2) plateau-associated with intromission, (3) orgasm, and (4) resolution, the maximum demonstrable physiological responses appear in phases 3 and 4. These consist of transient tachycardia, hypertension, and hyperventilation. These parameters progressively increase from phase 1 through phase 3 and decline equally rapidly following orgasm. This sequence occurs and reaches almost identical intensity regardless of the technique of sexual stimulation.

In subjects with underlying heart disease, there has long been concern about sudden death during intercourse, "la mort d'amour," but documentation of such episodes is remarkably sparse. Hellerstein and Friedman have estimated the physiologic stress of sexual intercourse to be 6–8 kilocalories/min, so that the patient who can walk briskly, complete the Master 2-step test, or bicycle on the ergometer at 600 kpm without symptoms, can presumably participate safely in sexual intercourse. Later investigators have confirmed these data in determining when a patient can safely resume his precoronary sexual activities. Most caution that intercourse in strange surroundings, during illicit relationships, or with other cause for uncertainty or feelings of guilt, may increase the hazard.

CORONARY INSUFFICIENCY

Renewed attention to the role of coronary artery spasm in the genesis of angina pectoris accompanies the realization that the supply–demand imbalance concept as the sole cause of angina is no longer tenable. In a group of patients subject to angina, a 12-minute stressful quiz resulted in positive responses (at least 1 mm ST segment depression) in one-third of the group [18]. The same patients showed the response at a lesser double product (heart rate × blood pressure) than was required to induce it by exercise stress testing, suggesting it was not caused by an increased physical work load. Similar conclusions were reached by others who measured coronary sinus blood flow in patients with coronary artery disease while doing difficult mental arithmetic in time to a clicking metronome. The possible mechanisms underlying transient coronary insufficiency and coronary arterial vasospasm will be examined in detail in other sections of this book.

REFERENCES

1. Abboud, F. M. and P. G. Schmid, Circulatory adjustments to heart failure. In *Heart Failure*, ed. A. P. Fishman, Washington, D.C. Hemisphere, 1978, pp. 249– 260.

2. Cannon, W. B., *Bodily Changes in Pain, Hunger, Fear and Rage*, New York, D. Appleton, 1929.
3. Chalmers, J. P., Brain amines and models of experimental hypertension, *Circ. Res. 36*: 469–480, 1975.
4. Engle, G., Sudden and rapid death during psychological stress: folklore or folk wisdom? *Ann. Int. Med. 74*: 771–782, 1971.
5. Goldblatt, H., J. Lynch, R. F. Nanzal, W. W. Summerville, Studies on experimental hypertension: I. Production of persistent elevation of systolic blood pressure by means of renal ischemia, *J. Exp. Med. 59*: 347–379, 1934.
6. Guyton, A. C., T. G. Coleman, A. W. Cowley, K. W. Scheel, R. D. Manning, R. A. Norman, Arterial pressure regulation. Overriding dominace of the kidneys in long-term regulation and hypertension, *Am. J. Med. 52*: 584–594, 1972.
7. Julius, S. and M. A. Schork, Borderline Hypertension—A critical review. *J. Chron. Diseases 23*: 723–754, 1971.
8. Lipton, J. M., *Fever*, Raven Press, New York, 1980.
9. Norwegian Multicenter Study Group, Timolol-induced reduction in mortality and reinfarction in patients surviving acute myocardial infarction, *N. Eng. J. Med. 304*: 801–807, 1981.
10. Okamoto, K. and K. Aoki, Development of a strain of spontaneously hypertensive rats, *Jap. Circ. J. 27*: 282–293, 1963.
11. Pantridge, J. F. and J. S. Geddes, A mobile intensive-care unit in management of myocardial infarction, *Lancet 2*: 271–273, 1967.
12. Pavlov, J. P., Über centrifugalen Nerven des Herzens, *Arch. f. Physiologie (Leipzig)*: 498–569, 1887.
13. Randall, W. C., J. A. Armour, W. P. Geis, D. B. Lippincott, Regional cardiac distribution of the sympathetic nerves, *Fed. Proc. 31*: 1199–1208, 1972.
14. Reid, J. L., J. A. Zivin, I. J. Kopin, Central and peripheral adrenergic mechanisms in the development of deoxycorticosterone-saline hypertension in rats, *Circ. Res. 37*: 569–579, 1975.
15. Review panel on coronary-prone behavior, Coronary prone behavior and coronary heart disease: a critical review, *Circulation 63*: 1199–1215, 1981.
16. Richter, C. P., On the phenomenon of sudden death in animals and man, *Psychosomatic Med. 19*: 191–198, 1957.
17. Safar, M., Y. Weiss, J. Levenson, G. London, P. Milliez, Hemodynamic study of 85 patients with borderline hypertension, *Am. J. Cardiol. 31*: 315–319, 1973.
18. Schiffer, F. C., L. H. Hartley, C. L. Schulman, W. H. Abelmann, Evidence for emotionally induced coronary artery spasm in patients with angina pectoris, *Br. Heart J. 44*: 62–66, 1980.
19. Taggart, P., M. Carruthers, W. Somerville, Emotions, catecholamines, and the electrocardiogram, *Cardiology 7*: 103–124, 1978.
20. Wehrmacher, W. H., J. V. Talano, M. P. Kaye, W. C. Randall, The unbalanced heart. Animal models of cardiac dysrhythmias, *Cardiology 64*: 65–74, 1979.
21. Wehrmacher, W. H., The treatment of essential hypertension, *Comp. Therapy 1*: 16–21, 1975.
22. Weiss, S. M., Sudden cardiac death/arrhythmias. Task Force Group members working conference on Circulation, Neurobiology and Behavioral Medicine, Dept. Health and Human Services, 1981.

2

Anatomy of the Extrinsic Efferent Autonomic Nerves and Ganglia Innervating the Mammalian Heart

J. ANDREW ARMOUR and DAVID A. HOPKINS

The neural regulation of the mammalian heart has been extensively investigated [25] but knowledge of the anatomy of the innervation of the heart and great vessels remains incomplete. The gross anatomy of cardiopulomonary nerves has been described on numerous occasions [12,21,29,30,32–36,40,41,45,46,50]. Present knowledge of the intrinsic innervation of the heart has been well reviewed [1,25] and will not be discussed. This chapter is concerned primarily with recent analyses of the gross and microscopic anatomy of extrinsic cardiopulmonary nerves and the locations of the cells of origin of the efferent axons in each major cardiopulmonary nerve. Although pulmonary afferents and efferents are also present to varying degrees in the thoracic autonomic nerves [2], we will refer only to the cardiac functions of these nerves.

CANINE CARDIOPULMONARY NERVES

The dog has been used widely in physiological investigations of cardiac neural control since the turn of the century [12,21,47], but the number of cardiac nerves observed has varied in both physiological and anatomical reports. In some anatomical reports only a few presumed cardiac nerves were identified [36] while in others many were described [29,47,50]. Mizeres [32–34], by combining physiological analysis with gross anatomical descriptions, presented the first widely accepted study of canine cardiac innervation. We expanded his pioneering work and described both sympathetic and parasympathetic distributions to the heart [3,4,42–45]. Recently, employing similar physiological techniques as well as histological and neuroanatomical tracing techniques, we have extended our analysis of the gross anatomy of cardiac nerves and identified the location of the cells of origin [5,18].

Supported by: Special MRC Grant SG II, MRC Grant MA-7369, and a Nova Scotia Heart Foundation Grant.
The authors wish to acknowledge the typing assistance of Marea Jones.

Gross Anatomy

Right-Sided Canine Cardiopulmonary Nerves. The extrinsic nerves and sympathetic ganglia on the right side of a dog are shown in Fig. 2-1. Because of the variations in nerve interconnections, shapes of ganglia, and locations of nerve branches, Fig. 2-1 is a composite of the most common patterns seen in dissections. We have used Mizeres' terminology [32,33,34] with the addition of terms relating to the branches of nerves from the middle cervical ganglion [5]. This terminology is based on both the gross anatomy and histological reconstructions of the ganglia. It should be kept in mind that in the living state the nerves and ganglia are surrounded by extensive connective tissue so that the nerves may appear to be much larger than they really are.

The stellate ganglion is a fusion of the inferior cervical ganglion and the first thoracic ganglion. On the basis of tracing the origin of the rami, the T2 ganglion is also a part of the stellate ganglion (Figs. 2-1 and 2-2). This is also apparent in serial histological sections of this ganglion (see Fig. 2-9). Axons terminating in or passing through the stellate ganglion originate in preganglionic neurons in the spinal cord from the C7 to the T5 segments [22,26,37,54].

The right middle cervical ganglion is located cranially in the thorax, usually dorsomedial to the vagus on the right side as it enters the thorax. Histological analysis demonstrated that the middle cervical ganglion is intimately related to the vagal trunk and has a major nerve arising from its cranial pole—the cranial pole nerve (Figs. 2-6, 2-8 and 2-10). The vagal and sympathetic nerves cranial to the middle cervical ganglion form the vagosympathetic trunk [17]. The right superior cervical ganglion usually lies dorsomedial and slightly cranial to the right nodose ganglion. In addition to these major ganglia, smaller mediastinal ganglia were frequently encountered.

Although a number of authors describe nerves arising from the thoracic sympathetic chain which innervate the heart [29,36,47], none were found in our investigations (Fig. 2-1). On the right side the ansae subclavia originate close to each other at the cranial pole of the stellate ganglion. The ventral ansa courses ventral to the subclavian artery and interconnects with the thoracic vagus at the same level as the stellate ganglion. The dorsal ansa lies dorsal to the subclavian artery and courses cranially for a few centimeters before entering the middle cervical ganglion. The ventral ansa usually gives rise to three branches. The first branch is small. A small cluster of neurons is frequently located near its origin. This nerve and its associated ganglion may originate at variable positions along the length of the ventral ansa. It has previously been named the right stellate cardiac nerve and its course in the mediastinum has been described [3,34,45]. We have designated this nerve the right interganglionic nerve because of its origin and the fact that it contains axons from cell bodies in both the middle cervical and stellate ganglia [5]. Similar considerations have required the modification of terminology with respect to other nerves as well [5]. Another branch of the ventral ansa usually courses horizontally and dorsally behind the vagus, but it may on occasion lie ventral to the vagus. It unites with a vagal branch arising at the same level of the vagus and courses toward the heart between the superior vena cava and aorta as the cranial vagal nerve. The cranial vagal nerve contains both sympathetic [42,45] and parasympathetic [4] fibers, as shown by tracing the cells of origin of its axons (Table 2-1). A third branch of the ventral ansa courses cranially just lateral to the vagus with which it is interconnected. At the level of the middle cervical ganglion this portion of the ventral ansa usually, but not always, passes dorsal to the vagus before entering the middle cervical ganglion. Just cranial to this junction the dorsal ansa joins the ganglion. The right internal thoracic nerve arises from the middle cervical ganglion and courses laterally to associate with the internal thoracic artery. The right medial nerve courses medially to innervate medial mediastinal structures. The right

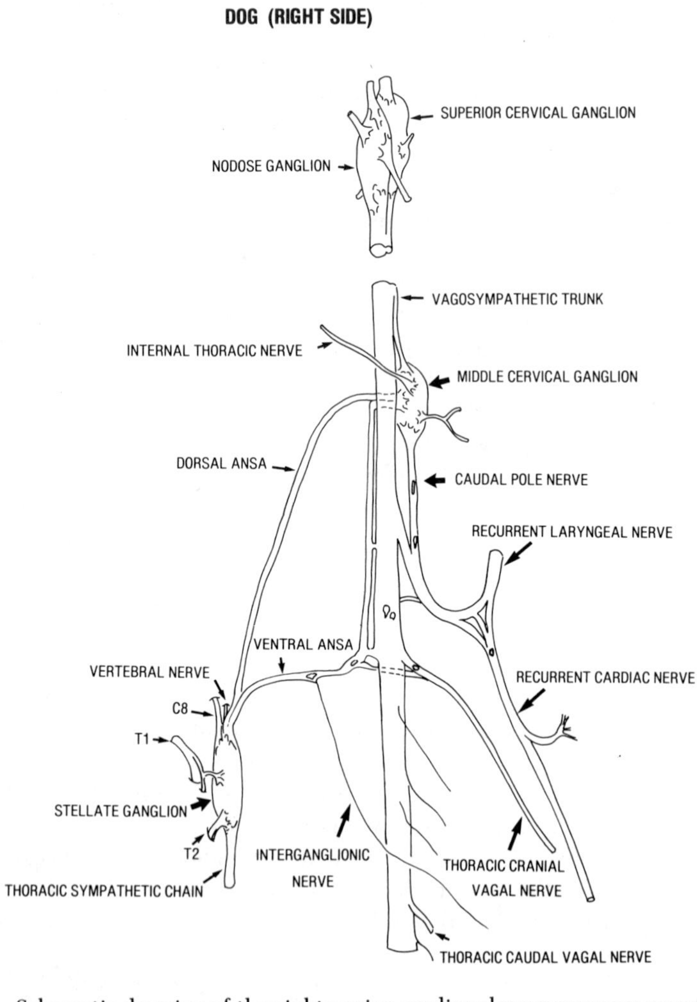

Fig. 2-1. Schematic drawing of the right canine cardiopulmonary nerves seen from the ventral aspect. The outlines of smaller ganglia are indicated in the nerves. This drawing represents a composite of the anatomy observed in many dogs.

cranial pole nerve (cervical sympathetic trunk) joins the vagus in a common sheath to form the vagosympathetic complex. The vagosympathetic complex extends cranially with substantial intermixing of vagal and sympathetic fibers occurring before it joins the nodose and superior cervical ganglia. A number of nerves arise from these structures [6,9].

The right recurrent cardiac nerve consists of a complex arrangement of nerves. The right caudal pole nerve arises from the caudal pole of the right middle cervical ganglion and often contains a ganglion one or two centimeters

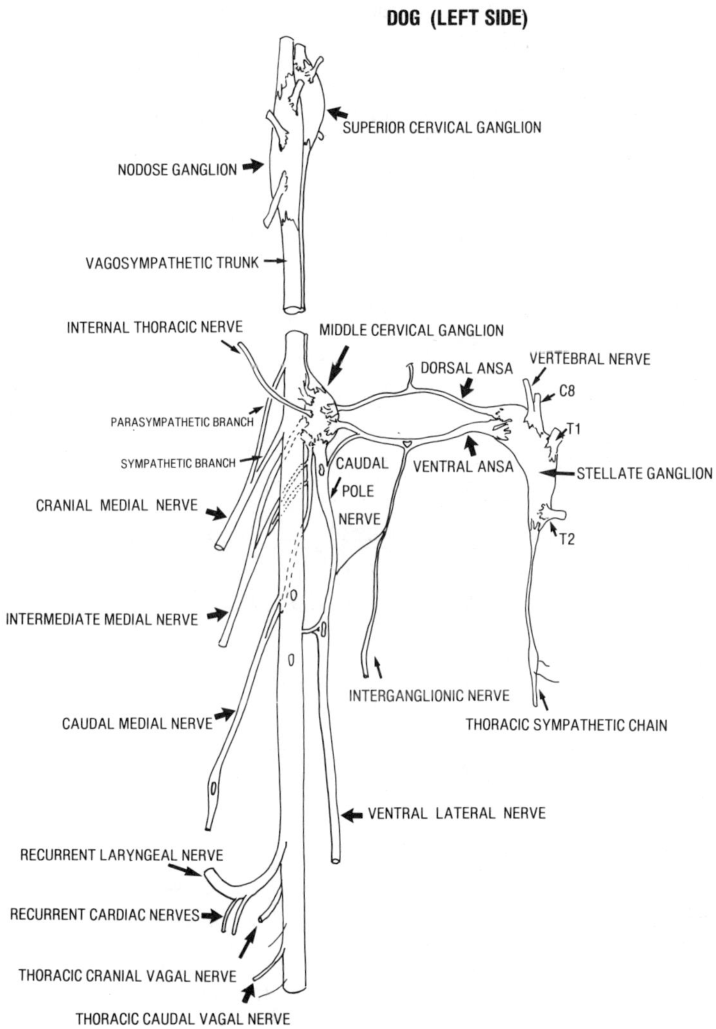

Fig. 2-2. Schematic drawing of the left canine cardiopulmonary nerves seen from the ventral aspect. Note the numerous interconnections between nerves and the presence of small ganglia in these nerves.

Table 2-1. Summary of injected nerves and distribution of retrogradely labeled neurons in the ipsilateral medulla oblongata and the major ipsilateral sympathetic ganglia

Injected cardiac nerve	Dog no.	HRP (μl)	Dorsal motor nucleus	Intermediate zone	Nucleus ambiguus
Left interganglionic nerve	45	11	0	0	0
Left cranial	19	25	0	0	0
medial nerve	49	10	0	0	0
Left caudal	27	20	+[a]	0	+
medial nerve	29	4	+	+	+
	41	15	++	0	++
	43	6	0	0	0
	46	10	0	0	0
Left caudal	33	10	0	0	0
pole nerve	44	20	0	0	0
	48	6	0	0	0
Left cranial	16	20	0	0	0
vagal nerve	21	15	++	0	++
	22	25	++	0	+++
	28	20	++	+	+++
	30	5	+	+	+
Left recurrent	17	25	+++	++	++++
cardiac nerve	18	10	+	0	0
	20	25	+++	++	++++
	23	10	0	0	++
	32	15	++	0	++
Right interganglionic nerve	35	5	0	0	0
	38	3	0	0	0
Right recurrent	2	15	++	+	++
cardiac nerve	4	10	0	+	++
(Caudal pole	5	8	+++	++	++
nerve and vagal	36	15	+	0	+
branches)	37	4	0	0	+
Right cranial	6	10	+	0	++
vagal nerve	7	10	0	0	+
	11	10	0	0	++
	14	15	0	+	++
	31	6	0	0	+
Right caudal	8	10	0	0	+
vagal nerve	10	3	0	0	++
	13	4	0	0	+
	15	3	++	+	++
	40	8	0	0	+

Cells per nucleus ganglion: [a]+, 1–10; [b]++, 10–100; [c]+++, 100–1000; [d]++++, over 1000; [e]—, tissue not obtained.

Ventrolateral nucleus ambiguus	Superior cervical ganglion	Middle cervical ganglion	Stellate ganglion ganglion	Caudal pole nerve ganglion	Mediastinal ganglion
0	0	+++	++++	0	+
0	++	++++	+++	—	—
0	+	+++[c]	+++	++	—
++[b]	—	++	0	0	0
++	+	++++[d]	++	—[e]	—
++	0	++++	++	—	—
0	+	+++	0	—	—
+	+	++++	++	0	—
0	0	++++	++	—	—
0	+	++++	++	++	—
0	++	++++	+++	+++	—
0	0	++	0	—	—
++	0	++	0	—	—
++	0	++	0	—	—
+++	0	0	0	—	—
++	+	+++	—	—	—
+++	0	++++	0	—	++
0	0	0	0	—	—
+++	—	0	0	—	—
++	0	0	0	—	—
++	+	++	—	—	—

0	0	++	+	0	—
+	0	+++	++	—	—
++	—	++++	—	—	—
+++	—	++	0	—	—
++	+	—	++	—	—
++	+	++++	++	++	—
++	++	++++	++	—	—
+++	0	0	0	—	—
++	0	0	0	—	—
+++	0	0	0	—	—
++	—	0	0	—	—
++	0	—	++	—	—
++	—	0	0	—	—
++	—	0	0	—	—
++	—	0	0	—	—
+++	—	0	0	—	—
++	+	++++	+++	—	—

from the middle cervical ganglion (Figs. 2-1 and 2-10; ref. 5). This nerve courses caudally and unites with sizeable branches originating from the recurrent laryngeal and vagus nerves. In keeping with this anatomical arrangement, physiological results show that both sympathetic and parasympathetic fibers are carried by the recurrent cardiac nerve [3]. Also an injection of HRP in this nerve labelled both vagal and sympathetic neurons (Table 2-1). The right caudal vagal nerve is a major branch which arises from the vagus caudal to the origin of the cranial vagal nerve and above the level of the azygous vein (Fig. 2-1). There are also a number of very small branches arising from the vagus between the level of the origin of the cranial vagal nerve to below the level of the azygous vein. Although these branches are small they can exert profound effects on the heart [4,43,44].

Left-Sided Canine Cardiopulmonary Nerves. The left-sided thoracic autonomic nerves and ganglia in the dog appear to differ from right-sided ones but with respect to their origins from the ganglia and their connections there are certain similarities. The left stellate ganglion is thick with an enlarged cranial region (Fig. 2-2). Because the majority of the left cardiopulmonary nerves arises from the middle cervical ganglion they have been named in accordance with their site of origin. This terminology describes their anatomy in the immediate vicinity of the middle cervical ganglion. Caudally the nerves unite to form the cardiopulmonary nerves which have considerable variability [3,32,33,36,45]. Major interconnections exist between the thoracic vagus and the middle cervical ganglion (Fig. 2-2). The thoracic vagus and middle cervical ganglion are usually bound within one sheath, the ganglion most frequently being dorsal and lateral to the vagus. Occasionally the left middle cervical ganglion is separate from the vagus and lies lateral to the vagus. The cranial pole nerve arises from the middle cervical ganglion and forms, with the thoracic vagus, the left cervical vagosympathetic complex. There are a number of interconnections between the vagus and nerves arising from the middle cervical ganglion. For instance, the left caudal pole nerve which arises from the caudal pole of the middle cervical ganglion often receives a contribution from the ventral ansa. Within one or two centimeters of the point of origin the caudal pole nerve, a ganglion is frequently present (Fig. 2-2; ref. 5). After interconnecting with the thoracic vagus a few centimeters from its origin, this nerve then courses toward the heart as the ventral lateral cardiac nerve. A ganglion is often present at the point where the vagal branch joins the caudal pole nerve. The caudal medial nerve normally unites with a vagal branch and may also have a ganglion along its course. Arising just cranial to the caudal medial nerve is the intermediate medial nerve. Finally, another nerve arises from the middle cervical ganglion cranial to the latter nerve, the cranial medial nerve. It usually unites with a distinct branch from the vagus (Fig. 2-2).

Microscopic Anatomy and Cells of Origin of Cardiopulmonary Nerves

Parasympathetic Preganglionic Neurons. Recent research in a variety of spe-

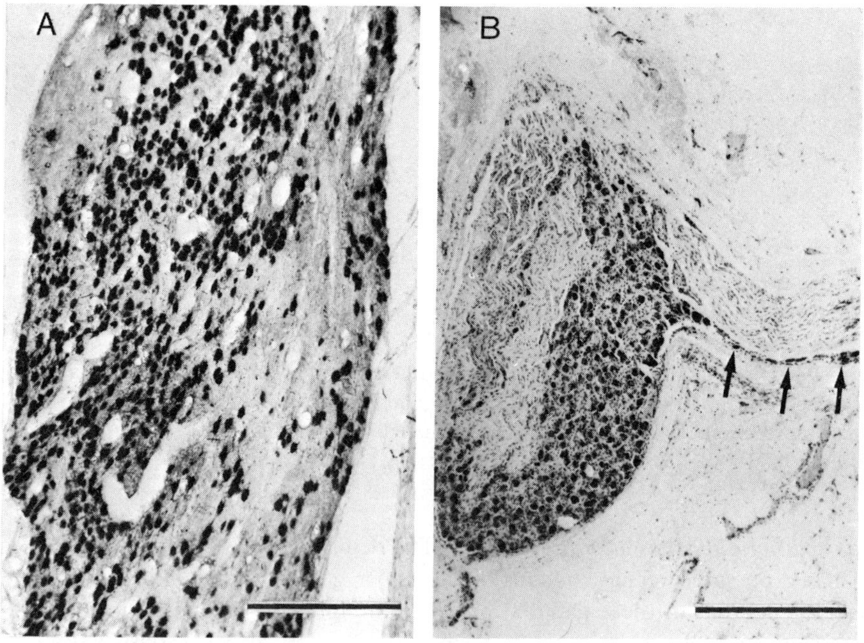

Fig. 2-3. (A) Photomicrograph of the right middle cervical ganglion following injection of HRP into the right recurrent cardiac nerve in dog 36. This section corresponds approximately to level 7 in Fig. 2-10. Neutral red counterstain. (B) Photomicrograph of a right mediastinal ganglion located near the origin of the cranial vagal nerve in a dog. Note the cell bodies tracking along a nerve (arrows). Cresyl violet stain. Calibration: A = 500 μm; B = 500 μm.

cies has shown that the medullary cells of origin of vagal fibers innervating the heart are located in four regions of the medulla oblongata [10,11,14–16,19,20,24,27,28,38,49,51]. These regions are the dorsal motor nucleus of the vagus nerve (DMV), an intermediate zone (IZ), the nucleus ambiguus (NA), and an area ventrolateral to the NA. Injections of horseradish peroxidase (HRP) into physiologically identified cardiac nerves has confirmed this general picture in the dog [18]. Table 2-1 summarizes the distribution in the medulla of the cells of origin of canine cardiac nerves identified physiologically in 38 separate experiments. These labeled cells were most numerous in the NA and a region ventrolateral to the NA, which we have designated the ventrolateral nucleus ambiguus (VLNA). In many cases more labeled neurons were located in the VLNA than in the NA, and the DMV was also labeled, as was an intermediate zone. Injection of HRP into some nerves, in which stimulation elicited both chronotropic and inotropic changes, resulted in labeling which was restricted to the NA and VLNA (Fig. 2-4). Therefore, it is likely that neurons in the NA and VLNA can control both chronotropism and inotropism.

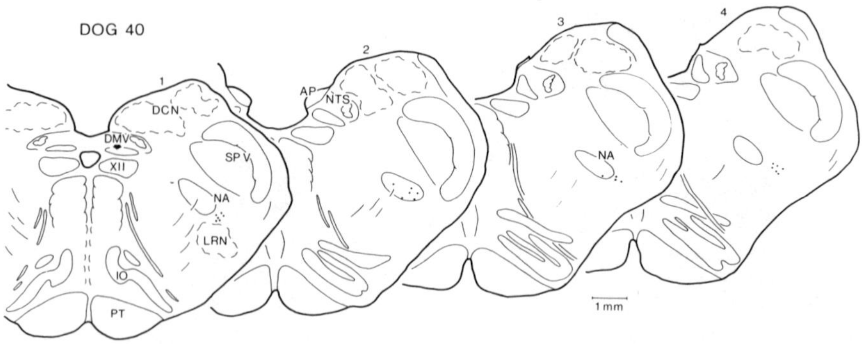

Fig. 2-4. Distribution of retrogradely labeled neurons in the medulla oblongata of dog 40. Each dot represents one labeled neuron and in each section the labeling in seven adjacent sections is represented. (Reproduced by permission of Brain Research Bulletin)

Sympathetic Postganglionic Neurons. The description in the following section is based on serial reconstructions of the major ganglia and the distribution of labeled neurons in those ganglia following the injection of horseradish peroxidase into physiologically identified cardiac nerves [5]. Serial reconstructions of the ganglia revealed details of the morphology and the locations of nerve branches. The right stellate ganglion is usually long and thin (Fig. 2-9), while the left one typically has an enlarged cranial pole (Fig. 2-2; ref. 5). The middle cervical ganglia are usually oblong in shape with major nerves arising from the cranial and caudal poles (Figs. 2-6, 2-8, and 2-10). These ganglia are generally intimately related to the thoracic vagus nerve, with which they have major interconnections (Figs. 2-6 and 2-10).

The sympathetic postganglionic neurons which project efferents into the cardiopulomonary nerves are located primarily in the middle cervical ganglia (Fig. 2-3A; Table 2-1), as has been suspected for some time [53]. Relatively few sympathetic neurons in the canine superior cervical ganglia are labelled following HRP injections into individual cardiopulmonary nerves. In the stellate ganglia

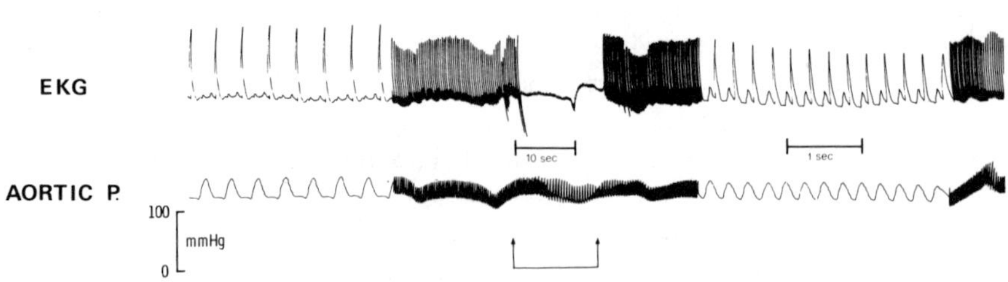

Fig. 2-5. Physiological responses obtained before, during (between arrows) and after stimulation of the right interganglionic nerve in dog 35. Note that the heart rate and the amplitude of the P wave increased.

labeled cells were clustered primarily in the cranial medial region (Fig. 2-8). Neurons which innervate the heart and lungs can be found in other thoracic neural elements as well. Previous anatomical investigations have reported the presence of neurons within the thoracic vagus [6], sympathetic nerves [31,45], or mediastinal ganglia [45], but studies of their connectivity or function have not been done. They have been detected by physiological investigations as well [8,52,53]. We located clusters of neurons in the caudal pole nerves (Figs. 2-2, 2-10 and 2-11) and at the site of origin of the interganglionic nerves (Figs. 2-1 and 2-2). Clusters of neurons have also been found in the right recurrent cardiac nerve, near the origin of the right cranial vagal nerve (Fig. 2-3B) and along the left medial nerves.

By combining physiological and neuroanatomical tracing techniques it is possible to relate function and anatomy of the extrinsic cardiac nerves. For example, the right interganglionic nerve increases heart rate and shifts the pacemaker (Fig. 2-5; refs. 3,42). Following injection of HRP into the right interganglionic nerve of one dog, labeled neurons were found scattered throughout the right middle cervical ganglion (Fig. 2-6) but only three labeled

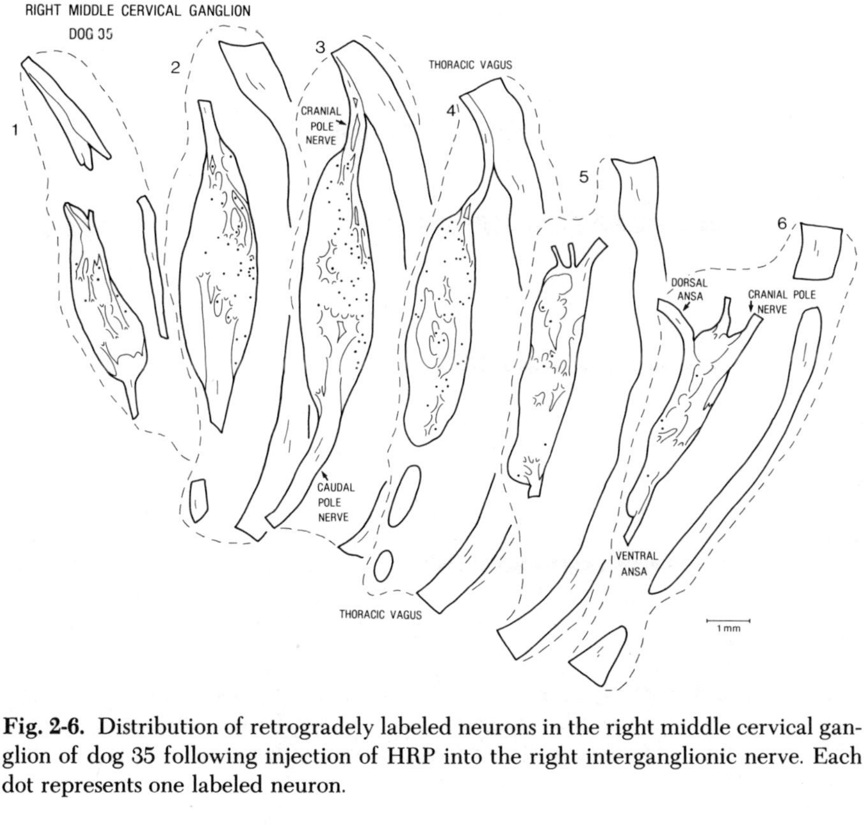

Fig. 2-6. Distribution of retrogradely labeled neurons in the right middle cervical ganglion of dog 35 following injection of HRP into the right interganglionic nerve. Each dot represents one labeled neuron.

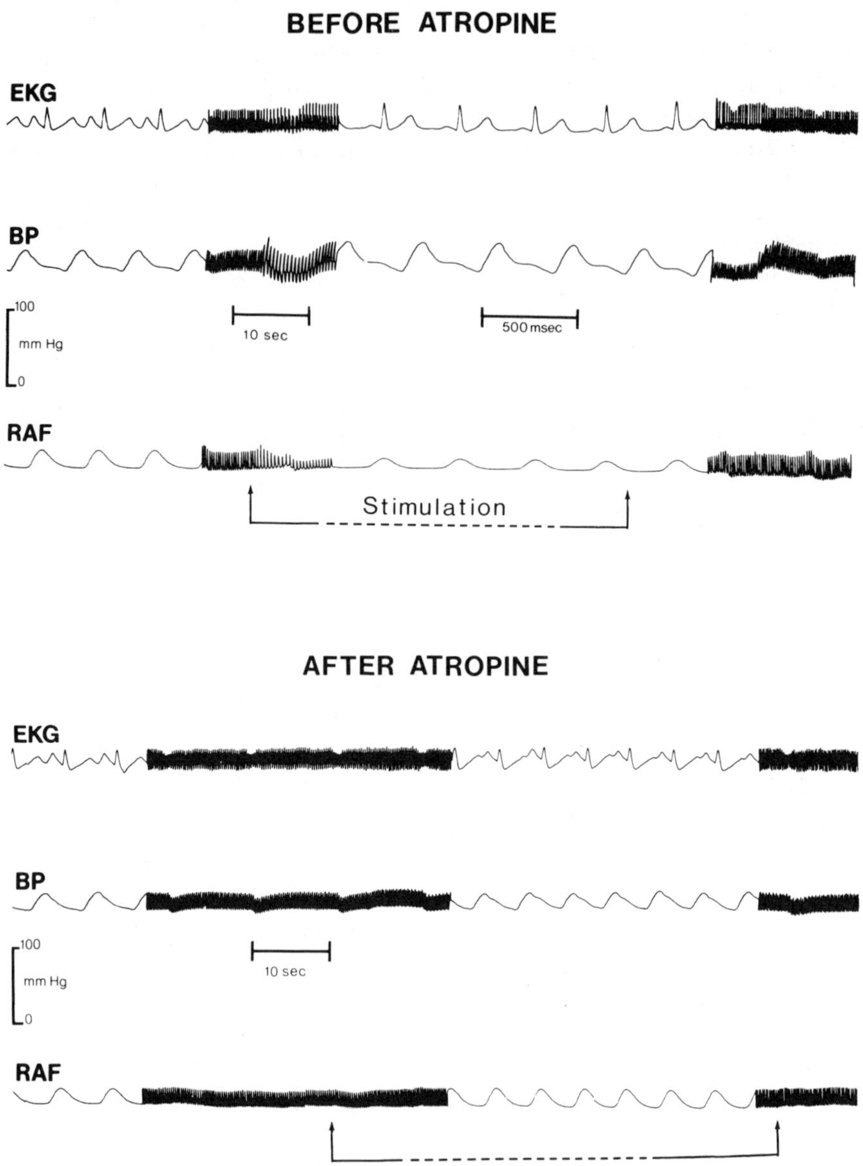

Fig. 2-7. Physiological responses obtained by stimulation (between arrows) of the right caudal vagal nerve before (upper panel) and after (lower panel) atropine in dog 40. This demonstrated the relative effects of the parasympathetic and sympathetic components in this nerve.

neurons were observed in the right stellate ganglion. Thus, although this nerve usually arises from the ventral ansa, frequently near the stellate ganglion [3,45], its cells of origin are in the ipsilateral middle cervical and stellate ganglia [5].

The right recurrent cardiac nerve axons arise from neurons predominantly in the middle cervical ganglion. Cells in small mediastinal ganglia and the stellate ganglion also contribute to the right recurrent cardiac nerve (Table 2-1; Fig. 2-10). When a mixed efferent nerve (sympathetic and parasympathetic), such as the right cranial vagal nerve, was stimulated, bradycardia and negative inotropism of the atrium were elicited. Following atropinization, stimulation of this nerve elicited tachycardia and atrial force augmentation (Fig. 2-7), as would be expected due to activation of sympathetic fibers in this nerve. An injection of HRP into this nerve resulted in labeled cells in the sympathetic ganglia and the medulla oblongata. Cells in the medulla were present mainly in the ipsilateral VLNA (Table 2-1). Labeled sympathetic cells were scattered throughout the right middle cervical ganglion (Fig. 2-8) and very few labeled neurons were present in the right stellate ganglion (Fig. 2-9).

When the left sided cardiopulmonary nerves were injected with HRP a similar picture emerged. Labeled cells were found primarily in the left middle cervical ganglion and the majority of cells in the stellate ganglion were located in its cranial medial portion [5]. The superior cervical ganglion contained a few labeled cells which were present primarily in the caudal pole. This distribution appears to be similar to that reported when the rat cervical sympathetic trunk was injected with HRP [7].

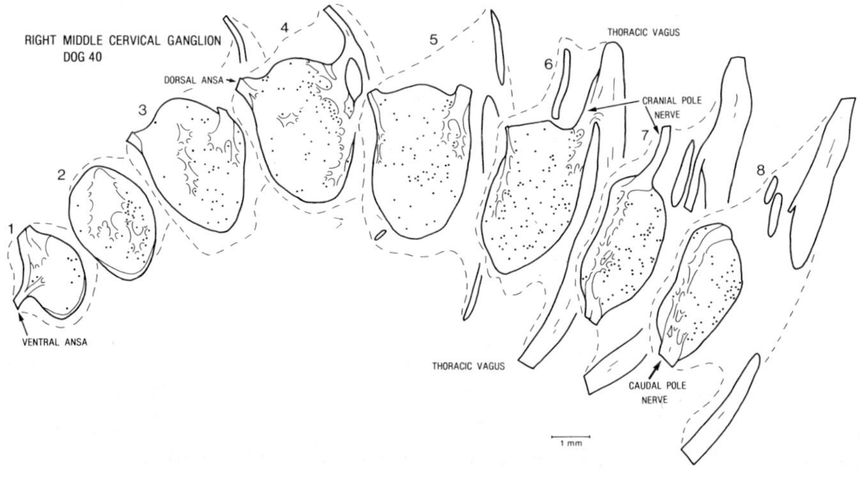

Fig. 2-8. Distribution of retrogradely labeled neurons in the right middle cervical ganglion of dog 40 following injection of HRP into the right caudal vagal nerve. (Reproduced by permission of the Journal of Comparative Neurology)

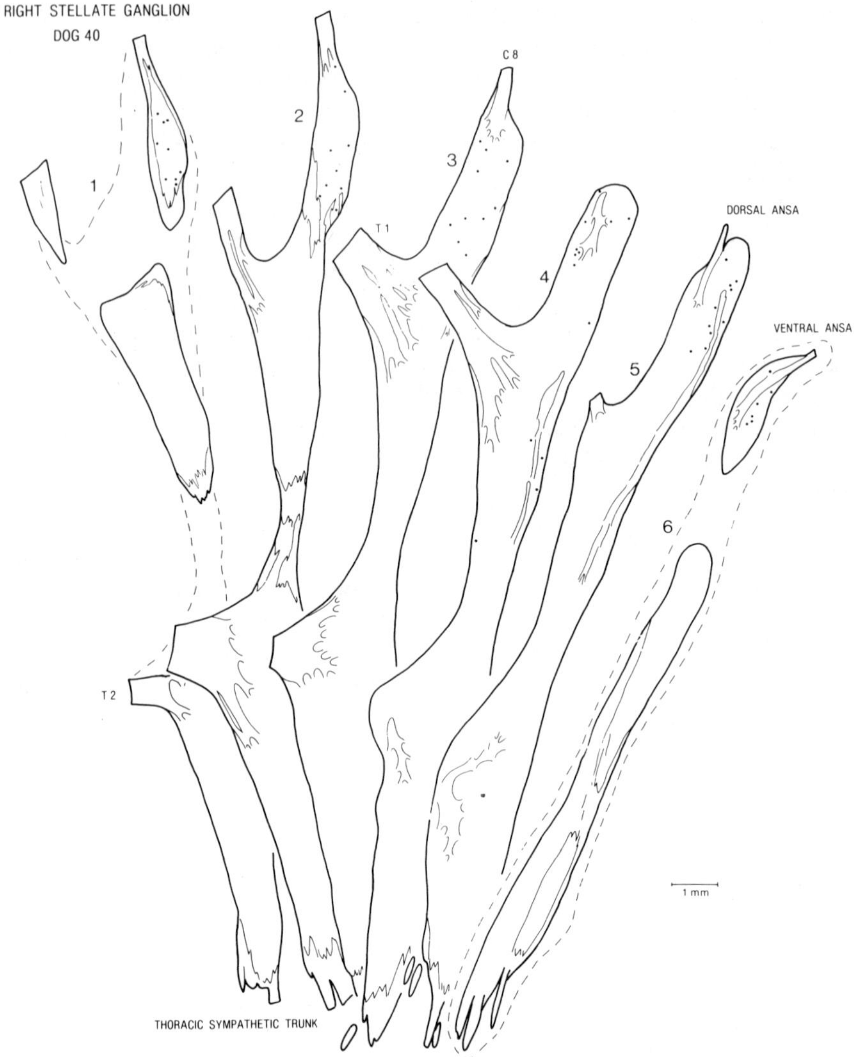

Fig. 2-9. Distribution of retrogradely labeled neurons in the right stellate ganglion in dog 40.

In summary, the majority of the vagal preganglionic neurons which innervate the canine heart and lung were located in the NA and VLNA. The majority of postganglionic sympathetic neurons were located in the middle cervical ganglia. Fewer were located in the stellate ganglia and relatively small numbers were located in the superior cervical ganglion. The most unexpected finding was the presence of labeled neurons outside these three major ganglia in mediastinal ganglia. No cells were located in contralateral ganglia.

Electrophysiology of Canine Cardiopulmonary Nerves

When thoracic neural elements (ganglia and nerves) are stimulated electrically, compound action potentials can be recorded from the various cardiopulmonary nerves. For instance when the caudal pole nerve was stimulated at different loci along its course, while recording with bipolar electrodes at its caudal end near the heart, changes in configuration and time of onset of evoked compound action potentials were recorded (Fig. 2-11). The decentralized middle cervical ganglion (MCG) was stimulated at its caudal pole (Fig. 2-11, site 1) while

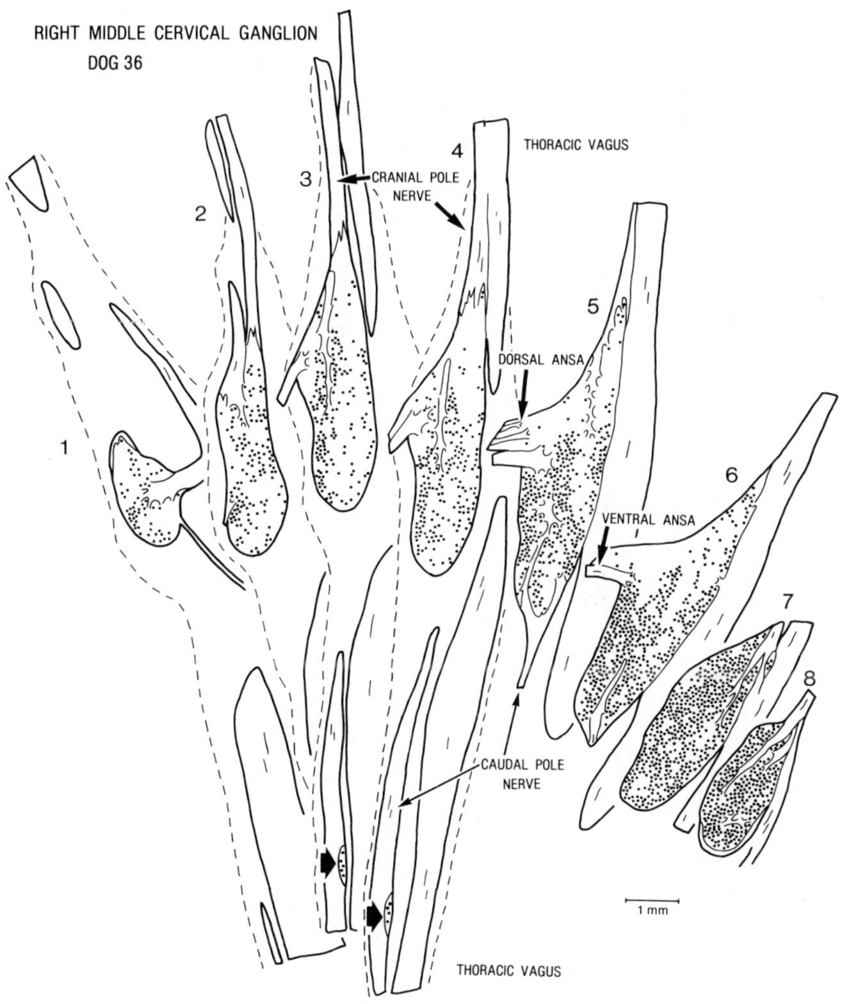

Fig. 2-10. Distribution of retrogradely labeled neurons in the right middle cervical ganglion in dog 36. Note the presence of labeled cells in the caudal pole nerve ganglion (large arrows). (Reproduced by permission of the Journal of Comparative Neurology)

recording from the caudal pole nerve 45 mm from the stimulation site. The onset of the single compound action potential occurred 50 msec after the stimulus (trace 1). The onset time of the compound action potential shifted slightly when the stimulus site was 29 mm from the recording site or 16 mm down the nerve from the caudal pole of the MCG (site 2). However, when the stimulus was moved a further 2 mm (site 3, 18 mm from the caudal pole of the MCG) the compound action potential had two peaks and the onset of the first one was about 36 msec after the stimulus. By stimulating another 2 mm down the nerve (site 4, 20 mm from the caudal pole of the MCG and 25 mm from the recording site) the compound action potential was more complex, its onset occurring after a delay of about 32 msec. When the nerve was stimulated another 2 mm closer to the recording site (site 5, 22 mm from the caudal pole of the MCG) the onset of the compound action potential occurred 28 msec after the stimulus. When the stimulus site was moved 28 mm from the caudal pole of the MCG and 17 mm from the recording site (site 6) the compound action potential started about

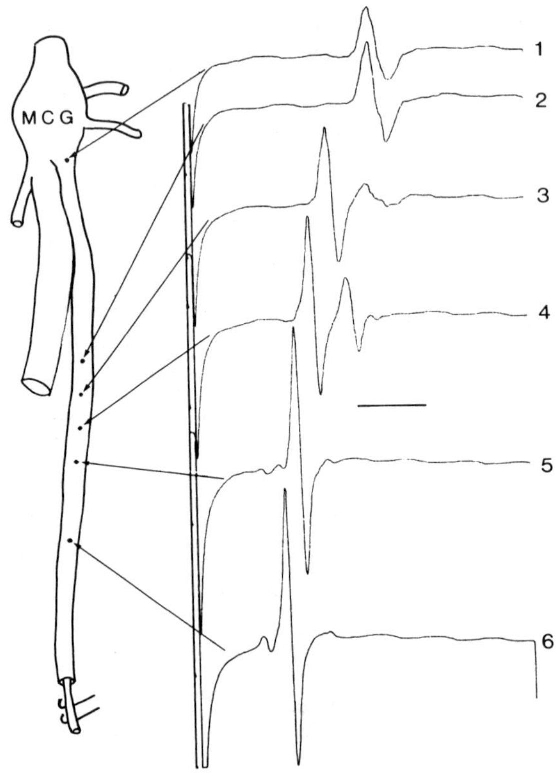

Fig. 2-11. Schematic diagram of the canine left middle cervical ganglion (MCG) and caudal pole nerve with records of compound action potentials obtained from the distal end of the left caudal pole nerve following stimulation of six sites along the nerve. Note that the compound action potentials changed configuration and latency as the stimulus site was moved along the nerve.

24 msec after the stimulus. The shifts of latencies of the onset of the compound action potentials were most evident between points 2 and 3, sites which were 2 mm apart. This experiment demonstrates that changes in latency and configuration of compound action potentials can be elicited by stimulation at different positions along a cardiac nerve. This suggests that complex electrophysiological responses can be elicited from one region of a cardiac nerve. When histology was performed on the nerve, neurons were found clustered in the center of the tissue between sites 2 and 5. They were not found in adjacent areas. These results confirm that ganglia exist in cardiopulmonary nerves and that they may be identified physiologically.

FELINE CARDIOPULMONARY NERVES

The gross anatomy of the cardiopulmonary nerves in the cat has been reported to be both complex [30] and relatively simple [36]. A complete anatomical assessment of these nerves correlated with physiological responses has yet to be performed. However, some physiological studies have incorporated analyses of right-sided [48] and left-sided [39] cat cardiopulmonary nerves, as well as the inferior cardiac nerve on the left side [8,13]. In our investigations we combined anatomical and physiological analyses as a preliminary to more detailed studies.

The gross anatomy of the feline cardiopulmonary innervation is shown in Figs. 2-12 and 2-13. Cat stellate ganglia are large but the middle cervical ganglia are small and relatively rostrally located. The right stellate ganglion joins with the right thoracic vagus via two or three ansae, the dorsal one sometimes having two components. The dorsal ansa or ansae travel cranially for a considerable distance before becoming closely associated with the thoracic vagus near the thoracic outlet, where the relatively small middle cervical ganglion is located. The recurrent laryngeal nerve gives rise to the recurrent cardiac nerve via two or three branches. This nerve exerts both parasympathetic and sympathetic control of the heart. Another major cardiopulmonary nerve, the right cranial vagal nerve, arises from the region of the junction of the ventral subclavian ansa and the thoracic vagus, which is similar to the pattern found in dogs. Vagal branches arise below this level and course toward the heart, also as in the dog.

The feline left stellate ganglion is also large (Fig. 2-13). The ventral one or two ansae join the vagus at the same level as the stellate ganglion. The dorsal ansa projects cranially to the thoracic outlet where it unites with the lateral aspect of the thoracic vagus. At this junction the relatively small middle cervical ganglion is located. This was called the vertebral ganglion by McKibben and Getty [30] because it lies ventral to the vertebral artery. Small ganglia also exist in the region where the ventral ansae unite with the thoracic vagus. Vagal branches arise from the thoracic vagus above the level of the aortic arch, as well as at and below the recurrent laryngeal nerve. The recurrent cardiac nerves arise from the recurrent laryngeal nerve. The ventral lateral nerve, arising from the ventral ansa, courses onto the lateral aspect of the heart behind the left atrial appendage. In this respect it is similar to the dog ventral lateral cardiac nerve.

The small stellate cardiac nerve, which varies in its site of origin, may arise from the stellate ganglion or the ventral ansa [13]. It is absent in some animals, as was also noted in the dog. The innominate nerve arises from the thoracic vagus high in the chest and exerts both parasympathetic and sympathetic control on the heart. There is usually another nerve, the ventromedial nerve which is formed from branches of the vagus, ventral ansae, and sometimes the caudal pole nerve. It exerts primarily sympathetic control of the heart.

Although the cat stellate and superior cervical ganglia have been shown to contain neurons which innervate the heart and lung [20], the middle cervical

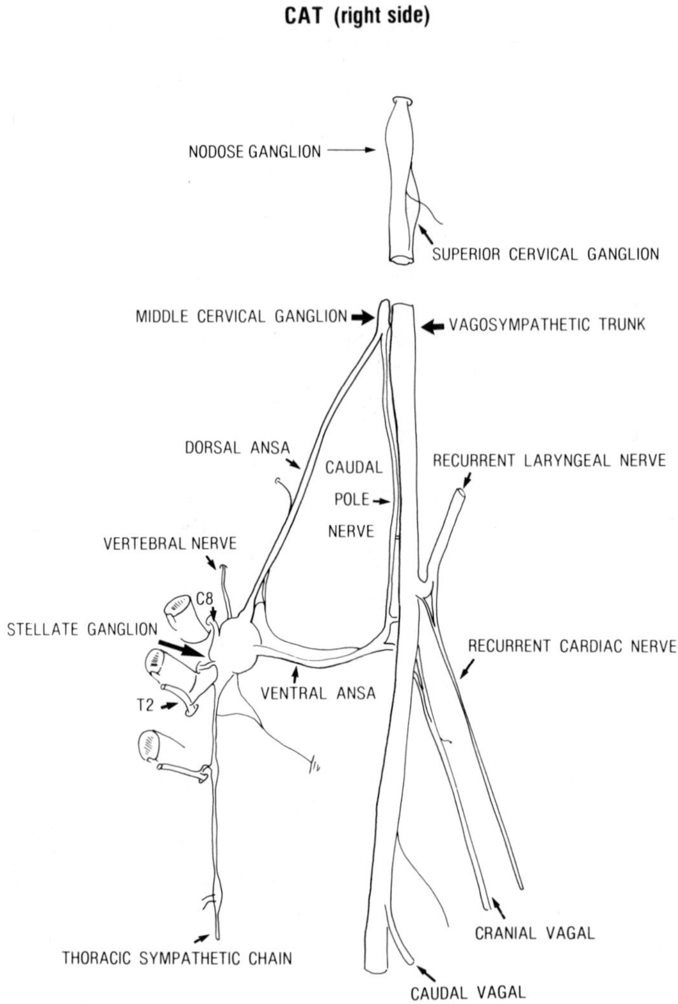

Fig. 2-12. Schematic drawing of the right feline cardiopulmonary nerves seen from the ventral aspect. Note the relatively large stellate ganglion.

ganglion was not examined so that comparisons with the dog and primate are not possible at the present time. The locations of cat vagal preganglionic cell bodies in the medulla have been studied extensively using both physiological [27,28] and anatomical [10,11,14,15,19,20,49,51] techniques. Vagal preganglionic neurons have been identified in the dorsal motor nucleus, the nucleus ambiguus and an intermediate zone, but it is becoming clear that the majority of the feline cells lie in or near the nucleus ambiguus [11,27,28,49].

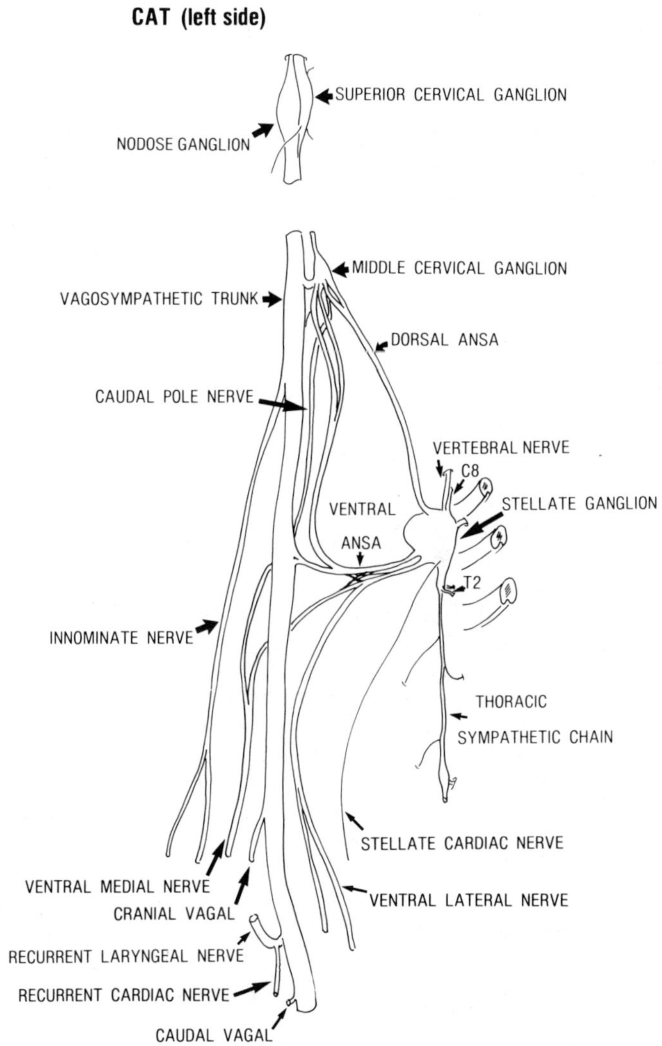

Fig. 2-13. Schematic drawing of the left feline cardiopulmonary nerves seen from the ventral aspect.

PRIMATE CARDIOPULMONARY NERVES

Gross Anatomy

The anatomy of the autonomic nerves innervating primate pulmonary and cardiac structures, particularly in humans, has been the subject of considerable investigation, [31,35,40,45]. As with other species, nonhuman primates have been described as having either few [23] or numerous [46] cardiopulmonary nerves. Cardiac nerves and variations of the major thoracic sympathetic ganglia have been described in the baboon, showing that specific cardiac nerves regulate specific regions of the heart [41]. The human vagi and their branches have been described as complex with numerous ganglia found along their course and branches [6]. The gross anatomy of the extrinsic cardiac nerves of man has been described elsewhere [45].

The gross anatomy in the rhesus monkey has also been briefly described [23,40]. We have investigated *Macaca mulatta* using the techniques described above. In the macaque the stellate ganglia are large. A group of quite small ganglia, which we refer to collectively as the middle cervical ganglia, are

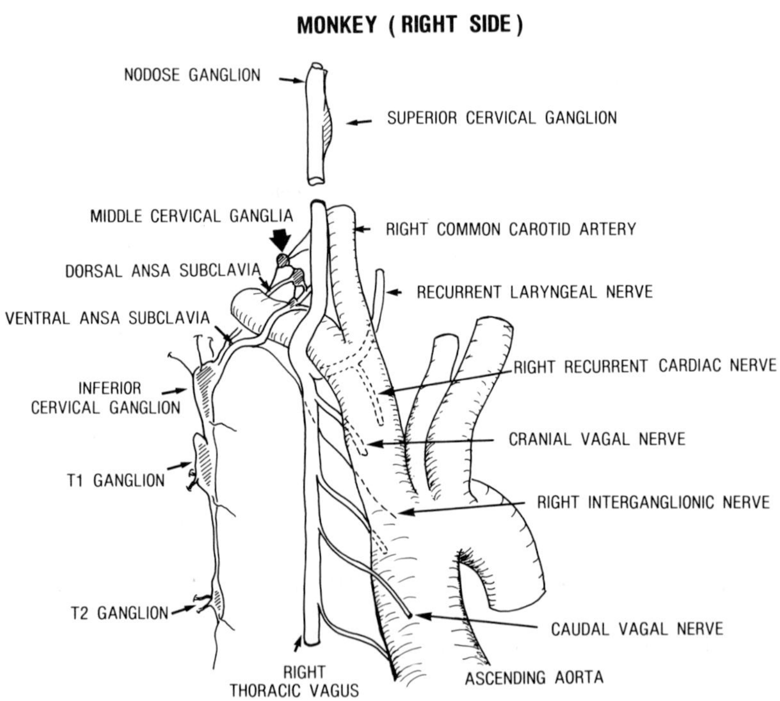

Fig. 2-14. Schematic drawing of the rhesus monkey right cardiopulmonary nerves seen from the ventral aspect. Note that there are a number of small ganglia which have been designated collectively as middle cervical ganglia. The major sympathetic ganglia are indicated by shading.

located just cranial to the subclavian arteries beside the thoracic vagi. This gross anatomy is like that found in the cat, where the stellate is the largest thoracic ganglion, in contrast to anatomy of the dog [3] and baboon [41] in which the middle cervical ganglia are well developed. In the rhesus monkey the right recurrent cardiac nerve arises from the recurrent laryngeal nerve. Cranial and caudal vagal nerves, as well as other smaller branches, arise from the thoracic vagus (Fig. 2-14).

On the left side a dorsal interconnecting branch, arising from the middle cervical ganglia, courses horizontally to join the vagus where another ganglion is usually located (Fig. 2-15). The vagosympathetic complex is formed by the vagus and contributions from the middle cervical ganglia. A nerve or nerves

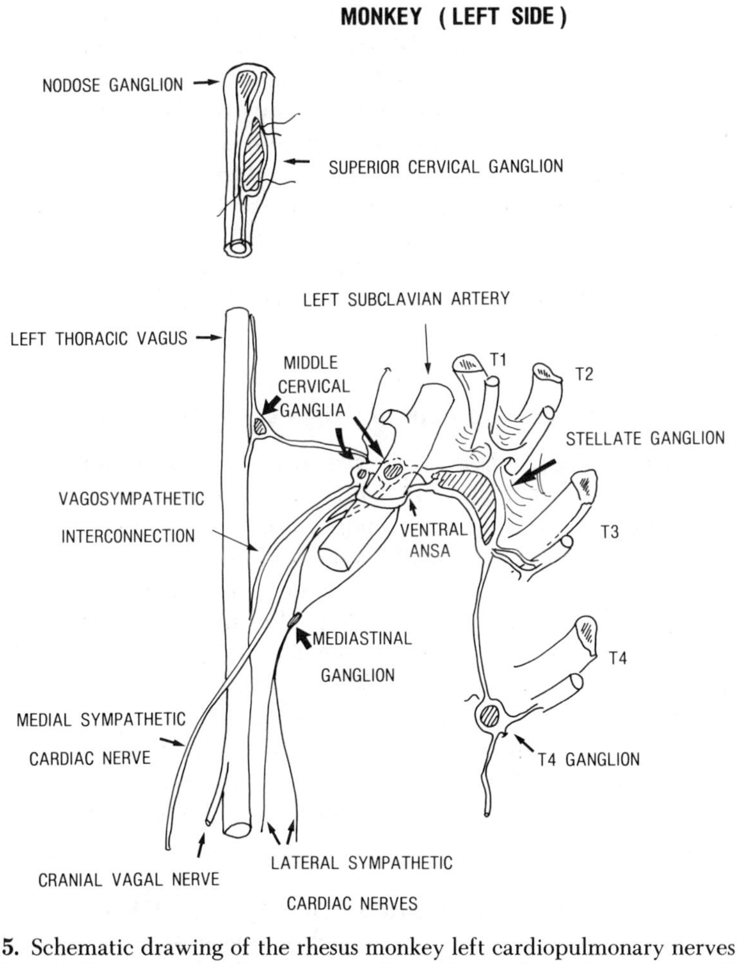

Fig. 2-15. Schematic drawing of the rhesus monkey left cardiopulmonary nerves seen from the ventral aspect. Note the presence of a mediastinal ganglion associated with the lateral sympathetic cardiac nerves.

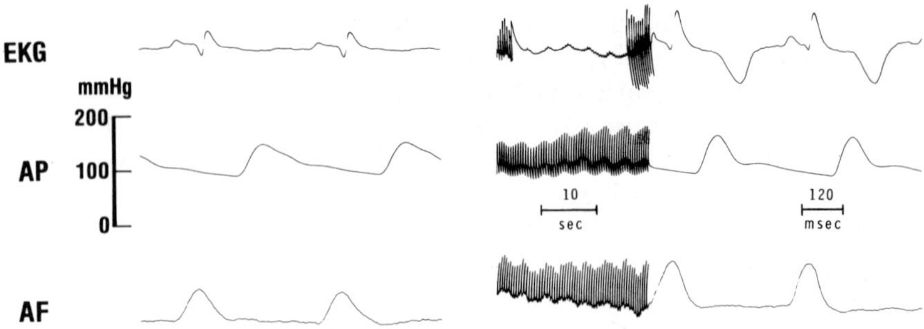

Fig. 2-16. Physiological responses obtained by stimulation of the left medial sympathetic cardiopulmonary nerve in rhesus monkey 32. Aortic pressure (AP) and left atrial force (AF) were augmented by the stimulation.

arising from the middle cervical ganglia also join the vagus, forming a caudal vagosympathetic interconnection. From these ganglia and a caudal vagosympathetic interconnection arises the relatively large medial sympathetic cardiac nerve. This nerve courses medially and caudally over the aortic arch to innervate the heart. The lateral sympathetic nerve(s) arise from branches of this medial sympathetic nerve and the ventral ansa. They course laterally to innervate the heart entering the pericardium near the left atrial appendage. This nerve appears to be the homologue of the ventral lateral nerve of the cat and dog. Vagal branches arise above, at, and below the level of the left recurrent laryngeal nerve. These exert predominantly parasympathetic influences on the heart.

Microscopic Anatomy of Cells of Origin of Cardiopulmonary Nerves

Parasympathetic Preganglionic Neurons. As far as we know there are no published studies on the medullary cells of origin of cardiac nerves in the primate using modern neuroanatomical techniques. Injection of HRP into individual physiologically identified vagal cardiopulmonary nerves in nine rhesus monkeys resulted in retrograde labeling in all four regions of the medulla, i.e., the DMV, intermediate zone, NA, and in the VLNA (Hopkins and Armour, in preparation). In contrast to the findings in the dog, all monkeys had labeling of a considerable number of neurons in the DMV, particularly in its lateral parts. In seven of the nine monkeys, labeling in the NA and VLNA was heavier than in the DMV. The intermediate zone had relatively few labeled neurons. In two of the nine animals a small number of neurons was labeled in the contralateral DMV and in one of these monkeys a single neuron was observed in the contralateral intermediate zone.

Sympathetic Postganglionic Neurons. Stimulation of a left medial cardiac nerve of the macaque resulted in slight tachycardia as well as considerable augmentation of left atrial force of contraction and blood pressure (Fig. 2-16). Following HRP injection into this nerve, labelled sympathetic neurons were rela-

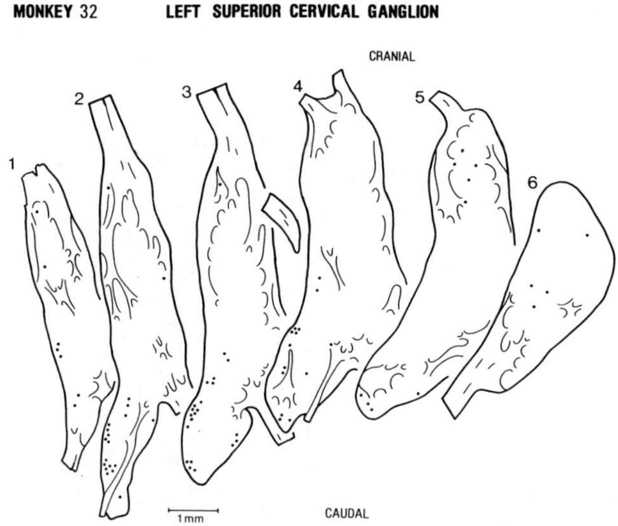

Fig. 2-17. Distribution of retrogradely labeled neurons in the left superior cervical ganglion following injection of the left medial sympathetic cardiopulmonary nerve in monkey 32. Anatomical orientation is indicated by the labels cranial and caudal.

tively evenly distributed among the superior and middle cervical ganglia and the stellate ganglion (Figs. 2-17, 2-18 and 2-19). The cells in the stellate ganglia were located craniomedially near the origin of the ventral ansa (Fig. 2-20B), as was found in the dog. In several other cases in which cardiac nerves were injected the superior cervical ganglion was very heavily labeled (Fig. 2-20A).

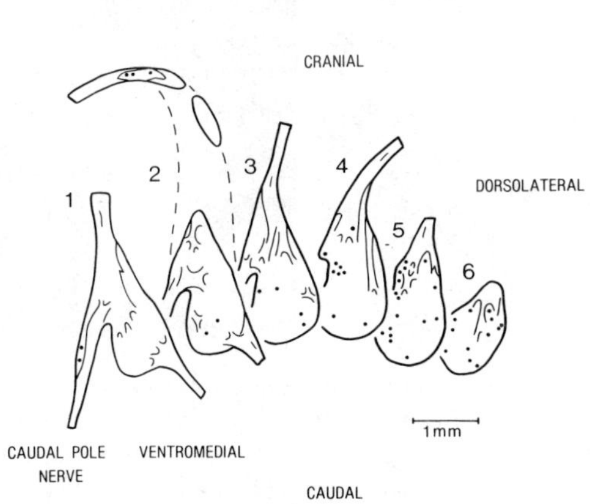

Fig. 2-18. Distribution of retrogradely labeled neurons in the left middle cervical ganglion in monkey 32. Note the presence of labeled neurons in the nerves branching from this ganglion.

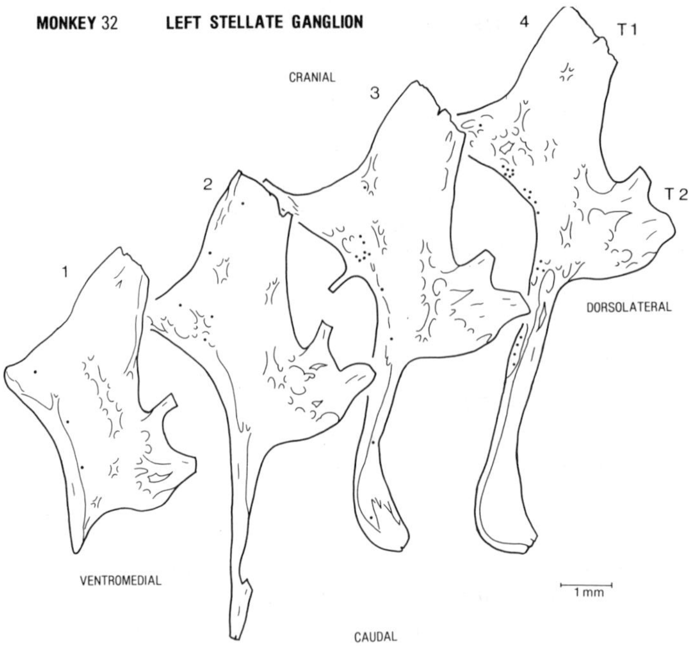

Fig. 2-19. Distribution of retrogradely labeled neurons in the left stellate ganglion in monkey 32. The labeled cells in level 3 are shown in the photomicrograph of Fig. 2-20B.

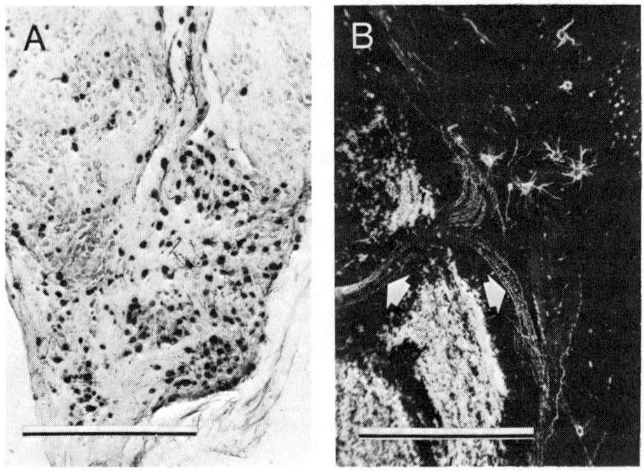

Fig. 2-20. (A.) Photomicrograph of the right superior cervical ganglion following injection of HRP into the right recurrent cardiac nerve in monkey 21. (B.) Dark-field photomicrograph of the left stellate ganglion following injection of HRP into the left medial sympathetic cardiopulmonary nerve in monkey 32. The two arrows indicate labeled axons in the ventral ansa and stellate ganglion. Calibration: A and B = 500 μm.

These results indicate that the superior cervical ganglion is relatively more important in the primate than it appears to be in dogs [5] or cats [20].

CONCLUSIONS

The gross anatomy of the dog, cat, and monkey demonstrates that each species has a large number of identifiable cardiac nerves, some of which appear to be comparable from species to species; however, ganglia vary in size in the three species.

The cells of origin of vagal efferent preganglionic fibers innervating the heart and lungs are located in four distinct regions of the medulla—the dorsal motor nucleus, an intermediate zone, the nucleus ambiguus, and the ventrolateral nucleus ambiguus. In the dog and the cat the majority of these neurons were located in the NA and the VLNA. In the primate the dorsal motor nucleus was also prominently labeled. The cells of origin of sympathetic postganglionic neurons were located in the three major ganglia, the superior and middle cervical ganglia and the stellate ganglion. In the dog the middle cervical ganglion was the major locus of these neurons. Other mediastinal ganglia also contained cardiac sympathetic neurons. In the monkey postganglionic cardiac sympathetic neurons appear to be more evenly distributed in the major ganglia, which is indicative of significant species differences. These findings are relevant to physiological studies of neural innervation of the heart. They imply that a simplistic approach to the anatomy of the neural innervation of the human heart, especially when applied to surgical interventions, is not justified.

REFERENCES

1. Abraham, A., *Microscopic Innervation of the Heart and Blood Vessels in Vertebrates Including Man,* Pergamon Press, Oxford, 1969.
2. Armour, J. A., Physiological behavior of thoracic cardiovascular receptors. *Am. J. Physiol. 225*: 177–185, 1973.
3. Armour, J. A. and W. C. Randall, Functional anatomy of canine cardiac nerves. *Acta Anat. 91*: 510–528, 1975.
4. Armour, J. A., W. C. Randall, S. Sinha, Localized myocardial responses to stimulation of small cardiac branches of the vagus. *Am. J. Physiol. 228*: 141–148, 1975.
5. Armour, J. A. and D. A. Hopkins, Localization of sympathetic postganglionic neurons of physiologically identified cardiac nerves in the dog. *J. Comp. Neurol. 202*: 169–184, 1981.
6. Botar, J., D. Afra, P. Moritz, J. Schiffmann, M. Scholz, Die Nervenzellen und Ganglien des N. Vagus. *Acta Anat. 10*: 284–314, 1950.
7. Bowers, C. W. and R. E. Zigmond, Localization of neurons in the rat superior cervical ganglion that project into different postganglionic trunks, *J. Comp. Neurol. 185*: 381–392, 1979.
8. Brown, A. M. Cardiac sympathetic adrenergic pathways in which synaptic transmission is blocked by atropine sulphate. *J. Physiol. (Lond.) 191*: 271–288, 1967.
9. Chase, M. R. and S. W. Ranson, The structure of the roots, trunk and branches of

the vagus nerve. *J.Comp. Neurol. 24*: 31–60, 1914.
10. Chen, H. I. and C. Y. Chai, Integration of the cardiovagal mechanism in the medulla oblongata of the cat. *Am. J. Physiol. 231*: 454–461, 1976.
11. Ciriello, J. and F. R. Calaresu, Medullary origin of vagal preganglionic axons to the heart of the cat. *J. Autonom. Nerv. Syst.* 5: 9–22, 1982.
12. Cyon, E., *Die Nerven des Herzens. Ihre Anatomie und Physiologie*. Verlag Springer, Berlin, 1907.
13. Emery, D. G., R. D. Foreman, R. E. Coggeshall, Categories of axons in the inferior cardiac nerve of the cat. *J. Comp. Neurol. 177*: 301–310, 1978.
14. Geis, G. S. and R. D. Wurster, Horseradish peroxidase localization of cardiac vagal preganglionic somata. *Brain Res. 182*: 19–30, 1980.
15. Geis, G. S., J. W. Kozelka, R. D. Wurster, Organization and reflex control of vagal cardiomotor neurons. *J. Autonom. Nerv. Syst. 3*: 437–450, 1981.
16. Gunn, C. G., G. Sevelius, M. J. Puiggari, F. K. Myers, Vagal cardiomotor mechanisms in the hindbrain of the dog and cat. *Am. J. Physiol. 214*: 258–262, 1968.
17. Heinbecker, P. and J. O'Leary, The mammalian vagus nerve—a functional and histological study. *Am. J. Physiol. 106*: 623–646, 1933.
18. Hopkins, D. A. and J. A. Armour, Medullary cells of origin of physiologically identified cardiac nerves in the dog. *Brain Res. Bull.*, in press.
19. Kalia, M., Brain stem localization of vagal preganglionic neurons. *J. Autonom. Nerv. Syst. 3*: 451–481, 1981.
20. Kalia, M. and M.-M. Mesulam, Brain stem projections of sensory and motor components of the vagus complex in the cat: II. Laryngeal, tracheobronchial, pulmonary, cardiac and gastrointestinal branches. *J. Comp. Neurol. 193*: 467–508, 1980.
21. Keng, L. B., On the nervous supply of the dog's heart. *J. Physiol. (Lond) 14*: 407–482, 1893.
22. Kostreva, D. R., E. J. Zuperku, J. F. Cusick, J. P. Kampine, Ventral root mapping of cardiac nerves in the canine using evoked potentials. *Am. J. Physiol. 232*: H590–H595, 1977.
23. Kuntz, A., The autonomic nervous system. In *The Anatomy of the Rhesus Monkey (Macaca mulatta), eds.* C. G. Hartman and W. L. Straus. Williams and Wilkins, Baltimore, pp. 328–338, 1933.
24. Lawn, A. M., The localization in the nucleus ambiguus of the rabbit, of the cells or origin of motor nerve fibers in the glossopharyngeal nerve and various branches of the vagus nerve by means of retrograde degeneration. *J. Comp. Neurol. 127*: 293–306, 1966.
25. Levy, M. N. and P. J. Martin, Neural control of the heart, In *Handbook of Physiology,* Sec. 2, *The Cardiovascular System*, Vol. 1, *The Heart,* eds. R. M. Berne, N. Speralakis, and S. R. Geiger. American Physiology Society, Bethesda, Maryland, 1979.
26. Lichtman, J. W., D. Purves, J. W. Yip, Innervation of sympathetic neurons in the guinea-pig thoracic chain. *J. Physiol. (Lond) 298*: 285–299, 1980.
27. McAllen, R. M. and K. M. Spyer, The location of cardiac vagal preganglionic motoneurons in the medulla of the cat. *J. Physiol. (Lond) 258*: 187–204, 1976.
28. McAllen, R. M. and K. M. Spyer, Two types of vagal preganglionic motoneurones projecting to the heart and lungs. *J. Physiol. (Lond) 282*: 353–364, 1978.
29. McKibben, J. S. and R. Getty, A comparative morphologic study of the cardiac innervation in domestic animals. I. The canine. *Am. J. Anat. 122*: 533–544, 1968.
30. McKibben, J. S. and R. Getty, A comparative morphologic study of the cardiac innervation in domestic animals. II. The feline. *Am. J. Anat. 122*: 545–553, 1968.

31. Mitchell, G. A. G., *Cardiovascular Innervation.* E. and S. Livingstone, London, 1956.
32. Mizeres, N. J., The anatomy of the autonomic nervous system in the dog. *Am. J. Anat. 96:* 285–318, 1955.
33. Mizeres, N. J., The course of the left cardioinhibitory fibers in the dog. *Anat. Rec. 127*: 109–116, 1957.
34. Mizeres, N. J., The origin and course of the cardioaccelerator fibers in the dog. *Anat. Rec. 132*: 261–279, 1958.
35. Mizeres, N. J., The cardiac plexus in man. *Am. J. Physiol. 112*: 141–151, 1963.
36. Nonidez, J. F., Studies on the innervation of the heart. I. Distribution of the cardiac nerves, with special reference to the identification of the sympathetic and parasympathetic preganglionics. *Am. J. Anat. 65*: 362–413, 1939.
37. Norris, J. E., R. D. Foreman, R. D. Wurster, Response of the canine heart to stimulation of the first five ventral thoracic roots. *Am. J. Physiol. 227*: 9–12, 1974.
38. Nosaka, S., T. Yamamoto, K. Yasunaga, Localization of vagal cardioinhibitory preganglionic neurons within rat brain stem. *J. Comp. Neurol. 186*: 79–92, 1979.
39. Peterson, D. F. and A. M. Brown, Pressor reflexes produced by stimulation of afferent fibers in cardiac sympathetic nerves of the cat. *Circ. Res. 28*: 605–610, 1971.
40. Pick, J., *The Autonomic Nervous System. Morphological, Comparative, Clinical and Surgical Aspects.* Philadelphia, Lippincott, 1970.
41. Randall, W. C., J. A. Armour, D. C. Randall, O. A. Smith, Functional anatomy of the cardiac nerves in the baboon. *Anat. Rec. 170*: 183–198, 1971.
42. Randall, W. C., J. A. Armour, W. P. Geis, D. B. Lippincott, Regional cardiac distribution of the sympathetic nerves. *Fed. Proc. 31*: 1199–1208, 1972.
43. Randall, W. C. and J. A. Armour, Complex cardiovascular responses to vagosympathetic stimulation. *Proc. Soc. Exp. Biol. Med. 145*: 493–499, 1974.
44. Randall, W. C. and J. A. Armour, Regional vagosympathetic control of the heart. *Am. J. Physiol. 227*: 444–452, 1974.
45. Randall, W. C. and J. A. Armour, Gross and microscopic anatomy of the cardiac innervation. In *Neural Regulation of the Heart,* ed. W. C. Randall. Oxford University Press, New York, pp. 13–41, 1977.
46. Riegle, L., Uber die Innervation der Hals-und Brustorgane bei einigen Affen. *Ztschr. f. Anat. u Entwich Ges. 80*: 777–858, 1926.
47. Schurawlew, A. N., Die Herznerven des Hundes. *Zeit. fur d. Ges. Anat. 86*: 654–695, 1928.
48. Shimizu, T., F. Peterson, V. S. Bishop, Reflex circulatory changes due to the afferent stimulation of cat pericoronary nerve. *Am. J. Physiol. 235*: H759-H766, 1978.
49. Sugimoto, T., K. Itoh, N. Mizuno, S. Nomura, A. Konishi, The site of origin of cardiac preganglionic fibers of the vagus nerve: an HRP study in the cat. *Neurosci. Lett. 12*: 53–58, 1979.
50. Tcheng, K. T., Innervation of the dog's heart. *Am. Heart J. 41*: 512–524, 1951.
51. Todo, K., Vagal preganglionic innervation of the cat heart. *Jap. Circ. J. 41*: 1341–1352, 1977.
52. Tollack, J., L. Grupp, W. C. Farr, Functional studies of right cardiac sympathetic nerves and ganglia in the dog. *Proc. Soc. Exp. Biol. Med. 137*: 772–775, 1971.
53. Wechsler, J. S., J. B. Pace, J. Goldberg, W. C. Randall, Location of synaptic connections in canine sympathetic cardiac innervation. *Am. J. Physiol. 217*: 1789–1794, 1969.
54. Wiesman, G. G., D. S. Jones, W. C. Randall, Sympathetic outflows from cervical spinal cord in the dog. *Science 152*: 381–382, 1966.

3

Selective Autonomic Innervation of the Heart

WALTER C. RANDALL

The relatively rich cardiac innervation is well documented by numerous outstanding articles and books published over tbe past 50 years [1,11,17,21–23,35]. Both light and electron microscopy have contributed importantly to this wealth of information. During the past 20 years, a plethora of physiological studies has led to insights into how overall cardiac performance comes under direct control by the central nervous system during reflexes arising from extrinsic sources, and even from stimuli arising within the heart itself. It is important to realize that the normal heart responds in a highly coordinated manner to carefully balanced inputs from both sympathetic and parasympathetic limbs of the autonomic system, with smoothly integrated effectiveness, while the normal body moves from quietly resting to grossly exaggerated stress-induced responsiveness. These changes in cardiac demand may represent extreme alterations in activity in either sympathetic or parasympathetic limbs with reciprocal adjustments within the opposite limb. Consider the common experience of rapid change from the quietly resting state when sympathetic drive to the heart is virtually "turned off" but vagal activity may be considerable, to sudden and violent muscular activity in which a diametrically opposite situation obtains.

The dynamic interactions between sympathetic and parasympathetic supply to the heart are dramatically illustrated in animals instrumented with pacing electrodes on the atrium. While standing quietly on the treadmill, unanesthetized animals were paced at 200/min to induce A-V block (Fig. 3-1A). Promptly upon initiation of exercise (signal), 1:1 conduction was quickly established and was sustained throughout the period of running. Block progressively returned upon cessation of exercise. Faster pacing increased severity of A-V block, but this too disappeared during exercise until extremely fast pacing was employed. Beta adrenergic blockade exerted little if any influence on conduction under

Experimental data reported was supported by grants from the National Institutes of Health, HL 08682, The Bane Charitable Trust of Chicago, and the James DePauw Fund of Chicago.

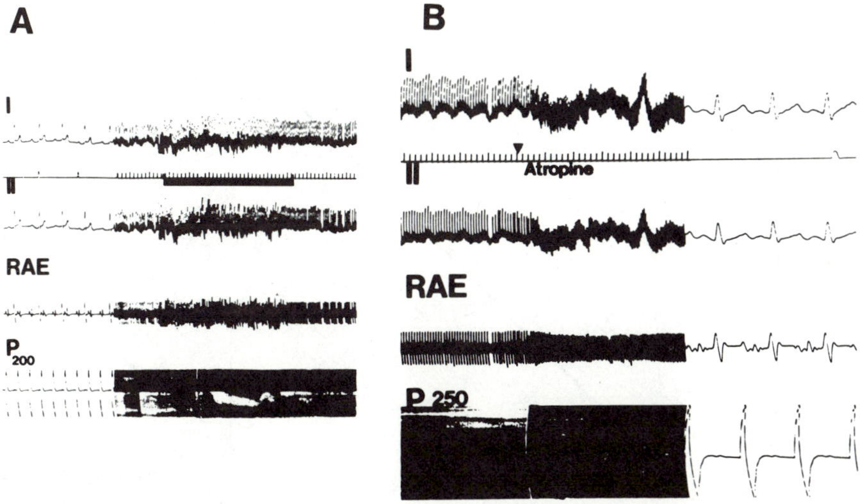

Fig. 3-1. Changes in A-V conduction during exercise (6 mph at 10% grade) and intravenous atropine (0.4 mg/kg) in the alert, conscious dog. Recording (RAE) and pacing (P) electrodes were chronically sutured upon the right atrium with lead wires exteriorized through the neck skin. Standard limb leads I and II of the electrocardiogram were also recorded.

quietly resting conditions, whereas cholinergic blockade (atropine, Fig. 3-1B) was markedly effective. Within a few seconds after intravenous injection, 1:1 conduction spontaneously occurred and remained even when pacing rates as high as 400/min were instituted [26].

Figure 3-2 graphically summarizes the widely differing influences of sympathetic and parasympathetic inputs to the heart of the normally responding, unanesthetized dog, instrumented for controlled atrial pacing. A straight line of identity relates atrial pacing rate (abscissa) and ventricular activation (ordinate) as detected by ventricular electrograms or by the QRS complex of the electrocardiogram. One-to-one conduction was maintained in the range of 100–140/min in the quietly resting dog, and this was increased to rates as high as 250–300 when the animal became alert or excited. A-V block often occurred at pacing rates below 100 while the animal was sleeping or undisturbed in his cage. Propranolol had little influence under these resting conditions. Barbiturates, probably due to their vagolytic action, markedly elevated pacing rates required to elicit block. Stellate stimulation elevated this pacing rate even higher. These data support the concept of dynamically changing autonomic influences on A-V junctional conduction in the awake, normally functioning animal [26,34].

The ability of the heart and its associated neural regulatory mechanisms to adjust are well recognized. The fact that such closely integrated control persists without significant interruption or default throughout the normal human lifespan is also well recognized. However, it is not generally realized that many of the intricate structure-functional relationships between the nervous system and the heart are still "black boxes." Such crucial facts as the precise distribution of

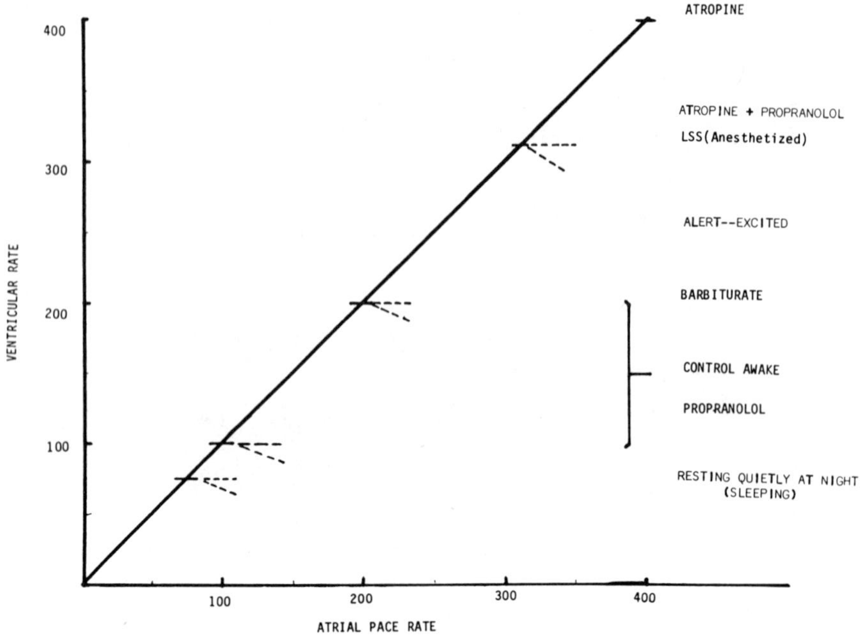

Fig. 3-2. Relationship between atrial pacing rate and ventricular activation in the conscious dog standing quietly in the laboratory. One-to-one conduction is represented by the straight line, with dashed lines indicating points of departure (A-V block). Physiological state is listed at the right.

either sympathetic or parasympathetic terminations around the effector cardiac cells remain unknown. With very few exceptions, investigators have not seen actual neuromyal junctions in the heart. While every medical student is certain of the almost instantaneous cardiac response to vagal stimulation, the most perceptive electron microscopist cannot securely describe the cholinergic terminal on specific pacemaker cells responsible for interruption of the heart beat. If the vagal stimulus is initiated in an appropriately timed portion of the cardiac cycle, it will dramatically alter the firing of (or conduction away from) the active pacemaker cell within that same cycle [14–15,19]. The time interval required for transduction of the electrical signal from the nerve terminal to acetylcholine release, diffusion, activation of receptors in the active pacemaker cells, and their subsequent effector response is incredibly short. It would appear essential that pacemaker cells be richly supplied with cholinergic terminals to accomplish this common event, but such coupling structures have not been found. The relatively longer time interval required for transduction of sympathetic adrenergic responses in the heart would not require such intimate neuromyal connections, but here too, clear pictures of the pertinent anatomical substrate are lacking.

At another level involving discrete distribution of both sympathetic and parasympathetic nerves to such critically important regions as the sinoatrial and atrioventricular nodal regions [25], precise information is almost totally lacking.

It is functionally clear, for example, that physiological demands for rapid acceleration in sinoatrial discharge frequency must be accompanied by concurrent improvement in conduction across atrioventricular junctional tissues, or A-V block will dissociate atrial from ventricular function. Both intrinsic and extrinsic neural integrations between concerted sinoatrial and atrioventricular regulation are recognized, and available details will be presented in chapter 4. The intricate reciprocal interactions between the central nervous system, as well as the peripheral distribution of nerve terminals to these two restricted portions of the heart remain obscure. These critically important research questions are highlighted here in the hope that carefully designed experimental protocols will be focused upon them by qualified and perceptive investigators within the near future. It seems highly probable that disturbances in autonomic physiology is involved in at least some of the severe cardiac dysrhythmias associated with some cardiac deaths in todays stressful environment. Such autonomic imbalance is presently only an attractive hypothesis [24]. Little or nothing is really known about its actual operation in normal and abnormal states. See also chapter 11.

This laboratory has expended much energy over many years in examining the selective distribution of both sympathetic and parasympathetic nerves to all portions of the heart, with particular attention to that of the sinoatrial (SAN) and atrioventricular (AVN) regions [8]. One approach has involved the classical procedures of electrical stimulation, with multiple response recordings from localized myocardial segments, before and after discrete interruption of individual branches of the cardiac nerves. These experiments culminated in the description of a surgical approach to the intrapericardial denervation of the canine heart [25]. The procedures were confined to intrapericardial regions in order to avoid interference with normal innervation of other thoracic and abdominal organs. With relatively simple recording technologies, completeness of denervation can be readily checked by repetition of nerve stimulations after completion of the surgical procedures. If positive responses occur in any portion of the heart to either sympathetic or parasympathetic stimulation, the appropriate anatomical reexploration and stimulation will reveal residual intact nerve connections, and these can be cut to assure completeness of denervation. Similarly, appropriately selective surgery can be performed to denervate restricted portions of the heart while leaving the remainder with essentially intact innervation. Thus we are capable of performing "*custom*" denervations in preparation of animal models for study under chronic conditions, with carefully designed protocols emphasizing specific environmental or intravascular pharmacologic stresses.

There is reason to anticipate that these intrapericardial interventions may have immediate implications for human patients sustaining severely restrictive, and life-threatening cardiac disease. The patient with demonstrable neurally mediated coronary vasospasm, for example, may be therapeutically restored, in theory at least, by transection of the alpha-adrenergic cardiac nerves, without interfering with the important systemic vasoconstrictor adjustments in the body as a whole. Also, in the patient with intractable ventricular tachycardia, reduction in ventricular automaticity by selective denervation may be life saving.

There is evidence that patients undergoing multiple vessel bypass surgery may enjoy added protection and extension in life expectancy by selective cardiac denervation [3,4]. Finally, there is experimental evidence accumulating that myocardial tissue subjected to severe ischemia sustains significantly less damage after chronic denervation than does tissue supplied with normal neural (presumably sympathetic) input [32]. These and other clinically pertinent outgrowths of fundamental studies of the cardiac innervation are detailed in other chapters of this book.

INTRAPERICARDIAL CARDIAC DENERVATION

Complete cardiac denervation of the canine heart is accomplished through a left thoracotomy between T4 and T5, with preparation of a pericardial cradle and isolation of sections of the right and left thoracic vagi and right and left stellate ganglia or ansae subclavia, for electrical stimulation [25,27]. Walton-Brodie strain gauge arches may be stitched to the myocardium of atria and ventricles for direct monitoring of contractile force changes, while simple electrocardiographic tracings provide adequate monitoring of chronotropic and dromotropic phenomena. The denervation procedure may be started by retraction of the left atrial appendage to permit clear visualization of the ventrolateral cardiac nerve (VLCN) as it penetrates the pericardium and crosses the left superior pulmonary vein (Fig. 3-3). The VLCN is sectioned at this level, and the dissection is extended to include the entire circumference of the superior pulmonary vein. With a retractor in the transverse sinus, the front wall of the left atrium is exposed, with extension of dissection from the VLCN toward the junction of left and right atria, sharply transecting the pericardial reflection over the

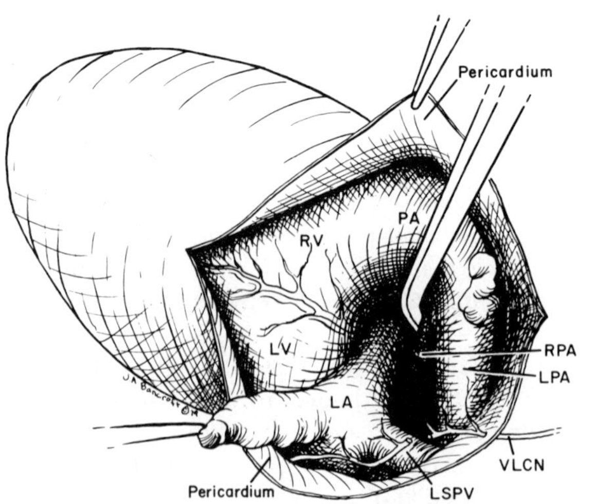

Fig. 3-3. Left side of the heart as viewed through pericardiotomy and left thoracotomy, to reveal the site of stage I of cardiac denervation. (Reproduced through courtesy of *J. Surg. Res.*, ref. 25).

cephalad surface of the left atrium and that portion of the right atrium within the transverse sinus. All tissues are cleaned from the bifurcation of the pulmonary artery and its right and left branches, with careful incision of the adventitia along the ventral surface to the root of the pulmonary artery. This completes stage I of the procedure.

Figure 3-4 illustrates the peripulmonary aspect of the dissection after removal of the fat pad between the pulmonary artery (PA) and the aorta. The aorta is retracted to the right while the PA is retracted to the left in order to visualize several relatively large nerves coursing along the dorsal surface of the PA. The latter are transected, and to interrupt any remaining small fibers passing by way of the pulmonary adventitia onto the heart, the latter is removed from the entire circumference of the main PA to complete stage II.

A ligature on the right atrial appendage is next directed caudally and the adventitia of the superior vena cava (SVC) is carefully dissected at the pericardial reflection (Fig. 3-5). Proceeding toward the heart, all connective and neural tissues are dissected from the SVC and the medial surface of the azygos vein, which is visualized, isolated, double tied, and divided. Care must be taken to avoid damage to the right vagus which passes extrapericardially in this area. As the dissection between the SVC and the aorta progresses, the right pulmonary artery is visualized and its surface is carefully cleared of all neural tissues. The dissection is continued to the intersection of the right and left atria, where the gauze sponge, inserted at the conclusion of stage I, is encountered, thus signaling completion of stage III.

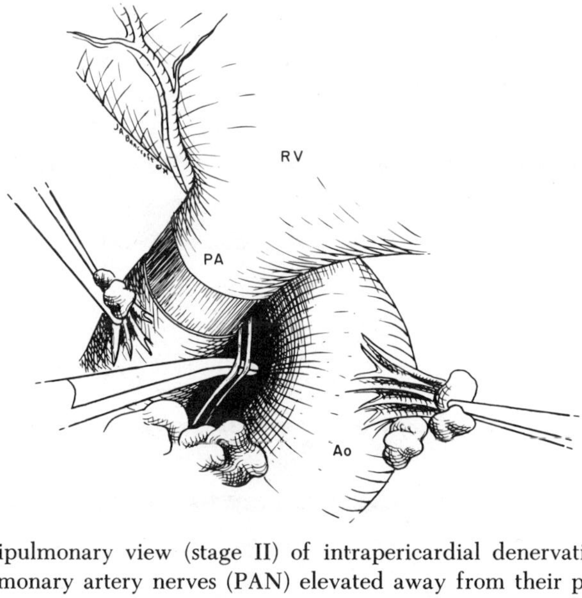

Fig. 3-4. Peripulmonary view (stage II) of intrapericardial denervation procedure revealing pulmonary artery nerves (PAN) elevated away from their position on the dorsal surface of the pulmonary artery. Also note removal of adventitia from circumference of pulmonary artery and dissection of fat and neural tissues between aorta and pulmonary artery (see credit, Fig. 3-3).

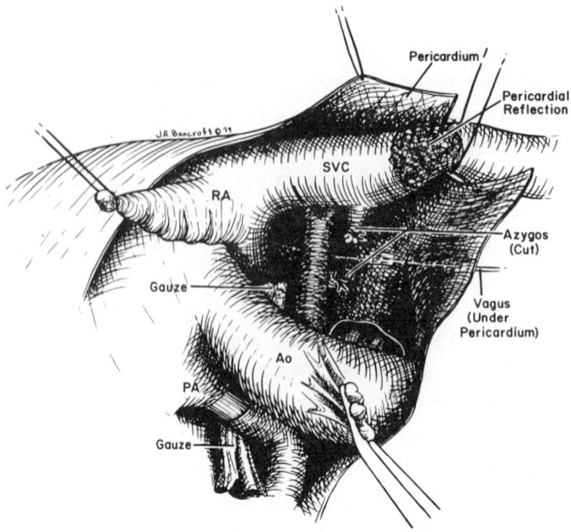

Fig. 3-5. Exposure of major vessels on right side of heart, with aorta retracted to left to permit visualization and dissection of superior vena cava, right pulmonary artery, and azygos vein. (See credit, Fig. 3-3).

Denervation is now complete and vagi and both sympathetic stimulation points are successively stimulated. If even slight changes in heart rate, contractile force, or shifts in pacemaker occur, the appropriate portions of each separate stage can be reexplored and any residual neural tissues transected, until one is satisfied the denervation is complete. Figure 3-6 provides convincing evidence

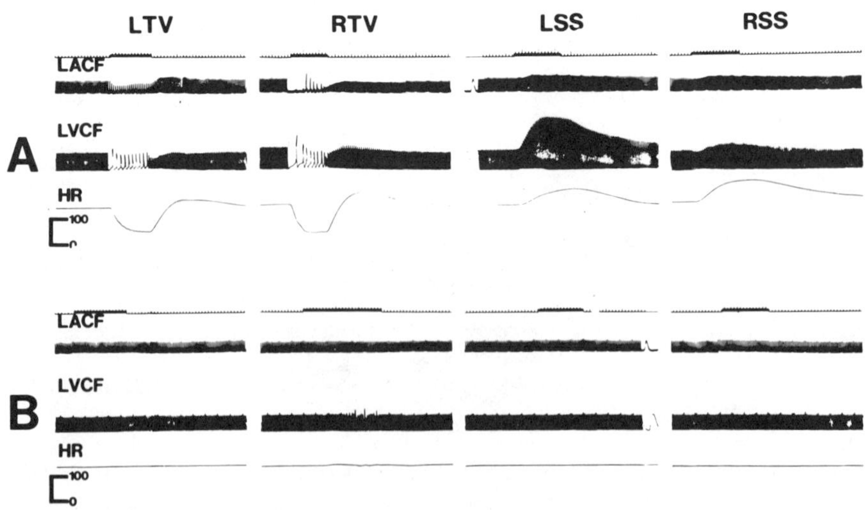

Fig. 3-6. Changes in inotropic, chronotropic, and dromotropic responses to both vagal and sympathetic stimulation before (A) and after (B) cardiac denervation. (See credit, Fig. 3-3).

for such completion. Pre- and postoperative stimulation records should prove total interruption of all efferent pathways. If instrumentation is to be installed for subsequent monitoring of cardiac performance, it may be done before the pericardium is loosely closed, the lungs expanded, and the chest closed in layers. The chest is carefully aspirated to remove residual air and the endotracheal tube removed as spontaneous breathing is restored. Postoperative antibiotic therapy is routinely employed.

During the course of these experiments, it became evident that one could test the relative amount of denervation accomplished during each stage of the procedure by repeating the stimulations of right and left vagi and sympathetic outflows after each separate stage. Thus, after stage I, (confined to the VLCN, superior left atrium, and projections across the pulmonary artery), the four stimulations of the proximal autonomic outflows to the heart were repeated.

Figure 3-7 illustrates the sequential deletion of functional responses to left (LTV) and right (RTV) vagal and left (LSS) and right (RSS) sympathetic stimulation during preoperative, control stimulations (panel A), after stage II (panel

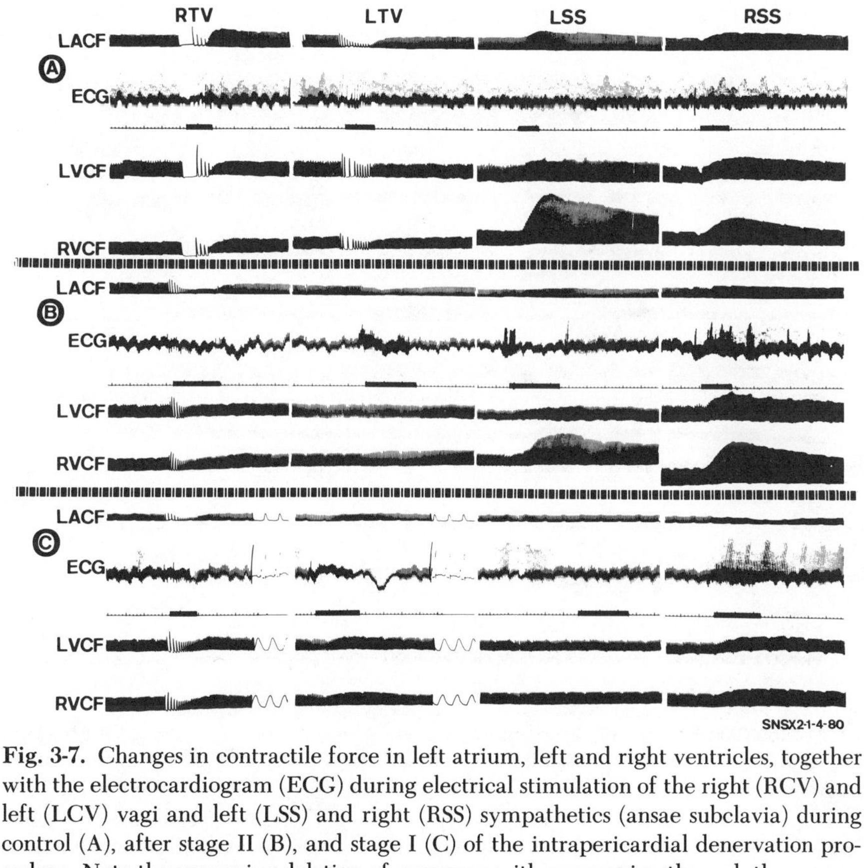

Fig. 3-7. Changes in contractile force in left atrium, left and right ventricles, together with the electrocardiogram (ECG) during electrical stimulation of the right (RCV) and left (LCV) vagi and left (LSS) and right (RSS) sympathetics (ansae subclavia) during control (A), after stage II (B), and stage I (C) of the intrapericardial denervation procedure. Note the successive deletion of responses with progression through these operative stages. (Reproduced through courtesy of *Am.J. Physiol.* ref. 27)

B), followed by stage I (panel C) of the denervation procedure. In addition to a standard limb lead II, contractile force (Walton-Brodie strain gauge arches) was recorded from the left atrium (LACF), and left (LVCF) and right (RVCP) ventricular surfaces. Marked bradycardia and suppression in atrial contractile force accompanied both left and right vagal stimulation, with slowing somewhat more pronounced during RTV. A-V block was complete during both stimulations. Contractile force was augmented during both LSS and RSS, more prominently in RVCF and during LSS. Heart rate, on the other hand, was accelerated more during RSS.

The fat pad was then removed from between the aorta and the pulmonary artery, and three relatively large nerves were gently lifted off the dorsal surface of the pulmonary artery, onto the stimulating electrodes. These nerves, shown schematically in Figure 3-4, have been called the pulmonary artery nerves (PAN). They were found in each of the animals, and invariably gave rise to profound changes in both ventricles and atria (Fig. 3-8). Their electrical stimulation produced marked augmentation in ventricular contractile force, often concurrently with inhibition in left atrial force. There was also an initial slight

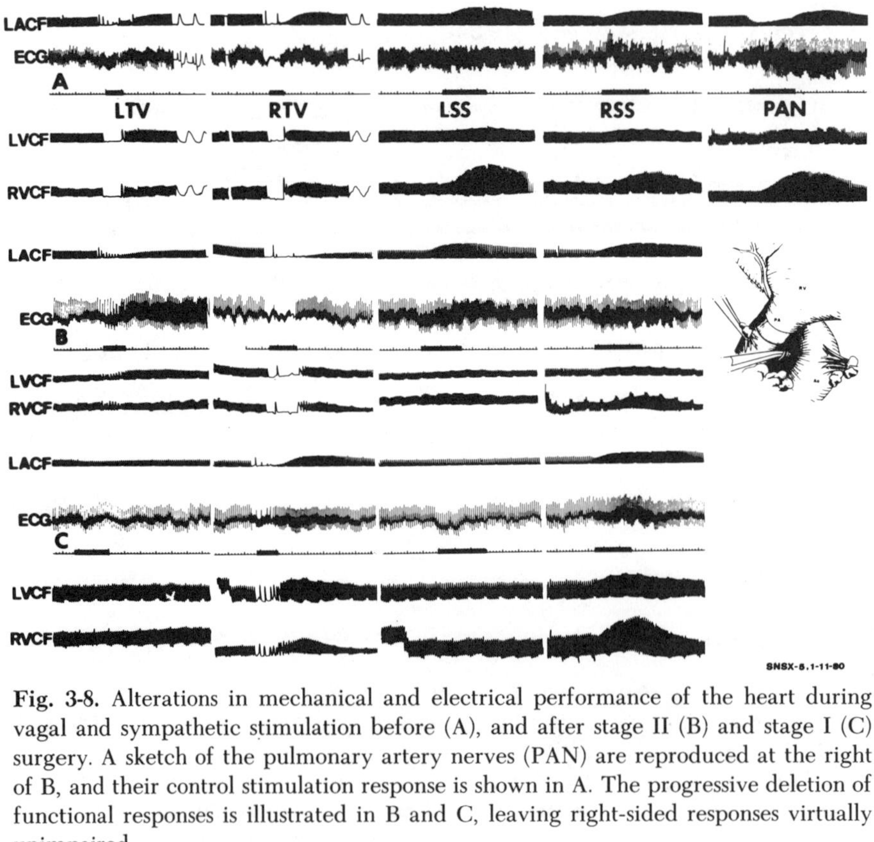

Fig. 3-8. Alterations in mechanical and electrical performance of the heart during vagal and sympathetic stimulation before (A), and after stage II (B) and stage I (C) surgery. A sketch of the pulmonary artery nerves (PAN) are reproduced at the right of B, and their control stimulation response is shown in A. The progressive deletion of functional responses is illustrated in B and C, leaving right-sided responses virtually unimpaired.

decrease in heart rate, and a rapid trace (not shown here) revealed shifting P-waves which were indicative of shifting pacemakers into the junctional region.

The PANs were transected (PAN-X), and the pulmonary arterial adventitia dissected (stage II). Panel B reveals significantly less negative chronotropism during LTV without marked change during RTV. Similarly, LSS induced distinctly less augmentation in ventricular contractile force than during control stimulation, but the chronotropic effects of RSS remained essentially undisturbed. Electrical stimulation of the distal end of the PANs elicited augmentation in ventricular contractile force, moderate acceleration in heart rate, and shifting P-wave. It did not elicit supression in atrial force, thus suggesting the negative chronotropic and inotropic responses in the left atrium of panel A were results of afferent nerve stimulation, with reflex feedback from brainstem nuclei to the heart. From these results, it is clear that Stage II interrupts efferent sympathetic pathways to both ventricles, without marked influences upon parasympathetic projections to the heart.

Stage I of the surgical denervation procedure was then performed, and the stimulation experiments repeated (panel C). This operative procedure ablated all effector responses to LTV and LSS, indicating complete ablation of the left autonomic input to the heart. While RTV responses were somewhat less profound (than control), significantly negative ino- and chronotropic responses remained. Also markedly positive chronotropic and inotropic changes persisted during RSS. Thus, Stages I and II totally ablated the left autonomic inputs without seriously jeopardizing right-sided inputs. The latter were completely eliminated in those experiments in which Stage III was subsequently done.

Figure 3-9 illustrates successive alterations in blood pressure, ECG, and contractile force sequentially following stage III and stage II of the denervation procedure. Panels 1 through 5 demonstrate the control responses to right and left thoracic vagal and sympathetic stimulation, as well as direct electrical excitation of the PAN nerves. In this animal, responses to RTV were more pronounced than during LTV, and while augmented responses during sympathetic stimulation were marked during both LSS and RSS, the chronotropic changes were greater during RSS. Stimulation of intact PANs again elicited marked augmentation in both right and left ventricular contractile force while eliciting suppression in atrial force. Stage III (panels 6 through 10), which is a right-sided procedure, resulted in total elimination of the negative chronotropic and inotropic actions of RTV, without seriously interrupting responses to LTV. LSS induced marked augmentation in contractile force but induced less positive chronotropic change in heart rate. The augmentor response during RSS was also changed in that the development of the positive inotropic response was slower and the chronotropic changes were attenuated. Stimulation of the intact PAN elicited responses qualitatively similar to those in the control panel. The PANs were then transected (stage IIa, PAN-X) and the stimulations repeated (panels 11 through 16). The distal end of the cut nerves elicited augmentation in ventricular contractile force plus modest acceleration in heart rate, but no suppression in atrial contractile force. Stimulation of the central end of the PANs, in contrast, reproduced the negative inotropic affect on left atrial force with only

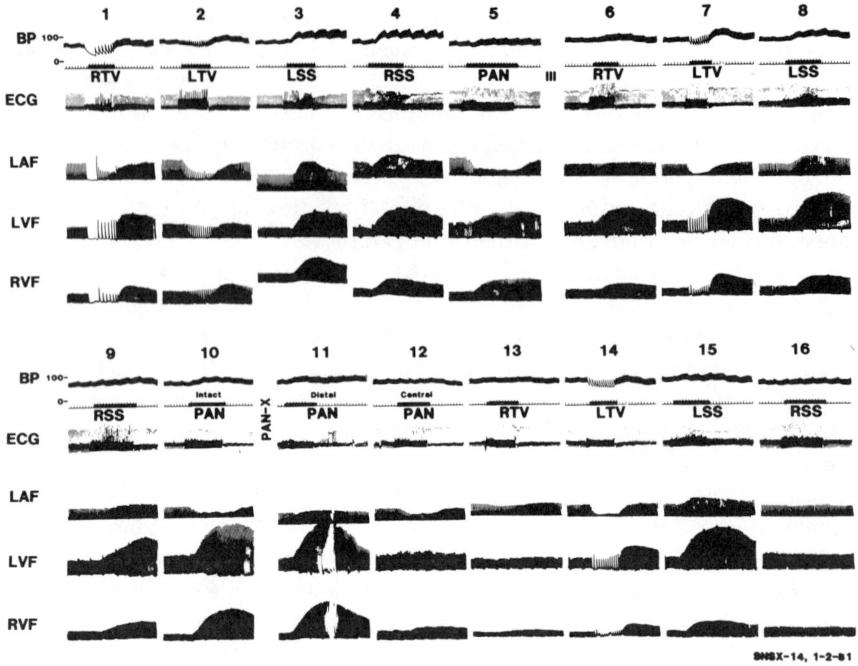

Fig. 3-9. Alterations in regional cardiac responses to vagal and sympathetic stimulation during control (panels 1–5), and after stages III (6–10) and II (11–16) of the intrapericardial denervation procedure.

slight actions on ventricular force. RTV no longer induced either parasympathetic (panel 1) or sympathetic (panel 6) changes, indicating complete denervation. LTV, in contrast, induced prominent inhibitory responses indicating little or no interruption of parasympathetic fibers from the left side. LSS also induced marked sympathetic changes (panel 15) while RSS demonstrated complete interruption of the right sympathetics. Here again, subsequent performance of stage I would be expected to completely denervate the heart.

These experiments demonstrate selective distribution of right and left autonomics to relatively restricted regions of the heart, and reveal potential ability to surgically ablate selected portions of the nerve supply to the heart.

SELECTIVE PARASYMPATHETIC DISTRIBUTION

The effects of acute bilateral cervical vagosympathectomy on the cardiovascular system have been well documented [20]. However, preparations of chronic animal models of parasympathetic cardiac denervation have been seriously complicated by mortality due to pulmonary and esophagogastric dysfunction [29–31]. Because of these extracardiac complications, Cooper et al. [7] devised a technique of intrathoracic selective cardiac vagotomy for the study of vagal influences on cardiac dynamics and coronary circulation. However, denervation proved to be incomplete in nearly one-half the original attempts with persistence of esophagogastric dysfunction.

From our early experience in mapping projections of the autonomic nerves onto the heart, it became apparent that the primary sympathetic nerves could be qualitatively isolated from the parasympathetic. However, due to intermingling of fibers from the two systems at the level of the caudal cervical ganglion (in the dog), it is probably impossible to preserve all of the cardiac sympathetic innervation while performing cardiac parasympathectomy. In 1975 however, we described a denervation technique permitting specific, total parasympathetic cardiac denervation with minimal interruption of sympathetic fibers and no residual pulmonary or esophagogastric complications [16].

The bulk of the parasympathetic fibers enter the canine heart between the right and left superior pulmonary veins and along the superior vena cava. Parasympathetic denervation was judged to be complete when, following dissection, supramaximal stimulation no longer elicited slowing in heart rate, depression in myocardial contractile force, or delayed conduction through the A-V junctional region. Verification of denervation was achieved in all animals in this series, and positive inotropic and chronotropic responses to vagosympathetic stimulation remained prominent *following* operation. The selectivity of the procedure was established by somewhat attenuated but still prominent inotropic and chronotropic responses to *sympathetic* stimulation following the operation.

Lazzara et al. [18] described two epicardial sites at which parasympathetic nerves enroute to the SA or AV nodal regions could be stimulated or blocked. Bipolar plunge electrodes were employed to explore the SA node, right atrium, coronary sinus region, and His bundle area [28]. An SA nodal stimulating site was located in the intercaval region of the right atrium, just posterior to the sulcus terminalis and near the pericardial reflection, at the anterior, superior border of a triangular fat pad. Selective stimulation of intracardiac nerves in this site produced slowing in sinus rate without change in intraatrial conduction, AV conduction, or refractory period of atrial muscle. An AV site was located in a pocket between the terminations of the inferior vena cava and coronary sinus on the posterior inferior right atrium. After atropinization, selective stimulation of these sites no longer produced sinus slowing or A-V block. These two sites coincide with our earlier impressions of major parasympathetic inputs to the heart [2,23,33].

From these experiments, we anticipated two primary projections of parasympathetic nerves onto the heart: (1) along the superior vena cava and over the superior right atrium, and (2) over the junction between inferior vena cava and inferior atria. We could not effectively predict whether vagal inputs to the SA and AV nodal regions could be separated. Since the classical demonstrations of Cohn and Lewis [5,6], more recently reinforced by Hondeghen [12], it has been known that the right vagus has a profoundly negative sinus chronotropic effect with relatively lesser affect on A-V conduction. Left vagal stimulation, in contrast, is generally thought to act primarily at the A-V junction. Irisawa et al, [13] reported that left vagal stimulation increased cardiac cycle length by 19.5% and the A-V interval by 17%. The right vagus, in contrast, increased cycle length by 34.5% but A-V interval by only 5.5%. However, Hamlin and Smith, in unpaced experiments, described approximately equal vagal restraints on SA and A-V nodal regions [10]. There is at present little real appreciation for the possibility of regional control of these two important conductile regions by vagal branches [2], and of selective interventions of cardiac performance. We therefore attempted to prepare canine models with restricted parasympathectomy of the SA nodal region while vagal supplies to the A-V nodal regions remained intact.

Following electrical excitation of the right and left vagi and the right and left stellate ganglia, concentrated phenol (90%) was applied in a fine line by camel's hair brush to each of eight epicardial segments of the heart. These areas were as follows, each approximately 2–3 mm wide and 2.0 to 3.0 cm long (Fig. 3-10): (1) superior surface of right atrium from appendage to superior vena cava and along its medial surface to the pericardial reflection, (2) circumference of the superior vena cava at the pericardial reflection, (3) from pericardial reflection along the lateral surface of the superior vena cava (intrapericardially) to the level of the right superior pulmonary vein, (4) medially from fat pad at level of superior pulmonary vein, across the sinoatrial nodal artery to the middle of the right atrial free wall, (5) from the end of paint number 4 rostrally to the superior edge of the right atrium (at this point, the sinoatrial node was completely encircled with phenol) (6) the junction of the inferior vena cava and the inferior atria, (7) posterior surface of the right atrium, and, finally (8) phenol was painted over the epicardial enclosure encompassed by paints 1 through 5, including the SA node. After each individual application of phenol, both cervical vagi and both stellate ganglia were electrically stimulated, while recording contractile force, heart rate, and atrioventricular conduction from multiple plunge electrodes in the right atrium.

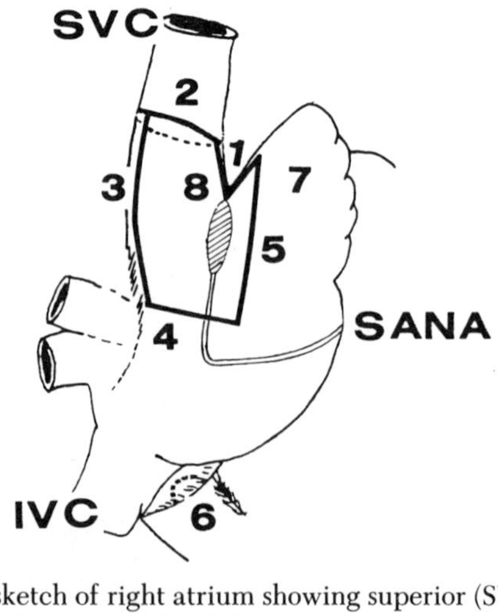

Fig. 3-10. Schematic sketch of right atrium showing superior (SVC) and inferior (IVC) venae cavae, course of the sinoatrial nodal artery (SANA), and location of the sinoatrial node (cross hatched zone). Numbers identify locations of phenol application.

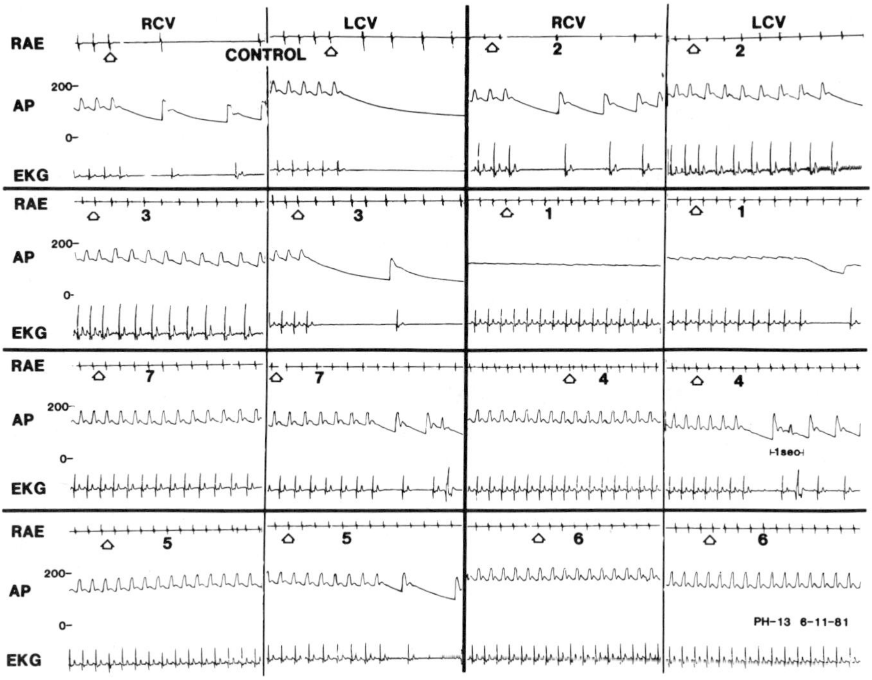

Fig. 3-11. Successive changes in electrical activation of atrium (RAE) and ventricle (R-wave of ECG), together with arterial blood pressure (AP) during electrical excitation of right (RCV) and left (LCV) cervical vagi before (control) and after each of seven successive applications of phenol (numbers at top of each panel identify location of phenol application as outlined in Fig. 3-10).

Figure 3-11 illustrates successive deletions in local cardiac responses to direct electrical stimulation of the right (RCV) and left (LCV) cervical vagi before and after each of seven separate applications of concentrated phenol to the epicardium. The first panel (upper left) shows alterations in the right atrial electrogram (RAE), arterial blood pressure (AP), and the EKG during electrical stimulation (20 Hz, 5 msec, 4–5 volts) under control conditions. Stimulation of the RCV induced marked bradycardia with virtually complete inhibition of sinus firing, but with partial block of A-V conduction. Stimulation of the LCV, on the other hand, induced less slowing in sinus firing rate, but produced complete A-V block, and was accompanied by no escape beats. The first application of phenol was by means of umbilical tape soaked in phenol and wrapped around the superior vena cava at the level of the pericardial reflection (paint no. 2). Right vagal stimulation then induced less sinus slowing (than during controls), and no evidence for A-V block. LCV stimulation elicited even less bradycardia than RCV, and significantly less than during the comparable control stimulation. It is apparent, therefore, that phenol destroyed some vagal pathways, coursing via both right and left sides, to the SAN and AVN regions. Phenol was then applied along the lateral surface of the superior vena cava and right atrium from the pericardial reflection to the level of the superior pulmonary vein (paint no. 3). Stimulation of RCV then revealed only slight cardiac slowing and no conduction block. LCV stimulation, on the other hand, induced little further change in sinus rate, but still showed marked A-V block. Phenol application along the superior right atrium and medial surface of the SVC totally ablated all right vagal input to the SAN region, but did not abolish left vagal influences on A-V conduction. Unfortunately, the blood pressure recording was damped. Phenolization of the posterior surface of the right atrium (paint no. 7) exerted no further influence on RCV, and also failed to abolish inhibitory fibers within the left vagus to the AV junctional region. Clear evidence for block appeared during later portions of the stimulation period. Similar results followed phenolization of area 4 (across right atrial free wall at caudal pole of the sinoatrial node); LCV again elicited varying degrees of A-V block. Paint number 5 completed the isolation of the SAN region by extending the tissue fixation between paints 1 and 4 (atrial side of SAN region, parallel to the right coronary artery). Again, A-V block was prominent during LCV. Finally, phenol was applied to the epicardium at the junction of the inferior vena cava and the inferior atria (area 6), with immediate elimination of left vagal induction of A-V block.

In another experiment, the sequence of phenol application was changed, with area 6 being painted first (Fig. 3-12). During controls, RCV stimulation induced prompt and complete cessation of firing of the pacemaker with consequent elimination of all atrial and ventricular electrical activity. LCV stimulation, on the other hand, only slowed sinus firing rate and this was associated with 1:1

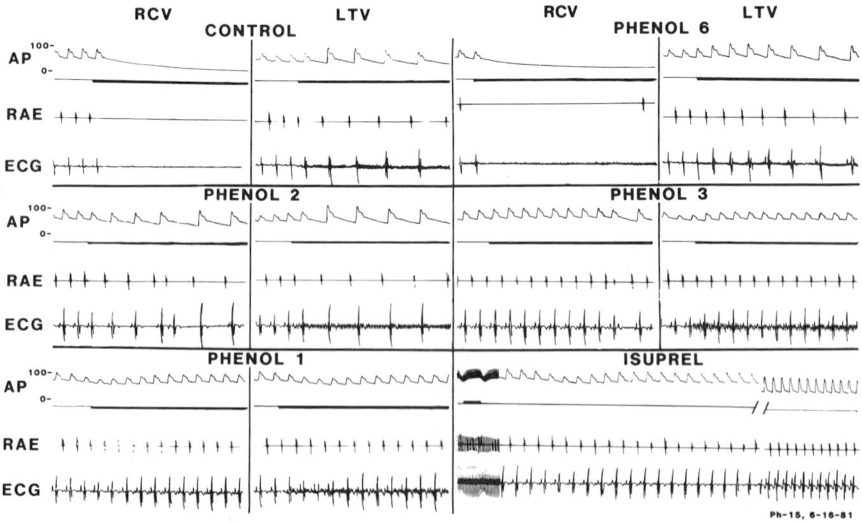

Fig. 3-12. Changes in activation of the atrium and ventricle during vagal stimulation after initial application of phenol to the inferior atrium (area 6) and subsequently to the superior atrium. Isuprel demonstrated the ability of sinus cells to respond after epicardial phenolization.

conduction to the ventricle. After phenol application to the junction of the inferior vena cava and inferior atria (area 6), RCV stimulation continued to exert complete inhibition of sinus firing rate without escape. Stimulation of LCV had fewer inhibitory effects on sinus rate than during control, and all atrial impulses were conducted to the ventricles. Phenol was then applied to the circumference of the superior vena cava (area 2), with consequent lesser inhibition of sinus firing rate during RCV. Left vagal stimulation revealed no further attenuation in its inhibition of either sinus firing or junctional conduction. Phenolization of the lateral surface of the superior vena cava and right atrium clearly interrupted right vagal input to the sinus region and its stimulation elicited no inhibition in sinus rate. Similarly, LCV stimulation failed to slow the atrial rate and conduction was 1:1. It is not surprising that application of phenol to area 1 had no additional influence, since all vagal input to the sinus region had been ablated by paints 2 and 3. Therefore, while areas 4 and 5 were phenolized, they induced no further change in either atrial firing rate or in conduction during either right or left vagal stimulation. A final experiment consisted of intravenous injection of isoproterenol (2.0 μg/kg) in order to confirm the functional integrity of the sinus node and its ability to respond to adrenergic stimulation. The left portion of the record reveals the time of injection at a control heart rate of 140/minute and a clear sinus rhythm. An 18 second segment was deleted from the illustration in order to show the maximum heart rate attained (235/min), with sinus origin and 1:1 conduction. This provided convincing evidence that the sinus node itself had not been damaged by the successive epicardial applications of phenol around its perimeter, and that failure to respond was indeed related to ablation of the parasympathetic branches from right and left vagi.

Vagal inhibition of sinus discharge masks negative dromotropic influences across the A-V junctional region. Atrial pacing is therefore necessary to reveal concurrent inhibition of impulse traffic to the ventricle. Figure 3-13 illustrates a different sequence of phenol application and also compares the effects of inputs from right (RCV) and left (LCV) cervical vagi on A-V conduction. Control records show maintenance of constant heart rate through pacing (right atrial pacing electrode) with immediate induction of complete A-V block and ventricular escape during both RCV and LCV stimulation. Phenol was then painted across the atrium at the level of the sharp rostral turn in the sinus nodal artery, to the lateral caval border, and rostrally to the SVC and its pericardial reflection (areas 4 and 3). RCV no longer induced A-V block but LCV elicited immediate and complete block (upper right). Phenol was next applied in a narrow band extending along the free wall to the superior border of the right atrium (area 5). RCV blocked two cycles during the 10-second stimulation period, while LCV elicited 4:1 block with ventricular escape. Phenol was then applied to the circumference of the SVC (area 2) with resultant ablation of all right vagal inhibitory affects on A-V conduction. In sharp contrast, LCV continued to induce complete A-V block, indicating lack of interruption of major vagal input to the junctional region from the left side. Phenolization of the superior border of the right atrium (area 1) was followed by complete absence of response to RCV, but LCV continued to induce complete block. Phenol was

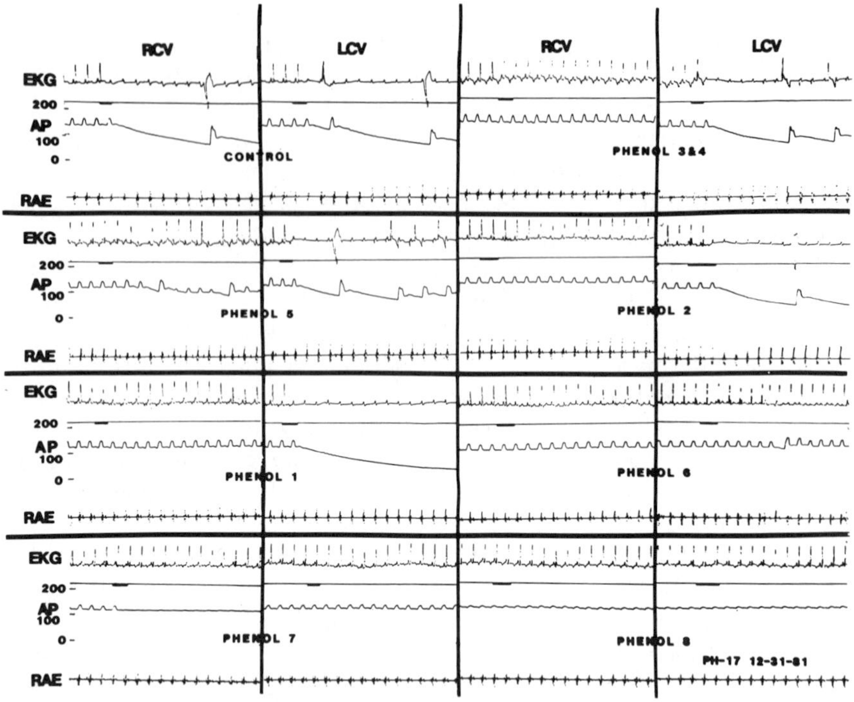

Fig. 3-13. Changes in electrical activity in the dog heart accompanying vagal stimulations following selective phenolization of the right atrium during atrial pacing.

then applied to tissues between the inferior vena cava and the inferior atrium (area 6), and was followed again by complete absence of block during RCV. Only four premature atrial systoles marred the regularity of conduction during the 15-second stimulation of LCV. Phenolization of areas 7 and 8 induced no further interruption of vagal input to the junctional region.

SELECTIVE DISTRIBUTION OF SYMPATHETICS

Both right and left stellate ganglia were also electrically stimulated before and after each individual phenol application. Figure 3-14 illustrates successive changes during right (RSS) and left (LSS) stellate stimulation after each phenol application. Control stimulations elicited marked acceleration in heart rate, more during RSS than during LSS. Note also the shift in P-wave during LSS but not during RSS. The positive chronotropic effect was clearly less after painting the superior surface of the right atrium (no. 1 and 2), but again, the P-wave did not shift during RSS. Phenolization of area 4 had little effect on either RSS or LSS, indicating few if any sympathetic fibers cross this portion of the atrium. Painting area 3, however, resulted in less acceleration during RSS and clearly was accompanied by shift in P-wave. LSS still induced a junctional tachycardia. Ablation of area 5 did not alter either response, and again suggests that few if

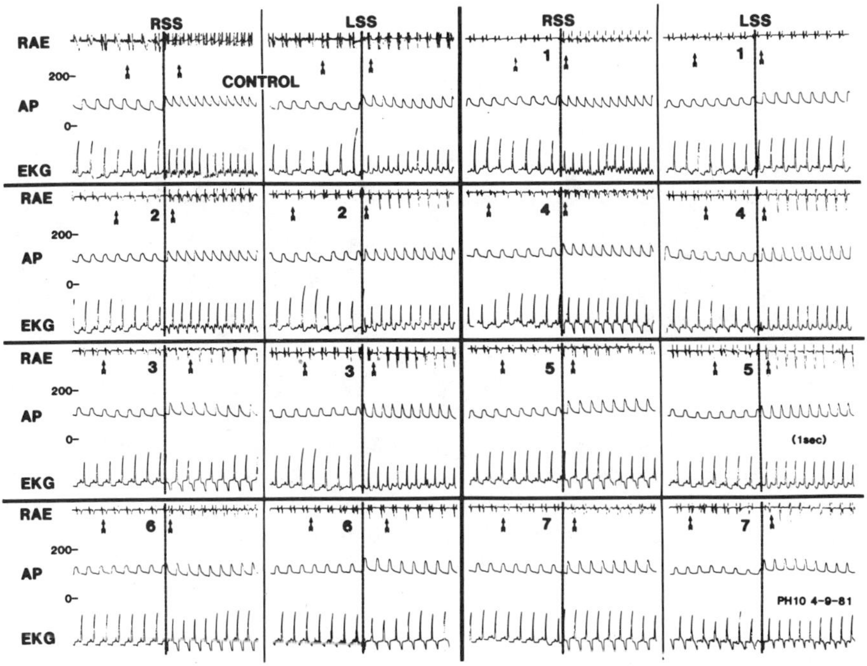

Fig. 3-14. Changes in right atrial electrogram (RAE), arterial blood pressure (AP), and electrocardiogram (EKG) accompanying right (RSS) and left (LSS) sympathetic stimulation, before (control) and after successive phenolization (numbers as in Fig. 3-10) of the right atrium. The first arrow represents onset and second arrow cessation of stimulation in each panel. A portion of the response has been removed from each separate procedure.

any sympathetic fibers cross this epicardial zone. Stimulations after painting areas 6 and 7 were still accompanied by junctional tachycardia, although of lesser magnitude than was observed during earlier stimulations. These experiments may be interpreted to indicate differential distribution of sympathetic fibers to both SAN and AVN regions, with some fibers following courses deep to the epicardium, since residual rate responses were consistently observed during sympathetic stimulation, even after ablation of all parasympathetic responses.

The experiments have been summarized in Fig. 3-15 with some reservations because of the use of successive applications of phenol to the eight different epicardial regions. Thus, the amount of atrial (sinus) or ventricular (AV nodal conduction) response during right or left vagal stimulation was related to the specific areas which had been phenolized before they were stimulated. Nevertheless, the figure reveals relationships worthy of emphasis. The data are expressed in terms of percent change in heart rate during right (RCV) or left (LCV) cervical vagal stimulation below the center baseline, and right (RSS) and left (LSS) stellate stimulation above the line. The stippled bars represent atrial rates while the solid bars represent ventricular responses. Successive applications

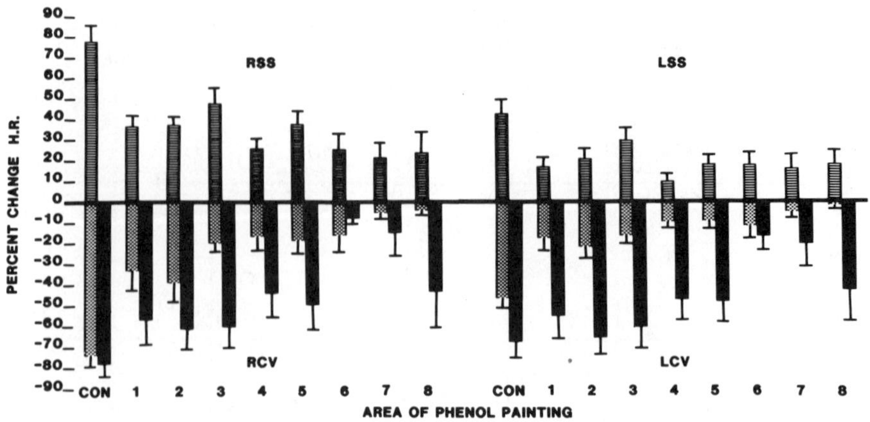

Fig. 3-15. Percent change in atrial (stippled bars) and ventricular (solid bars) rates during right (RCV) and left (LCV) vagal, and right (RSS) and left (LSS) sympathetic stimulation (ladder bars) before (con) and after each of eight separate applications of phenol to the right atrial epicardium. See Fig. 3-10 for precise location of each separate phenol strip. Negative chronotropic changes are shown below, while positive changes are shown above the center line.

of phenol (numbered 1–8 on abscissa, together with controls) were painted on the atria of 18 anesthesized dogs.

Right vagal stimulation consistently induced 75–80% slowing in atrial rate associated with simultaneous slowing in ventricular rate. Control stimulations of the left vagus, on the other hand, induced less slowing in sinus discharge rate, but consistently elicited A-V junctional conduction block. Experiments in which the right atrium was paced throughout the period of vagal stimulation, revealed simultaneous blockade of conduction across the junction during RCV, but on average, this was more prominent during LCV. Phenolization of areas 1, 2, and 3 (rostral portions of right atrium and the superior vena cava) markedly reduced the influence of the right vagus on sinus function with much less effect on A-V junctional conduction. Similarly, phenol painting of these three areas deleted nearly all vagal input to the SAN region from the left side, but again, failed to eliminate inhibition of junctional conduction. In contrast, phenol application to area 6 (junction of inferior vena cava and inferior atria) ablated a large majority of vagal fibers from both right and left sides to the junctional region, without seriously affecting vagal input to the sinoatrial nodal region. This was best shown in those experiments in which area 6 was painted early in the sequence of phenol applications. Phenolization of other areas surrounding the SAN (4 and 5) did not consistently alter the inhibitory effects of either right or left vagal stimulation, and it is concluded that relatively few fibers pass to the SAN region across these epicardial regions. Phenolization of area 7 (posterior right atrium) frequently resulted in elimination of inhibitory responses, suggesting the projection of vagal fibers from both right and left sides to the posterior surfaces of the atrium, with epicardial distribution to conductile regions. Area 8 consisted of epicardium overlying the SAN region, and was invariably painted last, in the event that a few fibers had not been reached by phenol applications elsewhere. This application completed the denervation, and indicates that few, if any, vagal fibers are distributed to the SAN region by routes deep to the epicardium and its immediately underlying (0.25 mm) tissue [9].

Heart rate responses to sympathetic stimulation are summarized above the center line, and reflect positive chronotropic changes during controls, and after each successive application of phenol. It is immediately evident that RSS induced significantly greater accelerations in heart rate than did LSS under control conditions. This relation also characterized most heart rate responses throughout the right sympathetic stimulations. Phenolization of the superior right atrium (paints 1, 2, and 3) clearly reduced the positive chronotropic response to both right and left sympathetic stimulation, but even painting of all regions failed to totally eliminate the heart rate response. An important point not illustrated by Fig. 3-15 is the fact that successive phenol applications to the superior right atrium interrupted sympathetic input to the SAN region, but did not generally interrupt all input to the AVN region. Thus, shifts in P-wave rarely occurred during control RSS, but commonly appeared after paints 1, 2, and 3. This indicates distribution of right sympathetic fibers to both SAN and AVN regions, but the accelerating effect at the sinus node generally overwhelms the lesser sympathetic drive at the junctional region. This is in sharp contrast to distribution of sympathetic fibers from the left side. Control LSS regularly resulted in shift of the P-wave with assumption of a junctional pacemaker. Sinus acceleration was significantly less during LSS, which we have interpreted to indicate significantly less innervation of the sinus region from the left sympathetics.

REFERENCES

1. Abraham, A., *Die Mikroskopische Innervation des Herzens und der Blutgefasse Von Verbraten*. Budapest:Akademiai Kiado, Verlag der Ungarischen Akademie der Wissenschaften, 1964.
2. Armour, J. A., W. C. Randall, S. Sinha, Localized myocardial responses to stimulation of small cardiac branches of the vagus. *Am. J. Physiol. 228*: 141–148, 1975.
3. Bertrand, M. E., J. M. Leblanche, M. F. Rousseau, H. H. Warembourg, C. Stankowtak, G. Soots, Surgical treatment of variant angina: use of plexectomy with aortocoronary bypass. *Circulation 61*: 877–882, 1980.
4. Bertrand, M. E., J. M. Leblanche, P. Y. Tilmant, Treatment of Prinzmetal's variant angina: role of medical treatment with Nifedipine and surgical coronary revascularization combined with plexectomy. *Am. J. Cardiol. 47*::174–178, 1981.
5. Cohn, A. E., On the differences in the effects of stimulation of the two vagus nerves on rate and conduction of the dog's heart. *J. Exp. Med. 16*: 732–757, 1912.
6. Cohn, A. E. and T. Lewis, The predominant influence of the left vagus nerve upon conduction between the auricles and ventricles in the dog. *J. Exp. Med. 18*: 739–747, 1913.
7. Cooper, T., W. Dagget, C. G. Nugent, C. R. Hanlon, Selective cardiac vagotomy. *J. Thoracic Cardiovasc. Surg.* 52: 761–768, 1966.

8. Geis, W. P., M. P. Kaye, W. C. Randall, Major autonomic pathways to the atria and SA and AV nodes of the canine heart. *Am. J. Physiol. 224*: 202–208, 1973.
9. Goldberg, J. M., J. H. Geesbreght, W. C. Randall, G. Brynjolfsson, Sympathetically induced pacemaker shifts following sinus node excision. *Am. J. Physiol. 224*: 1468–1474, 1973.
10. Hamlin, R. L., C. R. Smith, Effects of vagal stimulation on S-A and A-V nodes. *Am. J. Physiol. 215*: 560–568, 1968.
11. Hirsch, E. F., *The Innervation of the Vertebrate Heart*. C. C. Thomas, Springfield, Ill., 1971.
12. Hondeghen, L. M., E. Mouton, T. Stassen, H. DeGeest, Additive effects of acetylcholine released by vagal nerve stimulation on atrial rate. *J. Appl. Physiol. 38*: 108–113, 1975.
13. Irisawa, H., H. M. Caldwell, M. F. Wilson, Neural regulation of atrioventricular conduction. *Jap. J. Physiol. 21*: 15–25, 1971.
14. Jalife, J., G. K. Moe, Phasic effects of vagal stimulation on pacemaker activity of the isolated sinus node of the young cat. *Circ. Res. 45*: 595–607, 1979.
15. Jalife, J., A. J. Hamilton, V. R. Lamanna, G. K. Moe, Effects of current flow on pacemaker activity of the isolated kitten sinoatrial node. *Am. J. Physiol. 238*: H307–H316, 1980.
16. Kaye, M. P., G. R. Hageman, W. C. Randall, Selective parasympathectomy of the heart. *J. Appl. Physiol. 83*: 183–186, 1975.
17. Khabarova, A. Y. *The Afferent Innervation of the Heart*. Authorized translation from the Russian, B. Hagh, New York, Consultants Bureau, 1963.
18. Lazzara, R., B. J. Scherlag, M. J. Robinson, P. Samet, Parasympathetic control of canine SA and AV nodes. *Circ. Res. 32*: 393–401, 1973.
19. Levy, M. N. and P. J. Martin, Neural Control of the Heart. In *Handbook of Physiology*, Sec. 2, Vol. 1, ed. R. M. Berne. American Physiology Society, Bethesda, Md, pp. 581–620, 1979.
20. MacCanon, D. M. and S. M. Horvath, Effect of bilateral cervical vagotomy in the dog. *Am. J. Physiol. 189*: 569–572, 1957.
21. Nonidez, J. F., Studies on the innervation of the heart. I. Distribution of the cardiac nerves, with special reference to the identification of the sympathetic and parasympathetic preganglionics. *Am. J. Anat. 65*: 361–413, 1939.
22. Randall, W. C., *Nervous Control of the Heart*. Williams and Wilkins, Baltimore, 1965.
23. Randall, W. C., *Neural Regulation of the Heart*. Oxford University Press, New York, 1977.
24. Randall, W. C., D. E. Euler, H. K. Jacobs, W. H. Wehrmacher, M. P. Kaye, G. R. Hageman, Autonimic Neural control of cardiac rhythm: the role of autonomic imbalance in the genesis of cardiac dysrhythmia. *Cardiology 61*: 20–36, 1976.
25. Randall, W. C., M. P. Kaye, J. X. Thomas, M. J. Barber, Intrapericardial denervation of the heart. *J. Surg. Res. 29*: 101–109, 1980.
26. Randall, W. C. and J. X. Thomas, The selective autonomic innervation of the heart. In *Sidedness in the Neurovegetative Regulation of the Cardiovascular Appartus*, ed. F. Balsano and V. Marigliano. Edizioni L. Pozzi, S.r.1, Rome, pp. 114–132, 1981.
27. Randall, Walter C., J. X. Thomas, Jr., M. J. Barber, L. E. Rinkema, Selective denervation of the heart. *Am. J. Physiol., 244*: H607–H613, 1983.
28. Scherlag, B. J., B. D. Kosowsky, A. N. Damato, Technique for ventricular pacing from the His bundle of the intact heart. *J. Appl. Physiol. 22*: 584–587, 1967.

29. Sharpey-Schafer, E., Experiments on the cervical vagus and sympathetic. *Quart. J. Exp. Physiol. 12*: 231–301, 1919.
30. Shepard, R. S. and A. J. Whitty, Bilateral cervical vagotomy: a long time study on the unanesthetized dog. *Am. J. Physiol. 206*: 265–269, 1964.
31. Sloan, R. D., W. R. Webb, A. L. Meena, S. S. Tee, The cause of fatalities in bilateral vagotomies. *Surg. Forum 9*: 427–429, 1959.
32. Thomas, J. X., W. C. Randall, C. E. Jones, Protective effect of chronic versus acute cardiac denervation on contractile force during coronary occlusion. *Am. Heart J. 102*: 157–161, 1981.
33. Thomas, J. X., W. C. Randall, M. J. Barber, Intrapericardial localization of autonomics to the A-V node. *Fed. Proc. 37*: 790, 1978.
34. Thomas, J. X. and W. C. Randall, Autonomic influence on atrio-ventricular conduction in conscious dog. *Am. J. Physiol 244*: H102–H108, 1983.
35. Woolard, H. H., The innervation of the heart. *J.Anat. 60*: 345–373, 1925–26.

4

Parasympathetic Control of the Heart

MATTHEW N. LEVY and PAUL MARTIN

VAGAL CONTROL OF HEART RATE

Steady-State Control

The role of the vagus nerves in the control of cardiac rate and rhythm has been recognized for more than three centuries. During the seventeenth century, Richard Lower and Robert Boyle independently observed a transient period of cardiac standstill when they ligated the vagi in experimental animals [37]. Soon after electrical stimulating devices became available, the Weber brothers showed that vagal stimulation caused a reduction in the heart rate [37]. In 1897, Hunt carried out the first quantitative study of the effects of vagal stimulation on heart rate [41]. Rosenblueth [100] reported in 1932 that the change in heart rate evoked by vagal stimulation was a simple hyperbolic function of the stimulation frequency (Fig. 4-1). Since that study, the vagal control of heart rate has been analyzed in much greater detail, as more sophisticated measurement and modeling techniques have been developed [7–9,26,29,39,51,73,94, 118,120,121,123].

The chronotropic responses to stimulation of the cardiac sympathetic nerves tend to be slow in onset and to decay slowly upon cessation of stimulation [120]. In sharp contrast, the changes in heart rate elicited by a train of vagal stimuli (Fig. 4-2) appear after a brief latent period, reach a steady-state response within a few beats, and decay rapidly back to the control level when stimulation is discontinued [120]. This rapid decay is undoubtedly ascribable to the large quantities of acetylcholinesterase that are present in close proximity to the automatic cells in the S-A node [47]. Recent studies indicate that the chronotropic response to a constant train of vagal stimuli does not remain at a constant level, but tends to diminish somewhat over the next several beats before a steady-state level is attained [77,87]. This fading of the response may reflect the phenome-

Supported in part by the U.S. Public Health Grants HL 10951, HL 22484, and HL 15758.

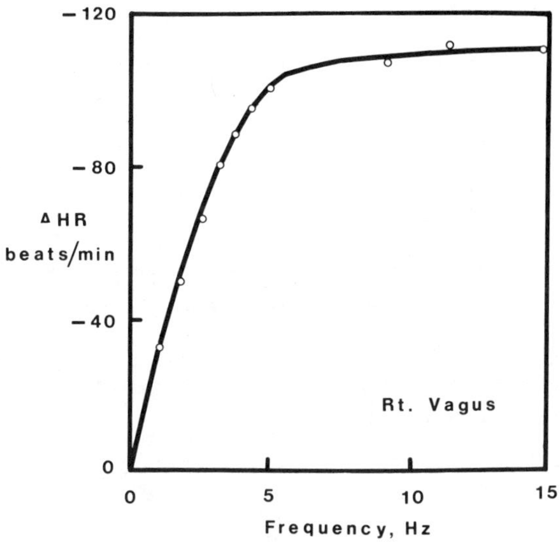

Fig. 4-1. The change in heart rate as a function of the frequency of right vagal stimulation in the cat. (Adapted from Rosenblueth, [100])

non of receptor or effector densensitization [77,87,45], which will be discussed below in the section on atrial contractility.

Effects of Brief Vagal Stimuli

Brown and Eccles [4,5] demonstrated in 1934 that a single stimulus or a brief burst of stimuli delivered to the vagus nerves influenced the heart rate for the next 10 to 15 seconds. The precise effect of such stimulation depended on the time in the cardiac cycle that the stimulus was applied. Their observations have

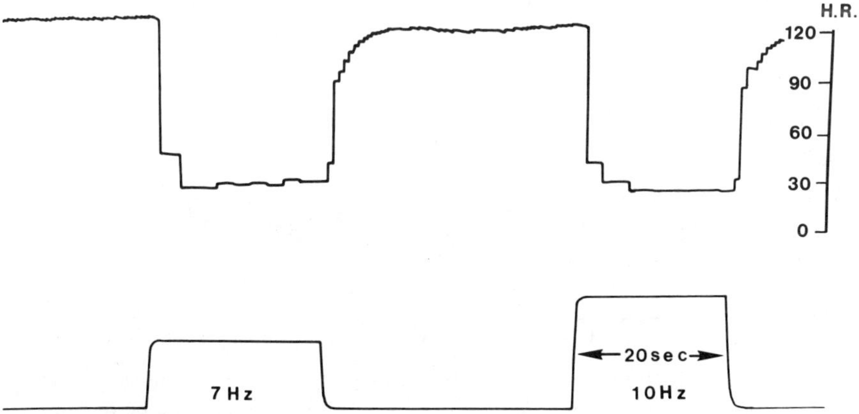

Fig. 4-2. The changes in heart rate evoked by trains of right vagal stimulation at frequencies of 7 and 10 Hz in a dog. (Adapted from Warner and Cox [120])

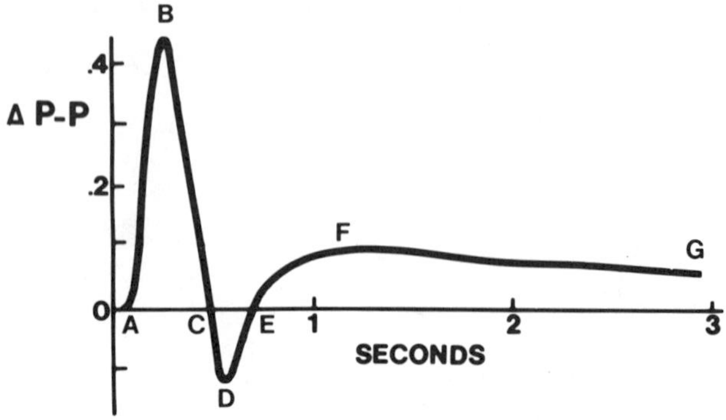

Fig. 4-3. Time course of the changes in P–P interval evoked by a brief burst of vagal stimuli in a dog. (Adapted from Iano et al. [42])

since been confirmed by many investigators [42,46,53,66,105,113,106], but some of the mechanisms underlying the response have only recently been elucidated.

A representative graph (Fig. 4-3) from a study by Iano et al. [42] shows the changes in cardiac cycle length (P–P interval) evoked by a brief vagal stimulus as a function of the time after the stimulus. Electrophysiological studies by Spear et al. [105] revealed that the initial prolongation of the P–P interval (the beginning of the first upstroke, AB) reflected a prolongation of the S-A conduction time rather than a true reduction in firing rate of the automatic cells in the S-A node. Their studies, as well as those of Jalife and Moe [46], also showed that the remainder of the primary phase of deceleration (ABC) was associated with a hyperpolarization of the automatic cells. Transmembrane potentials recorded from automatic cells in the S-A node are shown in Fig. 4-4 [46]. Shortly after a brief vagal stimulus was given (arrow), the cell membrane became hyperpolar-

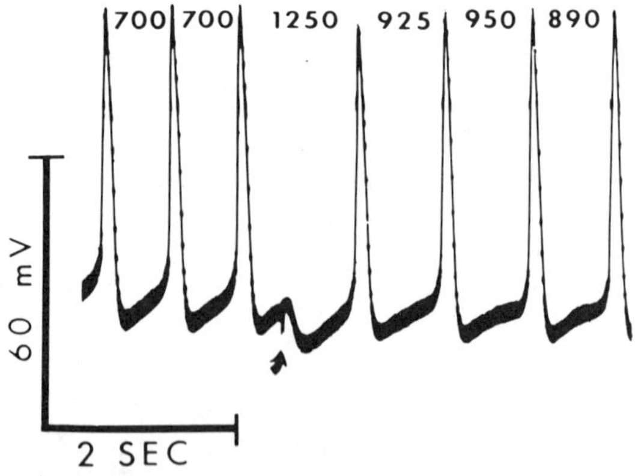

Fig. 4-4. Transmembrane action potentials recorded from the S-A node of a cat. A brief burst of vagal stimuli was given at the arrow. The numbers between the peaks of the action potentials indicate the cardiac cycle lengths, in msec. (Adapted from Jalife and Moe [46], with permission of the American Heart Association)

ized briefly. The acetylcholine (ACh) released at the vagal endings undoubtedly diminished the potassium conductance of the automatic cells [60], thereby evoking the hyperpolarization.

During the secondary phase of deceleration (EFG, Fig. 4-3), on the other hand, there was a reduction in the slope of the pacemaker potential [46,105], as shown in Fig. 4-4 (last three cardiac cycles). There was no detectable hyperpolarization during this secondary phase, which suggests that the ACh must have been almost completely hydrolyzed by the end of the primary phase of deceleration. Measurements made with a potassium-sensitive electrode indicated that the changes in cycle length during the secondary phase (EFG) were paralleled by changes in extracellular potassium concentration [105]. It is possible that such changes in potassium concentration are responsible for this secondary increase in cardiac cycle length.

The primary and secondary phases of deceleration are characteristically separated by a brief phase of relative or absolute cardiac acceleration (CDE, Fig. 4-3); that is, the dip in the curve may or may not extend below the prestimulation level of cardiac cycle length. During the brief acceleratory phase, the maximum diastolic potential of the pacemaker cells was found to rise slightly to a less negative value [105]. Hence, this transient acceleration might be ascribable to an evanescent increase in sodium conductance.

Phase-Dependent Effects of Repetitive Vagal Stimuli

If the cervical vagus nerves are stimulated once each cardiac cycle, the chronotropic response of the heart will depend on the timing of the stimuli relative to the phase of the cardiac cycle [66,99,113]. In the experiment illustrated in Fig. 4-5, one supramaximal pulse was delivered to the cardiac segments of the transected cervical vagi of an anesthetized dog each cardiac cycle [66]. When each stimulus (St) was delivered at the beginning of atrial depolarization (i.e. at a P–St interval of zero), the cardiac cycle length (P–P interval) increased to a value of 700 msec; the control value prior to vagal stimulation was 390 msec. As the stimuli were delivered at progressively later times in the cardiac cycle, the P–P interval continued to increase, until it reached a maximum value of 760 msec when the P–St interval was about 225 msec.

As the P–St intervals exceeded 225 msec (Fig. 4-5), the P–P interval progressively diminished. The minimum chronotropic response was obtained at a P–St interval of about 390 msec. When the nerves were stimulated at still later phases in the cycle, the chronotropic responses progressively increased again. Such a curve of the P–P intervals, plotted as a function of the P–St interval, constitutes a "phase–response curve" for the S-A node pacemaker cells. The precise phase–response relationship can be altered by other influences that affect automatic cell behavior, such as concomitant sympathetic activity [60] or the administration of glucagon [111].

The phase dependency of the chronotropic response to repetitive vagal stimulation confers a peculiar characteristic to such stimulation; i.e. such repetitive stimuli tend to entrain the S-A nodal pacemaker cells [66,99,113]. As a conse-

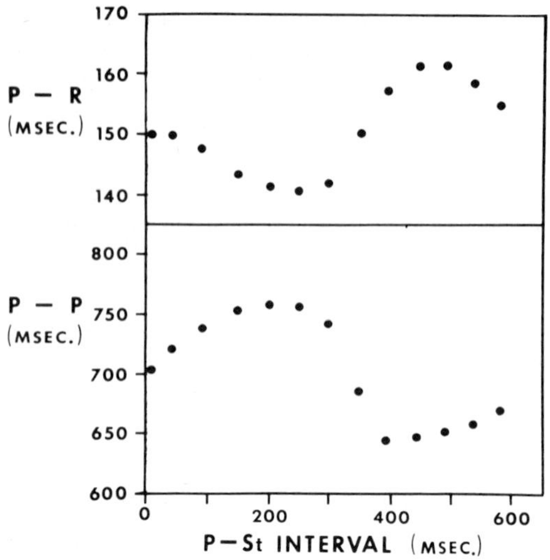

Fig. 4-5. The effects of vagal stimuli, delivered once each cardiac cycle, on the P–R and P–P intervals of the dog. The effects varied, depending on the P–St interval, which is the time after the onset of atrial depolarization (P wave). (From Levy et al. [66], with permission of the American Heart Association)

quence of such synchronization, as the frequency of vagal stimulation is changed within a critical range of frequencies, the heart rate takes on the same frequency as the vagal stimulation. Thus, within a limited range of frequencies, an increase in the frequency of vagal stimulation from f_1 to f_2 will cause an equal change in heart rate, from f_1 to f_2. This is a paradoxical response. Considering that the vagus nerves inhibit heart rate, an increase in stimulation frequency would be expected to induce a reduction in heart rate!

When the vagal stimulation consists of repetitive, brief bursts of pulses, rather than single, equally spaced pulses, the tendency for the S-A nodal cells to be synchronized by the vagal activity is augmented considerably [16,63]. The spontaneous activity recorded from efferent vagal fibers to the heart consists of such repetitive bursts of action potentials clustered within a discrete portion of each cardiac cycle [50,52,55].

Figure 4-6 illustrates the changes in cardiac cycle length (P–P interval) that occur when the vagi are stimulated by such repetitive bursts of pulses, and the frequency of those bursts is progressively increased [63]. It is evident that as the stimulation frequency was increased, there was an overall lengthening of the P–P interval; i.e. the P–P intervals near the right end of the record tended to be greater than those near the left end. This conforms to the well-established fact that the vagus exerts a negative chronotropic effect.

It is obvious, however, that the change in cycle length evoked by the vagal stimulation is not a continuous, monotonic function of the stimulation frequency, such as that shown in Fig. 4-1. Instead, the P–P interval tracing in Fig.

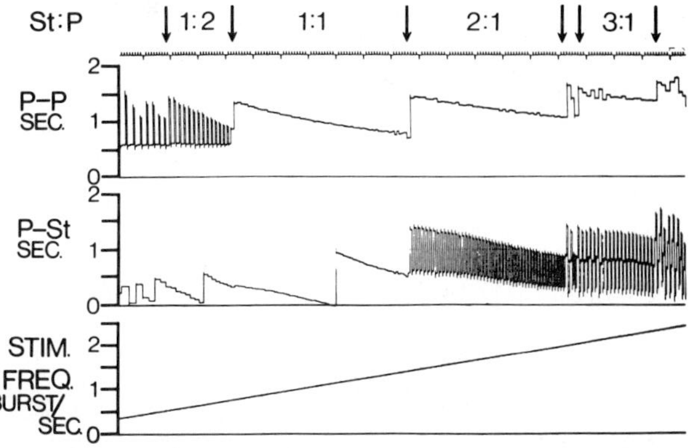

Fig. 4-6. Changes in P–P interval as the frequency of vagal stimulation was progressively increased in a dog. The P–St interval denotes the time after the beginning of atrial depolarization (P wave) that the vagal stimulus (St) happened to be given. The numbers between the arrows denote the ratio of vagal stimulus bursts to heart beats. (Adapted from Levy et al. [63], with permission of the American Heart Association)

4-6 discloses several discontinuities, such that a minute change in stimulation frequency may evoke a pronounced change in cardiac cycle length. Between each of the discontinuities (indicated by the arrows), the cardiac rate displayed a paradoxical response; i.e. the cardiac cycle length decreased (rather than increased) as the frequency of stimulation was raised. The ratios (St:P) that appear between the arrows denote the ratios of the number of stimulus bursts (St) to the number of atrial depolarizations (P waves). Between the arrows that signify an St:P ratio of 1:1, as the burst frequency was increased from 0.76 to 1.33 bursts/second, the P–P interval decreased from 1.32 to 0.75 second. When the P–P interval is converted to frequency, it becomes evident that the heart rate had increased from 0.76 to 1.33 beats/second, or from 46 to 80 beats/minute. This frequency was identical to the stimulation frequency, indicating that the heart had been beating once for each vagal stimulus burst over the entire frequency range from 0.76 to 1.33 Hz. Over other frequency ranges, synchronization had also prevailed, but in other St:P ratios (Fig. 4-6).

The same type of phase–response behavior that is characteristic of S-A nodal automatic cells is equally characteristic of automatic cells in the A-V junction [119]. Furthermore, in order to demonstrate such phasic effects of vagal activity on the cardiac pacemaker regions, the application of the stimuli need not be restricted to efferent vagal fibers. Stimulation of afferent fibers in the carotid sinus or aortic depressor nerves in dogs will evoke reflex effects on heart rate that depend on the time within the cardiac cycle that the stimuli are delivered [71,75]. Reflex vagal excitation by a neck suction device in human subjects has disclosed a similar phase–response relationship [18,19].

In the S-A node, the clusters of automatic cells are in poor communication; conduction velocity is very slow from one cluster to the next [34,48]. The pronounced synchronizing tendency of repetitive vagal activity probably serves to coordinate the automatic activity of such diverse cell clusters within the S-A node [48]. This mechanism probably also serves to synchronize the recipient S-A nodal rhythm with the donor heart rate in human cardiac transplant patients [109]. It may also be one of the ancillary mechanisms responsible for synchronizing the atrial and ventricular rhythms in experimental [74] and clinical [62] isorhythmic A-V dissociation.

VAGAL CONTROL OF ATRIOVENTRICULAR CONDUCTION

Steady-State Control

The vagi depress atrioventricular (A-V) conduction, whereas the cardiac sympathetic nerves facilitate it [17,36]. Continuous supramaximal trains of vagal stimulation prolonged A-V conduction time after a latency of less than 1 sec [43], and they induced bradydysrhythmias with fixed or variable degrees of heart block [31]. The prolongation of A-V conduction time was a monotonically increasing function of stimulus intensity. A-V block usually did not appear until the A-V conduction had been prolonged by 50–70% of control [43,33,93,66]. The degree of prolongation depended strongly on the concomitant degree of S-A nodal slowing [14,84,93]. That is, there was a strong interaction between the direct vagal inhibitory effect on the A-V node and the simultaneous indirect facilitatory effect on A-V conduction ascribed to the concomitant tendency for vagal activity to decrease the heart rate. Such a reduction in heart rate served to enhance A-V conduction. Consequently, quantitative conclusions about vagal control of A-V conduction are very tenuous in those studies where heart rate has not been held constant. This interaction between the direct and indirect influences of efferent vagal activity on A-V conduction will be discussed in detail below.

In an early study on dogs with atrial fibrillation, tbe opposing effects of simultaneous activity in the two autonomic divisions on A-V conduction were found to be algebraically additive [100]. We confirmed this result in dogs whose hearts were in normal sinus rhythm [73]. The change in A-V conduction time in response to activity in one autonomic division was independent of the level of activity in the other; i.e. there was no significant vagal-sympathetic interaction for A-V conduction. This is in sharp contrast to the control of S-A nodal function, where such an autonomic interaction is pronounced, as discussed below (Fig. 4-13).

In humans, autonomic blockade experiments have established that A-V conduction is normally under the influence of both autonomic divisions [1,101]. Nevertheless, when both divisions were blocked simultaneously and the heart was not paced, there was little change of A-V conduction time from control [96]. It was concluded that the effects of the two autonomic divisions were balanced in the control of A-V conduction. The problem with this interpretation, of course, is that the heart was not paced. Instead, the lack of change in A-V conduction may have been due to a balance between the direct and indirect vagal effects on cycle length discussed above.

Dynamic Control

The dynamics of the vagal control of A-V conduction are best studied with single stimuli or brief bursts of stimuli to the vagi. We found the effects of single stimuli to be extremely variable in experiments in which heart rate was not controlled by pacing. A-V conduction was shortened after some stimuli and prolonged after others, depending on the associated change in the cardiac cycle length of the preceding beat [66]. However, when the heart rate was held constant by pacing, single vagal stimuli always prolonged A-V conduction [82]. Just as for the S-A node, the phase of the cardiac cycle at the time the vagal impulse arrived at the A-V junction was an important determinant of its efficacy.

In order to quantify the effects of timing, we constructed "vagal effect curves" (Fig. 4-7), analogous to those devised by Brown and Eccles [4,5] in 1934 in their study of the vagal control of heart rate. The abscissa of these curves are the elapsed times from the vagal stimulus to the onsets of ventricular activation for several beats. The ordinates are the percent changes in AV conduction that occurred during each of these beats after the stimulus. A complete curve is generated by combining the responses to many individual stimuli that were applied at various times throughout the entire cardiac cycle.

The vagal effect curve in Fig. 4-7 shows that the change in A-V conduction depended on the time that had elapsed since the stimulation. The effect was most pronounced on the first beat after the stimulus (circles), and then it diminished on the second (squares), third, and fourth (triangles) beats. The atrial rate was also an important determinant of the magnitude of the response for a given stimulus. The upper and lower curves of Fig. 4-7 represent the data that were derived when the atria were paced at cardiac cycle lengths of 350 and at 450 msec, respectively. Note that when the atria were paced at the shorter cardiac

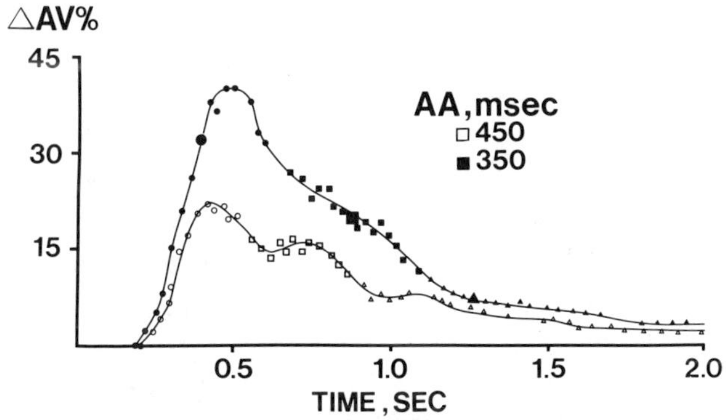

Fig. 4-7. Vagal effect curves from the dog in Fig. 4-6 at two different atrial pacing intervals. The abscissa indicates the time elapsed from a single vagal stimulus burst given at t = 0. The ordinate is the percent change in AV conduction time over a sequence of consecutive cardiac cycles with the circles, squares, and triangles measured in the first, second, and subsequent beats after the beat in which the stimulus is given. (From Martin [84] with permission)

cycle length the identical vagal stimulus induced a prolongation of A-V conduction twice the length of that induced when the atria were paced at the longer cycle length.

One mechanism responsible for this effect could be the fact that the relative refractory periods of the A-V conduction system [82,106] are longer than the durations of the associated action potential. As A-V conduction is prolonged (by vagal activity or otherwise) the action potential duration is increased in the A-V node due to electrotonic effects [38]. There is a concomitant lengthening of the relative refractory period, and thus the next impulse (during pacing) falls earlier in the relative refractory period [82,106]. This mechanism will likely lead to an additional increment in A-V conduction time, just as indicated in Fig. 4-7. This mechanism may also explain the A-V nodal Wenckebach phenomenon [67].

Persistent Effects of Vagal Stimulation

The cardiac responses to vagal stimulation are strongly dependent on the elapsed time between those stimuli [83,86]. We found that when the two identical vagal stimuli were separated by progressively greater time intervals the response to the second stimulus progressively decreased and it reached a value of about half the corresponding value of the first response when the time between stimuli was about 4 to 8 sec (Fig. 4-8). As the time between stimuli was increased further, the amplitude of the second response gradually increased to approach that of the first, but it did not reach that amplitude until about one minute had been allowed to elapse between stimuli. We recently extended these observations to include the chronotropic and intropic cardiac responses [86]. Figure 4-9, shows that the same time-dependency characteristic holds for all

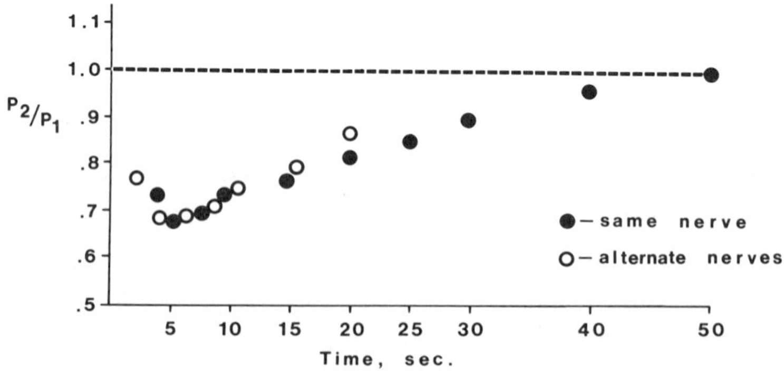

Fig. 4-8. Plot of ratio of second to first peak response amplitude (P2/P1) vs. time of separation; composite of 12 experiments. The standard errors are omitted for clarity, but the maximum standard error was 0.11. "Same nerve" denotes those points for which an ipsilateral vagus was used to produce both P1 and P2, "alternate nerve" denotes those points for which the nerve on one side was used for P1 and nerve on the alternate side for P2. (From Martin [84] with permission)

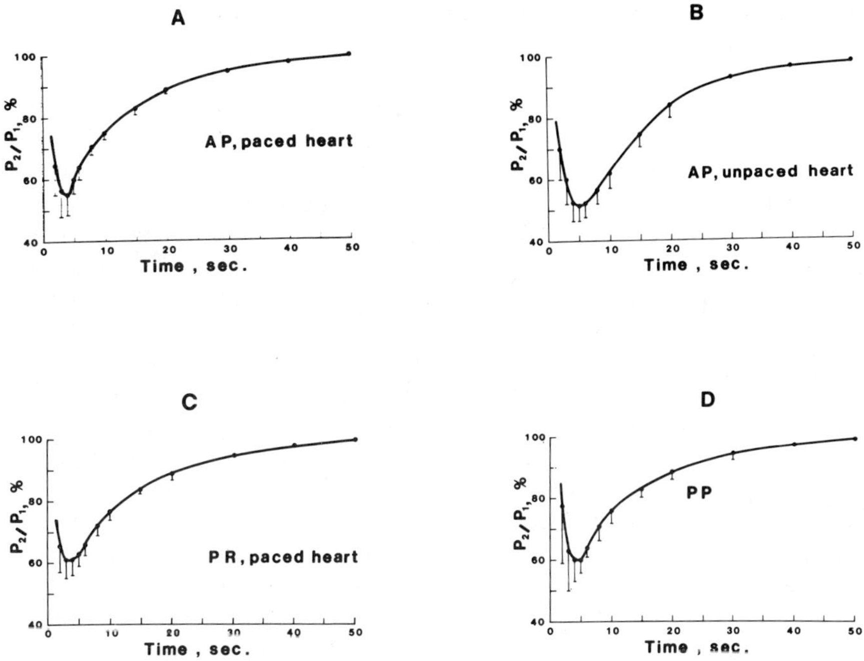

Fig. 4-9. Composite data plots of ratio of peak responses, P2/P1 vs. time of separation of stimuli for four cardiac variables measured: (A) atrial contractility (AP) in the paced heart preparation; (B) AP in the unpaced-heart preparation; (C) atrioventricular conduction, P–R interval in paced-heart preparation; (D) heart period, P–P. Points and vertical bars, means ± SE. (From Martin [86] with permission)

measured cardiac variables. Indeed, when these characteristics were normalized with respect to their maximal values, the four curves were virtually superimposable.

The mechanism of this time dependency of the neural effect has not been established. The attenuation of the second response does not depend on a decrease in the release of acetylcholine in response to the second stimulus, however. This was shown in experiments in which the first stimulus was given to one vagus and the second stimulus was given to the other vagus. The time dependency was similar to that observed when the two sequential stimuli were given to the same nerve (Fig. 4-8).

Vagal Effect–Cycle Length Interactions. In 1913 Cohn and Lewis [10] noted that the cardiac cycle length was an important determinant of A-V conduction time. Most who study the effect of direct neural stimulation on A-V function thus now use a paced-heart preparation. However, only a few investigators have attempted to characterize the interaction between the direct vagal effects on A-V conduction and the indirect vagal effects ascribable to the concomitant changes in heart rate [14,84,92]. Pavlov [93] used 5 second trains of vagal stimuli, and found that A-V conduction was maximally prolonged by weak stimuli, but stronger stimuli actually facilitated conduction. The weak stimuli scarcely affected heart rate, whereas the stronger stimuli caused a pronounced reduction in heart rate.

De Beer et al. [14] measured the effects of step changes in atrial pacing rate and of vagal stimulation on A-V conduction. They found that the change in A-V conduction time followed an exponential time course after a step change in pacing rate. Maximal vagal stimulation increased the time constant of the exponential function by a factor of four. These responses were independent of the level of background sympathetic activity. They were purely an A-V nodal phenomenon; changes in atrial or ventricular conduction did not contribute to the response.

We studied the interaction between the effects of heart rate and vagal activity on A-V conduction from a different perspective [84]. The combined effects of vagal stimulation and changes in heart rate on A-V conduction were first determined in spontaneously beating hearts. The change in the A-V conduction was thus the result of two oppositely directed influences: namely, the evoked decrease in heart rate acted to decrease the A-V conduction time during the next beat, whereas the acetylcholine released at the A-V junction acted directly to prolong A-V conduction. To measure the combined effect of these two factors, the vagi were stimulated when the heart was not paced. The beat-to-beat changes in A-V conduction time and cardiac cycle length were recorded in computer memory. To measure the direct effects per se, the atria were then paced at a constant rate, and the identical vagal stimulation was again applied. To measure the indirect effects of dynamic cycle length changes, the S-A node was first crushed. The identical sequence of cycle lengths that had previously been obtained during vagal stimulation when the heart was unpaced were now imposed on the heart through atrial pacing electrodes. This was done by "playing back" in real-time those sequences of cycle lengths previously stored in computer memory to trigger a stimulator connected to the atrial electrodes. The effects of the sequences of changes in cycle lengths on A-V conduction were thus assessed independently of the effects of vagal activity.

Figure 4-10 illustrates the results of a typical experiment. The vagal effect curve (U, dashed curve), top half of figure, shows the combined effects of vagal stimulation and changes in cycle length, and the solid curve (P) represents the effect of vagal stimulation when heart rate was held constant. It is evident that the response of the unpaced heart (U) first increased, then decreased, with time. At several time intervals the decreased conduction time is substantially less than control. However, when the heart rate was held constant by pacing (P), vagal stimulation produced only a prolongation of the A-V conduction time. The lower solid curve of the bottom panel (PB) depicts the effect on A-V conduction of inducing the same sequence of cardiac cycle lengths that had been obtained previously in the spontaneously beating heart during vagal stimulation. The data that produced curve PB were recorded, however, in the absence of vagal activity. The dashed curve (D) (lower half of figure) was obtained by subtracting curve P from curve U (i.e. $D = U - P$). This difference curve (D) represents the linear subtraction of the direct component from the total vagal effect

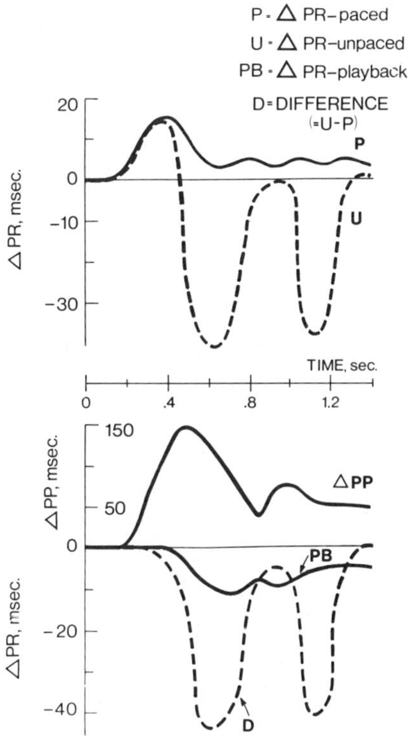

Fig. 4-10. Top: Vagal effect curves from the same preparation in which the vagus was stimulated and the heart was paced (P) or unpaced (U). Bottom: the effect of vagal stimulation on atrial rate (ΔPP) measured simultaneously with the unpaced heart curve (U) above. When these same sequences of changing atrial rates are used to pace the atrium without vagal stimulation, the effect on A-V conduction is measured as the curve labeled PB. The curve labeled D is the arithmetic difference between the unpaced and paced heart curves at each point in time. (From Martin [84] with permission)

(i.e., direct plus indirect) on A-V conduction. If the direct and indirect vagal effects were summated linearly, the P and D curves should have coincided. Figure 4-10 clearly shows that this hypothesis was not true, which indicated that the nonlinearities in the interaction between the direct and indirect effects were considerable.

Also, because the vagally induced increase in cycle length and the direct effect of the acetylcholine released in the A-V node have oppositely directed effects on A-V conduction, it was predicted that their combined influence would be intermediate between the effects of the direct and indirect influences acting independently. Figure 4-10 clearly shows that this prediction was incorrect. From the second through the fourth beat after the stimulus, the decrease in A-V conduction time evoked by a change in cycle length alone (curve PB) was less than that observed when the same sequence of cycle length changes had been induced by vagal stimulation (curve U). Paradoxically, the A-V conduction time was actually shorter in the presence than in the absence of vagal activity when the heart period underwent identical changes.

Two mechanisms were responsible for this unexpected result. Electrograms recorded from several atrial sites showed that the atrial activation patterns were radically altered by the vagal stimulus, which signified that there had been considerable shifts in the cardiac pacemaking site. It has since been amply demonstrated that many atrial sites are capable of subsidiary pacemaker function [22]. This mechanism did not account quantitatively for the entire difference between predicted and observed responses. Another component, less clearly defined, is related to the transmission properties of the A-V node or infranodal structures.

It is clear that increasing the cycle length ameliorates the depressive effects of acetylcholine on AV conduction [14,84,93]. It is also clear that the heart rate–vagal activity interactions are complex and much more work must be done before all the details of this phenomenon are understood. The application of microelectrode techniques could lead to insights in this area. It would be valuable to measure the transmembrane potentials of A-V nodal cells when the interval between depolarizations is suddenly varied during vagal stimulation or when acetylcholine is applied iontophoretically.

AUTONOMIC TONE AND CARDIAC REFRACTORY PERIODS

Vagal stimulation significantly reduces the atrial refractory period [126]. This effect is undoubtedly due to the significant shortening of the atrial action potential induced by acetylcholine [6].

The effect of ACh on ventricular refractory periods is not so clear, however. In both the dog [103] and human [30,160] atropine decreased the duration of such refractory periods. However, blockade of both autonomic divisions evoked negligible changes in refractory periods. Also, in the dog, vagal nerve stimulation significantly prolonged ventricular refractory periods, except when the dog was sympathectomized [89]. These findings suggest that ACh acted indirectly by antagonizing the sympathetic effects, rather than acting directly [30,89,103]. Reports of partial and total autonomic blockade experiments in humans, however, have established that resting vagal tone exerts a significant increase in ventricular refractoriness, and that the effect can occur in the presence of sympathetic blockade [96]. Also, the dominant pathway of the reflex control of ventricular refractory periods in cats was carried by the vagi, which required no sympathetic activity to exert such an effect [3]. Thus, the latter two studies are in conflict with the view that ACh acts only or primarily by antagonizing the effect of sympathetic activity. No obvious factors, based on possible differences in experimental methodologies, were found to explain these opposing views. It should be clarified that all evidence indicated that ACh antagonizes adrenergic effects; the dispute is over the degree of independent control of refractoriness by the vagi.

No matter what the mechanism, prolongation of refractory periods may prove beneficial in terminating arrhythmias. Many arrhythmias are sustained by a reentrant circuit. If the refractory periods of one limb of this circuit were prolonged, for example, the conduction through this limb may be stopped, or slowed sufficiently to interrupt the reentrant feedback that maintains the arrhythmia. Such a mechanism has been proposed to explain the effect of increased vagal activity in suppressing ventricular tachycardias [122].

CONTROL OF MYOCARDIAL CONTRACTILITY

Ventricular Contractility

Until the last decade it was commonly believed that the vagi had a negligible influence on ventricular function in mammals [58]. De Geest et al. [15] devised three separate experimental preparations in which the heart rate, preload, afterload, atrial transport function, and coronary perfusion pressure were rigorously controlled. When the vagi were maximally stimulated, ventricular contractility was significantly depressed by 15–25%.

These findings have been confirmed in a variety of canine preparations. Vagal stimulation caused the ventricular function curves to be shifted to the right [13,125], it significantly reduced the maximum ventricular dP/dt [13,24,35,76,92], and diminished the ventricular contractile force [12,21,35,60,91,97,98,107]. Randall et al. [98] have studied the regional effects of cardiac autonomic nerve stimulation in considerable detail. They found that the regional distribution of efferent vagal fibers was highly specific. Contractile force was more severely depressed at the base than at the apex of the ventricle by vagal stimulation.

Atrial Contractility

It is well established that the atria are much more sensitive than the ventricles to vagal influences. Wiggers [124] documented this in 1917, and Sarnoff et al. [102] later extended the concept with an analysis of the autonomic influences on cardiac function curves. The greater atrial sensitivity has been confirmed by many different types of observations, but perhaps in the most exquisite detail by the experiments of Randall et al. [97]. The atria have much higher cholinesterase concentrations and a much richer extrinsic [36,47] and intrinsic parasympathetic innervation than do the ventricles [95]. Hence, the onset and termination of atrial responses to vagal stimulation are more rapid than are those of the ventricles. In the atria, ACh has much shorter diffusion distances to effect an inotropic response. Furthermore, the response is terminated more rapidly in the atria due to the higher concentrations of cholinesterase. However, Priola et al. [95] have shown that these cannot be the sole factors because the ventricular responses to intracoronary injections of ACh have a slower onset and slower time course than do the atrial responses.

In previous studies of the atrial responses to vagal activity in mammals, long trains of stimuli were used and steady-state responses were measured. We recently studied the transient inotropic responses to single or brief vagal stimuli in canine atria [85]. Figure 4-11 shows the typical results of applying a single burst of 1, 2, or 3 pulses to the vagi while the heart was paced at one of two different rates. Note that a single vagal stimulus pulse reduced atrial contractile amplitude by 62% when the pacing interval was 600 msec. One burst of two or three pulses reduced the strength of the atrial contractions to almost zero for 2 to 8 seconds at this pacing interval. Pacing the heart at a shorter interval (500 msec) resulted in less reduction of the inotropic response to the identical stimuli.

Vagal effect curves were generated for the inotropic responses. The basic algorithm used was the same as that used previously for plotting the chronotropic and dromotropic responses. Figure 4-12 shows the vagal effect curves for the simultaneous changes in cardiac cycle length (PP) and atrial contractility. During the first high peak of the chronotropic response, there is no equivalent change in the inotropic response. The large-amplitude trough of the inotropic response is virtually a mirror image of the lower amplitude secondary peak of

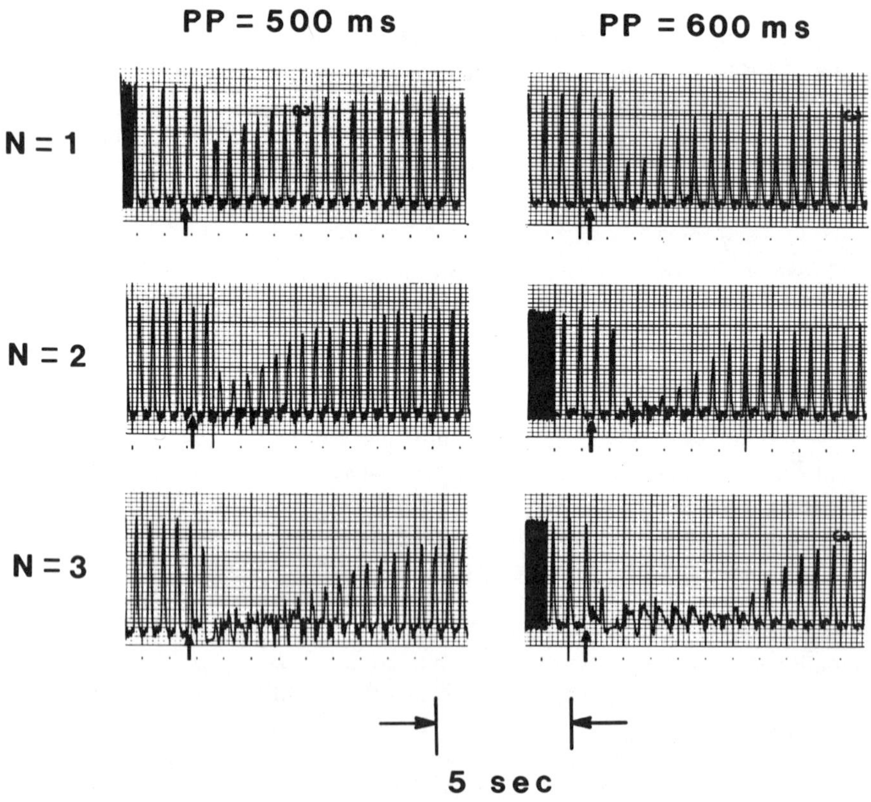

Fig. 4-11. Oscillograph tracings of atrial balloon pressure in response to 1, 2, or 3 stimuli per vagal burst (N), given at the time marked by arrow in each trace and with each set of stimuli at two different values of cardiac interval (PP) in paced heart. (From Martin [85] with permission)

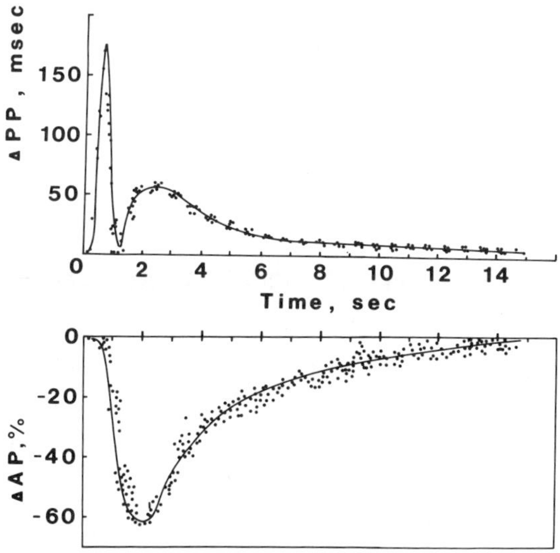

Fig. 4-12. Vagal effect curves for cardiac interval (PP), above in unpaced-heart preparation and atrial balloon pressure (AP, below) in paced-heart preparation. Curves represent data from sequence of stimulus bursts given at various P–St intervals in same experimental animal. Thus, the power curve is a summation of many responses, but plotted on common axes where the origin is the occurrence of stimulus. (From Martin [85] with permission)

the chronotropic response. That these separate inotropic and chronotropic response components have such a similar time course suggests that the mechanisms of action of these two components may be strongly related.

The functions of the S-A and A-V nodal regions are quite sensitive to the phase of the cardiac cycle at which a vagal stimulus burst is given as is atrial contractility [85]. That is, a sudden burst of vagal activity that occurs during one phase of the cardiac cycle may depress the next atrial contraction completely, whereas at a different phase, the same burst of activity may have relatively little effect. Such irregularities of timing may occur during certain arrhythmias and they may influence the atrial contribution to ventricular filling.

The negative inotropic responses to vagal stimulation in the paced-heart preparation were always lower in amplitude than the responses of the spontaneously beating heart to the identical stimuli. The clear and consistent differences between vagal effect curves for inotropic responses of paced- and unpaced-heart preparations could not be accounted for entirely by changes of preload, nor by the steady-state, frequency–force relationship of the atrial musculature. As the stimulus intensity was increased (more stimuli per burst), the differences between the responses in the paced and unpaced hearts diminished. One explanation for these phenomena involves the dynamic atrial frequency–force relationship. That is, there is probably a significant dynamic interaction between the direct vagal effect on atrial contractility and the indirect effect of

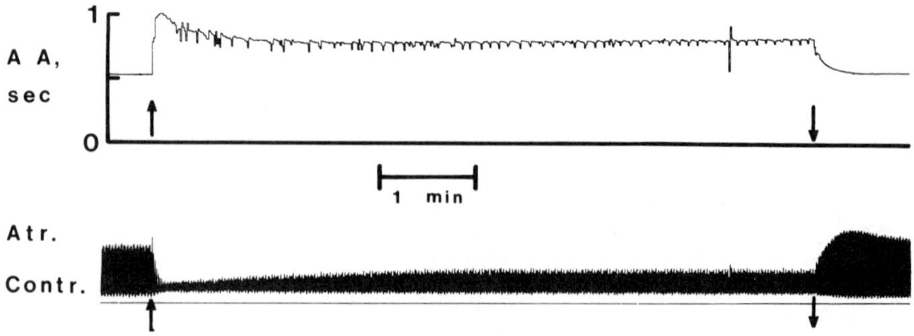

Fig. 4-13. Changes in heart period (AA, above) and atrial contractility (below) in response to a continuous train of vagal stimuli given between the arrows. Note that both the chronotropic and inotropic responses return back toward control from some initial maximal value, despite the continuous stimulation. (From Martin [87] with permission)

dynamically changing cardiac cycle lengths, as described above for A-V conduction. Further, this frequency–force relationship is probably quite different when measured on a beat-by-beat basis as opposed to the traditional steady-state characterization. Further study of the differences between the dynamic and the steady-state frequency–force relationships, and their interaction with the transient inotropic responses to vagal stimulation, is needed to unravel the underlying mechanisms.

Figure 4-13 shows the decay (or fading) of the cardiac responses during the application of a constant train of vagal stimuli. In these experiments, the fading of the chronotropic response reached a steady state in about 15–20 sec, whereas the fading of the inotropic response required 1–2 min. Others have reported recently that A-V conduction responses do not fade with continuous vagal stimulation [77]. Thus, different mechanisms may be responsible for the fading of different types of cardiac responses. Although a progressive reduction in the release of ACh cannot be entirely ruled out, other evidence suggests that receptor desensitization may be the principal mechanism [87,115]. Other investigators, using a variety of preparations, have reported similar phenomena [27,46,77] but no single mechanism seems to account for the diverse results.

VAGAL–SYMPATHETIC INTERACTIONS

In the walls of the heart many of the postganglionic vagal and sympathetic nerve endings lie close to each other [11,20,44,114]. As a consequence, complex interactions occur when both divisions of the autonomic nervous system are active at the same time. Several detailed reviews have been devoted to such peripheral autonomic interactions [17,36,59,104,60]. Various interactions have been described, but the principal type has been called "accentuated antagonism" [59]. Under its influence the inhibitory effect of a given level of vagal activity becomes more pronounced the greater the prevailing level of sympathetic activity.

Much has been learned about the mechanism responsible for accentuated antagonism over the past decade. The interaction is mediated at both presynaptic and postsynaptic levels; the synapse in question is that between the postganglionic sympathetic nerve ending and the cardiac effector cell. The presynaptic mechanism involves a cholinergically mediated inhibition of norepinephrine release from the postganglionic sympathetic nerve terminals. The postsynaptic mechanisms involve interactions at the level of the effector cell itself, and are probably mediated by the cyclic nucleotides, cAMP and cGMP. This section will deal with the cardiac manifestations of accentuated antagonism in the control of heart rate and myocardial contractility, and with the presynaptic mechanisms that are involved in the process. The postsynaptic aspects of this interaction will be described in chapters 5 and 6.

Accentuated Antagonism

The contribution of accentuated antagonism to the autonomic control of heart rate is illustrated in Fig. 4-14. In this experiment [73], supramaximal vagal stimulation at a frequency of 8 Hz (left) caused a reduction in heart rate of 80 beats/min (closed circles) when there was no concurrent sympathetic stimulation (S = 0). Stimulation of the cardiac sympathetic nerves alone at a frequency of 4 Hz (S = 4) caused the heart rate to increase by 80 beats/min (closed triangles). When vagal stimulation at 8 Hz was then added to this level of sympathetic stimulation (S = 4), the heart rate decreased by a total of 180 beats/min (closed triangles). Hence, the negative chronotropic effect of a given level of vagal activity was much more pronounced in the presence than in the absence of concomitant sympathetic activity.

The right side of Fig. 4-14 presents tbe same data from a different perspec-

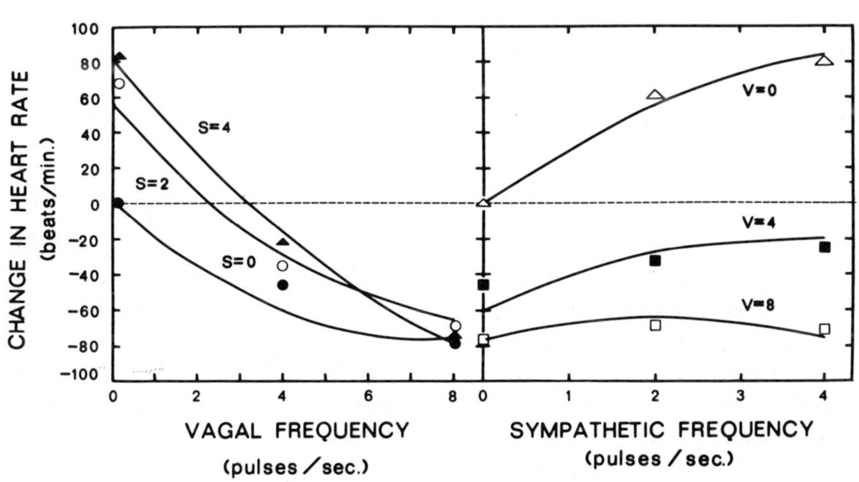

Fig. 4-14. Changes in heart rate elicited by simultaneous left vagal and right stellate stimulation in a dog. Symbols represent actual data, and the curves were derived by regression analysis. Numbers along the curves represent the frequencies (in Hz) of sympathetic (S) and vagal (V) stimulation. (From Levy and Zieske [73])

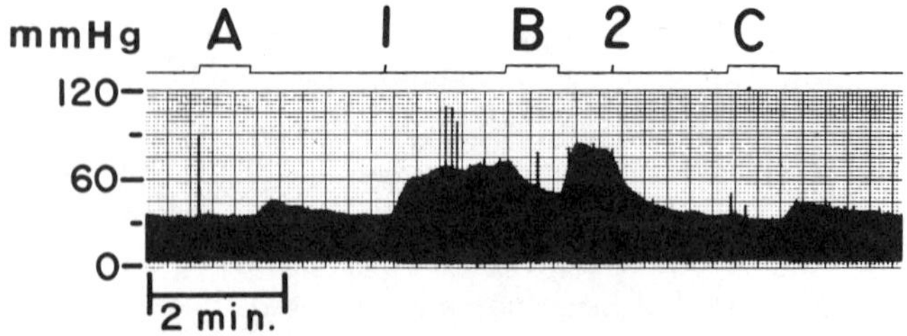

Fig. 4-15. The changes in left ventricular pressure in a paced, isovolumetric left ventricle preparation in response to vagal (during A, B, and C) and sympathetic (between 1 and 2) stimulation. (From Levy [59])

tive. Sympathetic stimulation at 4 Hz causes the heart rate to increase by 80 beats/min (open triangles) when there is no concurrent vagal activity (V = 0). However, during continuous vagal stimulation at 8 Hz (V = 8), varying the sympathetic stimulation frequency over the range from 0 to 4 Hz had virtually no influence on the heart rate (open squares).

The inhibitory effects of vagal activity on the atrial [110] and ventricular [59,61,69,71,88] myocardium are also accentuated as the level of sympathetic activity is progressively raised. In the experiment on an isovolumetric left-ventricle preparation in the dog shown in Fig. 4-15, vagal stimulation (event marks A and C) in the absence of concurrent sympathetic activity had virtually no effect on ventricular contractility, as gauged by the peak pressure generated by the left ventricle [59]. However, during a train of sympathetic stimulation (between marks 1 and 2), the same vagal stimulus (event mark B) had a pronounced depressant effect on ventricular contractility. These results suggest that the inhibitory effect of vagal activity on the ventricles is achieved in large part by antagonizing the prevailing level of sympathetic activity. The presynaptic mechanism involved in such antagonism is discussed in the next section.

Presynaptic Mechanism

Various receptors are located on the postganglionic sympathetic nerve endings in the heart. It has been postulated that such receptors are involved in the regulation of the release of norepinephrine (NE) from those nerve endings [108]. One of these is the muscarinic cholinergic receptor, which inhibits the release of NE during sympathetic neural activity [90,117]. Löffelholz and Muscholl [79,80] measured the quantity of NE released from an isolated, but innervated, atrial preparation in response to a standard train of sympathetic stimulation. They found that either the addition of cholinergic agonists or concurrent stimulation of the vagal nerves resulted in a substantial reduction in the quantity of NE released by the standard sympathetic stimulation.

Similarly, in anesthetized dogs, the rate of NE overflow into the coronary

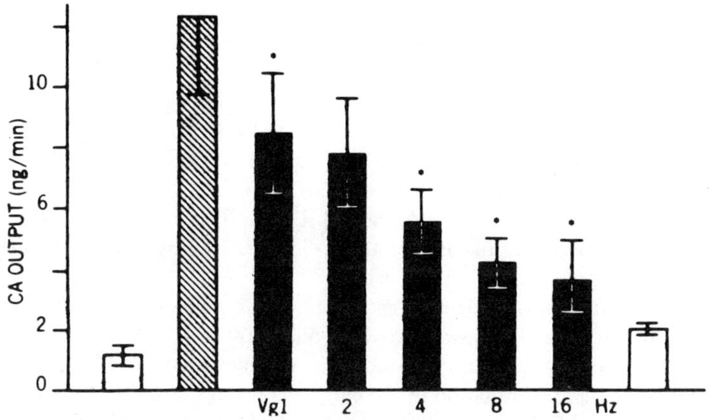

Fig. 4-16. The overflow of catecholamines (CA) into the coronary sinus blood in a dog, in response to cardiac sympathetic nerve stimulation alone (hatched bar) and during concurrent sympathetic and vagal stimulation (solid bars). The frequencies of vagal stimulation, in Hz, are denoted by the numbers below the solid bars. (Adapted from Lavallée et al. [57])

sinus blood evoked by cardiac sympathetic stimulation is substantially diminished by efferent vagal stimulation [57,61] or by reflexly induced increases in efferent vagal activity [56]. In an experiment recently conducted by Lavallée et al. [57], when a standard stimulus was applied to the cardiac sympathetic nerves (Fig. 4-16), the overflow of catecholamines (CA) into the coronary sinus blood amounted to 12 ng/min (hatched bar). The effects of concurrent vagal stimulation were frequency dependent (solid bars). Stimulation (Vg 1) at a frequency of only 1 Hz caused a 25% reduction in CA overflow. When the stimulation frequency was increased to 16 Hz, the CA output was diminished to about 30% of the output obtained in the absence of vagal stimulation. Such a marked suppression of NE release explains in part the pronounced vagally induced attenuation of the inotropic response to sympathetic stimulation, and the occurrence of a relatively weak negative inotropic effect of vagal stimulation when there is no background level of sympathetic activity (Fig. 4-15). However, part of the vagal–sympathetic interaction is undoubtedly mediated postsynaptically; i.e. at the level of the cardiac effector cell itself. Such postsynaptic mechanisms are described in detail in chapters 5 and 6.

REFERENCES

1. Akhtar, M., A. N. Damato, A. R. Caracta, W. P. Batsford, M. E. Josephson, S. H. Lau, Electrophysiologic effects of atropine on atrioventricular conduction studied by His bundle electrogram. *Am. J. Cardiol.* 33: 333–343, 1974.
2. Amlie, J. P. and H. Refsum, Vagus-induced changes in ventricular electrophysiology of the dog heart with and without β-blockade. *J. Cardiovas. Pharm.* 3: 1203–1210, 1981.

3. Blair, R. W., T. Shimizu, V. S. Bishop, The role of vagal afferents in the reflex control of the left ventricular refractory period in the cat. *Circ. Res. 46*: 378–386, 1980.
4. Brown, G. L. and J. C. Eccles, The action of a single vagal volley on the rhythm of the heart beat. *J. Physiol. (Lond.) 82*: 211–240, 1934.
5. Brown, G. L. and J. C. Eccles, Further experiments on vagal inhibition of the heart beat. *J. Physiol. (Lond.) 82*: 242–257, 1934.
6. Cagin, N. A., D. Kunstadt, P. Wolfish, B. Levitt, The influence of heart rate on the refractory period of the atrium and A-V conducting system. *Am. Heart J. 85*: 358–366, 1973.
7. Chess, G. F. and F. R. Calaresu, Frequency response model of vagal control heart rate in the cat. *Am. J. Physiol. 220*: 554–557, 1971.
8. Chess, G. F. and F. R. Calaresu, Model of dynamic behavior of heart period during bilateral vagal stimulation in the cat. *Am. J. Physiol. 221*: 593–596, 1971.
9. Chess, G. F. and F. R. Calaresu, A mathematical model of the vagus-heart period system in the cat. *IEEE Trans. Biomed. Eng. 21*: 21–27, 1974.
10. Cohn, A. E. and T. Lewis, The predominant influence of the left vagus nerve upon conduction between the auricles and ventricles of the dog. *J. Exp. Med. 18*: 739–747, 1913.
11. Cooper, T., Terminal innervation of the heart. In *Nervous Control of the Heart*, ed. W. C. Randall. Williams and Wilkins, Baltimore, 1965, pp. 130–153.
12. Cronin, R., J. A. Armour, W. C. Randall, Function of the in-situ papillary muscle in the canine left ventricle. *Circ. Res. 25*: 67–75, 1969.
13. Daggett, W. M., G. C. Nugent, P. W. Carr, P. C. Powers, Y. Harada, Influence of vagal stimulation on ventricular contractility, 0_2 consumption, and coronary flow. *Am. J. Physiol. 212*: 8–18, 1967.
14. De Beer, E. L., H. B. K. Boom, B. Naafs, The combined influence of the stimulus frequency of the vagal nerves and the atrial stimulus interval on the atrioventricular conduction time. *Cardiovas. Res. 11*: 47–54, 1977.
15. De Geest, H., M. N. Levy, H. Zieske, R. I, Lipman, Depression of ventricular contractility by stimulation of the vagus nerves. *Circ. Res. 17*: 222–235, 1965.
16. Dong, E., Jr. and B. A. Reitz, Effects of timing of vagal stimulation on heart rate in the dog. *Circ. Res. 27*: 635–646, 1970.
17. Duchêne-Marullaz, P. Effets de l'innervation cholinergique sur le coeur de mammifêre. Le tonus cardiomoderateur. *J. Physiol. (Paris) 66*: 373–397, 1973.
18. Eckberg, D. L., Temporal response patterns of the human sinus node to brief carotid baroreceptor stimuli. *J. Physiol. (London) 258*: 769–782, 1976.
19. Eckberg, D. L., Nonlinearities of the human carotid baroreceptor-cardiac reflex. *Circ. Res. 47*: 208–216, 1980.
20. Ehinger, B., B. Falck, B. Sporrong, Possible axo-axonal synapses between peripheral adrenergic and cholinergic nerve terminals. *Z. Zellforsch 107*: 508–521, 1970.
21. Endoh, M. and K. Hashimoto, Pharmacological evidence of autonomic nerve activities in canine papillary muscle. *Am. J. Physiol. 218*: 1459–1463, 1970.
22. Euler, D. E., S. B. Jones, W. P. Gunnar, J. M. Loeb, D. K. Murdock, W. C. Randall, Cardiac arrhythmias in the conscious dog after excision of the sinoatrial node and crista terminalis. *Circulation 59*: 468–475, 1979.
23. Freeman, S. E. and R. J. Turner, Effects of temperature change and adrenaline on sinoatrial and atrioventricular nodal potentials. *Cardiovas. Res. 8*: 443–450, 1974.

24. Furnival, C. M., R. J. Linden, H. M. Snow, The inotropic effect on the heart of stimulating the vagus in the dog, duck and toad. *J. Physiol. (Lond.) 230*: 155–170, 1973.
25. Furukawa, Y., M. Kobayashi, S. Chiba, A pharmacologic analysis of chronotropic and inotropic responses to direct electrical stimulation of the isolated, blood-perfused canine atrium. *Jap. Heart J. 21*: 873–882, 1980.
26. Gersche, W. and E. Dong, Jr., A note on Warner's vagus heart rate model. *IEEE Trans. Biomed. Eng. 20*: 145–148, 1973.
27. Gertjegerdes, W., U. Ravens, A. Ziegler, Time courses of carbachol-induced responses in guinea pig atria under the influence of ouabain, calcium, and rate of stimulation. *J. Cardiovasc. Pharmacol. 1*: 235–243, 1979.
28. Goldberg, J. M., Intra-SA-nodal pacemaker shifts induced by autonomic nerve stimulation in the dog. *Am. J. Physiol. 229*: 1116–1123, 1975.
29. Greco, E. C., Jr. and J. W. Clark, Jr. A mathematical model of the vagally driven SA nodal pacemaker. *IEEE Trans. Biomed. Eng. 23*: 191–199, 1976.
30. Guss, S. B., J. A. Kastor, M. E. Josephson, D. L. Scharf, Human ventricular refractoriness. Effects of cycle length, pacing site and atropine. *Circulation 53*: 450–455, 1976.
31. Hageman, G. R., W. C. Randall, J. A. Armour, Direct and reflex cardiac bradydysrhythmias from small vagal nerve stimulations. *Am. Heart J. 89*: 338–348, 1975.
32. Hahn, N., W. Kau, B. Falke, R. Sharif, P. Brinckmann, The influence of the vegetative nerve system on the maximal conduction velocity in the atrioventricular bundle and in the cardiac ventricles measured by the differential quotient of QRS. Investigations in dogs. *Bas. Res. Cardiol. 69*: 228–242, 1974.
33. Hamlin, R. L. and C. R. Smith, Effects of vagal stimulation on S-A and A-V nodes. *Am. J. Physiol. 215*: 560–568, 1968.
34. Hariman, R. J., B. F. Hoffman, R. E. Naylor, Electrical activity from the sinus node region in conscious dogs. *Circ. Res. 47*: 775–791, 1980.
35. Harmon, M. A. and T. J. Reeves, Effect of efferent vagal stimulation on atrial and ventricular function. *Am. Physiol. 215*: 1210–1217, 1968.
36. Higgins, C. B., S. F. Vatner, E. Braunwald, Parasympathetic control of the heart. *Pharmacol. Rev. 25*: 120–155, 1973.
37. Hoff, H. E., Vagal stimulation before the Webers. *Ann. Med. Hist. 8*: 138–144, 1936.
38. Hoffman, B. F. and P. F. Cranefield, *Electrophysiology of the Heart*. McGraw-Hill, New York, 1960, p. 132–174.
39. Hondeghem, L. M., E. Mouton, T. Stassen, H. DeGeest, Additive effects of acetylcholine released by vagal nerve stimulation on atrial rate. *J. Appl. Physiol. 38*: 108–113, 1975.
40. Hoskins, E. J., D. V. Priola, G. K. Weiss, Vagal stabilization of the ischemic canine ventricle. *Circ. Shock 5*: 393–406, 1978.
41. Hunt, R., Experiments on the relation of the inhibitory to the accelerator nerves of the heart. *J. Exp. Med. 2*: 252–279, 1897.
42. Iano, T. L., M. N. Levy, M. H. Lee, An acceleratory component of the parasympathetic control of heart rate. *Am. J. Physiol. 224*: 997–1005, 1973.
43. Irisawa, H., W. M. Caldwell, M. F. Wilson, Neural regulation of atrioventricular conduction. *Jap. J. Physiol. 21*: 15–25, 1971.

44. Jacobowitz, D., T. Cooper, H. B. Barner, Histochemical and chemical studies of the localization of adrenergic and cholinergic nerves in normal and denervated cat hearts. *Circ. Res. 20*: 289–298, 1967.
45. Jalife, J., A. J. Hamilton, G. K. Moe, Desensitization of the cholinergic receptor at the sinoatrial cell of the kitten. *Am. J. Physiol. 238*: H439–H448, 1980.
46. Jalife, J. and G. K. Moe, Phasic effects of vagal stimulation on pacemaker activity of the isolated sinus node of the young cat. *Circ. Res. 45*: 595–608, 1979.
47. James, T. N., Cardiac innervation: anatomic and pharmacologic relations. *Bull. N.Y. Acad. Med. 43*: 1041–1086, 1967.
48. James, T. N., The sinus node as a servomechanism. *Circ. Res. 32*: 307–313, 1973.
49. Janse, M. J., Influence of the direction of the atrial wave front on A-V nodal transmission in isolated hearts of rabbits. *Circ. Res. 25*: 439–449, 1969.
50. Jewett, D. L., Activity of single efferent fibres in the cervical vagus nerve of the dog, with special reference to possible cardio- inhibitory fibres. *J. Physiol. (Lond.) 175*: 321–357, 1964.
51. Katona, P. G., P. J. Martin, F. Jih, Neural control of heart rate: a conciliation of models. *IEEE Trans. Biomed. Eng. 23*: 164–166, 1976.
52. Katona, P. G., J. W. Poitras, G. O. Barnett, B. S. Terry, Cardiac vagal efferent activity and heart period in the carotid sinus reflex. *Am. J. Physiol. 218*: 1030–1037, 1970.
53. Koepchen, H. P., H. D. Lux, P. H. Wagner, Untersuchungen uber Zeitbedarf and zentrale Verarbeitung des pressoreceptorischen Herzreflexes. *Pfluegers Arch. Ges. Physiol. 273*: 413–430, 1961.
54. Kolman, B. S., R. L. Verrier, B. Lown, Effect of vagus nerve stimulation upon excitability of the canine ventricle. Role of sympathetic-parasympathetic interactions. *Am. J. Cardiol. 37*: 1041–1045, 1976.
55. Kunz, D. L., Reflex discharge patterns of cardiac vagal efferent fibers. *J. Physiol. (Lond.) 222*: 1–15, 1972.
56. Lavallée, M., J. deChamplain, R. A. Nadeau, Reflexly induced inhibition of catecholamine release through a peripheral muscarinic mechanism. *Can. J. Physiol. Pharmacol. 58*: 1334–1341, 1980.
57. Lavallée, M., J. deChamplain, R. A. Nadeau, N. Yamaguchi, Muscarinic inhibition of endogenous myocardial catecholamine liberation in the dog. *Can. J. Physiol. Pharmacol. 56*: 642–49, 1978.
58. Levy, M. N., Parasympathetic control of the heart. In *Neural Regulation of the Heart*, ed. W. C. Randall. Oxford University Press, New York, 1977, pp. 95–130.
59. Levy, M. N., Neural control of the heart: sympathetic-vagal interactions. In *Cardiovascular System Dynamics*, ed. J. Baan, A. Noordergraaf, J. Raines. MIT Press, Cambridge, 1978, pp. 365–370.
60. Levy, M. N., Neural control of cardiac rhythm and contraction. In *Cardiac Therapy*, ed. B. F. Hoffman and M. R. Rosen. Martinus Nighoff, Boston, 1983, in press.
61. Levy, M. N. and B. Blattberg, Effect of vagal stimulation on the overflow of norepinephrine into the coronary sinus during cardiac sympathetic nerve stimulation in the dog. *Circ. Res. 38*: 81–85, 1976.
62. Levy, M. N. and J. Edelstein, Mechanism of synchronization in isorhythmic A-V dissociation. II. Clinical studies. *Circulation 42*: 689–699, 1970.
63. Levy, N. N., T. Iano, H. Zieske, Effects of repetitive bursts of vagal activity on heart rate. *Circ. Res. 30*: 286–295, 1972.
64. Levy, M. N. and P. J. Martin, Neural control of the heart, In *Handbook of Physiology*, Sec. 2, *The Cardiovascular System*, Vol. 1, *The In Heart*, eds. R. M.

Berne, N. Speralakis, and S. R. Geiger. American Physiological Society, Bethesda, Md., 1979. Chap. 16, pp. 518–620.

65. Levy, M. N., P. J. Martin, J. Edelstein, L. B. Goldberg, The AV nodal Wenckebach phenomenon as a positive feedback mechanism. *Prog. Cardiovasc. Dis. 26*: 601–613, 1974.
66. Levy, M. N., P. J. Martin, T. Iano, H. Zieske, Paradoxical effect of vagus nerve stimulation heart rate in dogs. *Circ. Res. 25*: 303–314, 1969.
67. Levy, M. N., P. J. Martin, T. Iano, H. Zieske, Effects of single vagal stimuli on heart rate and atrioventricular conduction. *Am. J. Physiol. 218*: 1256–1262, 1970.
68. Levy, M. N., P. J. Martin, S. L. Stuesse, Neural regulation of the heart beat. *Ann. Rev. Physiol. 43*: 443–453, 1981.
69. Levy, M. N., M. Ng., P. Martin, H. Zieske, Sympathetic and parasympathetic interactions upon the left ventricle of the dog. *Circ. Res. 19*: 5–10, 1966.
70. Levy, M. N. and T. W. Simmons, The phasic effects of aortic nerve stimulation on heart rate in anaesthetized dogs. In *Arterial Baroreceptors and Hypertension*, ed. Peter Sleight. Oxford University Press, NY, Toronto, 1980. Chap. 59, pp. 383–388.
71. Levy, M. N. and H. Zieske, Effect of enhanced contractility on the left ventricular response to vagus nerve stimulation in dogs. *Circ. Res. 24*: 303–311, 1969.
72. Levy, M. N. and H. Zieske, Comparison of the cardiac effects of vagus nerve stimulation and of acetylcholine infusions. *Am. J. Physiol. 216*: 890–897, 1969.
73. Levy, M. N. and H. Zieske, Autonomic control of cardiac pacemaker activity and atrioventricular transmission. *J. Appl. Physiol. 27*: 465–470, 1969.
74. Levy, M. N. and H. Zieske, Mechanism of synchronization in isorhythmic dissociation. I. Experiments on dogs. *Circ. Res. 27*: 429–443, 1970.
75. Levy, M. N. and H. Zieske, Synchronization of the cardiac pacemaker with repetitive stimulation of the carotid sinus nerve in the dog. *Circ. Res. 30*: 634–641, 1972.
76. Linden, R. J. and Snow, H. M., Application of an assessment of inotropic changes in intact heart: responses to infusions of catecholamines and stimulation of nerves. *Proc. Roy. Soc. Med. 65*: 548–550, 1972.
77. Loeb, J. M., D. P. Dalton, J. M. Moran, Sensitivity differences of SA and AV node to vagal stimulation: attenuation of vagal effects at SA node. *Am. J. Physiol. 241*: H684–H690, 1981.
78. Löffelholz, K., Release of acetylcholine in the isolated heart. *Am. J. Physiol. 240*: H431–H440, 1981.
79. Löffelholz, K, and E. Muscholl, A muscarinic inhibition of the noradrenaline release evoked by postganglionic sympathetic nerve stimulation. *Naunyn-Schmiedebergs Arch. Pharmacol. 265*: 1–15, 1969.
80. Löffelholz, K. and E. Muscholl, Inhibition by parasympathetic nerve stimulation of release of adrenergic transmitter. *Naunyn-Schmiedebergs Arch. Pharmacol. 267*: 181–184, 1970.
81. Mancia, G., O. Bonazzi, L. Pozzoni, A. Ferrari, M. Gardumi, L. Gregorini, R. Perondi, Baroreceptor control of atrioventricular conduction in man. *Circ. Res. 44*: 752–758, 1979.
82. Martin, P. J., Dynamic vagal control of atrial-ventricular conduction: theoretical and experimental studies. *Ann. Biomed. Eng. 3*: 275–295, 1975.
83. Martin, P. J., Depression of atrioventricular sensitivity in the dog by successive brief bursts of vagal stimulation. *Circ. Res. 38*: 448–453, 1976.

84. Martin, P., The influence of the parasympathetic nervous system on atrioventricular conduction. *Circ. Res. 41*: 593–599, 1977.
85. Martin, P., Atrial inotropic responses to brief vagal stimuli: frequency-force interactions. *Am. J. Physiol. 239*: H333–H341, 1980.
86. Martin, P., Time-dependent heart period and contractility responses to successive brief vagal stimuli. *Am. J. Physiol. 239*: H494–H500, 1980.
87. Martin, P., M. N. Levy, and Y. Matsuda, Fade of the cardiac responses during tonic vagal stimulation. *Am. J. Physiol., 243*: H219–H225, 1982.
88. Martin, P. J., M. N. Levy, H. Zieske, Analysis and simulation of the left ventricular response to autonomic nervous activity. *Cardiovasc. Res. 3*: 396–410, 1969.
89. Martins, J. B. and D. P. Zipes, Effects of sympathetic and vagal nerves on recovery properties of the endocardium and epicardium of the canine left ventricle. *Circ. Res. 46*: 100–110, 1980.
90. Muscholl, E., Peripheral muscarinic control of norepinephrine release in the cardiovascular system. *Am. J. Physiol. 239*: H713–H720, 1980.
91. Musgrave, G. E., C. E. Branch, D. S. Beckett, Relative sensitivity of the canine sinus node and atrioventricular node to acetylcholine. *Can. J. Physiol. Pharmacol. 59*: 1058–1062, 1981.
92. Pace, J. B., W. C. Randall, J. W. Wechsler, D. V. Priola, Alterations in ventricular dynamics induced by stimulation of the cervical vagosympathetic trunk. *Am. J. Physiol. 214*: 1213–1218, 1968.
93. Pavlov, V., Dependence of the atrioventricular conduction on the cardiac rate upon increased vagal activity. *Agressologie 16B*: 9–13, 1975.
94. Penaz, J., Frequency response of the cardiac chronotropic action of the vagus in the rabbit. *Arch. Int. Physiol. Biochem. 70*: 636–650, 1962.
95. Priola, D. V., Intrinsic innervation of the canine heart. Effects on conduction in the atrium, atrioventricular node, and proximal bundle branch. *Circ. Res. 47*: 74–79, 1980.
96. Prystowsky, E. N., W. M. Jackman, R. L. Rinkenberger, J. J. Heger, D. P. Zipes, Effect of autonomic blockade on ventricular refractoriness and atrioventricular nodal conduction in humans. *Circ. Res. 49*: 511–518, 1981.
97. Randall, W. C. and J. A. Armour, Complex cardiovascular responses to vagosympathetic stimulation. *Proc. Soc. Expl. Biol. Med. 145*: 493–499, 1974.
98. Randall, W. C., J. B. Wechsler, J. B. Pace, M. Szentivanyi, Alterations in myocardial contractility during stimulation of the cardiac nerves. *Am. J. Physiol. 214*: 1205–1212, 1968.
99. Reid, J. V. O., The cardiac pacemaker: effects of regularly spaced nervous input. *Am. Heart J. 78*: 58–64, 1969.
100. Rosenblueth, A., The chemical mediation of autonomic-nervous impulses as evidenced by summation of responses. *Am. J. Physiol. 102*: 12–38, 1932.
101. Sapire, D. W., J. J. Shah, I. F. S. Black, Prolonged atrioventricular conduction in young children and adolescents. The role of increased vagal tone. *S. Afr. Med. J. 55*: 669–673, 1979.
102. Sarnoff, S. J., S. K. Brockman, J. P. Gilmore, R. J. Linden, J. H. Mitchell, Regulation of ventricular contraction. Influence of cardiac sympathetic and vagal nerve stimulation on atrial and ventricular dynamics. *Circ. Res. 8*: 1108–1122, 1960.
103. Schwartz, P. J., R. L. Verrier, B. Lown, Effect of stellectomy and vagotomy on ventricular refractoriness in dogs. *Circ. Res. 40*: 536–540, 1977.

104. Schwegler, M., Sympathetic-parasympathetic interactions on the ventricular myocardium: possible role of cyclic nucleotides. *Basic Res. Cardiol.* 3: 215–221, 1974.
105. Spear, J. F., K. D. Kronhaus, E. N. Moore, R. P. Kline, The effect of brief vagal stimulation on the isolated rabbit sinus node. *Circ. Res.* 44: 75–88, 1979.
106. Spear, J. F. and E. N. Moore, Influence of brief vagal and stellate nerve stimulation on pacemaker activity and conduction within the atrioventricular conduction system of the dog. *Circ. Res.* 32: 27–41, 1973.
107. Stanton, H. C. and R. L. Vick, Cholinergic and adrenergic influences on right ventricular myocardial contractility in the dog. *Arch. Int. Pharmacodyn. Ther.* 176: 233–248, 1968.
108. Starke, K. Regulation of noradrenaline release by presynaptic receptor systems. *Rev. Physiol. Biochem. Pharmacol.* 77: 1–24, 1977.
109. Stinson, E. B., J. S. Schroeder, R. B. Griepp et al., Observations on the behavior of recipient atria after cardiac transplantation in man. *Am. J. Cardiol.* 30: 615–622, 1972.
110. Stuesse, S. L., D. W. Wallick, M. N. Levy, Autonomic control of right atrial contractile strength in the dog. *Am. J. Physiol.* 236: H860–H865, 1979.
111. Stuesse, S. L., M. N. Levy, H. Zieske, Effects of glucagon on cardiac chronotropic response to vagal stimulation in the dog. *Am. J. Physiol.* 242: H4–H12, 1982.
112. Stull, J. T. and S. E. Mayer, Biochemical mechanisms of adrenergic and cholinergic regulation of myocardial contractility. *Handbook of Physiology*, Section 2, *The Cardiovascular System*. American Physiological Society, Waverly Press, Bethesda, Md. 1979. Chap. 21, p. 741–774.
113. Suga, H. and M. Oshima, Modulation-characteristics of heart rate by vagal stimulation. *Jap. J. Med. Elec. Biol. Eng.* 6: 465–471, 1968.
114. Thoenen, H. and J. P. Transer, Chemical sympathectomy by selective destruction of adrenergic nerve endings with 6-hydroxydopamine. *Naunyn-Schmiedebergs Arch. Pharmacol.* 261: 271–288, 1968.
115. Tokimasa, T., H. Hasuo, K. Koketsu, Desensitization of the muscarinic acetylcholine receptor of atrium in bullfrogs. *Jap. J. Physiol.* 31: 83–97, 1981.
116. Vallin, H. O., Autonomic influence on sinus node and AV node function in the elderly without significant heart disease: assessment with electrophysiological and autonomic tests. *Cardiovasc. Res.* 14: 206–216, 1980.
117. Vanhoutte, P. M. and M. N. Levy, Prejunctional cholinergic modulation of adrenergic neurotransmission in the cardiovascular system. *Am. J. Physiol.* 238: H275–H281, 1980.
118. Versprille, A. and M. E. Wise, Quantitative effect of vagal stimulation on heart interval in newborn and older rabbits. *Pfluegers Arch.* 325: 61–76, 1971.
119. Wallick, D. W., M. N. Levy, D. S. Felder, H. Zieske, Effects of repetitive bursts of vagal activity on atrioventricular junctional rate in dogs. *Am. J. Physiol.* 237: 275–81, 1979.
120. Warner, H. R. and A. Cox, A mathematical model of heart rate control by sympathetic and vagus efferent information. *J. Appl. Physiol.* 17: 349–355, 1962.
121. Warner, H. R. and R. O. Russell, Jr. Effect of combined sympathetic and vagal stimulation on heart rate in the dog. *Circ. Res.* 24: 567–573, 1969.
122. Waxman, M. B. and R. W. Wald, Termination of ventricular tachycardia by an increase in cardiac vagal drive. *Circulation* 56: 385–391, 1977.

123. Weaver, C. S. and E. Dong, Jr., A phase-sensitive vagal heart-rate control model. *J. Theor. Biol.* *36*: 291–311, 1972.
124. Wiggers, C. J., Physiology of the mammalian auricle. II. Influence of the vagus nerves on the fractionate contraction of the right auricle. *Am. J. Physiol.* *42*: 133–140, 1917.
125. Wildenthal, K., D. S. Mierzwiak, H. L. Wyatt, J. H. Mitchell, Influence of efferent vagal stimulation on left ventricular function in dogs. *Am. J. Physiol.* *216*: 577–581, 1969.
126. Zipes, D. P., M. J. Mihalick, G. T. Robbins, Effects of selective vagal and stellate ganglion stimulation on atrial refractoriness. *Cardiovasc. Res.* *8*: 647–655, 1974.

5

Adrenergic Receptors in the Heart: Pre- and Postsynaptic Mechanisms

JARL E. S. WIKBERG and ROBERT J. LEFKOWITZ

Cardiac function is regulated by the sympathetic nervous system and by circulating catecholamines of adrenal medullary origin. Postganglionic adrenergic nerve fibers seem to reach all parts of the heart but the densest innervation is found in the sinus and atrioventricular nodes. The atria are also richly innervated by adrenergic fibers. In the ventricles the adrenergic innervation is less dense and it shows a marked regional variation. The Purkinje system appears to be only sparsely innervated by sympathetic fibers [33,131,149]. Norepinephrine released from the sympathetic nerves and catecholamines diffusing from the bloodstream interact with adrenergic receptors on heart cells which leads to alterations in their physiological performance. Also, the sympathetic system itself appears to be regulated by "presynaptic" receptors which either inhibit or facilitate transmitter release. The present chapter is devoted to a discussion of adrenergic receptors in the heart. Their location, function, and regulation will be reviewed. Adrenergic receptors in other tissues will be discussed when they seem relevant to understanding the role of these receptors in the heart.

One of the most important and fruitful hypotheses on the mode of action of the catecholamines was the theory that they acted through two different receptors which were termed alpha and beta [4]. Before selective alpha and beta agonists and antagonists were used experimentally, only slow progress was made toward the understanding of the physiological and biochemical events induced by sympathetic nerve stimulation or catecholamines. Subsequently, it was suggested that beta receptors could be further subclassified into $beta_1$ and $beta_2$ types [89] and alpha receptors into $alpha_1$ and $alpha_2$ types [17,166]. It is not within the scope of this chapter to provide an extensive review on the classifi-

The experimental portions of research reported were supported by grant 14X-05957 from The Swedish Medical Research Council and grant HL20339 from the National Institute of Health. Dr. Wikberg is the recipient of a Fogarty International Fellowship (#1F05 TW03055-01) and a Fellowship from The Swedish Medical Research Council (#04F-6289).

cation of adrenergic receptors. However, in order to facilitate the discussion which follows, a brief outline will be given. For more extensive coverage the reader is referred to recent reviews of the classificaion of beta receptors [25,34,52,62,107,110] and alpha receptors [139,167].

ADRENERGIC RECEPTORS

The classification of adrenergic receptors into alpha and beta types by Ahlquist [4] was based on the observation that the order of potencies of some sympathetic amines differed when tested on smooth muscle and the heart. For the "alpha" effect the order of potencies of some of these amines was: epinephrine $>$ norepinephrine $>$ isoprenaline whereas for the "beta" effect the order was: isoprenaline $>$ epinephrine $\geq$ norepinephrine. Lands and co-workers [89] then classified the beta receptors into $beta_1$ and $beta_2$ based on the observation that the order of potencies of a series of 12 agonists fell into two distinct categories when tested on beta receptors in different tissues. Among these agonists epinephrine and norepinephrine were approximately equipotent on beta receptors in the heart and adipose tissue and these receptors were classified as $beta_1$. By contrast, in vascular and bronchial smooth muscles epinephrine was approximately tenfold more potent than norepinephrine and the beta receptors mediating these responses were classified as $beta_2$. Later studies seemed to substantiate this classification of beta receptors when selective $beta_1$ and $beta_2$ agonists and antagonists were introduced (i.e. salbutamol ($beta_2$) [23], and practolol ($beta_1$) [44].

However, the view that only two types of beta receptors existed did not become generally accepted since a wide variety of specificities of the beta selective drugs was observed when they were tested in different tissues [5,19,22,52]. It appears now that these discrepancies can be explained by the presence of both $beta_1$ and $beta_2$ receptors which mediate the same type of responses. It was initially observed that the physiological effects of selective beta agonists were differentially blocked by selective beta antagonists in the heart and some smooth muscles [26,53,78]. Then it was demonstrated by radioligand binding that both $beta_1$ and $beta_2$ receptors could be detected simultaneously in tissues such as heart, brain, and lung [14,38,67,70,105,106].

The knowledge that alpha receptors do not comprise a homogeneous population has been acquired fairly recently. It was first observed that alpha receptors which mediate inhibition of transmitter release from adrenergic and cholinergic neurons ("presynaptic alpha receptors") differed pharmacologically from those mediating contraction of smooth muscles and positive inotropic effects in the heart ("postsynaptic alpha receptors") [43,136,169]. Several studies later confirmed and extended these results (see 167 and references therein). The differences between pre- and postsynaptic alpha receptors seemed to be so generally present that the terms pre- and postsynaptic came to be used to refer to both the anatomic location and the pharmacological characteristics of alpha receptors. However, it then became evident that alpha receptors which showed properties similar to the presynaptic ones could be located on structures other

Table 5-1. Alpha$_1$ and alpha$_2$ selective drugs

	Agonists	Antagonists
Alpha$_1$ selective		
	Phenylephrine	Prazosin
	Methoxamine	Indoramin
		Corynanthine
Alpha$_2$ selective		
	Clonidine	Yohimbine
	Tramazoline	Rauwolfscine
	Xylazine	
	Guanfacine	
	Azepexole	
	B-HT 920	

than nerve terminals. Therefore, the nomenclature alpha$_1$ and alpha$_2$ was adopted to distinguish between the pharmacological properties of alpha receptors [17,166]. The initial subclassification of alpha receptors relied solely on functional studies with a number of selective alpha agonists and antagonists. More recently it has also become possible to distinguish between alpha$_1$ and alpha$_2$ receptors by radioligand binding techniques [77,168]. In Table 5-1 some alpha agonists and antagonists that have proven of value in distinguishing alpha$_1$ and alpha$_2$ receptors are listed. However, there is some controversy in the literature with regard to the selectivity of some of the agonists (see refs. 139 and 167) and the table should be interpreted with this in mind. In this context it should be borne in mind that an agonist may act selectively not only in binding to a receptor but also in the ability to stimulate it. (For a more complete discussion see ref. 168.)

Recent work indicates that the beta receptor signal arises from the interactions of three membrane-bound proteins, the beta receptor protein itself, a stimulatory guanine nucleotide regulatory protein (N_s)*, and the adenylate cyclase protein (C), when an agonist binds to the receptor unit [reviews 95,96,135,168]. The theories that have emerged account for the presence of high- and low-affinity states (beta$_H$ and beta$_L$) of agonist binding, the regulation of agonist binding by guanine nucleotides, and the dependence of beta receptor stimulated adenylate cyclase activity on the presence of GTP. The molecular mechanism of action of alpha receptors is less well understood. At least in some tissues, alpha$_2$ receptors may act in a fashion which is analogous to beta receptors except that their interaction with agonists leads to a diminished adenylate cyclase activity [104,167,168,170]. Otherwise, a number of similarities exist,

***Abbreviations:* N_s, stimulatory guanine nucleotide regulatory protein; C, adenylate cyclase; R_β, beta receptor unit; [^{3}H]DHE, [^{3}H]-dihydroergocryptine; 6-OHDA, 6-hydroxydopamine; 6-OHDOPA, 6-hydroxydopa; Gpp(NH)p, guanyl-5′-yl-imidodiphosphate; cAMP, cyclic adenosine 3′,5′ monophosphate; cGMP, cyclic guanosine 3′,5′ monophosphate.

such as the formation of $alpha_{2H}$ and $alpha_{2L}$ states for agonist binding and regulation of the receptors by guanine nucleotides. The mechanism of action of $alpha_1$ receptors is only poorly understood at present although it has been suggested that the receptor may be dependent on the calcium ion for its function in the cell membrane [167,168].

ADRENERGIC RECEPTOR CONTROL OF CARDIAC NEURONS

Considerable evidence has accumulated that chemical neurotransmission can be regulated by a variety of effectors which either facilitate or inhibit transmitter release. Many of these effectors seem to act on presynaptic receptors located on the axon terminals. For example, catecholamines, acetylcholine, prostaglandins, adenosine, and angiotensin may all act on such presynaptic receptors in sympathetic neurons in the heart. Several recent reviews treat various aspects of presynaptic control of neurotransmission [90,137,138,157,165] and the reader is referred to these for a more general treatment of the subject. Here only a summary of the evidence for the existence of adrenergic receptor control of sympathetic and parasympathetic neurotransmission in the heart will be provided.

Sympathetic Neurons

Several methodological approaches have been used. If a drug is given to an animal in vivo an effect on sympathetic neurotransmission may be monitored by a change in heart rate or contractile force. However, from such experiments it is generally difficult to decide if the drug affects the central nervous system directly or if its effects arise secondarily, due to some autonomic reflex, for example by a change in blood pressure. In order to exclude such mechanisms during in vivo experiments some type of decentralization may be induced, such as pithing the animal or vagotomy. In most in vivo studies the activity of the sympathetic nerves has been monitored only indirectly by measuring heart rate and contractile force. Therefore the effects might also have been caused by postsynaptic regulation of heart cells. In some studies the preganglionic fibers of the cardioaccelerans nerve were stimulated and in these experiments a ganglionic effect of drugs cannot be excluded.

Another experimental approach has been to remove the heart together with its nerve supply and study it in vitro. Viability may be preserved by perfusion or incubation in physiological buffer solutions. When this model is used the sympathetic nervous activity can be monitored either indirectly as above or by measuring the release of the sympathetic transmitter. (The efflux of norepinephrine can be estimated either by measuring the release of tritium in hearts preloaded with $[^3H]$norepinephrine or by measuring the release of the endogenous transmitter.)

Since all sympathetic fibers of the heart are believed to be postganglionic, an effect on transmitter release might be assumed to be induced by an action on the neurons themselves, e.g., in the case of adrenergic drugs by a presynaptic receptor. However, there is also some evidence that transsynaptic mechanisms may be operating which modulate sympathetic neurotransmission.

Alpha Receptor Mediated Inhibition of Sympathetic Neurotransmission

The knowledge that alpha receptors may modulate the release of norepinephrine from sympathetic neurons gradually evolved from observations of different tissues. It was first observed that the alpha adrenolytic drug dibenamine enhanced transmitter release on sympathetic nerve stimulation in the cat spleen [24] and this observation was later followed by similar observations with β-haloalkylamines and other alpha blocking drugs in the cat [46], mouse [47], guinea pig [3,103,121], and rabbit hearts [136,142,146,162] as well as in a number of other peripheral adrenergically innervated tissues. Initially it was believed that the alpha blockers caused this action by inhibiting the neural uptake of norepinephrine or otherwise interfering with its metabolic elimination. However, it soon became clear that this effect could only partially account for the increase in transmitter release, in some of the tissues, when high concentrations of some of the adrenolytic drugs were used [137,165]. Since it was also found that alpha adrenergic agonists such as phenylephrine, xylazine, clonidine, naphazoline, and oxymetazoline induced the opposite effect as the alpha adrenolytic drugs on the stimulation-induced release of norepinephrine in the heart and other tissues, it was suggested that alpha receptors controlled the release of the adrenergic transmitter [103,121,136,161]. The effects of exogenously applied alpha agonists could in general also be blocked by administration of an alpha blocking drug, which supports this notion. Two theories have emerged to explain these observations: (1) the presynaptic hypothesis and (2) the transsynaptic hypothesis (Fig. 5-1). Most authors have favored the presynaptic hypothesis but it has

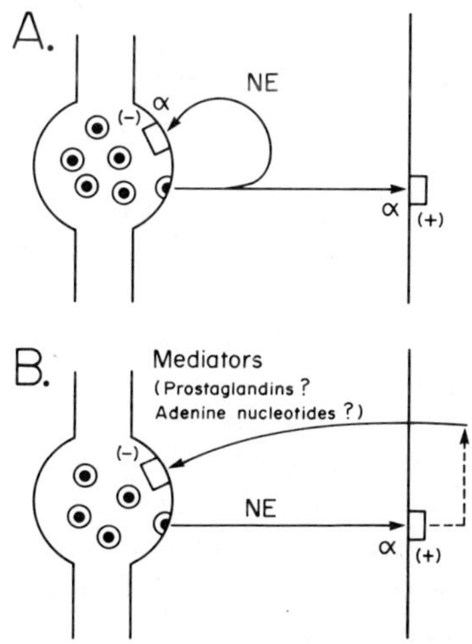

Fig. 5-1. Models for alpha receptor control of sympathetic neurotransmission. (A.) Presynaptic hypothesis. (B.) Transsynaptic hypothesis. NE = norepinephrine.

proven to be exceedingly difficult to distinguish unequivocally between the two possibilities. The anatomic location of the alpha receptor mediating inhibition of norepinephrine release will be discussed further below. Meanwhile it will be referred to as "presynaptic," based solely on its effect on sympathetic neurotransmission.

Classification of Presynaptic Alpha Receptors in the Heart

The first observation that pre- and postsynaptic alpha receptors might differ pharmacologically was made in the heart. Starke [136] observed that phenylephrine, oxymetazoline, and naphazoline depressed stimulation-evoked release of norepinephrine from the perfused rabbit heart by stimulating alpha receptors. By contrast only phenylephrine induced a positive inotropic effect in the same preparation by stimulating postsynaptic alpha receptors, the imidazolines being completely ineffective at concentrations that maximally depressed norepinephrine release. Thus, these results indicated that oxymetazoline and naphazoline preferentially activated the presynaptic alpha receptors of the sympathetic neurons. Drew [40] observed that the order of potency of some alpha agonists for inhibition of the chronotropic effect of preganglionic stimulation of the cardioaccelerans nerve vs. their blood pressure increasing effect in the pithed rat was: xylazine > clonidine > oxymetazoline > naphazoline > phenylephrine > methoxamine. Similar observations were made by Pichler and Kobinger [118] in the pithed rat. They found that the corresponding order of potency was: clonidine > oxymetazoline > methoxamine. In the vagotomized dog Lokhandwala et al. [99] found that the order of potency for the inhibition of the tachycardic effect on postganglionic stimulation of the cardioaccelerans nerve vs. the blood pressure increasing effect of some sympathetic amines was alpha-methylnoradrenaline > phenylephrine $\doteq$ noradrenaline. These results are similar to a number of findings on other tissues when pre- and postsynpatic alpha receptors have been compared [139,167] and indicate that the alpha receptors mediating inhibition of sympathetic neurotransmission in the heart are of the $alpha_2$ type as described by agonists. Antagonist data are also compatible with the view that these receptors are of the $alpha_2$ type. Thus, for example, yohimbine was much more potent than thymoxamine in antagonizing the presynaptic actions of clonidine on the cardioaccelerans nerve in the pithed rat [40]. During similar experimental conditions indoramine seemed to be virtually ineffective, even though it blocked postsynaptic pressor responses to alpha-receptor stimulation [7]. In the vagotomized dog yohimbine was also more potent than prazosin in antagonizing the presynaptic actions of clonidine on the accelerans nerve [32]. Thus, these results fully support the idea that the presynaptic alpha receptors in sympathetic neurons of the heart are of the $alpha_2$ type (Table 5-1). Interestingly, however, Roach et al. [122] found that prazosin and phentolamine were approximately equally effective in antagonizing the bradycardic effect of clonidine during sympathetic nerve stimulation in the spinal cat and dog, whereas prazosin was almost ineffective in comparison to phentolamine in the pithed rat. Thus, these results seem to indicate that the effect of drugs on the presynaptic alpha receptor in the sympathetic neurons of the heart is species selective.

Location of Alpha Receptors Mediating Inhibition of Sympathetic Neurotransmission

The presynaptic hypothesis proposes that the alpha receptors are located on the axon terminals and mediate a direct inhibition of transmitter release (Fig. 5-1A). Either exogenously applied alpha agonists or endogenous norepinephrine would act on these receptors and restrict the release of norepinephrine evoked by action potentials traveling down to the terminal varicosities. The action of endogenous norepinephrine would constitute a negative feedback loop that restricts further transmitter release. The ability of alpha blockers to enhance transmitter release is explained by assuming that they prevent endogenous norepinephrine from exerting this negative feedback by blocking the presynaptic alpha receptors.

The transsynaptic hypothesis assumes that alpha receptors are located at postsynaptic sites; e.g., in the myocytes and that on stimulation they induce the release of some mediator(s) which diffuses over to the nerve varicosities and there causes inhibition of transmitter release (Fig. 5-1B). Several lines of evidence have been provided in support of both hypotheses [48,66,73,139,165]. In support of the presynaptic hypothesis it was claimed that alpha-receptor-mediated feedback inhibition could be observed in tissues where postsynaptic alpha receptors were lacking. This was said to be the case in the heart [165]. Clearly, however, since $alpha_1$ receptors can be demonstrated in the myocardium physiologically and by radioligand binding techniques respectively (see below), this is not the case. On the other hand, if the transsynaptic hypothesis is the only explanation for the observed relations, there must be postsynpatic $alpha_2$ receptors which modulate the release of the transsynaptic modulator(s) and such receptors have not yet been demonstrated.

When radioligand binding techniques for alpha receptors became available it was hoped that the question of alpha receptor location could be solved. However, most studies thus far reported have produced equivocal results. Guicheney et al. [64] found that [^{3}H]DHE bound to two different sites in membranes isolated from the rat heart. It was stated that the binding to the high-affinity site was selectively displaced by the "postsynaptic alpha blocker" ARC 239 whereas the binding to the low-affinity site was selectively displaced by the "presynaptic alpha blocker" yohimbine. Furthermore, the low-affinity site was said to show positive homeotropic cooperativity for the [^{3}H]DHE binding. Accordingly these investigators suggested that the high-affinity site represented postsynaptic alpha receptors and the low-affinity site represented presynaptic alpha receptors. However, in a number of other studies these results were not confirmed since it was reported that [^{3}H]DHE bound to only one site in cardiac membranes [102,129,173–175]. Furthermore, [^{3}H]DHE appeared to label only $alpha_1$ receptors since prazosin was 1000-fold more potent than yohimbine in inhibiting its binding [173]. In fact, $alpha_2$ receptors could not be detected at all since [^{3}H]clonidine did not bind specifically to the heart membranes.

Another experimental approach has been to induce sympathetic denervation with 6-OHDA. Thus, it was reported that chemical denervation induced a 60–70% decrease in the [^{3}H]DHE binding sites of rat hearts, which supported the loss of a corresponding amount of presynaptic alpha receptors [128,147]. In one of these studies it was also found that the K_D of [^{3}H]DHE decreased from 11.3 nM to 2.6 nM on 6-OHDA treatment [147]. However, these studies are open to criticism. Since a rather long time (14 days) was used to induce denervation, it is also possible that a change in postsynaptic alpha receptors, due to some trophic interaction, could have occurred which gave rise to the loss of [^{3}H]DHE binding sites. In these studies no attempts were made to classify the type of receptor that was labeled by [^{3}H]DHE, a procedure that could have shed more light on the question of whether presynaptic $alpha_2$ receptors were abolished by the denervation procedure. As mentioned above, the data from other studies indicate that [^{3}H]DHE probably exclusively labels $alpha_1$ receptors in the heart [173].

Although results on the heart have been equivocal, data on other tissues indicate that presynaptic receptors are in fact a reality. For example, Vogel et al. [158] found that in cultured superior ganglionic cells the stimulation-evoked release of norepinephrine was enhanced by phenoxybenzamine. Since these cells show axonal sprouts which are devoid of postsynaptic elements these results strongly indicate that a negative feedback inhibition of transmitter release by presynaptic alpha receptors was present. However, further studies of this type are warranted since it cannot, for example, be excluded that phenoxybenzamine acted by its ability to block reuptake of norepinephrine.

Another elegant approach was recently reported by Laduron [88]. After making a ligature of the splenic sympathetic nerve of the dog, he detected an accumulation of muscarinic receptors, evident as [^{3}H]dexetimide binding sites on both sides of the ligature. These results show that both an anterograde and a retrograde transport of muscarinic receptors take place in the axon. (For reviews on axoplasmic transport of macromolecules see refs. 42 and 86.) It seems quite probable that by the anterograde transport, muscarinic receptors, synthesized in the perykaryon, are transported down to the axon terminals where they can fulfill their physiological functions. There is much evidence from physiological studies that muscarinic cholinergic receptors inhibit the release of the adrenergic transmitter in a similar way to the $alpha_2$ adrenergic receptors [137,138,165]. To date, however, no attempts have been undertaken to investigate whether alpha receptors can be transported in a similar way to the muscarinic receptors.

In summary, extant data seem to support the existence of presynaptic alpha receptors in adrenergic neurons of the heart and elsewhere. However, in many cases the evidence is rather indirect and further studies will be necessary to provide definite proof.

Theoretically transsynaptic regulation may function in several ways. One possibility is that mediators which exert a tonic influence at the presynaptic site are continuously released from the postsynaptic elements unaffected by the neurotransmitter (or any other factor originating from the nerves). Alternatively, the postsynaptic actions of the transmitter may directly affect the release of the mediators which then feed back control of further release of transmitter. Two candidates have been proposed as transsynaptic mediators, namely prostaglandins (mainly PGE_2) and adenine nucleotides (mainly adenosine) [50,51,72]. The role of prostaglandins as a negative feedback modulator of norepinephrine release was supported by the observation that either sympathetic nerve stimulation or exogenous catecholamines increased the release of prostaglandins from the heart and other tissues [75,85,163; further refs. in 72 and 165]. In some tissues the stimulation-evoked release of prostaglandins could be prevented by alpha blockers [37,54,75], which supported the theory that alpha receptors mediate feedback inhibition, at least partly, by stimulating prostaglandin release. By contrast, in the heart, a beta blocker (sotalol) was found to be effective in blocking the release of prostaglandins upon sympathetic nerve stimulation [8], which rather strongly speaks against the prostaglandin hypothesis for alpha inhibition in this tissue. However, the most serious objection to the prostaglandin hypothesis comes from the observation that prostaglandin synthesis inhibitors, such as indomethacin, did not block the alpha effects on transmitter release in heart and other tissues [71,141]. However, prostaglandins may still exert a tonic inhibitory effect on norepinephrine release since indomethacin alone enhanced the stimulation-evoked release of transmitter [71,72,141,165].

The suggestion that adenine nucleotides act as transsynaptic modulators comes from observations similar to those for prostaglandins. In the rabbit heart adenosine inhibited stimulation-evoked release of norepinephrine [74]. On nerve stimulation of the same preparation adenosine was released in quantities that could have been active on transmitter release [51]. Studies on other tissues indicate similar relations [73]. At present it seems that further data will be required to assess the hypothesis that the feedback regulation of norepinephrine release by alpha receptors is mediated via adenosine. Theoretically, both a presynaptic and a transsynaptic mechanism could act in parallel and the balance between them could vary under different conditions. Perhaps the use of selective $alpha_1$ and $alpha_2$ drugs may prove to be useful in finding answers to these questions. It would seem reasonable to assume that the presynaptic pathway acts via $alpha_2$ receptors whereas a transsynaptic pathway, if it exists, acts via $alpha_1$ receptors.

Physiological Role of Alpha Adrenoceptor Mediated Negative Feedback Regulation of Sympathetic Neurotransmission in the Heart

The question whether feedback inhibition of norepinephrine secretion is a regulatory mechanism that occurs physiologically has given rise to a great deal of controversy. In the presynaptic alpha receptor hypothesis one must assume that a critical concentration of norepinephrine must be released before the inhibition of further norepinephrine release can take place, and the question then arises whether such concentrations are ever reached physiologically. And if such negative feedback inhibition occurred, one would expect it to be more active during rapid neural discharge activity and perhaps not at all active during very low neural activity. Other factors may also be of importance. The concentration of norepinephrine in the vicinity of the nerve terminal may depend not only on the amount released but also on its rate of elimination, i.e., by diffusion and by tissue reuptake. The responsiveness of the nerve terminal itself to alpha receptor stimulation is of importance as well. It seems quite probable that these factors vary in different tissues and species and it is therefore not surprising that controversies have developed. Also the inability of researchers to define "physiological" and "unphysiological" conditions as well as the fact that alpha blockers may have effects other than blocking alpha receptors seem to have added to the confusion.

The question of a physiological role of feedback inhibition has been studied mainly in the heart. It was argued that if presynaptic inhibition by endogenous norepinephrine was important, its blockade by alpha antagonists should lead to an increased release of transmitter which in turn could be monitored by measuring the heart rate since the chronotropic response on nerve stimulation is mediated mainly by beta receptors [91]. The hypothesis was tested in a spontaneously contracting guinea pig atrium-nerve preparation. Stimulation of the accelerans nerve with short trains of pulses (20 volleys at 0.5 Hz) induced a chronotropic response which was potentiated approximately 1.5 fold by low concentrations of phentolamine. Under the same conditions [^{3}H]norepinephrine release was also potentiated about threefold. Subsequently a number of investigators used similar approaches to test the hypothesis that feedback inhibition is a physiological phenomenon [10,148; 41 for further refs.]. The findings were inconsistent. It is likely that the discrepancies are due to species differences as well as differences in the experimental conditions. Thus, for example, the combined data on guinea pig atria indicate that feedback inhibition cannot be observed after only a few volleys (1–4) of stimulation whereas it is readily observed after a moderate number (16 volleys at 2 Hz) of stimulating pulses (cf. 10,91,148].

The possibility that alpha-receptor-mediated feedback inhibition could take place in vivo was elegantly demonstrated by Cavero et al. [29]. They found that in the spinal vagotomized dog infusion of either phentolamine or prazosin potentiated the chronotropic response as well as the increase in plasma norepinephrine in the coronary sinus on electrical stimulation of the cardioaccelerator nerve (see Fig. 5-2). The alpha blockers did not modify the chronotropic response to exogenous norepinephrine, thus clearly indicating that the observed potentiation of the chronotropic effect probably was due to the increased release of endogenous norepinephrine.

Beta Receptor Mediated Facilitation of Sympathetic Neurotransmission

A number of studies indicate that beta adrenoceptors can increase the release of norepinephrine from sympathetic neurons. This relation has been found both

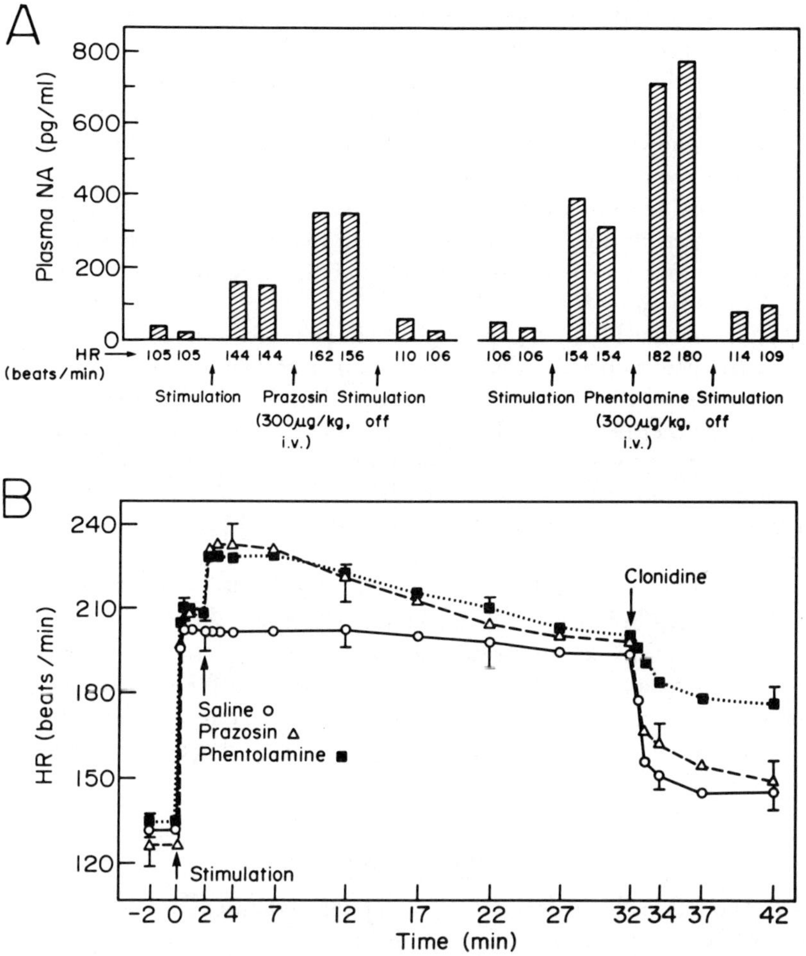

Fig. 5-2. (A.) Effects of electrical stimulation of the cardioaccelerans nerve and drugs on the plasma norepinephrine content (NA) in coronary sinus and the heart rate in the anesthetized dog. (B.) Effect of electrical stimulation of the accelerans nerve and drugs on the heart rate in the dog during similar conditions as in part A. The drugs were given intravenously for phentolamine and prazosin 300 μg/kg and for clonidine 20 μg/kg. The accelerans nerve was stimulated at a rate of 1H_z in both experiments. (HR = heart rate). (Reproduced by courtesy of *Br. J. Pharmacol.* 67: 283–292, 1979)

in adrenergic neurons of the heart and elsewhere. Several aspects of this topic have recently been reviewed by others [90,137,165] and will therefore only be briefly summarized here. For example, in guinea pig atria it was found that low concentrations of isoprenaline enhanced the stimulation-evoked release of norepinephrine [3]. However, some investigators did not find this effect following beta receptor stimulation. Thus, for example, Farnebo and Hamberger [47] failed to demonstrate any effect on transmitter release by isoprenaline in the mouse atria. Such discrepant findings have been explained by assuming that facilitative beta receptors were not ubiquitously present. Also the possibility must be considered that presynaptic alpha receptors could be stimulated by high concentrations of beta agonists which could prevent the facilitative effect from being observed [137]. It was recently observed that the ability of isoprenaline to enhance norepinephrine release in rat atria was more pronounced after blocking alpha receptors with phentolamine and less pronounced in the presence of norepinephrine. This might indicate that the degree of activation of presynaptic alpha receptors determines the ability of a presynaptic beta effect to be expressed physiologically [100].

The physiological role of presynaptic beta receptors is uncertain at present. Some investigators observed that the stimulation-evoked release of norepinephrine from the heart and other tissues was reduced by beta-adrenolytic drugs [3,183; for further refs. see 90,137], which might indicate that presynaptic beta receptors were activated by endogenous norepinephrine. On the other hand, inhibition of norepinephrine release by beta blockers has not been observed in several other studies, even though beta agonists caused an increase in transmitter release [137].

Recently Kalsner et al. [79] reported that (+) and (−) propranolol were equally effective in blocking the facilitative effect of isoprenaline on noradrenergic neurotransmission in the guinea pig atria. Thus, these results could indicate that isoprenaline did not act via typical beta receptors. However, more extensive studies are needed to settle this question. In other tissues stereoselective actions of beta agonists and antagonists on presynaptic beta receptors were reported [90].

Cholinergic Neurons

There is considerable evidence that cholinergic and adrenergic neurotransmission may be regulated in a similar fashion by different types of presynaptic receptors [157]. Starke [136] observed that the bradycardic response to vagal stimulation of the isolated rabbit heart was diminished by administration of the alpha agonist oxymetazoline. By contrast, the bradycardic effect of exogenous acetylcholine was not similarly affected. Thus, these results suggest that stimulation of alpha receptors inhibits cholinergic neurotransmission in the heart. Studies on other tissues (brain, intestine, and trachea) also indicate that $alpha_2$ receptors exert an inhibitory control of cholinergic neurotransmission [63,167].

Postsynaptic Cardiac Adrenergic Receptors

According to Ahlquist's initial classification, catecholamines caused their inotropic effect on the heart by interacting with beta receptors [4]. This notion found much support when it was demonstrated that dichloroisoproterenol, the first beta blocking agent, inhibited the catecholamine effects in the heart [108]. However, further studies, particularly those utilizing the more alpha-selective agonist, phenylephrine, indicated that activation of alpha receptors could also have a role in eliciting the inotropic effects [16,59,60,164]. A large number of studies later confirmed these results on different heart preparations from several mammalian species (for references see 15,114) and it seems now to be generally accepted that alpha receptors play a role in controlling the contractile force of the heart. Catecholamines were also found to exert profound influences on the electrophysiological behavior of heart cells and it was shown that both alpha and beta receptors participated in eliciting these effects (see below). With the advent of radioligand binding techniques it has become possible to directly identify both alpha and beta receptors in the myocardium. These techniques have made possible the study of several new aspects of adrenergic receptor function, i.e. their regulation during normal and pathological conditions.

Physiological Effects of Adrenoceptor Stimulation of the Myocardium

The inotropic effects of catecholamines and their analogues may be mediated by activation of both alpha and beta receptors. However, following the initial observations indicating such a role for alpha receptors, subsequent studies revealed conflicting results. Thus alpha inotropic effects were observed in atrial and/or ventricular muscles from frogs, guinea pigs, humans, rabbits, rats, and cats by some investigators [130,159,160; for further refs. see 114] whereas others failed to observe this effect (for refs. see 130). There may be several reasons for these discrepant results. For example, there might be regional, age, strain, species, or seasonal variations in the myocardial adrenergic receptor densities. Some of these possibilities have already found support from studies by radioligand binding techniques (see below). Another reason may be that certain experimental conditions precluded the observation of an alpha inotropic effect. Thus, for example, the beta effect of adrenergic agonists, even that of some predominantly alpha selective ones like phenylephrine, may overshadow any activation of alpha receptors and the alpha effect may not become apparent unless the beta receptors are blocked or a more alpha selective drug is used. That this might indeed be the case is illustrated by the experiments shown in Fig. 5-3 by Simpson and McNeil [132]. In the rat atria neither propranolol nor phenoxybenzamine alone blocked the inotropic effect of phenylephrine, but when a combination of both blockers was used complete inhibition was achieved. By contrast, when methoxamine was used, phenoxybenzamine alone was sufficient for blockade. These results indicate that (1) phenylephrine stimulates both alpha and beta receptors, (2) weak additivity exists for alpha and beta stimulation for this preparation, and (3) methoxamine is a more selective alpha agonist than phenylephrine. The ability to observe a positive inotropic alpha effect may also depend on other experimental factors, such as the contraction frequency of the myocardium. In the rat and guinea pig atria, both the potency and maximal effect of methoxamine to increase the contractile force by activating alpha receptors were much greater at low (0.5 Hz) than at high (2 Hz) stimulation frequencies [130].

There are distinct differences in alpha and beta inotropic effects. In general the alpha effect seems to develop more slowly [15], although the contrary has

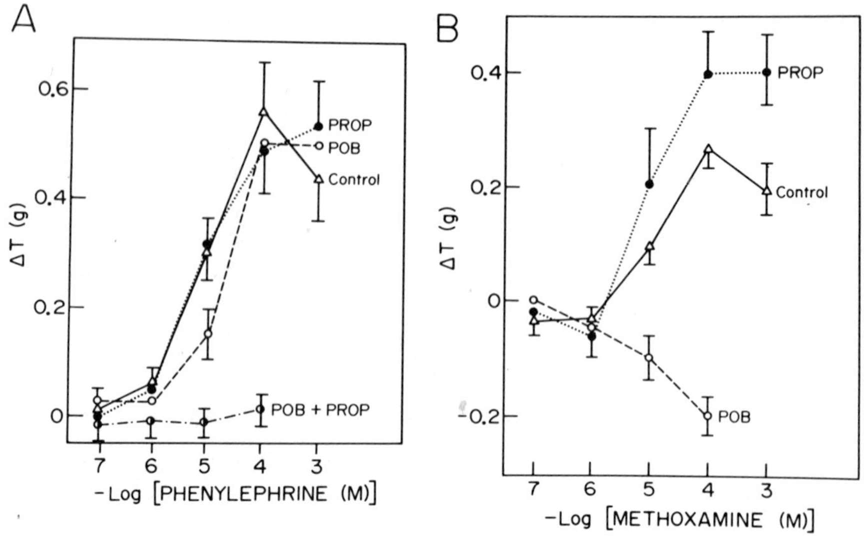

Fig. 5-3. (A.) Effects of phenylephrine on the contractile force in the spontaneously contracting rat right atrium for controls and in the presence of 10^{-6}M phenoxybenzamine (POP) and propranolol (PROP), respectively. (B.) Effect of methoxamine on the same type of preparation. (Reproduced by courtesy of *Advances in Myocardiol. 1*: 412–435, 1980)

also been observed [60]. In the rat heart, but not in several other species, the effect of alpha stimulation was triphasic: an initial short-lasting increase in contractile force followed by a plateau or a decrease which again was followed by a more long-lasting increase [115,116]. This relation was found in both atrial and ventricular muscle (perfused heart and papillary preparation). By contrast, the beta effect was always uniphasic. The triphasic response indicates that stimulatory as well as inhibitory alpha receptors could be present in the myocardium.

The contraction-relaxation cycle is also differentially affected by alpha and beta stimulation. The beta inotropic effect is accompanied by a shortening of the mechanical systole; the time to peak tension is shortened and the onset of the relaxation starts earlier than in the normal state. The alpha effect mainly uniformly increases the force of contraction [116]. The different patterns indicate that different mechanisms are operating to link alpha and beta receptor activation to effects on the myocardial contractile proteins (see below).

Catecholamines as well as sympathetic nerve stimulation exert distinct effects on transmembrane potentials in myocardial cells. Both alpha and beta receptors seem to participate in eliciting these electrophysiological effects. In general, catecholamines seem to affect mainly (1) the slope of the slow diastolic depolarization of pacemaker cells and (2) the slope of the plateau phase of the electrical systole (phase 2 of repolarization) and its duration. However, the extent of these changes may vary between different regions of the heart. Slow diastolic depolarizations are normally observed in the cells of the sinus and AV nodes, atrial fibers in the mitral valve leaflet, and the Purkinje system. In general, catecholamines appear to increase the rate of this depolarization which may lead to increased pacemaker activity (increased automaticity) [176]. In atrial cells, catecholamines may also induce diastolic depolarization even though it was absent previously [176]. The increased rate of diastolic depolarization seems to be mediated by beta receptors since the electrophysiological as well as the chronotropic response resulting from the electrophysiological changes are selectively affected by beta agonists and antagonists [124,153].

A closer analysis of the catecholamine effects revealed that in low doses they could sometimes have the opposite effect on automaticity in cardiac Purkinje fibers [119,124]. This effect seems to be mediated by stimulation of alpha receptors [124]. Similar changes on alpha-receptor stimulation were also reported for specialized conducting fiber cells in the human right atrium [101]. However, the alpha effect on automaticity seems not to be expressed as a decrease in heart rate [15]. Rather, the contrary, an increased heart rate has sometimes been observed on stimulation of alpha receptors (e.g. in hypothyroid hearts) [132]. In the ventricular cells spontaneous diastolic depolarization is not present and may not be induced by stimulation with catecholamines [176].

The effects of catecholamines on the action potentials of myocardial cells have been studied mainly in Purkinje fibers and atria. In general the catecholamines decreased the rate of repolarization during the plateau phase of electrical systolic (i.e., rendered it more positive) [28,56,117,155,156]. The catecholamines also either shortened or prolonged the duration of the action potential. A closer analysis of these effects indicates that beta receptor stimulation may increase the amplitude of the plateau phase and concomitantly shorten the duration of the action potential. To the contrary, the alpha effect may predominantly be to increase the duration of the action potential [56,117]. Stimulation of alpha and beta receptors also respectively increased and decreased the atrial functional refractory period [61], as might be anticipated from the electrophysiological effects. In ventricular myocytes the action of the catecholamines on the characteristics of the action potential has not been extensively characterized but some data indicate that stimulation of adrenergic receptors probably induces changes similar to those in Purkinje or atrial cells [28,111,176].

The molecular basis for the effects of catecholamines on the myocardium has been the subject of intense investigations during the last decades. We do not intend to give an extensive review on this topic. The reader is instead referred to some excellent reviews [81,114,115,154]. Following the initial discovery of cAMP and its relation to the actions of the catecholamines, much effort was devoted to prove or disprove the hypothesis that the nucleotide is the second messenger of the catecholamines in the heart. Although some data suggesting dissociation between the physiological effects of catecholamines on the one hand and cAMP on the other was reported, the overwhelming evidence suggests that cAMP is indeed the second messenger of the beta-adrenergic receptor in this tissue. It is probable that cAMP by virtue of its action on cAMP-dependent protein kinases triggers phosphorylation reactions of proteins which directly or indirectly may increase the transmembranal influx of Ca^{2+}; cAMP may affect fluxes of other ions as well, which accounts for the changes in the electrophysiological behavior of the myocardial cells. The intracellular translocation of Ca^{2+} is also affected. The most prominent of the later effects is the phosphorylation of a sarcoplasmic-reticulum-bound protein, phospholamban, which in its phosphorylated form increases the ability of sarcoplasmic reticulum to accumulate Ca^{2+}, by activating a calcium transport ATPase. These direct changes in calcium metabolism and the indirect changes that they may lead to seem to account for the mechanical changes observed in the contraction-relaxation cycle. Also, direct effects on the contractile proteins, by virtue of phosphorylation of troponin-I (a protein subunit within troponin that controls calcium sensitivity of the contractile elements), may be of importance.

By contrast, the molecular basis for the actions of the myocardial alpha receptors are only incompletely understood. It seems clear, however, that the alpha receptors do not act by elevating the intracellular cAMP [114,115] and cGMP does not seem to act as the second messenger for alpha receptors in the heart [15,114]. It is possible that the alpha receptors cause an increased influx of calcium from the extracellular space, but the experimental data supporting this hypothesis seem to be fairly limited. It has been observed that the alpha effect was more sensitive to blockade by calcium channel blockers than was the beta effect [45,94].

Classification of Myocardial Alpha Receptors

Radioligand binding studies clearly indicate that a majority of the myocardial alpha receptors are of the $alpha_1$ type. In Table 5-3 selected data from binding studies are presented. [^{3}H]DHE (nonselective), [^{3}H]prazosin ($alpha_1$ selective), and [^{3}H]WB4101 (predominantly $alpha_1$ selective) bind specifically to guinea pig or rat heart membranes and the order of potency of some $alpha_1$ and $alpha_2$ selective drugs to displace these ligands clearly show that they all bind predominantly to $alpha_1$ receptors. (The data are very similar to the findings of Stark [139] for [^{3}H]prazosin and [^{3}H]WB4101 binding to $alpha_1$ receptors in a number of other peripheral and central tissues.) As previously discussed, the $alpha_2$ receptors have not yet been detected in the myocardium by binding studies. Naturally, that does not necessarily mean that $alpha_2$ receptors are not present. Instead their densities probably are too low to allow detection with available techniques.

By physiological methods the alpha receptors in the myocardium have been shown to be predominantly $alpha_1$, but further studies are warranted before this question can be finally settled. For example, the $alpha_1$ selective agonists phenylephrine and methoxamine have generally caused a positive inotropic effect in heart preparations [for refs. see 114], whereas a number of imidazoline alpha agonists such as oxymetazoline, naphazoline, xylometazoline, or clonidine were ineffective [136,143]. At least some of the latter agonists may show preferential activity at $alpha_2$ receptors (clonidine, oxymetazoline, naphazoline), although this has not always been the case for some (oxymetazoline) [167]. The imidazolines might be ineffective because of a combination of low intrinsic activity and a low efficiency of myocardial alpha receptors to affect mechanical tension (i.e. total absence of "receptor reserve"). With respect to antagonists, no systematic studies have been performed. However, Skomedal et al. [133] found that the pA_2 of prazosin for inhibition of the positive inotropic effect of phenylephrine in the rat papillary muscle was 10.4, which is highly indicative of an $alpha_1$ type receptor [167]. As mentioned above, in the rat heart, stimulation of alpha receptors causes a triphasic response. Interestingly, prazosin was found to be less effective in inhibiting the negative than the positive response to phenylephrine. Phentolamine was equally effective on both responses [133]. These observations might indicate that besides $alpha_1$ receptors, another class, possibly $alpha_2$, might be present in the myocardium.

Recently it was suggested that atrial alpha receptors differed from other postsynaptic alpha receptors because the natural catecholamines, epinephrine and norepinephrine, did not stimulate the atrial type [143]. However, this suggestion seems to be premature. The ability to demonstrate an alpha component of an adrenergic agonist clearly depends on two factors: (1) the balance between alpha and beta activity of the drug and (2) the sensitivity of the tissue to alpha and beta stimulation. Thus, the inability to detect an alpha effect may be due to the fact that the beta effect has overwhelmed the alpha effect. The alpha component may become apparent only after blockade of the beta receptors. Thus, for example, Wagner et al. [160] found that in the human atrium the dose-response curve of epinephrine (inotropic effect) was shifted approximately tenfold to the left by 1×10^{-8}M pindolol (a beta blocker). By addition of 3×10^{-6}M phentolamine, a further threefold shift was induced. By contrast, the dose response curve of norepinephrine was shifted only by pindolol (approximately tenfold) but not by the addition of phentolamine. These results clearly indicate that epinephrine significantly stimulated alpha receptors but they do not necessarily indicate that norepinephrine was completely devoid of alpha activity. Ligand binding data indicate that norepinephrine appears to be tenfold less potent than epinephrine at $alpha_1$ receptors in the heart (Table 5-2), and if one assumes that the beta stimulatory activity of the two transmitters is

Table 5-2. Dissociation constants (K_I) and IC_{50} values for some adrenergic agonists and antagonists determined from the displacement of tritiated alpha antagonists in heart membranes

Species	guinea pig[a] [80]	rat[b] [173]	rat[c] [182]
Ligand	[^{3}H]prazosin	[^{3}H]DHE	[^{3}H]WB4101
	K_I (nM)	IC_{50} (nM)	K_I (nM)
Prazosin	0.33	0.35	0.18
WB4101	1.2	–	0.20
Indoramin	3.7	–	–
Phentolamine	126	37	5.32
Yohimbine	59,480	918	421
(−)Epinephrine	3,700	2,300	90
(−)Norepinephrine	37,200	2,700	723
(−)Phenylephrine	59,400	22,000	1,170
Clonidine	–	1,300	369

[a]K_D of [^{3}H]prazosin = 0.58 nM. [b]K_D of [^{3}H]DHE = 1.5 nM. [c]K_D of [^{3}H]WB4101 = 0.2 nM.

about equal, it seems likely that the relative contribution of alpha stimulation by norepinephrine, even after 1×10^{-8}M pindolol, is too low to be detected. In addition, some investigators have found alpha inotropic effects of norepinephrine as well as of epinephrine in both the atrial and ventricular myocardium from several species [for refs. see 114].

Classification and Distribution of Myocardial Beta Receptors

Lands and co-workers [89] assigned beta receptors in the heart to the $beta_1$ category. However, a few years later Carlsson et al. [26] presented evidence that both $beta_1$ and $beta_2$ receptors mediated chronotropic responses in the cat. Recent studies with radioligand binding techniques have given clear support to the notion that $beta_1$ and $beta_2$ receptors coexist in the heart. Furthermore, recent physiological studies indicate that the $beta_1$ receptors may be predominantly linked to the inotropic response, whereas both $beta_1$ and $beta_2$ receptors are linked to the chronotropic response. The presence and distribution of beta receptor subtypes was studied in the guinea pig and cat hearts by Hedberg et al. [70]. By analyzing the displacement curves of the nonselective beta receptor ligand [^{125}I]hydroxybenzylpindolol by several $beta_1$ and $beta_2$ selective drugs, it was revealed that in the right atria both receptor subtypes were present. To the contrary, in the left ventricles almost exclusively $beta_1$ receptors were detected (Fig. 5-4). Furthermore, in the cat, the $beta_2$ selective agonist terbutaline was more effective in increasing heart rate than it was in inducing an inotropic effect, whereas the $beta_1$ selective agonist prenalterol (H 80/62) was equally

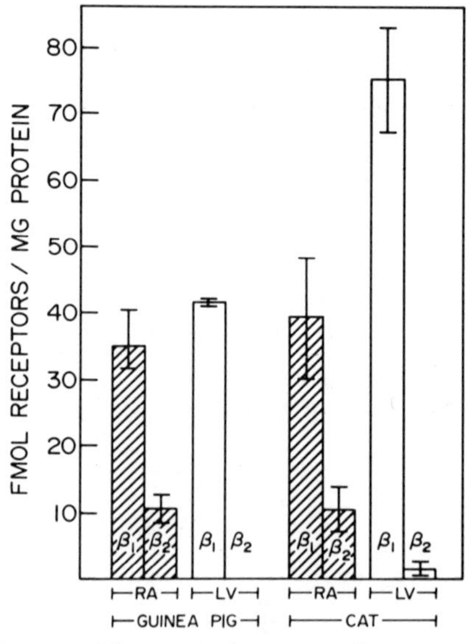

Fig. 5-4. Densities of $beta_1$ and $beta_2$ receptors in right atrium (RA) and left ventricle (LV) of the guinea pig and cat estimated by radioligand binding. (Reproduced by courtesy of *J. Pharmacol. Exp. Ther. 212*: 503–508, 1980)

effective on both responses [27,69]. Thus, these results seem to be compatible with the notion mentioned above that different beta receptor subtypes are coupled to different physiological responses in the heart. These results also fit nicely with the binding data. The ventricular beta$_1$ receptors would predominantly affect force, whereas some of the atrial beta$_1$ and beta$_2$ receptors may be located in pacemaker cells.

Additional studies also support the idea that different beta receptor subtypes mediate different physiological responses. Thus, in man the beta blocking agent mepindolol was found to be much more effective in counteracting the chronotropic response to isoprenaline than in counteracting the increase in stroke volume whereas propranolol was approximately equally effective [20]. In the spontaneously contracting rabbit atria the beta blocker PS-6 was found to be 50-fold more potent in inhibiting the isoproterenol-induced inotropic effect than it was in counteracting its chronotropic effect [134].

REGULATION OF MYOCARDIAL ADRENERGIC RECEPTORS

Considerable evidence has accumulated that hormone and neurotransmitter receptors are subject to dynamic regulation by a variety of stimuli. Historically, many studies dealt with receptor supersensitization and desensitization, but not

Table 5-3. Regulation of myocardial beta-adrenergic receptors

Factor	Receptor Density	Classification	References
Propranolol	Increase	Homologous	57
Guanethidine	Increase	Homologous	58
Isoproterenol[a]	Decrease	Homologous	151
6-OHDOPA or 6-OHDA	Increase	Homologous	113,181
Indomethacin	Decrease	Homologous (?)	49
Thyroid hormone	Increase	Heterologous	13,30,83,102,127, 144,150,152,172
Hypothyroidism	Decrease	Heterologous	13[b],30[c],102[c],144[b]
Ischemia[d]	Increase	Unknown	109
Abdominal aortic constriction[a]	Increase	Homologous (?)	97
Hypertension	Decrease	Homologous	18[e],98[e],123[e],177[e], 178[f,g],179[g],180[f]
Diabetes	Decrease	Heterologous	126[h]
Maturation	Decrease	Unknown	12,18
Desmethylimipramine	Decrease[i]	Homologous	76
Adrenalectomy	Increase	Heterologous	2

[a]Isoproterenol and abdominal aortic constriction induced cardiac hypertrophy.
[b]Hypothyroidism induced by thyroidecomy.
[c]Hypothyroidism induced by propylthiouracil.
[d]Ischemia induced by ligation of coronary artery.
[e]Spontaneously hypertensive rats.
[f]Hypertension induced by deoxycorticosterone/salt treatment.
[g]Renal hypertensive rats.
[h]Diabetes induced by streptozotocin.
[i]Decrease observed only in animals treated with thyroxine. 6-OHDA = 6-hydroxydopamine. 6-OHDOPA = 6-hydroxydopa. For further details see text.

until radioligand binding techniques became available has it become possible to investigate the exact role of changes in the receptor densities in such phenomena. Several recent studies do indicate that both increases and decreases of adrenergic receptor number may take place. Some relevant studies on myocardial beta receptors are given in Table 5-3. However, change in receptor number is theoretically not the only possible regulation mechanism. For example, the beta receptor protein (referred to as R_β) is intimately related to two other membrane-bound proteins, the stimulatory guanine nucleotide regulatory protein (N_s) and the enzyme adenylate cyclase (C); changes in the concentrations or functions of these proteins may affect the efficiency of the membrane transduction process (i.e. the process by which an extracellular chemical signal—the agonist—is converted to an intracellular signal—increased formation of cAMP). It is now possible to test these possibilities experimentally and recent studies indicate that changes in the concentrations of the N_s and C units may take place as well [92,145]. Data are still lacking on the heart, but indirect evidence indicates that such changes may take place in this tissue.

Homologous Regulation of Myocardial Beta Receptors

Receptor regulation is often described as either homologous (the ability of the receptor's own agonist to regulate the receptor number) or heterologous (all other types of regulation). There is firm evidence that myocardial beta receptors are subjected to homologous regulation. Thus, prolonged stimulation with exogenous isoprenaline leads to "down regulation" of the beta receptors. Also, drugs which either increase the release of endogenous norepinephrine (indomethacin) or prevent its uptake (desmethylimipramine) may have a similar effect. On the other hand drugs that either block the action of endogenous catecholamines (propranolol) or prevent the release of the adrenergic neurotransmitter (guanethidine, 6-OHDA) may have the opposite effect (Table 5-3). These changes were usually observed without changes in the affinities of the antagonist ligands used to estimate the beta receptor numbers. (We are inclined to believe that indomethacin enhances norepinephrine release in the heart [141], although a homologous mechanism was not favored by Feuerstein and co-workers [49] since indomethacin induced a decrease in the plasma norepinephrine concentrations. However, the possibility still remains that a local or phasic elevation of catecholamines was present in the heart. On the other hand, the possibility of a heterologous regulation of beta receptors via the prostaglandin system deserves further studies.)

Detailed analysis of homologous regulation indicates that other membrane changes may also take place. First, prolonged treatment with isoprenaline induced a decrease in basal, sodium fluoride, and isoprenaline stimulated adenylate cyclase activity in the heart [151]. Second, the isoprenaline treatment induced an increase in the ED_{50} of isoprenaline to displace [^{3}H]dihy droalprenolol bound to beta receptors in cardiac membranes. The effect of guanylylimidodiphosphate (Gpp(NH)p) is also to increase the ED_{50} of the isoprenaline displacement curves, and in the desensitized hearts the ED_{50} was increased to approximately the same absolute values as in the controls by the GTP analogue [151]. The first observations indicate that a decrease in the ability of beta receptors to activate adenylate cyclase is present. Part of this effect may result from the decreased beta receptor number, but since basal and fluoride-stimulated activity was diminished, other changes must also have taken place. The basal activity (in the presence of MG^{2+} ATP) may reflect the activity of both free C units and preformed N_sC-complexes. On the other hand, fluoride seems to depend on the presence of N_s for its activity and therefore F^- stimulation may reflect the system's ability to form N_sC complexes. Therefore, these results imply either a decrease in the number of N_s units or a change in their function. (Changes in the C unit cannot be completely ruled out from these observations, however.) The second observation would also support this notion. The overall affinity of a beta agonist is determined from the $beta_H$ (high affinity) and $beta_L$ (low affinity) sites. By detailed computer-aided analysis it has been shown that the $beta_L$ site probably reflects the agonist binding to the R_β unit, whereas the $beta_H$ site probably reflects its binding to the $R_\beta N_s$ complex [39]. In the presence of guanine nucleotides, such as Gpp(NH)p, only the $beta_L$ site can be observed. The increased ED_{50} of isoprenaline together with the observed effect of Gpp(NH)p support a diminished affinity and/or a diminished amount of $beta_H$ sites. These changes speak, in turn, for a diminished agonist-promoted formation of the $R_\beta N_s$ complex in the desensitized heart membranes. (Similar observations have been made on the desensitized frog erythrocyte beta receptors, and in this tissue the changes were thoroughly documented by computer modeling techniques [84]). It seems quite probable that all these effects can be explained by a decrease in the amount of the N_s protein in the cardiac membranes after isoprenaline treatment, but it is necessary to make direct measurements to confirm this.

It is possible that some pathological conditions may be associated with changes in cardiac beta receptors due to homologous regulation. A number of studies indicate that experimental hypertension is accompanied by a decrease in myocardial beta receptors (Table 5-3). The down regulation of beta receptors has generally been attributed to the increased plasma norepinephrine concentrations or increased sympathetic neural activity observed in the different hypertensive models [178,180]. Some investigators have observed lesions in the cAMP system in spontaneous hypertensive rat hearts [18], which are similar to those mentioned above for isoprenaline desensitization. Also, a decrease in the ability of isoprenaline to compete for [^{3}H]dihydroalprenolol was observed in the spontaneous hypertensive rats [18]. Thus, these observations would support the notion that the hypertensive state gives rise to beta receptor down regulation by a mechanism similar to that of isoprenaline treatment. Thus far, no studies have been undertaken to investigate the role of antihypertensive diseases. This is of interest since the majority of these agents interact with the adrenergic system.

Considerable interest has been devoted to the so-called propranolol withdrawal syndrome and the possibility that regulation of beta receptors plays a role in its development. The syndrome was described by Alderman et al. [6]

who observed that following cessation of propranolol treatment in patients with stable angina pectoris, a worsening of their symptoms occurred and in some even myocardial infarction or sudden death. In later experimental studies it was observed that during propranolol withdrawal in humans an increased cardiac responsiveness to infused isoprenaline took place [21,112]. In view of the observation that propranolol treatment in an animal model gave rise to "up regulation" of myocardial beta receptors, this mechanism may be of clinical importance in man [57]. Treatment of human subjects with propranolol leads to an increase in the number of beta-adrenergic receptors on their lymphocytes [1].

Another condition, myocardial hypertrophy, induced by abdominal aortic constriction, was associated with an increased number of beta receptors. This effect was attributed to the decreased adrenergic innervation observed in the hypertrophied hearts, and thus to a homologous up regulation by a diminished influence of endogenous norepinephrine [97]. Naturally it is difficult to exclude other possibilities. It is interesting to note that hypertrophy induced by isoproterenol is associated with the opposite regulation of beta receptors [151]. In experimental hypertension a similar relation was observed, i.e. left ventricular hypertrophy and a decrease in beta receptor densities [180]. Normal growth of the heart is associated with a decrease of the beta receptor density, although the total number of beta receptors per heart is increased [12].

Heterologous Regulation of Myocardial Beta Receptors

At present the best documented heterologous type regulation of myocardial beta-adrenergic receptors is by the influence of thyroid hormones. Thus, hyperthyroidism induced by exogenous thyroxine or triiodothyronine leads to an increase in beta receptor density, whereas hypothyroidism induced either surgically or pharmacologically had the opposite effect (Table 5-3). In general these changes were noted without any effects on the affinities of the antagonist ligands used to assay the beta receptors. The "up regulation" of beta receptors by thyroid hormones is associated with an increased sensitivity for the inotropic and chronotropic effects of beta receptor stimulation [68,152,171]. Also the ability of isoprenaline to stimulate adenylate cyclase was potentiated in the hyperthyroid state whereas, on the other hand, the basal and NaF stimulated activity remained unchanged [152]. Recently Stiles and Lefkowitz [144] found that the affinity of isoproterenol for the $beta_H$ state was increased in triiodothyronine pretreated rats, which might indicate that agonists shcw an increased ability to form the $R_\beta N_s$ complex in the hyperthyroid state. At present it is difficult to interpret this observation in molecular terms. It is also possible that the density of the N_s protein might be affected by thyroid hormones in a similar way as the beta receptor protein itself. This has been demonstrated in reticulocytes from hypothyroid rats [145].

The effect of thyroid hormone is exerted directly on the heart since it was observed in both cultured heart cells and on heart slices in vitro [83,150]. Kempson and co-workers [83] found that the effect of thyroid hormones occurred in two phases during in vitro stimulation of heart slices. The short-term effect (1.5–

2 h), to increase beta receptors, could not be blocked by either of the protein synthesis inhibitors, cycloheximide or puromycin. The long-term effect (15 h), on the other hand, was abolished by cycloheximide. These results might indicate that thyroid hormones have multiple sites of action on the myocytes. One effect is to increase the de novo synthesis of beta receptor protein, and this effect is blocked by protein synthesis inhibitors. The other effect might be related to some posttranscriptional event, such as the assembly of functional beta receptor units (i.e. the glycosylation of the receptor protein) or their transport and incorporation into the sarcolemma. Interestingly, Kempson and co-workers found that the addition of a mixture of 20 amino acids was necessary to obtain a good response to thyroid hormones both for the short- and the long-term effects in their in vitro model.

Much attention has been paid to the clinical relevance of these findings and the possibility that "up regulation" of cardiac beta receptors may account for adrenergic supersensitivity in clinical hyperthyroidism. At present it is difficult to directly assess the status of myocardial beta receptors in humans by binding, but recent data suggest that clinical and experimental thyrotoxicosis is associated with an elevated number of leukocyte beta receptors [9,55].

The myocardial beta receptors are presumably under trophic control by factors other than the thyroid hormones, but too little data are currently available to allow for a satisfactory analysis of these effects. However, Abrass and Scarpace [2] found that adrenalectomy of rats led to an increase in cardiac beta receptors and that this effect was prevented by the administration of cortisol. By contrast, Davies et al. [35] found adrenalectomy to have no effect on the cardiac beta-adrenergic receptor number in rats. Instead, these investigators noted a decrease in the ability of agonists to form the high-affinity state (i.e. the $beta_H$ state). Thus, the effects of corticoid hormones might be composite in cardiac tissue. Gluco- and mineralocorticoids were also found to potentiate the inotropic and arrhythmogenic effects of beta receptor stimulation in the heart [65,82], but it is not known whether this effect is caused by an alteration in the efficiency of receptor coupling in the cell membrane or by some effect distal to the membrane transduction process. Corticoids appear to be tissue specific, since different patterns of beta-adrenergic receptor regulation were found in different organ systems [36]. Thus, further experimentation will be required before the role of the corticoid hormones in the regulation of myocardial beta receptors can be elucidated.

Experimental diabetes was found to be associated with a decrease in myocardial beta receptors [126]. The decrease was accompanied by a bradycardia, which might be related to the decreased cardiac performance observed in diabetic patients [125]. The mechanism by which the diabetic state causes a down regulation of beta receptors is unknown, although it was postulated that it might result from a hypothyroid disease state [126]. However, at present there seems to be fairly little evidence to support this. Instead the down regulation might be due to a decrease in protein synthesis which has been observed in the diabetic state [11], but further studies will be necessary to evaluate this possibility.

Another condition, cardiac ischemia, induced by coronary occlusion, is associated with an up regulation of beta receptors [109]. Although the mechanism by which this effect is induced is completely unknown, the increase in beta receptors might be of great clinical importance in view of the fact that one of the major causes of death during myocardial infarction is arrhythmias, which in turn might have been caused by a sensitization of the myocardium to catecholamines.

Regulation of Myocardial Alpha Receptors

Comparatively few data are available on the regulation of myocardial alpha receptors and some of these results are contradictory. A number of laboratories have reported that alpha receptors decreased on treatment with thyroid hormones [30,87,102,129,175]. In some studies it was reported that the affinity of [^{3}H]DHE was reduced by thyroid hormone treatment. Thus, Williams and Lefkowitz [175] observed a significant increase in the K_D of [^{3}H]DHE, from 2.5 nM in control rat hearts to 4.0 nM in hyperthyroid hearts. Likewise Ciaraldi and Marinetti [31] found an increase of K_D from 4.5 nM in controls to 18.5 in hearts from hyperthyroid animals. By contrast several other investigators found no changes in affinity in the hyperthyroid state either for [^{3}H]DHE or [^{3}H]WB4101 [87,102,129]. With respect to hypothyroidism, Ciaraldi and Marinetti [30,31] found a drastic decrease in alpha receptor densities (reduction by approximately 60–80%) in propylthiouracil treated rats. McConnaugh et al. [102] similarly also reported a 30% decrease in propylthiouracil treated rats. By contrast, Williams and Lefkowitz [175] found a slight increase of alpha receptors in rats made hypothyroid by propylthiouracil treatment. Thus, at present it is difficult to make any definite conclusions on the effects of thyroid status on the myocardial alpha receptors.

In the renal hypertensive rat the myocardial alpha receptor density, assayed as [^{3}H]DHE binding sites, was decreased [179]. Also in the deoxycorticosterone/salt hypertensive rat the alpha receptor content, measured as [^{3}H]WB4101 sites, was decreased [180]. Thus, these results suggest, as did the regulation of beta receptors in the hypertensive states, that a homologous down regulation of alpha receptors due to an adrenergic hyperactivity could have taken place. Chemical denervation by 6-OHDA was found to increase the specific binding of [^{3}H]WB4101 in the rat heart [181] which may support the notion of regulation of alpha receptors in the heart by the adrenergic system. However, by contrast, Kunos et al. [87] found that chemical denervation with 6-OHDA, in the thyroidectomized rat, reduced the [^{3}H]WB4101 binding sites by more than 50%. Furthermore, denervation with 6-OHDA induced a decrease in the [^{3}H]DHE binding sites of rat hearts [128,147]. Although the latter investigators suggested that the decrease was due to a loss of presynaptic alpha receptors, we think, for reasons discussed in a previous paragraph, that this interpretation is unlikely. Instead the combined data suggest that either a more complex and not yet fully recognized regulation of postsynaptic myocardial alpha receptors occurs or otherwise that some of the contradictory results are due to experimental inadequacies.

REFERENCES

1. Aarons, R. D., A. S. Nies, J. Gal, L. R. Hegstrand, P. B. Molinoff, Elevation of beta-adrenergic receptor density in human lymphocytes after propranolol administration. *J. Clin. Invest.* *65*: 949–952, 1980.
2. Abrass, I. B. and P. J. Scarpace, Glucocorticoid regulation of myocardial beta-adrenergic receptors. *Endocrinol.* *108*: 977–980, 1981.
3. Adler-Graschinsky, E. and S. Z. Langer, Possible role of a beta-adrenoceptor in the regulation of noradrenaline release by nerve stimulation through a positive feedback mechanism. *Br. J. Pharmacol.* *53*: 43–50, 1975.
4. Ahlquist, R. P., Studies of the adrenotropic receptors. *Am. J. Physiol.* *153:* 586–600, 1948.
5. Ahlquist, R. P. Adrenergic beta-blocking agents. *Prog. Drug Res.* *20*: 27–42, 1976.
6. Alderman, E. L., D. J. Coltart, G. E. Wettach, D. C. Harrison, Coronary artery syndrome after sudden propranolol withdrawal. *Ann. Int. Med.* *81*: 625–627, 1974.
7. Algate, D. R. and J. F. Waterfall, Action of indoramine on pre- and postsynaptic alpha-adrenoceptors in pithed rats. *J. Pharm. Pharmacol.* *30*: 651–661, 1978.
8. Amin, D. V., R. B. Doctor, A. O. Girdhar, U. H. Shah, The effect of beta-adrenergic stimulation and blockade on the efflux of PGE_1-like material from the isolated perfused rabbit heart. *Experientia* *36*: 1410–1411, 1980.
9. Andersson, R. G. G., O. R. Nilsson, J. F. Kuo, Beta-adrenoceptor-cyclic AMP system in human leukocytes before and after treatment for hyperthyroidism. In preparation.
10. Angus, J. A. and P. I. Korner, Evidence against presynaptic alpha-adrenoceptor modulation of cardiac sympathetic transmission. *Nature* *286*: 288–291, 1980.
11. Arnqvist, H. J. and K. Norrby, Effect of insulin in vivo and in vitro on incorporation of amino acid into protein in normal and diabetic rat aorta. *Horm. Metab. Res.* *12*: 15–19, 1980.
12. Baker, S. P. and L. T. Potter, Cardiac beta-adrenoceptors during normal growth of male and female rats. *Br. J. Pharmacol.* *68*: 65–70, 1980.
13. Banerjee, S. P. and L. S. Kung, Beta-adrenergic receptors in rat heart: effect of thyroidectomy. *Eur. J. Pharmacol.* *43*: 207–208, 1977.
14. Barnett, D. B., E. L. Rugg, S. R. Nahorski, Direct evidence of two types of beta-adrenoceptor binding sites in lung tissue. *Nature* *273*: 166–168, 1978.
15. Benfey, B. G., Cardiac alpha-adrenoceptors. *Can. J. Physiol. Pharmacol.* *58*: 1145–1157, 1980.
16. Benfey, B. G. and D. R. Varma, Interactions of sympathomimetic drugs, propranolol and phentolamine on atrial refractory period and contractility. *Br. J. Pharmacol. Chemother.* *30*: 603–611, 1967.
17. Berthelson, S. and W. A. Pettinger, A functional basis for classification of alpha-adrenergic receptors. *Life Sci.* *21*: 595–606, 1977.
18. Bhalla, R. C., R. V. Sharma, S. Ramanathan, Ontogenic development of isoproterenol subsensitivity of myocardial adenylate cyclase and beta-adrenergic receptors in spontaneously hypertensive rats. *Biochem. Biophys. Acta* *632*: 497–506, 1980.
19. Boissier, J. R., C. Advenier, J. F. Guidicelli, P. Viars, Studies on the nature of the bronchial beta-adrenoceptors. *Eur. J. Pharmacol.* *57*: 101–109, 1971.
20. Bonelli, J., D. Magometschnigg, G. Hitzenberger, G. Kaik, A model for distinguishing between $beta_1$-receptors which mediate a specific effect on the heart rate

and those which mediate a positively inotropic effect. *Int. J. Clin. Pharmacol. 15*: 381–383, 1977.

21. Boudolas, H., R. P. Lewis, R. E. Kates, G. Dalamangus, Hypersensitivity to adrenergic stimulation after propranolol withdrawal in normal subjects. *Ann. Int. Med. 87*: 433–436, 1977.
22. Bristow, M., T. R. Sherod, R. D. Green, Analysis of beta receptor drug interactions in isolated rabbit atrium, aorta, stomach and trachea. *J. Pharmacol. Exp. Ther.* 171: 52–61, 1970.
23. Britain, R. T., J. B. Farmer, D. Jack, L. E. Martin, W. T. Simpson, Alpha-[(t-bytylamino)methyl]-4-hydroxy-m-xylene α^1 α^3-diol (AH 3365); a selective beta-adrenergic stimulant. *Nature 219*: 862–863, 1968.
24. Brown, G. L. and J. S. Gillespie, Output of sympathin from the spleen. *Nature 178*: 980–981, 1956.
25. Carlsson, E., On the classification and distribution of beta-adrenoceptors. *Acta Pharmacol. Toxicol. 44, suppl. II*: 17–20, 1979.
26. Carlsson, E., B. Åblad, A. Brändström, B. Carlsson, Differential blockade of the chronotropic effects of various adrenergic stimuli in the cat heart. *Life Sci. 11*: 953–958, 1972.
27. Carlsson, E., C.-G. Dahlöf, A. Hedberg, H. Persson, B. Tångstrand, Differentiation of cardiac chronotropic and inotropic effects of beta-adrenoceptor agonists. *Naunyn-Schmiedebergs Arch. Pharmacol. 300*: 101–105, 1977.
28. Carmeliet, E. and J. Vereecke, Adrenaline and the plateau phase of the cardiac action potential. *Pflugers Arch. 313*: 300–315, 1969.
29. Cavero, I., T. Dennis, F. Lefevre-Borg, P. Perrot, A. G. Roach, B. Scatton, Effects of clonidine, prazosin and phentolamine on heart rate and coronary sinus catecholamine concentration during cardioaccelerator nerve stimulation in spinal dog. *Br. J. Pharmacol. 67*: 283–292, 1979.
30. Ciaraldi, T. and G. V. Marinetti, Thyroxine and propylthiouracil effects in vivo on alpha and beta adrenergic receptors in rat heart. *Biochem. Biophys. Res. Commun. 74*: 984–991, 1977.
31. Ciaraldi, T. P. and G. V. Marinetti, Hormone action at the membrane level. VIII. Adrenergic receptors in rat heart and adipocytes and their modulation by thyroxine. *Biochem. Biophys. Acta 541*: 334–346, 1978.
32. Constantine, J. W., R. A. Weeks, W. K. McShane, Prazosin and presynaptic alpha-receptors in the cardioaccelerator nerve of the dog. *Eur. J. Pharmacol. 50*: 51–60, 1978.
33. Dahlström, A., K. Fuxe, M. Mya-Tu, B. E. M. Zetterström, Observations on adrenergic innervation of dog heart. *Am. J. Physiol. 209*: 689–692, 1965.
34. Daly, M. J. and Levy, G. P., The subclassification of beta-adrenoceptors: evidence in support of the dual beta-adrenoceptor hypothesis. In *Trends in Autonomic-Pharmacology*, Ed. D. Kalsner. Urban and Schwartzenberg, Baltimore and Munich, Vol. 1, pp. 347–385, 1979.
35. Davies, A. O., A. De Lean, R. J. Lefkowitz, Myocardial beta-adrenergic receptors from adrenalectomized rats: impaired formation of high-affinity agonist-receptor complexes. *Endocrinology 108*: 720–722, 1981.
36. Davies, A. O. and R. J. Lefkowitz, Regulation of adrenergic receptors. In *Receptors and Recognition,* ed. R. J. Lefkowitz. Chapman, London, Ser. B, Vol. 13, pp. 84–120, 1981.
37. Davies, B. N., and E. W. Horton, and P. G. Withrington, The occurrence of prostaglandins E_2 in splenic venous blood of the dog following splenic nerve stimulation. *Br. J. Pharmacol. 32*: 127–135, 1968.

38. De Lean, A., A. Hancock, R. J. Lefkowitz, Validation and statistical analysis of a computer modelling method for quantitative analysis of radioligand binding data for mixtures of pharmacological receptor subtypes, *Mol. Pharmacol. 21*: 5–16, 1982.
39. De Lean, A., J. M. Stadel, and R. J. Lefkowitz, A ternary complex model explains the agonist-specific binding properties of the adenylate cyclase-coupled beta-adrenergic receptor. *J. Biol. Chem. 255*: 7108–7117, 1980.
40. Drew, G. M., Effects of alpha-adrenoceptor agonists and antagonists on pre- and postsynaptically located alpha-adrenoceptors. *Eur. J. Pharmacol. 36*: 313–320, 1976.
41. Drew, G. M., Presynaptic modulation of heart rate responses to cardiac nerve stimulation in pithed rats. *J. Cardiovasc. Pharmacol. 2*: 843–856, 1980.
42. Droz, B., Synthetic machinery and axoplasmic transport: maintenance of neuronal connectivity. In *The Nervous System*, ed. D. B. Tower. Vol. 1, *The Basic Neurosciences*, Ed. R. O. Brody. Raven Press, New York, pp. 111–127, 1975.
43. Dubocovich, M. L. and S. Z. Langer, Negative feedback regulation of noradrenaline release by nerve stimulation in the perfused cat's spleen: differences in potency of phenoxybenzamine in blocking the pre- and postsynaptic adrenergic receptors. *J. Physiol. (London) 237*: 505–519, 1974.
44. Dunlop, D. and R. G. Shanks, Selective blockade of adrenoceptive beta receptors in the heart. *Br. J. Pharmacol. Chemother. 32*: 201–218, 1968.
45. Endoh, M., H. J. Schumann, N. Krappitz, B. Hillen, Alpha-adrenoceptors influence of temperature on the positive inotropic effects mediated by alpha and beta-adrenoceptors in the isolated rabbit papillary muscle. *Naunyn-Schmiedebergs Arch. Pharmacol. 287*: 61–72, 1975.
46. Farah, M. G. and S. Z. Langer, Protection by phentolamine against the effects of phenoxybenzamine on transmitter release elicited by nerve stimulation in the perfused cat heart. *Br. J. Pharmacol. 52*: 549–557, 1974.
47. Farnebo, L.-O. and B. Hamberger, Influence of alpha and beta-adrenoceptors on the release of noradrenaline from field stimulated atria and cerebral cortex slices. *J. Pharm. Pharmacol. 26*: 644–646, 1974.
48. Farnebo, L.-O. and T. Malmfors, [^{3}H]Noradrenaline release and mechanical response in the field stimulated mouse vas deferens. *Acta Physiol. Scand., Suppl. 371*: 1–18, 1971.
49. Feuerstein, G., T. Torda, I. J. Kopin, Effect of indomethacin on cardiac beta-adrenergic receptors. *Eur. J. Pharmacol. 67*: 469–472, 1980.
50. Fredholm, B. B. and P. Hedqvist, Presynaptic inhibition of transmitter release by adenosine and its antagonism by theophylline. In *Adv. Biosci. Presynaptic Receptors*, Vol. 18, Eds. S. Z. Langer, M. Dubocovitch, K. Starke. Pergamon, Oxford, pp. 281–286, 1979.
51. Fredholm, B. B., P. Hedqvist, L. Vernet, Release of adenosine from the rabbit heart by sympathetic nerve stimulation. *Acta Physiol. Scand. 106*: 381–382, 1979.
52. Furchgott, R. F., The classification of adrenoceptors. In *Handbook of Experimental Pharmacology*, Vol. 33, Eds. H. Blaschko and E. Muscholl. Springer, Berlin, pp. 283–335, 1972.
53. Furchgott, R. F., Postsynaptic adrenergic receptor mechanisms in vascular smooth muscle. In *Vascular Neuroeffector Mechanisms*, Eds. J. Bevan et al. S. Karger, Basel, pp. 131–141, 1976.
54. Gilmore, N., J. R. Vane, J. H. Wyullie, Prostaglandin release by the spleen. *Nature 218*: 1135–1140, 1968.

55. Ginsberg, A. M., W. E. Clutter, S. D. Shah, P. E. Cryer, Triiodothyronine-induced thyrotoxicosis increases mononulear leukocyte beta-adrenergic receptor density in man. *J. Clin. Invest. 67*: 1785–1791, 1981.
56. Giotti, A., F. Ledda, P. F. Manncioni, Effects of noradrenaline and isoprenaline in combination with alpha and beta-receptor blocking substances, on the action potential of cardiac purkinje fibres. *J. Physiol. 229*: 99-113, 1973.
57. Glaubiger, G. and R. J. Lefkowitz, Elevated beta-adrenergic receptor number after chronic propranolol treatment. *Biochem. Biophys. Res. Commun. 78*: 720–725, 1977.
58. Glaubiger, G., B. S. Tsai, R. J. Lefkowitz, B. Weiss, E. M. Johnson, Chronic guanethidine treatment increases cardiac beta-adrenergic receptors. *Nature 273*: 240–242, 1978.
59. Govier, W. C., A positive inotropic effect of phenylephrine mediated through alpha adrenergic receptors. *Life Sci. 6*: 1361–1365, 1967.
60. Govier, W. C., Myocardial alpha adrenergic receptors and their role in the production of a positive inotropic effect by sympathomimetic agents. *J. Pharmacol. Exp. Ther. 159*: 82–90, 1968.
61. Govier, W. C., N. C. Mosal, P., Whittington, A. H. Broom, Myocardial alpha and beta adrenergic receptors as demonstrated by atrial functional refractory-period changes. *J. Pharmacol. Exp. Ther. 154*: 255–263, 1966.
62. Grana, E., A. Lucchelli, F. Zonta, Selectivity of beta-adrenergic compounds, III. Classification of beta-receptors. II. *Farmaco Ed. Sc. 79*: 786–792, 1974.
63. Grundström, N., R. G. G. Andersson, J. E. S. Wikberg, Prejunctional $alpha_2$ adrenoceptors inhibit contraction of tracheal smooth muscle by inhibiting cholinergic neurotransmission. *Life Sci. 28*: 2981–2986, 1981.
64. Guicheney, P., R. P. Garay, C. Levy-Marchal, P. Meyer, Biochemical evidence for presynaptic and postsynaptic alpha-adrenoceptors in rat heart membranes: positive homotropic cooperativity of presynaptic binding. *Proc. Natl. Acad. Sci. USA 75*: 6285–6289, 1978.
65. Guideri, G., M. Green, D. Lehr, Potentiation of isoproterenol cardiotoxicity by corticoids. *Res. Commun. Chem. Phatol. Pharmacol. 21*: 197–212, 1978.
66. Häggedal, J. Some further aspects on the release of the adrenergic transmitter. *Bayer-Symposium II*. Springer, Berlin, pp. 100–109, 1970.
67. Hancock, A., A. L. De Lean, and R. J. Lefkowitz, Quantitative resolution of beta-adrenergic subtypes by selective ligand binding: application of a computerized model fitting technique. *Mol. Pharmacol. 16*: 1–9, 1979.
68. Hashimoto, H. and M. Nakashima, Influence of thyroid hormone on the positive inotropic effects mediated by alpha and beta-adrenoceptors in isolated guinea pig atria and rabbit papillary muscles. *Eur. J. Pharmacol. 50*: 337–347, 1978.
69. Hedberg, A., Studies on $beta_1$ and $beta_2$ adrenoceptor mechanisms in the mammalian heart with special reference to the action of prenalterol. Thesis, Gothenburg, 1980.
70. Hedberg, A., K. P. Minneman, P. B. Molinoff, Differential distribution of $beta_1$ and $beta_2$ adrenergic receptors in cat and guinea pig heart. *J. Pharmacol. Exp. Ther. 213*: 503–508, 1980.
71. Hedqvist, P., Role of the alpha-receptor in the control of noradrenaline release from sympathetic nerves. *Acta Physiol. Scand. 90*: 158–165, 1974.
72. Hedqvist, P., Basic mechanisms of prostaglandin action on autonomic neurotransmission. *Ann. Rev. Pharmacol. Toxicol. 17*: 259–279, 1977.
73. Hedqvist, P., Autoinhibition versus transsynaptic control of noradrenaline secretion in the rabbit kidney. *Acta Physiol. Scand. 110:* 441–443, 1980.

74. Hedqvist, P. and B. B. Fredholm, Inhibitory effect of adenosine on adrenergic neuroeffector transmission in the rabbit heart. *Acta Physiol. Scand. 105*: 120–122, 1979.

75. Hedqvist, P., L. Gustafsson, P. Hjemdahl, and K. Svanborg, Aspects of prostaglandin action on autonomic neuroeffector transmission. *Adv. Prostaglandin Thromboxane Res. 8*: 1245–1248, 1980.

76. Hess, M. E., K. A. Reynolds, A. Frazer, D. Viscusi, Inhibitory effects of desmethylimipramine on the action of thyroxine on cardiac beta-receptors and myocardial phosphorylase. *J. Cardiovasc. Pharmacol. 2*: 867–87, 1980.

77. Hoffman, B. B., A. De Lean, C. L. Wood, D. D. Schocken, R. J. Lefkowitz, Alpha-adrenergic receptor subtypes: quantitative assessment by ligand binding. *Life Sci. 24*: 1739–1746, 1979.

78. Johansson, S. R. M., R. G. G. Andersson, J. E. S. Wikberg, Comparison of $beta_1$ and $beta_2$ receptor stimulation in oestrogen or progesterone dominated rat uterus. *Acta Pharmacol. Toxicol. 47*: 252–258, 1980.

79. Kalsner, S., The effects of (+) and (−)-propranolol on [^{3}H]transmitter efflux in guinea pig atria and the presynaptic beta-adrenoceptor hypothesis. *Br. J. Pharmacol. 70*: 491–498, 1980.

80. Karliner, J. S., P. Barnes, C. A. Hamilton, C. T. Dollery, $Alpha_1$-adrenergic receptors in guinea pig myocardium. *Biochem. Biophys. Res. Commum. 90*: 142–149, 1979.

81. Katz, A. M., Role of the contractile proteins and sarcoplasmic reticulum in the response of the heart to catecholamines: an historical review. *Adv. Cycl. Nucl. Res. 11*: 303–342, 1979.

82. Kauman, A. J., Potentiation of the effects of isoprenaline and noradrenaline by hydroxortison in cat heart muscle. *Naunyn-Schmiedebergs Arch. Pharmacol. 273*: 134–153, 1972.

83. Kempson, S., G. V. Marinetti, A. Shaw, Hormone action at the membrane level. VII. Stimulation of dihydroalprenolol binding to beta-adrenergic receptors in isolated rat heart ventricles by triiodothyronine and thyroxine. *Biochem. Biophys. Acta 540*: 320–329, 1978.

84. Kent, R. S., A. De Lean, R. J. Lefkowitz, A quantitative analysis of beta-adrenergic receptor interactions: resolution of high and low affinity states of the receptor by computer modeling of ligand binding data. *Mol. Pharmacol. 17*: 14–23, 1980.

85. Khan, M. T. and K. U. Malik, Sympathetic nerve stimulation of the isolated rat heart: release of a prostaglandin-like substance and the inhibitory effect of prostacyclin on the output of [^{3}H]norepinephrine. *Adv. Prostaglandin Thromboxane Res. 8*: 1241–1243, 1980.

86. Kristensson, K., Retrograde transport of macromolecules in axons. *Ann. Rev. Pharmacol. Toxicol. 18*: 97–110, 1978.

87. Kunos, G., L. Mucci, S. O'Regan, The influence of hormonal and neuronal factors on rat heart adrenoceptors. *Br. J. Pharmacol. 71*: 371–386, 1980.

88. Laduron, P., Axoplasmic transport of muscarinic receptors. *Nature 286:* 287–288, 1980.

89. Lands, A. M., F. P. Luduena, H. H. Buzzo, Differentiation of receptors responsive to isoproterenol. *Life Sci. 6*: 2241–2249, 1967.

90. Langer, S. Z., Presynaptic regulation of the release of catecholamines. *Pharmacol. Rev. 32*: 337–362, 1981.

91. Langer, S. Z., E. Adler-Graschinsky, O. Giorgi. Physiological significance of alpha-adrenoceptor-mediated negative feedback mechanism regulating noradrenaline release during nerve stimulation. *Nature 265*: 648–750, 1977.

92. Larner, A. C. and E. M. Ross, Alteration in the protein components of catecholamine-sensitive adenylate cyclase during maturation of rat reticulocytes. *J. Biol. Chem. 256*: 9951–9557, 1981.
93. Ledda, A. G. and P. F. Mannaioni, Effects of noradrenaline and isoprenaline, in combination with alpha and beta receptor blocking substances, on the action potential of cardiac purkinje fibres. *J. Physiol. 229*: 99–113, 1973.
94. Ledda, F., P. Marchetti, M. Mugelli, Studies on the positive inotropic effect of phenylephrine: a comparison with isoprenaline. *Br. J. Pharmacol. 54*: 83–90, 1975.
95. Lefkowitz, R. J., M. G. Caron, J. Stadel, Biochemical mechanisms of hormone receptor-effector coupling: the beta-adrenergic receptor and adenylate cyclase, *Fed. Proc.*, 1982, in press.
96. Levitzki, A., The beta-adrenergic receptor and its mode of coupling to adenylate cyclase. *Crit. Rev. Biochem. 10*: 81–112, 1981.
97. Limas, C. J., Increased number of beta-adrenergic receptors in the hypertrophied myocardium. *Biochem. Biophys. Acta 588*: 174–178, 1979.
98. Limas, C. and C. J. Limas, Reduced number of beta-adrenergic receptors in the myocardium of spontaneously hypertensive rats. *Biochem. Biophys. Res. Commun. 83*: 710–714, 1978.
99. Lokhandwala, M. F., J. T. Coats, J. P. Buckely, Effects of several catecholamines on sympathetic transmission to the myocardium: role of presynaptic alpha-adrenoceptors. *Eur. J. Pharmacol. 42*: 257–265, 1977.
100. Majewski, H. and M. J. Rand, An interaction between prejunctional alpha-adrehnoceptors and prejunctional beta-adrenoceptors. *Eur. J. Pharmacol. 69*: 493–498, 1981.
101. Mary-Rabine, L., A. J. Hordof, F. O. Bowman, J. R. Malm, M. R. Rosen, Alpha and beta effects on human atrial specialized conducting fibres. *Circulation 57*: 84–90, 1978.
102. McConnaughey, M. M., L. R. Jones, A. M. Watanabe, H. R. Besch, L. T. Williams, R. J. Lefkowitz. Thyroxine and propylthiouracil effects on alpha- and beta-adrenergic receptor number, ATPase activities, and sialic acid content of rat cardiac membrane vesicles. *J. Cardiovasc. Pharmacol. 1*: 609–623, 1979.
103. McCulloch, M. W., M. J. Rand, D. F. Story, Inhibition of [^{3}H]noradrenaline release from sympathetic nerves of guinea-pig atria by a presynaptic alpha-adrenoceptor mechanism. *Br. J. Pharmacol. 46*: 523–624P, 1972.
104. Michel, T., B. B. Hoffman, R. J. Lefkowitz, M. G. Caron, Different sedimentation properties of agonist and antagonist-labeled alpha$_2$ adrenergic receptors. *Biochem. Biophys. Res. Commun. 100*: 1131–1136, 1981.
105. Minneman, K. P., A. Hedberg, P. B. Molinoff, Comparison of beta-adrenergic receptor subtypes in mammalian tissues. *J. Pharmacol. Exp. Ther. 211*: 502–508, 1979.
106. Minneman, K. P., L. R. Hegstrand, P. B. Molinoff, Simultaneous determination of beta$_1$ and beta$_2$ adrenergic receptors in tissues containing both receptor subtypes. *Mol. Pharmacol. 16*: 34–46, 1979.
107. Minneman, K. P. and P. B. Molinoff, Classification and quantitation of beta-adrenergic receptor subtypes. *Biochem. Pharmacol. 29*: 1317–1323, 1980.
108. Moran, N. C. and M. E. Perkins, Adrenergic blockade of the mammalian heart by a dichloro analogue of isoproterenol. *J. Pharmacol. Exp. Ther. 124*: 223–237, 1958.

109. Mukherjee, A., T. M. Wong, L. M. Buja, R. J. Lefkowitz, J. T. Willerson, Beta-adrenergic and muscarinic cholinergic receptors in canine myocardium. Effects of ischemia. *J. Clin. Invest.* *64*: 1423–1428, 1979.
110. Nahorski, S. R. Identification and significance of beta-adrenoceptor subtypes. *TIPS.* *2*: 95–98, 1981.
111. Nathan, D. and G. W. Beele, Electrophysiological correlates of the inotropic effects of isoproternol in canine myocardium. *J. Mol. Cell. Cardiol.* *7*: 1–15, 1975.
112. Nattel, S., R. E. Rango, G. Van Loon, Mechanism of propranolol withdrawal phenomena. *Circulation* *59*: 1158–1164, 1979.
113. Nomura, Y., H. Kajiyama, T. Swgawa, Hypersensitivity of cardiac beta-adrenergic receptors after neonatal treatment of rats with 6-hydroxydopa. *Eur. J. Pharmacol.* *66*: 225–232, 1980.
114. Osnes, J.-B., Cyclic AMP dependent and independent inotropic effects of adrenergic amines. Thesis, Oslo, 1978.
115. Osnes, J.-B. and I. Øye, Relationship between cyclic AMP metabolism and inotropic response of perfused rat hearts to phenylephrine and other adrenergic amines. *Adv. Cycl. Nucl. Res.* Vol. 5, ed. G. I. Drummond and G. A. Robison. Raven, New York, pp. 415–433, 1975.
116. Osnes, J.-B., H. Refsum, T. Skomedal, I. Øye, Qualitative differences between beta-adrenergic and alpha-adrenergic inotropic effects in rat heart muscle. *Acta Pharmacol. Toxicol.* *42*: 235–247, 1978.
117. Pappano, A. J. Propranolol-insensitive effects on action potential repolarization in electrically driven atria of the guinea pig. *J. Pharmacol. Exp. Ther.* *177*: 85–95, 1971.
118. Pichler, L. and W. Kobinger, Presynaptic activity at peripheral adrenergic sites and blood pressure effects of alpha-adrenoceptor stimulating drugs. *Eur. J. Pharmacol.* *52*: 287–295, 1978.
119. Posner, P., E. L. Farrar, C. R. Lambert, Inhibitory effects of catecholamines in canine cardiac purkinje fibres. *Am. J. Physiol.* *231*: 1415–1420, 1976.
120. Powell, C. E. and I. H. Slater, Blocking of inhibitory adrenergic receptors by a dichloro analog of isoproterenol. *J. Pharmacol. Exp. Ther.* *122*: 480–488, 1958.
121. Rand, M. J., D. F. Story, G. S. Allen, M. W. McCulloch, Pulse to pulse modulation of noradrenaline release through a prejunctional alpha-receptor auto-inhibitory mechanism. In *Frontiers in Catecholamine Research,* Eds. E. Usdin and S. H. Snyder. Pergamon, New York, pp. 519–581, 1973.
122. Roach, A. G., F. Lefevre, I. Cavero, Effects of prazosin and phentolamine on cardiac presynpatic alpha-adrenoceptors in the cat, dog and rat. *Clin. Exp. Hypertension* *1*: 87–101, 1978.
123. Robberecht, P., J. Winand, P. Chatelain, P. Poloczek, J.-C. Camus, P. De Neef, J. Christophe, Comparison of beta-adrenergic receptors and the adenylate cyclase system with muscarinic receptors and guanylate cyclase activities in the heart of spontaneously hypertensive rats. *Biochem. Pharmacol.* *30*: 385–387, 1981.
124. Rosen, R., A. J. Hordof, J. P. Ilvento, P. Danilo, Effects of adrenergic amines on electrophysiological properties of neonatal and adult canine purkinje fibres. *Circulation Res.* *40*: 390–400, 1977.
125. Rufler, S., M. Reza, M. Sajadi, M. H. Araoyl, F. D. Hoeford, Noninvasive estimation of myocardial performance in patients with diabetes. *Diabetes* *27*: 127–134, 1978.
126. Savarese, J. J. and B. A. Berkowitz, *Beta-adrenergic receptor decrease in diabetic rat hearts. Life Sci.* *25*: 2075–2078, 1979.

127. Scarpace, P. J. and I. B. Abrass, Thyroid hormone regulation of beta-adrenergic receptor number in aging rats. *Endocrinology 108*: 1276–1278, 1981.
128. Sharma, V. K. and S. P. Banerjee, Pre-synaptic alpha-, beta-adrenergic and muscarinic cholinergic receptors in rat peripheral tissues. *Fed. Proc.* 37: 346, 1978.
129. Sharma, V. K. and S. P. Banerjee, Alpha-adrenergic receptors in rat heart: effect of thyroidectomy. *J. Biol. Chem. 253*: 5277–5279, 1978.
130. Shibata, S., D. G. Seriguchi, S. Iwadare, Y. Ishida, T. Shibata, The regional and species differences on the activation of myocardial alpha-adrenoceptors by phenylephrine and methoxamine. *Gen. Pharmac. 11*: 173–180, 1980.
131. Shindler, R., C. Harakal, R. W. Lewy, Catecholamine content of sinoatrial node and right atrial tissue. *Proc. Soc. Exp. Biol. Med. 128*: 798–800, 1968.
132. Simpson, W. W. and J. H. McNeil, Effect of adrenergic agonists on tension development and rate in atria from euthyroid and hypothyroid rats. *Adv. Myocardial Res. 1*: 417–435, 1980.
133. Skomedal, T., J.-B. Osnes, I. Øye, Competitive blockade of alpha-adrenergic receptors in rat heart by prazosin. *Acta Pharmacol. Toxicol. 47*: 217–222, 1980.
134. Somani, P., P. Guse, P. Toscano, A. L. Bassett, Myocardial transmembranes potentials and adrenergic receptors. *Adv. Myocardiol.* Vol. 1, ed. M. Tajuddin, P. K. Das, M. Tariq, N. S. Dhalla. University Park Press, Baltimore, pp. 189–207, 1980.
135. Stadel, J. M., A. De Lean, R. J. Lefkowitz, Molecular mechanisms of coupling in hormone receptor-adenylate cyclase systems. *Adv. Enzymol. 53*: 1–43, 1982.
136. Starke, K. Alpha sympathomimetic inhibition of adrenergic and cholinergic transmission in the rabbit heart. *Naunyn-Schmiedebergs Arch. Pharmacol. 274*: 18–45, 1972.
137. Starke, K. Regulation of noradrenaline release by presynaptic receptor systems. *Rev. Physiol. Biochem. Pharmacol. 77*: 1–124, 1977.
138. Starke, K., Presynaptic receptors. *Ann. Rev. Pharmacol. Toxicol. 21*: 7–30, 1981.
139. Starke, K., Alpha-adrenoceptor subclassification. *Rev. Physiol. Biochem. Pharmacol. 88*: 199–236, 1981.
140. Starke, K. and K. P. Altmann, Inhibition of adrenergic neurotransmission by clonidine: an action on prejunctional alpha-receptors. *Neuropharmacology 12*: 339–347, 1973.
141. Starke, K. and H. Montel, Sympathomimetic inhibition of noradrenaline release: mediated by prostaglandins? *Naunyn-Schmiedebergs Arch. Pharmacol. 278*: 11–116, 1973.
142. Starke, K., H. Montel, H. J. Schumann, Influence of cocaine and phenoxybenzamine on noradrenaline uptake and release. *Naunyn-Schmiedebergs Arch. Pharmacol. 270*: 210–214, 1971.
143. Stene-Larsen, G., Characterization of the atrial alpha-receptor of the rat as a subgroup of the postsynaptic alpha-adrenoceptor. *Gen. Pharmacol. 11*: 575–581, 1980.
144. Stiles, G. L. and R. J. Lefkowitz, Thyroid hormone modulation of agonist-beta-adrenergic receptor interactions in the rat heart. *Life Sci. 28*: 2529–2536, 1981.
145. Stiles, G. L., J. M. Stadel, A. De Lean, R. J. Lefkowitz, Hypothyroidism modulates beta-adrenergic receptor-adenylate cyclase interactions in rat reticulocytes. *J. Clin. Invest. 68*: 1450–1455, 1981.
146. Stjarne, L. and A. Wennmalm, Quantitative estimation of secretion and reuptake of adrenergic transmitter in the rabbit heart. *Acta Physiol. Scand. 81*: 286–288, 1971.

147. Story, D. D., M. S. Briley, S. Z. Langer, The effects of chemical sympathectomy with 6-hydroxydopamine on alpha-adrenoceptor and muscarinic cholinoceptor binding in rat heart ventricle. *Eur. J. Pharmacol.* 57: 423–426, 1979.

148. Story, D. F., M. W. McCulloch, M. J. Rand, C. A. Stanford-Starr, Conditions required for the inhibitory feedback loop in noradrenergic transmission. *Nature 293*: 62–65, 1981.

149. Thaemert, J. C., Atrioventricular node innervation in ultrastructural three dimensions. *Am. J. Anat. 128*: 239–263, 1970.

150. Tsai, J. S. and A. Chen, Effect of L-triiodothyronin on (−)[^{3}H]dihydroalprenolol binding and cyclic AMP response to (−)adrenaline in cultured heart cells. *Nature 275*: 138–140, 1978.

151. Tse, J., J. R. Powell, C. A. Baste, R. E. Priest, J. F. Kuo, Isoproterenol-induced cardiac hypertrophy: modifications in characteristics of beta-adrenergic receptors, adenylate cyclase and ventricular contraction. *Endocrinology 105*: 246–255, 1979.

152. Tse, J., R. W. Wrenn, J. F. Kuo, Thyroxin-induced changes in characteristics and activities of beta-adrenergic receptors and adenosine 3′,5′-monophosphate and guanosine 3′,5′-monophosphate systems in the heart may be related to reputed catecholamine supersensitivity in hyperthyroidism. *Endocrinology 107*: 6–16, 1980.

153. Tsien, R. W., Effects of epinephrine on the pacemaker potassium current of cardiac purkinje fibres. *J. Gen. Physiol. 64*: 293–319, 1974.

154. Tsien, R. W., Cyclic AMP and contractile activity in heart. *Adv. Cycl. Nucl. Res. 8*: 363–420, 1977.

155. Tsien, R. W., W. Giles, P. Greengard, Cyclic AMP mediates the effects of adrenaline on cardiac purkinje fibres. *Nature New Biol. 240*: 181–183, 1972.

156. Vassort, G., O. Rougier, D. Garnier, M. P. Sauviat, E. Coraboeuf, Y. M. Garoull, Effects of adrenaline on membrane inward currents during the cardiac action potential. *Pflugers Arch. 309*: 70–81, 1969.

157. Vizi, E. S., Presynaptic modulation of neurochemical transmission. *Prog. Neurobiol. 12*: 181–290, 1979.

158. Vogel, S. A., S. D. Silberstein, K. R. Berv, I. J. Kopin, Stimulation-induced release of norepinephrine from rat superior cervical ganglion in vitro. *Eur. J. Pharmacol. 20*: 308–311, 1972.

159. Wagner, J. and O.-E. Brodde, On the presence and distribution of alpha-adrenoceptors in the heart of various mammalian species. *Naunyn-Schmiedebergs Arch. Pharmacol. 302*: 239–254, 1978.

160. Wagner, J., H. J. Schumann, A. Knorr, N. Rohm, J. C. Reidemeister, Stimulation by adrenaline and dopamine but not by noradrenaline of myocardial alpha-adrenoceptors mediating positive inotropic effects in human atrial preparations. *Naunyn-Schmiedebergs Arch. Pharmacol. 312*: 99–102, 1980.

161. Wasserman, M. A. and B. Levy, Selective beta-adrenergic receptor blockade in the rat. *J. Pharm. Exp. Ther. 182*: 256–263, 1972.

162. Wennmalm, A., Quantitative evaluation of release and reuptake of adrenergic transmitter in the rabbit heart. *Acta Physiol. Scand. 82*: 532–538, 1971.

163. Wennmalm, A., Prostaglandin release and mechanical performance in the isolated rabbit heart during induced changes in the internal environment. *Acta Physiol. Scand. 93*: 15–24, 1975.

164. Wenzel, D. G. and J. L. Su, Interactions between sympathomimetic amines and blocking agents on the rat ventricle strip. *Arch. Int. Pharmacodyn. Ther. 160*: 379–389, 1966.

165. Westfall, T. C., Local regulation of adrenergic neurotransmission. *Physiol. Rev. 57*: 659–728, 1977.

166. Wikberg, J. E. S., Pharmacological classification of adrenergic alpha receptors in the guinea pig. *Nature 273*: 164–166, 1978.

167. Wikberg, J. E. S., The pharmacological classification of adrenergic $alpha_1$ and $alpha_2$ receptors and their mechanisms of action. *Acta Physiol. Scand. Suppl. 468:* 1-99, 1979.

168. Wikberg, J. E. S., Adrenergic receptors: classification, ligand binding and molecular properties. *Acta Medica Scand.* 1982, in press.

169. Wikberg, J. E. S., J. R. Andersson, X. X. Lundholm. Differentiation of adrenergic alpha-receptors in guinea pig intestine and rabbit aorta. *Blood Vessels 12*: 383–384, 1975.

170. Wikberg, J. E. S., L. Johansson, S. Hedman, Properties of pre and postsynaptic alpha receptors. In *Modulation of Neurochemical Transmission*, ed. E. S. Vizi. Pergamon, Budapest, pp. 47–56, 1980.

171. Wildenthal, K. Studies of fetal mouse hearts in organ culture: influence of prolonged exposure to triiodothyronine on cardiac responsiveness to isoproterenol, glucagon, theophyllin, acetylcholine and dibutyryl cyclic 3′,5′ adenosine monophosphate. *J. Pharmacol. Exp. Ther. 190*: 272–279, 1974.

172. Williams, L. T., R. J. Lefkowitz, A. M. Watanabe, D. R. Hathaway, H. R. Besch, Thyroid hormone regulation of beta-adrenergic receptor number. *J. Biol. Chem. 252*: 2787–2789, 1977.

173. Williams, R. S., D. F. Dukes, R. J. Lefkowitz, Subtype specificity of alpha-adrenergic receptors in rat heart. *J. Cardiovasc. Pharmacol.* 3: 522–531, 1981.

174. Williams, R. S. and R. J. Lefkowitz, Alpha-adrenergic receptors in rat myocardium: identification by binding of [^{3}H]dihydroergocryptine. *Circ. Res. 43*: 721–727, 1978.

175. Williams, R. S. and R. J. Lefkowitz, Thyroid hormone regulation of alpha-adrenergic receptors: studies in rat myocardium. *J. Cardiovasc. Pharmacol. 1*: 181–189, 1979.

176. Wit, A. L., B. F. Hoffman, M. R. Rosen, Electrophysiology of cardiac arrythmias IX. Cardiac electrophysiologic effects of beta-adrenergic receptor stimulation and blockade. Part A. In *Appraisal and Reappraisal of Cardiac Therapy*, Eds. DeGraff and Frieden. *Am. Heart J. 90*: 521–533, 1975.

177. Woodcock, E. A., J. W. Funder, and C. I. Johnston, Decreased cardiac beta-adrenoceptors in hypertensive rats. *Clin. Exp. Pharmacol. Physiol. 5*: 545–550, 1978.

178. Woodcock, E. A., J. W. Funder, and C. I. Johnston, Decreased cardiac beta-adrenergic receptors in deoxycorticosterone-salt and renal hypertensive rats. *Circ. Res. 45*: 560–565, 1979.

179. Woodcock, E. and C. I. Johnston, Changes in tissue alpha and beta-adrenergic receptors in renal hypertension in the rat. *Hypertension 2*: 156–161, 1980.

180. Yamada, S., H. I. Yamamura, W. R. Roeske, Alterations in central and peripheral adrenergic receptors in deoxycorticosterone/salt hypertensive rats. *Life. Sci. 27*: 2405–2416, 1980.

181. Yamada, S. Y., H. I. Yamamura, W. R. Roeske, Alterations in cardiac autonomic receptors following 6-hydroxydopamine treatment in rats. *Mol. Pharmacol. 18*: 185–192, 1980.
182. Yamada, S., H. I. Yamamura, W. R. Roeske, Characterization of alpha$_1$ adrenergic receptors in the heart using [^{3}H]WB4101: effect of 6-hydroxydopamine treatment. *J. Pharmacol. Exp. Ther. 215*: 176–185, 1980.
183. Yamaguchi, N., J. De Champlain, R. A. Nadeau, Regulation of norepinephrine release from cardiac sympathetic fibres in the dog by presynaptic alpha and beta-receptors. *Circ. Res. 41*: 108–117, 1977.

6

Cellular Mechanisms of Muscarinic Regulation of Cardiac Function

AUGUST M. WATANABE

The importance of the parasympathetic nervous system in regulating cardiac function has been well known to physiologists, pharmacologists, and clinicians for many years. Many commonly used clinical maneuvers of diagnostic or therapeutic importance are based on manipulating vagal nervous system tone to the heart. For example, in patients who have supraventricular tachyarrhythmias, the ventricular rate can be slowed and sometimes the supraventricular tachyarrhythmia terminated, by massage of the carotid sinus. The use of pressor agents in attempting to terminate supraventricular tachyarrhythmias also depends on the activity of the parasympathetic nervous system. Both of these techniques reflexly activate vagal tone to the heart and the resultant increased vagal tone then terminates the arrhythmia because of effects on the atria or atrioventricular node (the latter resulting in slow ventricular rate). The pharmacological effects of certain chronically administered cardiac drugs, such as digitalis glycosides, depend in part on modification of vagal influences on the heart. The therapeutic effects of anticholinergic agents like atropine are due to blockade of muscarinic receptors in the heart. Some of the side effects of certain cardiac drugs, such as quinidine and disopyramide, are due to unwanted anticholinergic actions.

Parasympathetic control over the heart is of obvious importance in normal physiological states. High vagal tone is largely responsible for the slow resting heart rate of conditioned athletes. It may also be of protective value in patients who suffer myocardial infarction. In animal models of myocardial ischemia, high vagal tone protects against the development of lethal ventricular arrhythmias.

Despite the profound importance of parasympathetic control of the heart in

The author's research cited in this chapter was supported by the Herman C. Krannert Fund; by grants HL08795, HL06308, HL07182 from the National Heart, Lung, and Blood Institute, National Institutes of Health; and by the American Heart Association, Indiana Affiliate. The excellent secretarial assistance of Terri Butcher is gratefully acknowledged.

normal and pathological states and in the actions of numerous drugs, the cellular and subcellular mechanisms by which activation of the parasympathetic nervous system modifies cardiac function are only partially understood, and much of the available insight has been acquired only recently. In this chapter, I will review the current theories regarding this regulatory mechanism.

BIOCHEMISTRY AND MOLECULAR PHARMACOLOGY OF MUSCARINIC CHOLINERGIC RECEPTORS

Acetylcholine released from parasympathetic nerve endings interacts with muscarinic receptors on the plasma membrane of cardiac myocytes. A large body of information regarding the physiology and pharmacology of muscarinic receptors has come from classical pharmacological studies, based on physiological experiments combined with analysis of structure–activity relationships [41]. These studies have yielded physiological evidence on the tissue distribution of muscarinic receptors and on the determinants of agonist and antagonist activity of drugs that interact with the receptor [41]. While these types of classical pharmacological studies have yielded very important physiological insights, only with the recent development of radioligand binding assays, which allow the direct study of muscarinic receptors, have there been new discoveries regarding the biochemistry and molecular pharmacology of muscarinic receptors [10,27,47,106,122]. This section will review some of the major findings derived from radioligand binding studies which are particularly relevant to the cardiovascular pharmacology of drugs that modify parasympathetic nervous system function.

Radioligand binding studies of muscarinic receptors were first performed by Paton and Rang who studied the interaction of [^{3}H]-atropine with muscarinic receptors on guinea pig gastrointestinal smooth muscle [95]. In subsequent years, investigators have used a variety of antagonist ligands to study muscarinic receptors in various tissues [10,27,106]. [^{3}H]Quinuclidinyl benzilate ([^{3}H]-QNB) is the ligand that has been used most widely to study cardiac muscarinic receptors [19,29,30,32,65,88,125,131].

Three major criteria are generally applied to radioligand binding studies to establish that binding of the ligand represents specific interaction with the receptor. These criteria are saturability, specificity, and localization of binding. Receptors exist in a finite number; therefore specific binding should saturate with increasing concentrations of the radioligand. As shown in Fig. 6-1A, with progressively higher concentrations of [^{3}H]-QNB the amount of ligand bound to canine cardiac muscarinic receptors increases until all sites are filled (at about 1 pmol/mg protein in this example) and at greater concentrations no more [^{3}H]-QNB is bound. If radioligands are binding to true muscarinic receptors, this binding should be inhibited by appropriate concentrations of drugs known from physiological studies to interact with the receptor and should not be modified by drugs which do not interact with the receptor; i.e. the binding should fulfill the criterion of pharmacological specificity. This is illustrated in Fig. 6-1B. The muscarinic antagonists QNB, dexetemide, and atropine and the agonists oxotre-

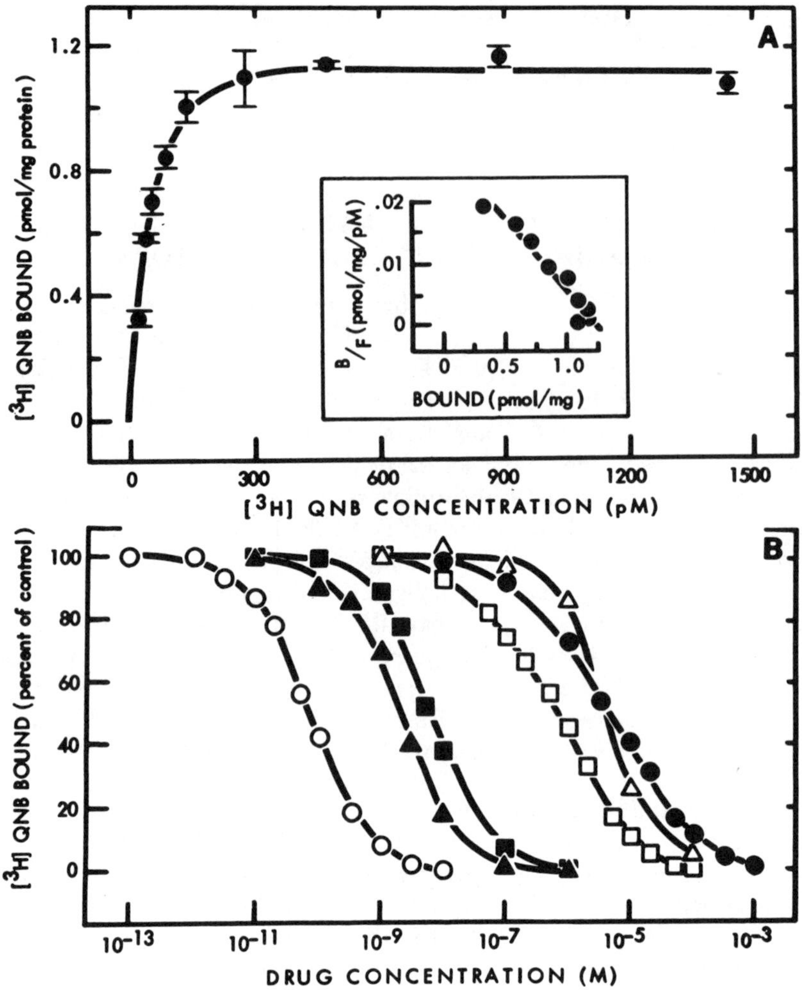

Fig. 6-1. Saturation of [^{3}H]QNB binding (A) and agonist and antagonist competition curves for [^{3}H]QNB binding (B) to muscarinic receptors in membrane vesicles derived from canine ventricular myocardium. Inset in panel A is a Scatchard plot of the saturation data. In B, data from separate experiments performed in purified membrane preparations are presented, with binding expressed as a percent of control binding in the absence of competing drug. For all curves, [^{3}H]QNB concentration was approximately 80 pM. Drugs are QNB (○), dexetimide (▲), atropine (■), oxotremorine (□), methacholine (●), and levetimide (△). (Reprinted with permission from ref. 88)

morine and methacholine compete with [^{3}H]-QNB for binding to muscarinic receptors in the same rank order of potency that these agents exhibit in intact tissue pharmacological studies. Note also in Fig. 1B that the interaction of [^{3}H]-QNB with muscarinic receptors is stereoselective, as inferred from competition studies. The pharmacologically more effective dexetemide competes much more potently with [^{3}H]-QNB binding to muscarinic receptors than the less effective isomer levetemide. Finally, saturable binding of muscarinic radioligands should occur only in tissues known from pharmacological studies to possess muscarinic receptors. Each of these criteria has been fulfilled in radioligand binding studies of muscarinic receptors in cardiac tissues [10,19,27.29, 30,32,65,88,125].

Tissue and Subcellular Distribution of Muscarinic Receptors in Heart. From classical pharmacological analysis in intact tissues or whole animals, muscarinic receptors in the heart are thought to be located postjunctionally on the innervated tissues and also on prejunctional sympathetic nerve terminals. Although the presence of muscarinic receptors on prejunctional sympathetic nerve terminals is strongly suggested by results from physiological experiments [67,70,77,78], the few studies that have attempted to demonstrate this directly by radioligand binding assays do not agree [105,109,130]. Three different groups have attempted to demonstrate the presence of prejunctional muscarinic receptors by comparing the density of specific binding sites in hearts from normal animals with the density in hearts from animals subjected to chemical sympathectomy with 6-OH-dopamine. One study showed a 30% reduction in specific binding of [^{3}H]-QNB in particulate fractions derived from hearts of 6-OH-dopamine treated animals [105]. The conclusion was that in hearts from untreated animals [^{3}H]-QNB was binding both to postjunctional muscarinic receptors on myocardial cell membranes and to receptors on prejunctional sympathetic nerve terminals. The 30% reduction in [^{3}H]-QNB binding after sympathectomy was attributed to loss of those sites originally on sympathetic nerve terminals [105]. However, two other studies that used the same method of sympathectomy did not show any change in the number of [^{3}H]-QNB binding sites in heart [109,130]. As the presence of muscarinic receptors on prejunctional sympathetic nerve terminals seems firmly established from intact tissue and whole animal studies [67,70,77,78], the reasons for this discrepancy are not apparent. The failure to verify the presence of these receptors with binding studies may reflect limits of the sensitivity of the assay and/or problems with the method of sympathectomy. Perhaps the percentage contribution of neural binding sites to total cardiac binding sites is so small that the assay cannot detect the loss of sites resulting from destruction of sympathetic nerves. Alternatively, 6-OH-dopamine may produce nonspecific effects that alter the total number of bindings sites and thus obscure any change that may have been produced by denervation.

Muscarinic receptors have been demonstrated in various regions of the heart by radioligand binding studies. The localization of these receptors by binding assays agrees well with physiological evidence for their distribution [125]. Binding studies of muscarinic receptors in various organs indicate that they are associated with membrane and are probably predominantly or exclusively located in the plasma membrane [1,55,64,65,125]. We studied localization of muscarinic binding sites in purified sarcolemma and sarcoplasmic reticulum isolated from dog hearts by the method of Jones [55]. [^{3}H]-QNB binding activity copurified

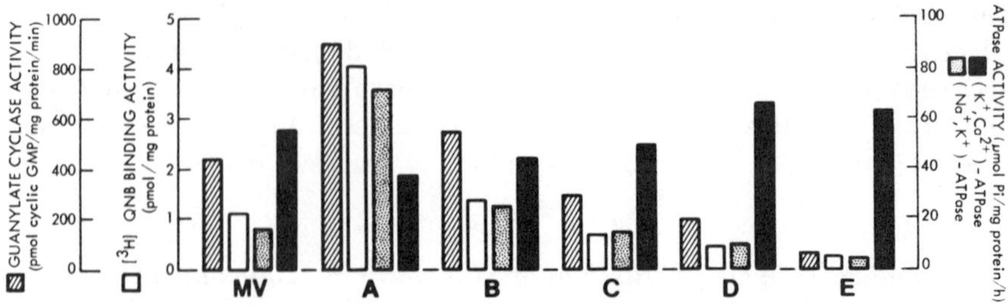

Fig. 6-2. Copurification of particulate guanylate cyclase activity and [^{3}H]QNB binding activity with sarcolemmal (Sl) Na^+,K^+-ATPase activity. Ca^{2+}-ATPase activity, the marker for sarcoplasmic reticulum (SR) membranes, is also shown. Membrane vesicles (MV) which contain both sarcolemmal and sarcoplasmic reticulum membranes were prepared. This relatively crude MV fraction was then preloaded with Ca^{2+}-oxalate to selectively increase the density of SR vesicles and the MV was subfractionated by density gradient centrifugation as described previously by Jones [59]. Fraction A is most enriched in Na^+,K^+-ATPase activity, with remaining fractions having progressively less enrichment [59]. By contrast, Ca^{2+}-ATPase activity progressively increases to maximal levels in fractions D and E [59]. Guanylate cyclase and [^{3}H]QNB binding activities copurify with with Na^+,K^+-ATPase activity. All enzyme activities were in the presence of activating agents: sodium dodecyl sulfate for Na^+,K^+-ATPase, lubrol PX for guanylate cyclase and A23187 for Ca^{2+}-ATPase.

with the sarcolemmal marker Na^+,K^+-ATPase and away from the sarcoplasmic reticulum marker Ca^{2+}-ATPase (Fig. 6-2) [55,79]. Furthermore, [^{3}H]-dihydroalprenolol binding activity also copurified with Na^+,K^+-ATPase activity [55,79,122]. Therefore, both beta-adrenergic and muscarinic receptors are localized to the sarcolemma in dog myocardium [79]. Such a location would be optimal for accessibility of neurotransmitters to the receptors and for intracellular interaction between the two branches of the autonomic nervous system at the level of the receptors and their effectors.

Regulation of Muscarinic Receptors. The affinity of muscarinic receptors for antagonists appears to be similar in a wide variety of tissues from various mammalian species [10]. The affinity constants determined by antagonist binding assays agree well with those derived from classical pharmacological analyses of antagonism of whole tissue responses to muscarinic stimulation. Antagonists appear to bind to a single, homogenous class of muscarinic receptors [10].

In contrast to analyses of antagonist–receptor interactions, the assessment of agonist interaction with muscarinic receptors by binding studies is more complex [10,27,122]. The pharmacological efficacy of an agonist in evoking a response in intact functioning tissues may not necessarily correspond to the affinity of the receptor for that agonist. Among the reasons for this is the presence of multiple intervening steps, each of which might be regulatable, between agonist interaction with the receptor and the measured physiological response. In addition, binding studies have revealed that muscarinic receptors exist in multiple states, and more than one state may interact with agonists

[7,8,10,26,27]. The same binding sites (i.e., muscarinic receptors) which interact with antagonists in a uniform manner, interact with agonists heterogenously. This was first recognized by analysis of the curves relating the occupancy of muscarinic receptors to the concentration of muscarinic agonists added to the receptors. The binding curves relating antagonist occupation of receptors to antagonist concentration are of the form predicted by the application of the law of mass action to the interaction of a ligand with a uniform set of binding sites [10] (Fig. 6-1B). In contrast, the pattern of agonist binding curves deviates substantially from this simple mass action relationship [8,10,27] (Fig. 6-1B). These agonist curves are shallower than antagonist binding curves (Fig. 6-1B). Note in Fig. 6-1B that the curves for oxotremorine and methacholine are shallower than those for QNB, dexetemide, and atropine. Several alternative explanations for this anomalous binding pattern for agonists have been considered [8]. The most plausible explanation appears to be that muscarinic receptors exist in multiple states in terms of their interaction with agonists [8,10,27]. Three different classes of muscarinic binding sites, each with a different affinity for agonists, have been described in rat brain membranes [8]. At least two binding sites (high and low affinity) for agonists have been described in several other organs including heart [3,31,98,126,127]. These different affinity binding sites are noninterconvertible in the binding assay, and therefore the slopes describing occupancy as a function of agonist concentration represent the sum of the interaction of ligand with multiple binding sites. This explains the shallow slopes for oxotremorine and methacholine in Figure 6-1B.

An explanation for this phenomenon has come from studies of the regulation of muscarinic receptors by guanine nucleotides. Cardiac muscarinic receptors, like beta and alpha adrenergic, dopaminergic, and opiate receptors, can be regulated by guanine nucleotides [3,31,98,126,127]. Study of muscarinic receptors in cardiac membrane preparations, from which endogenous guanine nucleotides have been removed, yields the shallow binding curves described above (Fig. 6-1B). However, if exogenous guanine nucleotides are added, the curves become steeper, which is compatible with the interaction of ligand with a single, homogenous class of binding sites [6]. At the same time the affinity of the receptor for agonists is reduced substantially [3,31,98,126,127]. These data show a guanine nucleotide-induced conversion of receptors in a high-affinity state into a low-affinity state [6], analogous to the situation with guanine nucleotide regulation of beta-adrenergic receptors [59,122]. Thus, with added guanine nucleotide, binding curves become steeper (representing a single class of binding sites) and shift to the right because most or all of the receptors are in a low affinity state. The physiological significance of these phenomena remains to be elucidated. It has been suggested that the different agonist affinity states of the receptor are coupled to different membrane responses [10]—e.g. altered cation fluxes, altered phospholipid turnover, inhibition of adenylate cyclase—or that the different states represent varying degrees of receptor–effector coupling, the low affinity state being "coupled" to an effector such as a guanine nucleotide binding protein [6]. However, these speculations must be verified by appropriate in vitro studies.

The properties of muscarinic receptors as assessed by in vitro binding studies also can be shown to be modified by cations. Divalent cations (Mg^{2+} or Ca^{2+}) increased the affinity of muscarinic receptors for agonists and enhanced the guanine nucleotide-induced decrease in receptor affinity for agonists [127]. The effects of both guanine nucleotides and divalent cations were abolished by treatment of membranes with *N*-ethylmaleimide, suggesting the involvement of sulfhydryl groups in the effects of these agents [127]. Monovalent cations decreased the affinity of muscarinic receptors for agonists [6,9,98]. This effect is small and appears to be related primarily to ionic strength rather than any specific regulatory interaction of monovalent cations with the receptor [9].

The density of cardiac muscarinic receptors varies in response to the ambient concentrations of muscarinic agonists. This was first demonstrated in cultured chick embryo heart cells exposed to carbamylcholine for various time periods [32]. Cultured heart cells exposed to the choline ester had a diminished negative chronotropic response to muscarinic agonists associated with a substantial reduction in receptor density [32]. More detailed analysis revealed a biphasic pattern to this agonist-induced receptor alteration, a rapid phase (occurring over one minute) associated with a reduced affinity of receptors for agonists followed by a slower phase (occurring over several hours) reflecting a true reduction in measurable receptor binding [31]. The agonist-induced reduction in cardiac muscarinic receptor density has been confirmed in vivo. Carbachol was administered to chicks in ovo. The negative chronotropic response to carbachol of hearts removed from these chicks was diminished compared to hearts from control chicks, and the density of muscarinic receptors in homogenates of these hearts was markedly reduced [43].

Hormones or neurotransmitters other than acetylcholine may modify the properties of muscarinic receptors; i.e. they can be heterotropically regulated. Thyroidectomy increased the density of cardiac muscarinic receptors as assessed by [^{3}H]-QNB binding [104]. On the other hand, treatment with triiodothyronine resulted in a modest decrease in density of receptors [104]. These effects of thyroid state on muscarinic receptors are exactly the opposite of the effects on beta-adrenergic receptors. Hyperthyroidism increases the density [129] whereas hypothyroidism decreases [81] the density of beta-adrenergic receptors in cardiac tissues. Thus, the tachycardia of hyperthyroid animals and the bradycardia of hypothyroid animals may reflect a reciprocal alteration in the density of receptors of both divisions of the autonomic nervous system.

In summary, a substantial amount of new information about the biochemistry and the biochemical and molecular pharmacology of muscarinic receptors has resulted from radioligand binding assays. These observations confirm and are complementary to conclusions based on physiological and classical pharmacological approaches. However, many fundamental questions remain to be answered. For example, the nature of the coupling of muscarinic receptors to intracellular effectors and the nature and identity of intracellular messengers that mediate the effects of muscarinic activation remain either unknown or only partially understood, as will be discussed in the next section. The application of radioligand binding assays in combination with other biochemical and molecular approaches will yield further insight into these areas of investigation.

INTRACELLULAR EFFECTORS COUPLED TO MUSCARINIC RECEPTORS

The intracellular mechanisms by which activation of muscarinic receptors lead to alterations in cardiovascular function have been only partially elucidated. It has been known for years, from electrophysiological and radioisotopic studies, that activation of muscarinic receptors in cardiac tissues results in an augmentation of outward K^+ currents [114]. However, it is not known if the muscarinic receptor is linked directly to K^+ channels or if intermediate steps occur between the receptor and K^+ channels. Moreover, what these tentative intermediate steps are remains to be established. Similarly, the intracellular mediators for the other cardiac effects (e.g. negative inotropic effects, antiadrenergic effects) of muscarinic agonists are unknown. Some of the candidates are cyclic GMP, cyclic AMP, and inositol phospholipids. Although there is substantial evidence in noncardiac tissues for a role of inositol phospholipids in mediating some effects of muscarinic agonists [84], few studies have demonstrated this in cardiac tissues [96]. The discussion in this section will be limited to cation channels and the cyclic nucleotides.

Cation Channels. The tissues of the mammalian heart show marked variability in response to muscarinic receptor activation [46,48,71,91,101]. These differences are manifest in the contractile, electrophysiological, and biochemical responses of supraventricular (nodal tissues and atria) and ventricular structures. Activation of muscarinic receptors in atria caused marked shortening of action potential duration associated with negative inotropic effects [48,49,112,114]. By contrast, muscarinic activation alone produced little or no effect on action potential duration [2] or contractility [120] of isolated ventricles. The electrophysiological and inotropic effects of muscarinic activation of mammalian atria are associated with an increase in outward K^+ current [16,112,114]. This increase results in earlier repolarization of the membrane and thus shortening of action potential duration and decreases in contractility [112]. The reduction in contractility is thought to be due to a secondary diminution in the slow inward current (I_{si}) [112]. Because action potential duration is shortened by increased outward currents, the plateau phase of the action potential during which time I_{si} occurs is abbreviated [112]. Whether this electrophysiological mechanism can account entirely for the negative inotropic effects of muscarinic activation or whether additional mechanisms (to be discussed later in this section) are operative remains to be established. Also, it is not known whether muscarinic receptors are coupled directly to K^+ channels or if intermediary steps (e.g., altered phospholipid turnover, increased cyclic GMP levels) must occur between activation of the receptors and increased K^+ current.

In mammalian atria, the effects of muscarinic activation on cation channels appears to depend on the concentration of muscarinic agonist used. With low concentrations of acetylcholine (sufficient to reduce twitch tension by 30–40%), the previously described effects of muscarinic activation on K^+ currents occurred [112]. At this concentration of acetylcholine the changes in I_{si} were secondary or "indirect"; i.e. these changes resulted from the shortening in plateau duration. With higher concentrations of acetylcholine (sufficient to reduce twitch tension by 70–90%) a direct effect on I_{si} also was observed with voltage clamp studies [112]. Thus, with high concentrations of muscarinic agonists, K^+ outward currents increased and I_{si} also decreased. These dual actions on ion flux would be expected to produce strong negative inotropic effects. As for K^+ channels, the nature of the coupling between muscarinic receptors and I_{si} channels remains unknown.

Tissue differences also exist in muscarinic effects on I_{si}. In mammalian atria high concentrations of acetylcholine directly reduced I_{si} [112]. However, in mammalian ventricular tissues activation of muscarinic receptors did not appear to produce a direct effect on I_{si} even with high concentrations of acetylcholine [2,52].

There is also species variability in muscarinic effects on cation channels. All of the foregoing observations regarding the relationship between muscarinic receptors and ion channels came from studies in mammals. Acetylcholine appeared to have a more potent effect on I_{si} in frog atrium [38] than in mammalian atria. Chick ventricular tissue behaved like either mammalian atria or ventricles, depending on the stage of development of the chick. Ventricles taken from embryonic chicks behaved like mammalian ventricles; i.e. muscarinic agonists did not have a direct effect on I_{si} [5]. By contrast, ventricles taken from chicks behaved like mammalian atria in that muscarinic agonists directly reduced I_{si} [5].

Thus, one well established effect of muscarinic activation is alterations in the properties of ion channels located in the sarcolemma of myocardial cells. It seems unlikely that these changes can account for all the multiple intracellular effects of muscarinic receptor activation. Other possible mediators will be discussed below.

Cyclic GMP. It was first shown in cardiac tissue that cyclic GMP levels could be elevated by activation of muscarinic cholinergic receptors [36]. Subsequently, many studies in a variety of different tissues have shown that activation of muscarinic receptors leads to increases in the tissue concentration of cyclic GMP [40]. However, the role of cyclic GMP in modifying the physiological properties of these tissues has not yet been firmly established [40]. Moreover, the biochemical mechanisms by which changes in tissue cyclic GMP levels might alter function are unknown [40].

The original observation of muscarinic-induced increases in cyclic GMP levels in cardiac tissue [36] was confirmed and extended by subsequent studies of hearts from a variety of species [33,37,67,69,80,85,111,120]. Thus, there is no question that under appropriate conditions, possibly related to the concentration of Ca^{2+} in the extracellular medium, activation of muscarinic receptors can increase myocardial tissue cyclic GMP levels. However, whether this muscarinic-induced elevation in cyclic GMP levels has any physiological role remains controversial [76].

When assessing the possible role of an intracellular mediator of muscarinic effects, it must be considered that muscarinic receptors might be coupled to multiple cellular effectors which may or may not themselves interact. As mentioned, there is good evidence that muscarinic receptors are somehow coupled with K^+ and I_{si} channels [16,38,112]. As will be discussed in detail, muscarinic receptors are coupled to adenylate cyclase [123]. Muscarinic agonists also can antagonize the intracellular effects of cyclic AMP by an as yet unexplained mechanism (see below) [123]. In noncardiac tissues, activation of muscarinic receptors results in changes in the rate of turnover of phosphotidylinositol [17], and this may also occur in cardiac tissues [96]. Therefore, before a role for cyclic GMP in mediating muscarinic effects can be ruled in or out, each of the specific known effectors of muscarinic activation (cation flux, antagonism of cyclic AMP effects, phosphotidylinositol turnover) must be examined.

The original studies which attempted to demonstrate a physiological role for cyclic GMP correlated a physiological response (e.g. contractile state) with tissue cyclic GMP levels. In these studies, acetylcholine was added to cardiac preparations in various concentrations for different durations, the mechanical or electrophysiological responses of the hearts were observed, and cyclic GMP levels determined [34,36,37,72,111]. Although there appeared to be a fairly good correlation between tissue cyclic GMP levels and the measured physiological response [36,72], these studies could be regarded as inconclusive because a sufficiently detailed concentration-response analysis was not performed [37,72]. In addition, the direct negative inotropic effects of muscarinic stimulation are in general small, although the rat heart may be an exception to this rule [36,37,72].

The bulk of the additional evidence supporting a role for cyclic GMP in mediating some of the physiological effects of muscarinic activation comes from studies utilizing analogues of cyclic GMP to attempt to increase directly the intracellular levels of the nucleotide. Analogues (e.g. dibutyryl cyclic GMP or 8-bromo-cyclic GMP) are used because they are less susceptible to degradation during superfusion or perfusion, and because they are thought to penetrate the sarcolemma more readily than does cyclic GMP. It is reasoned that if intracellular cyclic GMP levels can be increased directly with these agents, and if these agents mimic the action of acetylcholine, then this is evidence that cyclic GMP mediates that action of acetylcholine. A similar rationale has been applied to studies utilizing analogues of cyclic AMP to establish the role of this nucleotide in mediating a given effect of a hormone or neurotransmitter [97]. When using analogues of either cyclic nucleotide, the results must be interpreted cautiously, because the time course of action of these agents is generally slower than that of neurotransmitters and because relatively large concentrations are needed (in view of the low endogenous concentrations of these cyclic nucleotides) to produce the expected physiological effects. Bearing these caveats in mind, many laboratories have utilized these analogues to generate substantial data pertinent to the question of the role of cyclic GMP in cardiac regulation.

Analogues of cyclic GMP have been shown to mimic certain of the electrophysiological effects of acetylcholine. Dibutyryl cyclic GMP slowed the spontaneous beating rate of isolated cultured rat heart cells and dibutyryl cyclic AMP increased the spontaneous beating rate [63]. Cyclic GMP injected directly into sinoatrial nodal cells by iontophoresis decreased the slope of spontaneous diastolic depolarization [113]. Acetylcholine administered by this same route had no effect, presumably because the choline ester must interact with muscarinic receptors on the outside of the sarcolemma to produce its effects [113]. Like acetylcholine, 8-bromocyclic GMP inhibited atrial slow response action potentials [60], an indirect assessment of I_{si}. Associated with this inhibition of the slow response action potential there was a negative inotropic effect [60]. 8-bromocyclic GMP mimicked the effects of acetylcholine on action potential configuration and contractile state of rat atria [90]. In this same study, 8-bromocyclic GMP decreased Ca^{2+} uptake by contracting atrial preparations but had no effect on K^+ content [90]. It was concluded that cyclic GMP might mediate the effects of muscarinic activation on I_{si} but not on K^+ channels [90].

Cyclic GMP has also been shown to mimic the negative inotropic effects of acetylcholine. Fibers of mouse ventricle in which the sarcolemma was chemically disrupted were used to study the inotropic effects of cyclic GMP [115]. Cyclic GMP applied to such fibers markedly reduced both the force and frequency of contractions [115].

Analogues of cyclic GMP have also been used to assess its possible role in the antiadrenergic effects of acetylcholine. Dibutyryl cyclic GMP mimicked the effect of acetylcholine and antagonized the positive inotropic effects of cate-

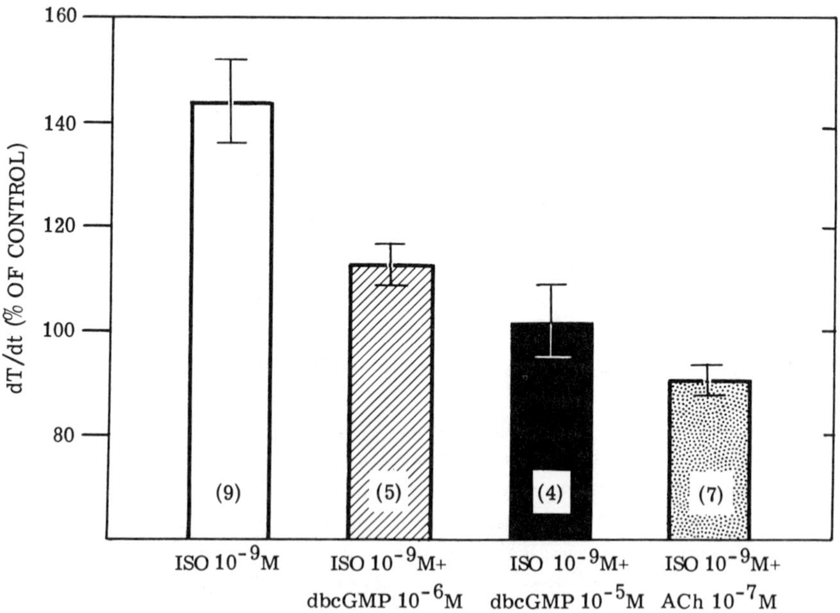

Fig. 6-3. Effect of dibutyryl cyclic GMP (dbcGMP) on isoproterenol (ISO)-induced increases in contractility (dT/dt). Dibutyryl cyclic GMP was perfused for 15 minutes prior to the administration of isoproterenol. The effect of isoproterenol on contractility was measured after a 2-minute infusion (dibutyryl cyclic GMP infusion was also continued). Values are means ± SE for the number of hearts noted at the bottom of the bars. (ACh) acetylcholine. (Reprinted with permission from ref. 120)

cholamines in isolated cardiac tissues [120] (Fig. 6-3). These results have been confirmed by other laboratories [76,103,128]. Like acetylcholine, dibutyryl cyclic GMP also attenuated the positive inotropic effects of isoproterenol in hearts from hyperthyroid rats [121]. Cyclic GMP analogues also mimic acetylcholine in antagonizing certain of the electrophysiological effects of catecholamines or cyclic AMP. Isoproterenol antagonized the inhibition of 8-bromo-cyclic GMP of slow responses in guinea pig atria [60]. This can be thought of as the reciprocal of cyclic GMP antagonism of isoproterenol-induced augmentation of slow responses. Cyclic GMP analogues also mimicked the cholinergic antagonism of the cardiac metabolic effects of catecholamines [121]. Hearts from hyperthyroid rats were hyperresponsive to the metabolic effects of beta agonists compared to those from euthyroid animals [121]. Acetylcholine antagonized isoproterenol-induced activation of phosphorylase in such hearts [121]. Dibutyryl cyclic GMP mimicked these effects of acetylcholine without lowering cyclic AMP levels [121]. Thus, it has been shown that analogues of cyclic GMP can mimic the effects of acetylcholine in antagonizing the electrophysiological, inotropic, and metabolic actions of beta agonists.

Cardiac cyclic GMP levels can be increased independently of stimulating muscarinic receptors by other means. One agent widely used to accomplish this is Na nitroprusside, which will be discussed later. Another agent that we have used is the divalent cation ionophore A23187 [74]. This drug produces complex effects on guinea pig ventricles. When given alone A23187 caused histamine release, presumably from tissue mast cells. The net result of A23187 administration was therefore elevation in cyclic AMP levels (presumably from histamine stimulation of H_2 receptors) and increases in cyclic GMP levels (presumably from the ionophore-induced transport of Ca^{2+} to guanylate cyclase (Fig. 6-4). The increase in cyclic AMP levels could be blunted substantially by blockade of H_2 receptors with metiamide (Fig. 6-4). The noteworthy finding from these studies was that a given level of cyclic AMP seemed to be relatively ineffective in causing positive inotropic effects or activating phosphorylase. Cyclic AMP levels had to exceed 1.0 pmol/mg wet weight before contractility or percent phosphorylase were increased (Fig. 6-4). This is in marked contrast to the efficacy of a given level of cyclic AMP when the levels are increased by catecholamines or agents such as histamine. In such cases, increasing cyclic AMP levels to .6 or .7 pmol/mg wet weight produced prominent inotropic [119] and metabolic [121] effects. One possible explanation for this apparent lack of efficacy of cyclic AMP was the fact that cyclic GMP levels in the same hearts were markedly elevated (Fig. 6-4). Thus, it was hypothesized that cyclic GMP generated in response to the direct ionophoric effects of A23187 antagonized the intracellular effects of cyclic AMP generated in response to H_2 receptor activation [74].

If cyclic GMP is involved in mediating some of the effects of muscarinic receptor stimulation in the heart, the biochemical mechanism by which this occurs remains unknown. One hypothesis is that, as in the cyclic AMP-protein kinase system, cyclic GMP interacts with a specific protein kinase which in turn phosphorylates certain substrates to alter protein function. A cyclic GMP-

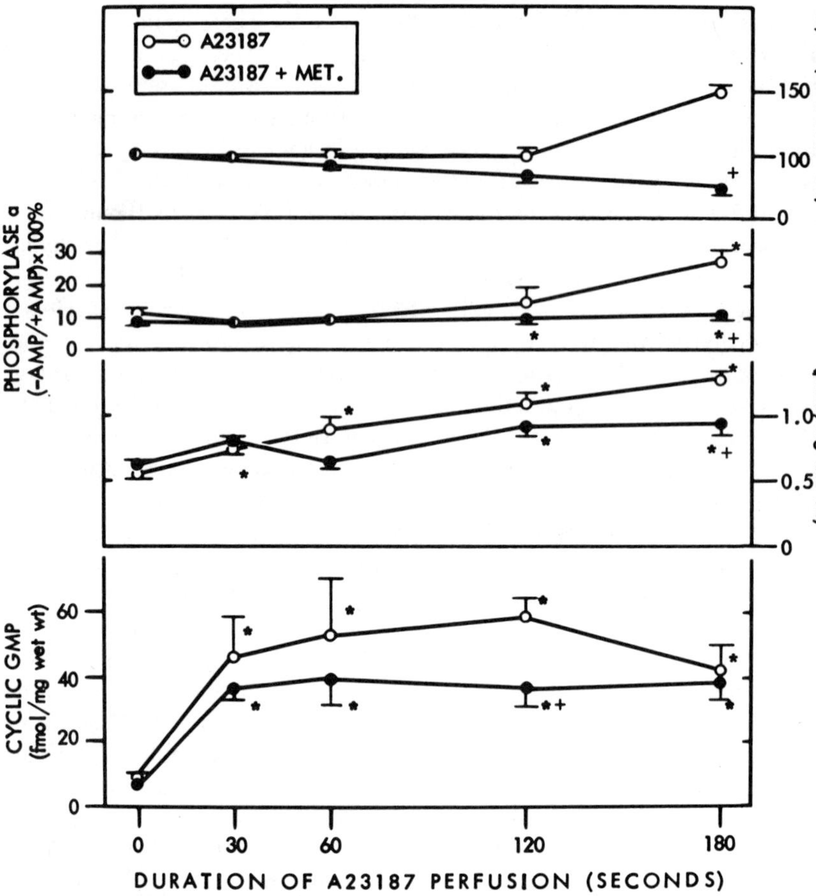

Fig. 6-4. Effect of 1.0 μM A23187 alone and combined with metiamide (10 μM) on the contractile and biochemical properties of isolated guinea pig ventricles. Values are means ± SE of 4 to 6 hearts. (*)p < 0.05 compared to basal. (+)p < 0.05 compared to absence of metiamide. (Adapted with permission from ref. 74)

dependent protein kinase has been identified in various tissues including heart [62,72,73]. Recently, an assay has been developed for studying the activity of cyclic GMP-dependent protein kinase in cardiac tissues [72,73]. This has shown for the first time that administration of acetylcholine to intact rat heart results in increases in cyclic GMP-dependent protein kinase activity ratios associated with elevations in cyclic GMP levels [72,73]. Both of these biochemical responses were associated with a negative inotropic effect in the same hearts. Na nitroprusside also increased cyclic GMP levels, in fact to much greater levels than that caused by acetylcholine. However, Na nitroprusside did not increase cyclic GMP-dependent protein kinase activity ratios nor did it change force of contraction [72,73]. These results: (1) suggest a possible mechanism by which cyclic GMP, which fluctuates in response to muscarinic stimulation, might modify protein function and the physiological properties of the heart; (2) support the notion, already suggested by others [93], that cyclic GMP and its intracellular effectors might be compartmentalized; and (3) demonstrate the hazards of using agents other than muscarinic agonists to elevate cyclic GMP levels, which may lead to inaccurate conclusions about the role of cyclic GMP if these agents do not mimic the choline esters [76].

There is a body of evidence that has been interpreted to show that cyclic GMP does not have a role in cardiac regulation [76]. One concentration–response study showed a dissociation between inotropic and cyclic GMP elevating effects of low concentrations of carbachol [12]. Low concentrations of carbachol (.03–1.0 μM) decreased contractility, whereas only high concentrations (2 or 10 μM) elevated cyclic GMP levels [12]. Also, by using a low concentration of carbachol, a dissociation in time of response was demonstrated. With 0.3 μM carbachol, contractility fell but cyclic GMP levels did not change [12]. These data were interpreted as evidence that cyclic GMP does not have a role in regulating the contractile state of atria. However, an alternative interpretation is that the contractile state of atria, as modified by muscarinic agonists, is determined by more than one factor, and cyclic GMP regulates only one of those factors. It was shown by voltage clamp studies that low concentrations of acetylcholine increased K^+ outward currents, whereas high concentrations reduced I_{si} and also increased outward currents in mammalian atria [112]. Even low concentrations (that only modified K^+ currents) produced negative inotropic effects, presumably because I_{si} was indirectly abbreviated owing to the shortened duration of the action potential [112]. High concentrations produced more marked negative inotropic effects presumably because I_{si} was directly inhibited as well as being abbreviated due to the shortened action potential. Thus, it is possible that with low concentrations of muscarinic agonists, negative inotropic effects occur independently of cyclic GMP and with high concentrations a second mechanism (e.g. inhibition of I_{si}) becomes operative and that this second mechanism involves cyclic GMP. Such a conclusion would be compatible with studies that showed that cyclic GMP modulates I_{si} or slow responses [60,90].

Another approach to test the cyclic GMP hypothesis is to elevate cyclic GMP with drugs which do not interact with muscarinic receptors. Because of its potency in elevating tissue cyclic GMP levels, Na nitroprusside has been widely used for such studies. It has been shown that Na nitroprusside did not mimic the inotropic [24,57,76], electrophysiological [85,111], metabolic [57], or antiadrenergic [15,57,73] effects of acetylcholine, even though it markedly increased cyclic GMP levels [24,57,73,76,85]. However, because Na nitroprusside elevates cyclic GMP levels in heart without producing physiological effects, it does not necessarily follow that cyclic GMP has no role in mediating the effects of acetylcholine. Immunohistochemical evidence in noncardiac [93] and cardiac [87] tissues has shown that cyclic GMP can be compartmentalized within the cell and that muscarinic agonists and Na nitroprusside affect the concentrations of this nucleotide in different compartments. The recent observations that acetylcholine, but not Na nitroprusside, activates cyclic GMP-dependent protein kinase in rat hearts provides further evidence for different compartments, or pools, of cyclic GMP, each of which can be selectively regulated and which has different intracellular effectors [72,73]. Analogous evidence has been provided for compartmentalization of cyclic AMP and differential regulation of cyclic AMP levels in different pools in myocardial cells [45].

Perhaps the most convincing evidence against a role for cyclic GMP in mediating certain physiological effects are the observations that over a range of concentrations of muscarinic agonist certain physiological effects can be induced without changing tissue cyclic GMP levels. Acetylcholine decreased automaticity and shortened action potential duration of guinea pig atria and these changes appeared to occur without any relationship to tissue cyclic GMP levels [85]. Muscarinic agonists antagonized the positive inotropic effects of agents that elevate cyclic AMP levels (catecholamines, phosphodiesterase inhibitors, cholera toxin) without elevating cyclic GMP levels [15,94]. These results could be interpreted as evidence for eliminating the role of cyclic GMP in the electrophysiological or antiadrenergic effects of muscarinic agonists. However, the following considerations are reiterated: (1) muscarinic receptors might be linked to multiple responses; only one or a few of these may be regulated by cyclic GMP; each must be examined carefully before ruling out in blanket fashion any physiological role for cyclic GMP; (2) cyclic GMP might be compartmentalized and small undetectable (by available assays) changes in levels might have occurred in experiments that appeared to show no change in the levels of the nucleotide.

In arguing against a physiological role for cyclic GMP in the antiadrenergic effects of muscarinic agonists, the data with analogues of cyclic GMP have been discounted because other agents such as verapamil also have antiadrenergic effects [76]. This conclusion is not valid. The fact that negative inotropic agents exist which can produce antiadrenergic effects by nonspecific or generalized negative inotropic mechanism does not justify the conclusion that cyclic GMP analogues also act in such a nonspecific or generalized manner. Agents such as verapamil antagonize the positive inotropic effects of various agents in addition to catecholamines. Before discarding the results with cyclic GMP analogues, it must be shown that they are indeed as nonspecific in their antiadrenergic action as agents such as verapamil.

To summarize, substantial evidence exists both for and against the concept that cyclic GMP plays a role in mediating certain cardiac effects of muscarinic receptor stimulation. It is clear that this is an unresolved issue. Further experiments must be done to establish or completely eliminate a role for this cyclic nucleotide in cardiac regulation.

Guanylate Cyclase. Cyclic GMP levels are regulated by two enzymes, guanylate cyclase and cyclic GMP phosphodiesterase [40]. Guanylate cyclase occurs as both a membrane-associated and soluble enzyme in cardiac tissues. The membrane-bound form is located in sarcolemma, which also contains the muscarinic receptors (Fig. 6-2). The two forms of the enzyme in cardiac muscle are regulated differentially: nonionic detergents stimulated the particulate enzyme without modifying the activity of the soluble one, whereas Na nitroprusside stimulated only the soluble enzyme (Figs. 6-5 and 6-6). These results, which show differential activation of the two forms of the enzyme, provide further support for the notion of different intracellular pools of cyclic GMP that can be modified selectively by certain agents. Acetylcholine presumably increases cyclic GMP levels by stimulating guanylate cyclase. As noted, both muscarinic receptors and particulate guanylate cyclase are located in sarcolemma (Fig. 6-2). However, except for rare reports [35], investigators have failed to show any effect of muscarinic agonists on guanylate cyclase activity in broken cell preparations [40]. In intact tissues Ca^{2+} is required for muscarinic-induced elevations in cyclic GMP levels [85,102]. The divalent cation ionophore A23187 increased cyclic GMP levels in guinea pig ventricles, presumably by elevating Ca^{2+} in certain critical areas of the myocardial cell [74] (Fig. 6-4). Ca^{2+} has been shown to stimulate particulate guanylate cyclase activity [118]. Based on these and similar results, it has been suggested that Ca^{2+} might in some way function as an intermediary between the muscarinic receptor and guanylate cyclase. However,

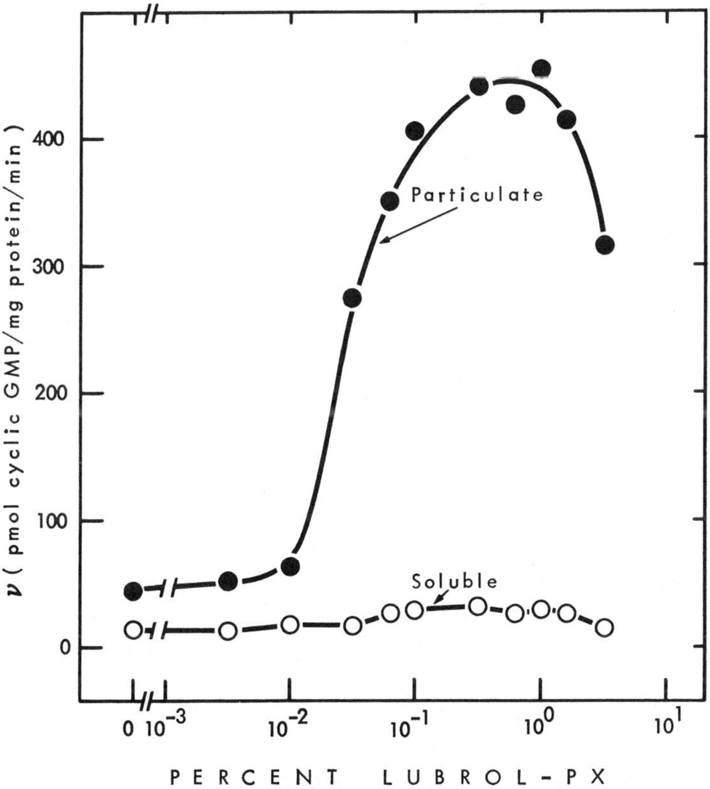

Fig. 6-5. Concentration effect of Lubrol PX on soluble (○) and particulate (●) guanylate cyclase activities. Reaction mixtures contained 1 mM GTP, 2 mM $MnCl_2$, and the indicated percent (w/v) of Lubrol-PX.

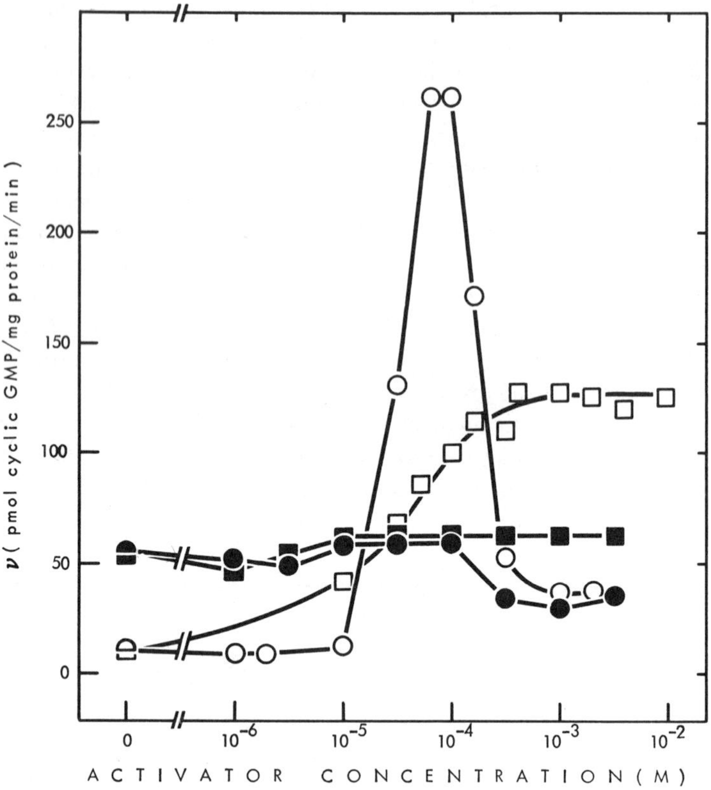

Fig. 6-6. Concentration effect of sodium nitroprusside (circles) and sodium azide (squares) on soluble (open symbols) and particulate (closed symbols) guanylate cyclase activities. All incubation mixtures contained 1 mM GTP and 2 mM $MnCl_2$ and the indicated concentrations of activators. Catalase (10 μg) was required in the reaction mixtures containing sodium azide for azide stimulation. No azide stimulation was observed in the absence of catalase.

other studies have shown Ca^{2+} inhibition of guanylate cyclase [92]. In cardiac muscle, although Ca^{2+} is required for muscarinic-induced increases in cyclic GMP levels, the physiological response to muscarinic stimulation is either no change or a decrease in contractile state [74,85]. These mechanical effects suggest that muscarinic agonists do not produce a generalized increase in intracellular Ca^{2+} concentration. If activation of muscarinic receptors leads to mobilization of Ca^{2+}, this must occur in discrete intracellular pools (presumably in the region of guanylate cyclase) because contractile proteins and other intracellular enzymes (e.g. phosphorylase kinase) do not appear to be affected.

MUSCARINIC MODULATION OF BETA-ADRENERGIC EFFECTS ON THE HEART

Physiological Studies. Studies in intact animals clearly demonstrate that vagus nerve activity attenuates the cardiac effects of circulating catecholamines. In conscious, chronically instrumented dogs, blockade of muscarinic receptors with atropine markedly augmented the positive inotropic effects of the catecholamines norepinephrine, isoproterenol, and dopamine [116]. The atropine-induced enhancement of catecholamine effects was abolished by vagotomy [116]. These results were interpreted as showing a vagal antagonism of the inotropic effects of circulating catecholamines. In the intact animal, tonic vagus nerve activity restrained the response of the myocardium to beta receptor stimulation by circulating catecholamines. Blockade of postjunctional muscarinic receptors removed this vagal restraint. Vagotomy removed the vagal restraint and therefore also rendered the muscarinic blockade ineffective. These results in conscious animals provide functional evidence for vagal innervation of the ventricles and suggest physiological relevance for this innervation. This is consistent with earlier studies in anesthetized dogs which showed that intracoronary administration of acetylcholine attenuated the inotropic effects of catecholamines infused into coronary arteries [50].

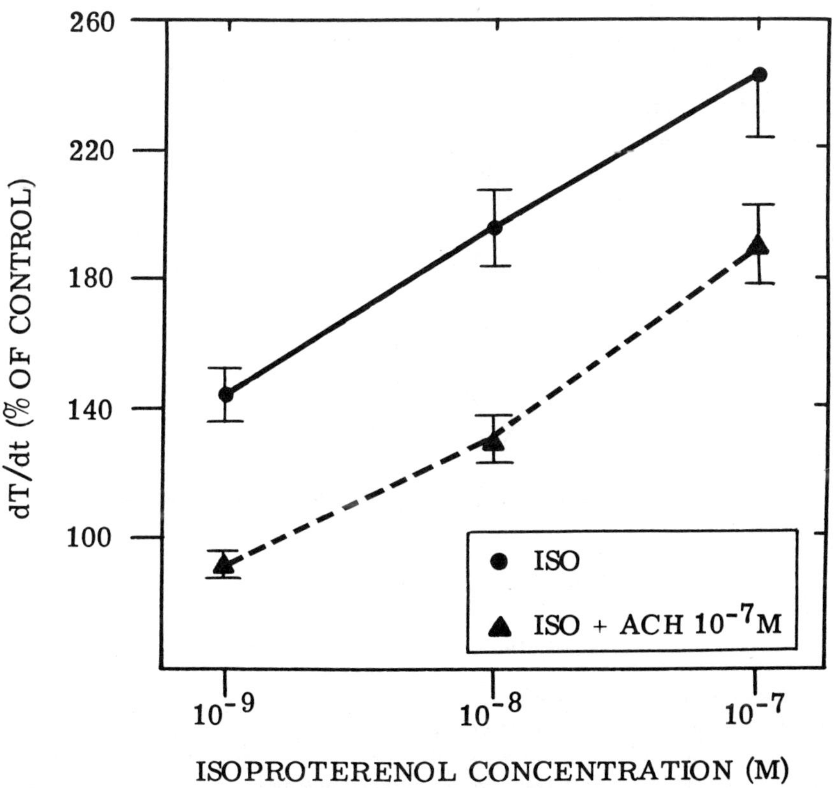

Fig. 6-7. Effect of acetylcholine (ACh) (10^{-7} M) on the positive inotropic effect of isoproterenol (ISO) in isolated, perfused guinea pig ventricles. Measurements were taken after hearts had reached a stable level of contractions after 2 minutes of continuous drug infusion. Note that the inotropic response to isoproterenol is markedly attenuated by acetylcholine. Values are means ± SE for 7–15 hearts. (Reprinted with permission from ref. 120)

The intracellular (postjunctional) interaction between the sympathetic and parasympathetic nervous systems has been documented by a wide variety of studies with isolated organs and tissues. In cardiac preparations from various mammalian species (guinea pig, rabbit, cat, dog, and rat) it has been shown clearly that choline esters antagonize the positive inotropic effects of beta receptor agonists [11,15,20,22,53,66,83,120] (Fig. 6-7). This antiadrenergic effect of choline esters was blocked by atropine, thus verifying that the effect was mediated via muscarinic receptors [22,66,83]. In most of these studies with isolated tissues, the negative inotropic effects of muscarinic agonists given alone were prominent and easily detectable in atria [15,66], but were small in ventricles [20,53,66,83,120]. Muscarinic antagonism of the positive inotropic effects of catecholamines was seen in both atria and ventricles. Thus, it appears that in atrial tissues muscarinic agonists produce negative inotropic effects both by a direct action and by antagonizing the effects of the beta receptor agonists. By contrast, in ventricles the predominant muscarinic effect appears to be inhibition of the inotropic effects of beta agonists.

In isolated cardiac preparations, muscarinic agonists also antagonize the electrophysiological effects of catecholamines. Choline esters attenuated the positive chronotropic effects of catecholamines on isolated atrial preparations [18,42,100], presumably by antagonizing the catecholamine-induced increase in spontaneous phase 4 depolarization [21]. Muscarinic agonists antagonize the electrophysiological effects of catecholamines on isolated Purkinje fibers or ventricular muscle. Acetylcholine inhibited isoproterenol-induced shortening of action potential duration in normally polarized paced cardiac Purkinje fibers [2] (Fig. 6-8). Acetylcholine also abolished isoproterenol-dependent slow responses

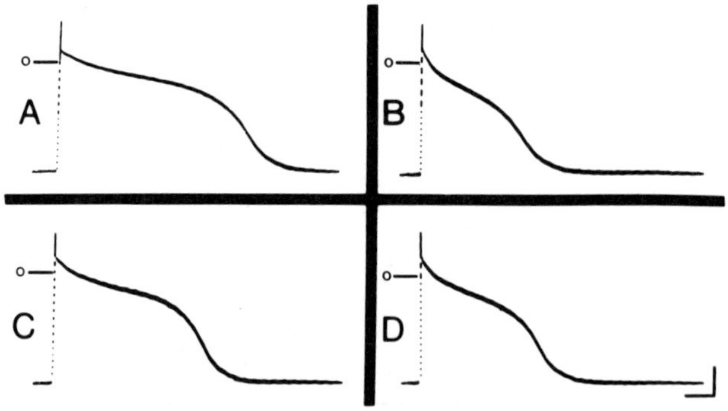

Fig. 6-8. Effect of acetylcholine on the shortening of action potential duration produced by isoproterenol in a canine cardiac Purkinje fiber. (A) A control cardiac Purkinje fiber action potential. (B) Shortening of action potential duration produced by isoproterenol (10^{-7} M). (C) The addition of acetylcholine (10^{-6} M) partially reversed the shortening of action potential duration effected by isoproterenol. (D) Atropine (10^{-6} M) attenuated the effects of acetylcholine, resulting in an action potential duration resembling that produced by the superfusion of isoproterenol alone. Zero potential indicated in each panel. Calibrations: horizontal bar = 50 msec; vertical bar = 25 mV. (Reprinted with permission from ref. 2)

in cardiac Purkinje fibers or guinea pig papillary muscles [2,52]. Muscarinic agonists also exerted antiarrhythmic effects in cats or dogs treated with a combination of hydrocarbon anesthetics and epinephrine [23,25].

Activation of muscarinic receptors also modulates the cardiac metabolic effects of beta-adrenergic receptor stimulation. Acetylcholine completely antagonized the glycogenolytic effect of epinephrine in isolated perfused guinea pig hearts [117]. Subsequent studies showed that this was due to a muscarinic antagonism of beta-adrenergic activation of glycogen phosphorylase [11,20,33,121] (Fig. 6-9). Acetylcholine also antagonized norepinephrine-induced stimulation of lipase in dog myocardium [39].

Thus, in isolated cardiac preparations there is abundant evidence for intracellular interaction between activation of beta-adrenergic and muscarinic receptors. In isolated ventricular tissues, it appears that modulation of sympathetic effects is a major mechanism by which the parasympathetic nervous system exerts its effect. Choline esters alone produced little or no change in the inotropic [11,66,120] electrophysiologic [2], or metabolic [11,117,121] properties of isolated ventricular tissues. Only when these physiological or metabolic

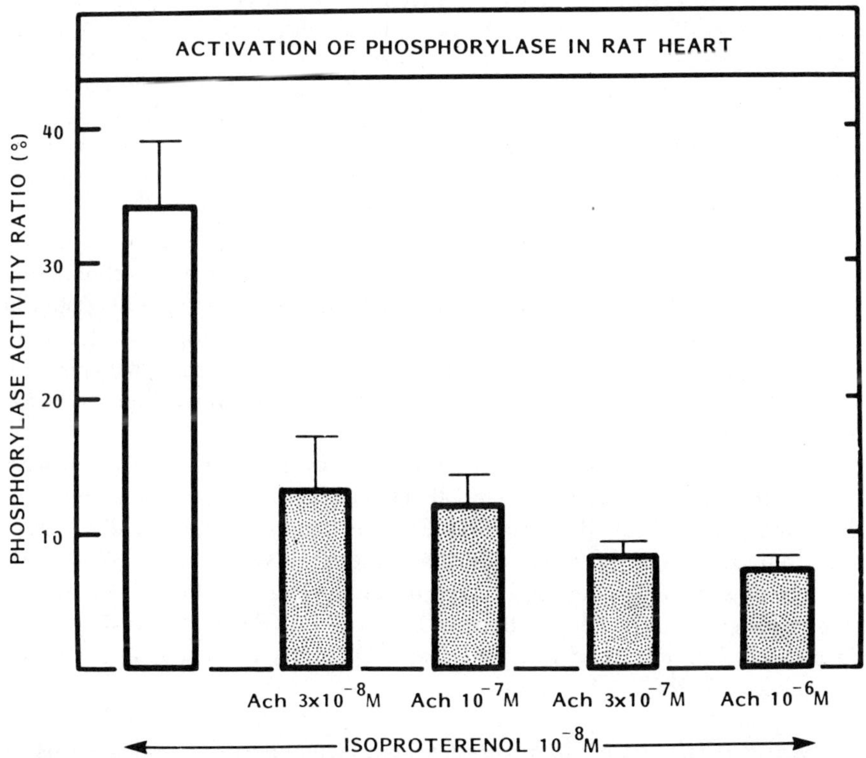

Fig. 6-9. Muscarinic cholinergic antagonism of isoproterenol activation of glycogen phosphorylase in isolated perfused hearts taken from hyperthyroid rats. Basal phosphorylase activity ratio was 8%. Values were mean ± SE of 6–8 hearts.

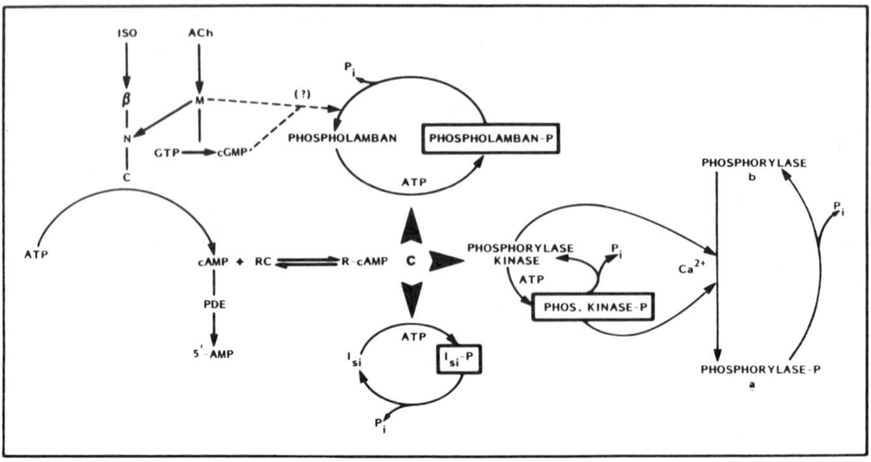

Fig. 6-10. Flow diagram of reactions thought to mediate intracellular effects of autonomic receptor stimulation. Catecholamines (ISO) activate beta-adrenergic (β) receptors which leads via a regulatory protein (N) to activation of the catalytic subunit (C) of adenylate cyclase. Cyclic AMP thereby generated interacts with cyclic AMP-dependent protein kinase (RC) to release the catalytic unit (C) which, in turn, catalyzes the phosphorylation of a variety of proteins, including phospholamban, phosphorylase kinase, and (possibly) slow inward current channels (I_{si}). One or more of these phosphorylation reactions may contribute to the inotropic and electrophysiological effects of beta agonists. Acetylcholine stimulates muscarinic receptors to inhibit adenylate cyclase activity. This reaction appears to occur via the N protein. In addition, muscarinic agonists can increase cyclic GMP levels and also block the effects of beta agonists at some point beyond cyclic AMP by as yet unknown mechanisms.

responses were altered by beta-adrenergic agonists did muscarinic cholinergic effects become readily apparent. In this situation, muscarinic agonists potently antagonized the beta-adrenergic alteration of these properties [2,11,66, 117,120,121]. The mechanisms for the intracellular interaction between the components of the sympathetic and parasympathetic systems will be discussed in this section.

Substantial evidence supports the notion that cyclic AMP mediates at least some of the physiological and metabolic effects of beta-adrenergic agonists on the heart [86,110,123]. If muscarinic agonists produce some or all of their antiadrenergic effects by modifying the cyclic AMP system, they could theoretically do so by acting at one or more of the steps in the cascade of reactions that mediates the intracellular effects of beta agonists (Fig. 6-10). Available evidence regarding effects of muscarinic agonists at each of these steps will be considered.

Muscarinic Inhibition of Adenylate Cyclase. A number of investigators using different types of cardiac preparations from various species have shown that muscarinic agonists can attenuate beta agonist-induced increases in steady state tissue cyclic AMP levels [5,13–15,33,51,58,66,68,80,121]. When physiological or metabolic responses were measured, the muscarinic attenuation of cyclic AMP generation paralleled the inhibition of the myocardial response to catecholamines. Muscarinic agonists inhibited catecholamine-induced increases in cyclic AMP levels and concomitantly attenuated the positive inotropic effects [5,14,15,51,58,66,80]. Muscarinic agonists also antagonized catecholamine-induced activation of phosphorylase while inhibiting cyclic AMP generation [33,58,121]. These results are consistent with the conclusion that the muscarinic inhibition of cyclic AMP generation is physiologically and metabolically important in cardiac cells, and that attentuation of cyclic AMP generation might be a contributing mechanism for the antiadrenergic effects of muscarinic agonists.

The mechanism for muscarinic attenuation of catecholamine-induced cyclic AMP generation involves inhibition of adenylate cyclase activity. It first was shown two decades ago, prior to any detailed knowledge regarding regulation of adenylate cyclase, that muscarinic agonists inhibited adenylate cyclase activity in crude preparations of dog myocardium [89]. Carbachol added to these preparations inhibited both basal and epinephrine stimulated adenylate cyclase activity [89]. These results were confirmed in similar experiments which used a crude myocardial preparation from rabbit hearts [66]. The biochemical mechanism for this muscarinic inhibition of adenylate cyclase activity began to be elucidated after substantial information regarding regulation of adenylate cyclase had been obtained from other systems [99]. Studies done largely in model systems revealed that hormone stimulated adenylate cyclase is comprised of at least three distinct components, the hormone receptor, the catalytic subunit, and a third component which "couples" the receptor to the catalytic subunit [99]. The third component has been referred to as the G/F or N protein because it possesses binding sites for and is regulated by guanine nucleotides such as GTP. In relatively purified membrane preparations devoid of endogenous GTP, exogenous guanine nucleotides must be added to the system to demonstrate hormone stimulation of adenylate cyclase activity [99]. Thus, guanine nucleotides must interact with the N protein for the receptor to activate the catalytic subunit. In some tissues like myocardium, guanine nucleotides can directly activate catalytic activity of adenylate cyclase even in the absence of hormone [124]. Guanine nucleotides acting on the N protein also can modulate the affinity of receptors for agonists. This is true for a variety of receptors including beta-adrenergic [47,122] and muscarinic [3,31,98,126,127] receptors. It has been theorized that this dual regulation by guanine nucleotides and the N protein of both the receptor and catalytic subunit is involved in mediating the receptor activation of adenylate cyclase [47,99]. Another property associated with the N protein is a GTPase activity which is thought to regulate GTP effects by hydrolyzing the guanine nucleotide to GDP [99].

As is the case with virtually all systems studied, adenylate cyclase activity in purified membranes from myocardial cells is not stimulated by hormones unless exogenous guanine nucleotides are added. Addition of exogenous guanine nucleotides stimulated the enzyme directly as well as facilitating hormone stimulation of the enzyme [124] (Fig. 6-11). Thus, guanine nucleotides can activate cardiac adenylate cyclase directly and are required for hormone activation of

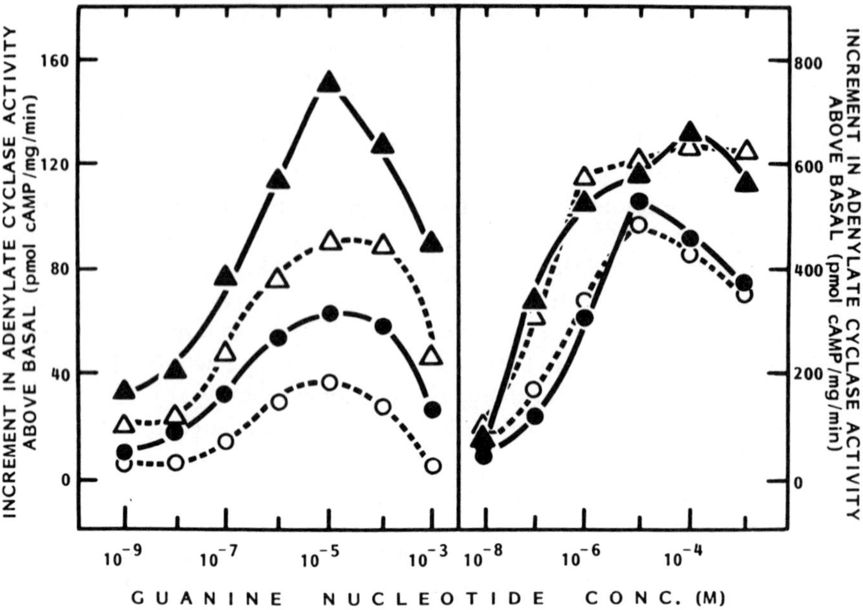

Fig. 6-11. Guanine nucleotide stimulation of adenylate cyclase activity in canine cardiac membrane vesicles. Guanine nucleotide added was GTP in left panel and Gpp(NH)p in right panel. Circles are values with guanine nucleotides alone and triangles with guanine nucleotides plus 10^{-7} M isoproterenol. Unfilled symbols designate the presence of 10^{-5} M methacholine in addition to guanine nucleotide alone or with isoproterenol. Note that methacholine significantly inhibits GTP or GTP plus isoproterenol activation of adenylate cyclase (left) but does not affect adenylate cyclase activity when the guanine nucleotide added is Gpp(NH)p (right).

the enzyme. In purified membrane preparations, muscarinic agonists had no effect on basal adenylate cyclase activity, i.e., that activity in the absence of added guanine nucleotides [124]. If GTP was added to the enzyme preparation, muscarinic agonists inhibited adenylate cyclase activity (Fig. 6-11, left panel). This was true whether GTP was added alone or together with a catecholamine (Fig. 6-11, left panel). In the earlier studies cited [66,89], because the membrane preparations were crude it is likely that endogenous GTP was present. Thus, in these earlier studies it is likely that muscarinic effects on adenylate cyclase activity were also dependent on GTP. This dependency was specific for this guanine nucleotide. Cardiac adenylate cyclase activity was also increased by the nonhydrolyzable guanine nucleotide Gpp(NH)p (Fig. 6-11, right). However, muscarinic agonists had no effect on enzyme activity in the presence of this nucleotide [124] (Fig. 6-11, right). Similarly, muscarinic agonists did not modify NaF stimulation of adenylate cyclase activity [124]. The effects of muscarinic agonists were blocked by atropine [124]. It was concluded that the interaction of both muscarinic and beta-adrenergic receptors with adenylate cyclase was regulated by the naturally occurring guanine nucleotide GTP. These studies have been confirmed subsequently [54]. Based on these findings and the data that show guanine nucleotide regulation of muscarinic receptor affinity for agonists [3,31,98,126,127], it is reasonable to hypothesize that an N protein, with which GTP interacts, is involved in "coupling" inhibitory muscarinic receptors to adenylate cyclase. Whether this is the same N protein that couples stimulatory receptors to the enzyme is unknown. The detailed biochemical mechanism by which activation of muscarinic receptors leads to reduction of the efficacy of GTP is also unknown. The fact that this inhibition does not occur when the nonhydrolyzable analog Gpp(NH)p is the guanine nucleotide suggests that muscarinic agonists increase the activity of an adenylate cyclase-associated GTPase. It has been shown in another system that muscarinic agonists can activate adenylate cyclase-associated GTPase activity [61]. In studies indirectly assessing GTPase activity, this mechanism is suggested for cardiac membranes [108]. Other mechanisms are also possible instead of or in addition to those postulated. Thus, the specific details regarding the biochemical and molecular mechanisms by which activation of muscarinic receptors inhibits adenylate cyclase remain to be elucidated. Nevertheless, it seems clear that muscarinic agonists can diminish tissue cyclic AMP levels by inhibiting catecholamine stimulation of adenylate cyclase.

Theoretically, muscarinic agonists could reduce steady-state tissue levels of cyclic AMP by activating phosphodiesterase (Fig. 6-10). Although the studies are limited, this possibility has been examined by a few laboratories [4,13,66]. With the experimental approaches used these studies failed to demonstrate any effect of muscarinic agonists on phosphodiesterase activity from myocardium [4,13,66].

Muscarinic Modulation of Cyclic AMP Effects Independent of Changes in Cyclic AMP Levels. The muscarinic attenuation of catecholamine-induced cyclic AMP generation cannot entirely account for the muscarinic antagonism of the cardiac effects of beta agonists. Under certain conditions, perhaps determined by species and buffer conditions (e.g. Ca^{2+} concentration), muscarinic agonists can potently inhibit the physiological and metabolic effects of catecholamines without changing cyclic AMP levels. Acetylcholine markedly antagonized the positive inotropic effects of isoproterenol in isolated perfused guinea pig ventricles [120] (Fig. 6-7). Cyclic GMP levels in the acetylcholine treated hearts were markedly elevated (Fig. 6-12). However, cyclic AMP levels in hearts receiving both acetylcholine and isoproterenol were not significantly different from those in hearts receiving isoproterenol alone [120] (Fig. 6-12). These results have been confirmed by several other investigators. It has been shown either that muscarinic agonists attenuated a physiological or metabolic response to catecholamines out of proportion to the magnitude of reduction in cyclic AMP [51,58] or that the inhibition of physiological response occurred without any change in cyclic AMP levels [15]. Additional evidence for muscarinic antagonism of catecholamine effects by mechanisms not involving cyclic AMP reduction comes from studies in which cyclic AMP levels are increased independently of stimulation of beta receptors. It was observed many years ago that acetylcholine blocked the positive inotropic effects of both epinephrine and theo-

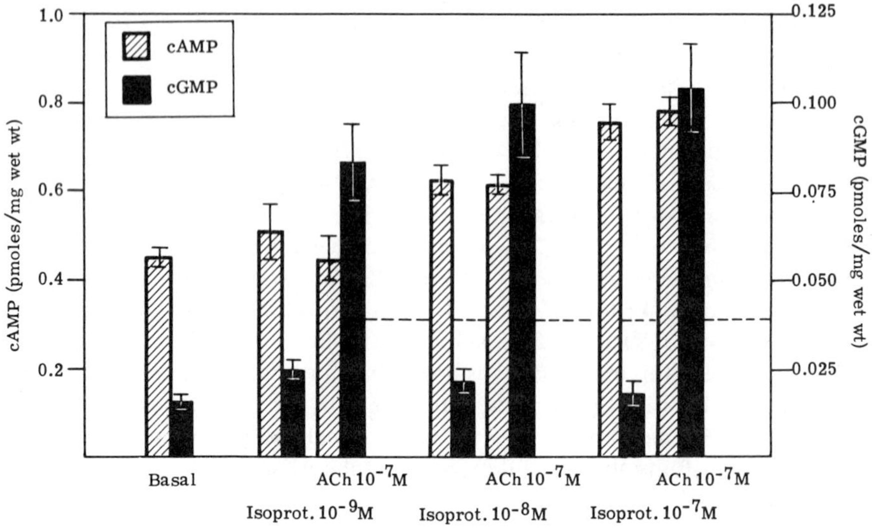

Fig. 6-12. Cyclic nucleotide levels in hearts receiving isoproterenol (Isoprot.) alone or combined with acetylcholine (ACh) for 2 minutes of continuous infusion. Values are means ± SE for 7–16 hearts. The horizontal dashed line is the mean value of cyclic GMP found in hearts receiving 10^{-7} M acetylcholine alone for 2 minutes. (Reprinted with permission from ref. 120)

phylline in isolated turtle hearts [83]. Although cyclic AMP levels were not measured, it is reasonable to conclude that the positive inotropic effects of both epinephrine and theophylline were mediated at least partially by cyclic AMP [83]. Subsequently, several investigators utilized phosphodiesterase inhibitors to produce positive inotropic effects and elevate cyclic AMP levels in cardiac preparations and then examined the effects of muscarinic agonists on these parameters. Methylisobutylxanthine (MIX) elevated cyclic AMP levels and augmented Ca^{2+}-dependent action potentials and contraction in chick ventricles [4]. Acetylcholine (10^{-6} M) abolished the MIX-induced increase in tension without reducing tissue cyclic AMP levels [4]. In isolated rat left atria, methacholine antagonized the positive inotropic effects of MIX without changing cyclic AMP levels [15]. Myocardial cyclic AMP levels also can be increased by treating the intact tissue with cholera toxin [13,14,94]. The presumed mechanism is that cholera toxin inhibits the adenylate cyclase-associated GTPase. Thus, the GTP concentration available to interact with the N protein is increased and adenylate cyclase is thereby activated. Cholera toxin elevated cyclic AMP levels [13,14,94] and increased contractions [94] of intact cardiac preparations. Muscarinic agonists inhibited the positive inotropic effect of cholera toxin without reducing cyclic AMP levels [94]. These results provide additional evidence that muscarinic agonists can antagonize the effects of cyclic AMP within the myocardial cell.

There are several potential sites beyond cyclic AMP where muscarinic agonists could act to interfere with the intracellular effects of the nucleotide (Fig.

6-10). One of these is cyclic AMP activation of cyclic AMP-dependent protein kinase. Experiments have been limited. However, the studies that attempted to examine the relationship failed to reveal any effect of acetylcholine [51,58]. That is, for a given level of cyclic AMP, cyclic AMP-dependent protein kinase was proportionately activated in the presence or absence of muscarinic agonists. Muscarinic agonists thus do not appear to interfere with cyclic AMP activation of protein kinase.

Another potential site where muscarinic agonists might interfere with the intracellular effects of cyclic AMP is at the level of phosphorylation of proteins which are thought to mediate the effects of hormones or drugs that elevate cyclic AMP concentrations. Several proteins, including troponin I [28], phosphorylase kinase [82], and phospholamban [75,123] have been shown to be phosphorylated in intact hearts with administration of beta-adrenergic agonists. It has been hypothesized, but not yet demonstrated, that slow inward current channels (I_{si}) are also phosphorylated when cyclic AMP levels are increased by catecholamines [86,107].

We have begun to examine possible effects of muscarinic agonists on phosphorylation of proteins by studying the protein phospholamban in intact guinea pig ventricles. Isoproterenol administered to isolated perfused guinea pig hearts which had been previously perfused with $^{32}P_i$ produced characteristic positive inotropic effects [75,123]. The hearts then were freeze clamped, membranes prepared, and then subjected to polyacrylamide gel electrophoresis. The incorporation of ^{32}P was assessed by autoradiography. Isoproterenol produced a time-dependent increase in ^{32}P incorporation into proteins with apparent molecular weights of 22,000 and 8,000–10,000 [75,123] (Fig. 6-13). On the basis of a variety of additional information, it is felt that the 22,000 molecular weight protein is phospholamban and the lower molecular weight protein is a component (perhaps a monomer) of phospholamban. The ^{32}P incorporation correlated very well temporally with the positive inotropic effects of isoproterenol. The muscarinic agonist acetylcholine potently attenuated the isoproterenol-induced increase in ^{32}P incorporation into phospholamban and also antagonized the positive inotropic effects of the catecholamine [123] (Fig. 6-13). Thus, muscarinic agonists can potently antagonize catecholamine-induced phosphorylation of a myocardial cell protein which may be involved in mediating the positive inotropic effects of catecholamines. It is not yet known whether this attenuation of protein phosphorylation can be accounted for entirely by muscarinic reduction in cyclic AMP levels and thus in protein kinase activity. In view of the earlier studies mentioned this seems unlikely. Rather, it seems more likely that cyclic AMP may have been reduced somewhat and that this partially accounts for the reduced phosphorylation. However, some additional mechanism was also operative to produce the ultimate observed inhibition of ^{32}P incorporation. One reasonable hypothesis is that muscarinic agonists somehow activate a protein phosphatase (Fig. 6-10). There are, however, no available experiments that address this question specifically.

Thus, muscarinic agonists appear to act at more than one level in the cascade of reactions mediating the intracellular effects of beta receptor stimulation.

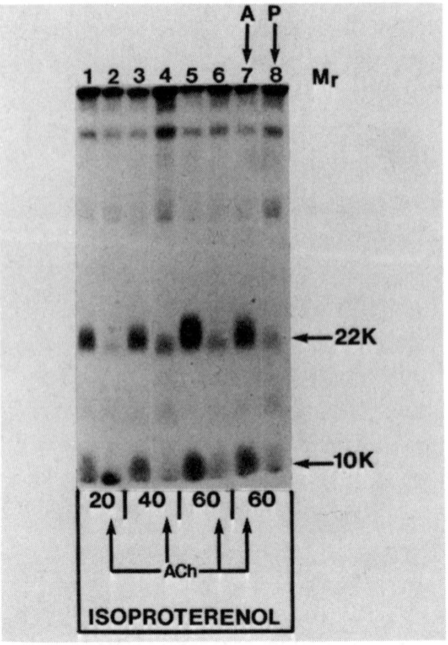

Fig. 6-13. Autoradiogram of guinea pig ventricles perfused with $^{32}P_i$ and then treated with isoproterenol (10^{-8} M) alone or isoproterenol plus acetylcholine (10^{-7} M) for 20, 40, and 60 seconds. After perfusion with drugs for the respective time periods, ventricles were freeze-clamped and then membrane vesicles were prepared. Vesicles were subjected to gel electrophoresis and this autoradiogram was subsequently obtained. Acetylcholine was perfused simultaneously with and for the same duration as isoproterenol. Hearts in lanes 1, 3, and 5 received isoproterenol plus acetylcholine. Heart in lane 7 received atropine in addition to isoproterenol and acetylcholine, and heart in lane 8 received propranolol in addition to isoproterenol. Note that isoproterenol produces a time-dependent increase in ^{32}P incorporation into the 22,000- and 8,000- to 11,000-M_r proteins (lanes 1, 3, and 5). Propranolol antagonizes this effect of isoproterenol (lane 8). Acetylcholine clearly attenuates the isoproterenol-induced increase in ^{32}P incorporation (lanes 2, 4, and 6). Atropine reverses the effect of acetylcholine (lane 7). (Reprinted with permission from ref. 123)

They can inhibit adenylate cyclase activity by somehow reducing the efficacy of GTP. In addition, they appear to be able to interfere with the intracellular effects of cyclic AMP. The mechanism for the latter effect is unknown.

CONCLUSIONS

The parasympathetic and sympathetic divisions of the autonomic nervous system are the primary systems extrinsic to the heart that regulate cardiac function. The parasympathetic nervous system regulates cardiac function by releasing the neurotransmitter acetylcholine from vagal nerve endings in the heart. Acetylcholine interacts with muscarinic receptors on the sarcolemma of myocytes to alter the physiological properties of cardiac tissues.

With the use of recently developed radiolabelled ligand binding studies, much new information about the biochemical and molecular properties of muscarinic receptors has become available. However, much remains to be learned. A major area of investigation that remains for further study is the mechanism by which the interaction of agonists with muscarinic receptors leads to changes in the properties of myocytes; that is, what is the nature of the "coupler" between the muscarinic receptor and intracellular effectors. Specific questions remaining to be answered include the following: Are muscarinic receptors directly coupled to ionic (e.g. potassium) channels? What is the role of phosphotidylinositol turnover in cardiac tissues in mediating muscarinic effects? What is the role of guanylate cyclase and cyclic GMP in mediating muscarinic effects? How do muscarinic receptors function as inhibitory regulators of adenylate cyclase activity? Do muscarinic agonists activate an adenylate cyclase-associated GTPase? Are there two different guanine nucleotide binding proteins, one for cyclase stimulating receptors and another for cyclase inhibiting receptors? What is the mechanism by which muscarinic agonists reduce phosphorylation of proteins putatively involved in mediating effects of agents that elevate cyclic AMP levels? Pursuit of these questions should result in exciting and fruitful research and the resulting answers should be of great interest to physiologists, pharmacologists, and clinicians.

REFERENCES

1. Alberts, P. and T. Bartfai, Muscarinic acetylcholine receptor from rat brain, *J. Biol. Chem. 251(6)*: 1543–1547, 1976.
2. Bailey, J. C., A. M. Watanabe, H. R. Besch, Jr., D. A. Lathrop, Acetylcholine antagonism of the electrophysiological effects of isoproterenol on canine cardiac Purkinje fibers. *Circ. Res. 44*: 378–383, 1979.
3. Berrie, C. P., N. J. M. Birdsall, A. S. V. Burgen, E. C. Hulme, Guanine nucleotides modulate muscarinic receptor binding in the heart, *Biochem. Biophys. Res. Commun. 87(4)*: 1000–1005, 1979.
4. Biegon, R. L., P. M. Epstein, and A. J. Pappano, Muscarinic antagonism of the effects of a phosphodiesterase inhibitor (methylisobutylxanthine) in embryonic chick ventricle. *J. Pharmacol. Exp. Ther. 215*: 348–356, 1980.
5. Biegon, R. L. and A. J. Pappano, Dual mechanism for inhibition of calcium-dependent action potentials by acetylcholine in avian ventricular muscle: relationship to cyclic AMP. *Circ. Res. 46*: 353–362, 1980.
6. Birdsall, N. J. M., C. P. Berrie, A. S. V. Burgen, E. C. Hulme, Modulation of the binding properties of muscarinic receptors: evidence for receptor-effector coupling. In *Receptors for Neurotransmitters and Peptide Hormones*. eds. G. Pepeu, M. J. Kuhar, and S. J. Enna, Raven Press, New York, pp. 107–116, 1980.
7. Birdsall, N. J. M., A. S. V. Burgen, E. C. Hulme, A study of the muscarinic receptor by gel electrophoresis. *Br. J. Pharmacol. 66*: 337–342, 1979.
8. Birdsall, N. J. M., A. S. V. Burgen, E. C. Hulme, The binding of agonists to brain muscarinic receptors. *Mol. Pharmacol. 14*: 723–736, 1978.
9. Birdsall, N. J. M., A. S. V. Burgen, E. C. Hulme, J. W. Wells, The effects of ions on the binding of agonists and antagonists to muscarinic receptors, *Br. J. Pharmacol. 67*: 371–377, 1979.

10. Birdsall, N. J. M. and E. C. Hulme, Biochemical studies on muscarinic acetylcholine receptors, *J. Neurochem.* *27*: 7–16, 1976.
11. Blukoo-Allotey, J. A., N. H. Vincent, S. Ellis, Interactions of acetylcholine and epinephrine on contractility, glycogen and phosphorylase activity of isolated mammalian hearts. *J. Pharmacol. Exp. Ther.* *170*: 27–36, 1969.
12. Brooker, G., Dissociation of cyclic GMP from the negative inotropic action of carbachol in guinea pig atria. *J. Cyclic Nucleotide Res.* *3*: 407–413, 1977.
13. Brown, J. H. Cholinergic inhibition of catecholamine-stimulable cyclic AMP accumulation in murine atria. *J. Cyclic Nucleotide Res.* *5(6)*: 423–433, 1979.
14. Brown, J. H. Depolarization-induced inhibition of cyclic AMP accumulation: cholinergic-adrenergic antagonism in murine atria. *Mol. Pharmacol.* *16*: 841–850, 1979.
15. Brown, B. S., J. B. Polson, J. J. Krzanowski, J. R. Wiggins, Influence of isoproterenol and methylisobutylxanthine on the contractile and cyclic nucleotide effects of methacholine in isolated rat atria. *J. Pharmacol. Exp. Ther.* *212*: 325–332, 1980.
16. Burgen, A. S. V. and K. G. Terroux, On the negative inotropic effect in the cat's auricle. *J. Physiol. (Lond.)* *120*: 449–464, 1953.
17. Canessa de Scarnatti, O., M. Sato, E. De Robertis, Muscarinic cholinergic stimulation of phosphatidyl inositol turnover in the CNS. *Adv. Exp. Med. Biol.* *83*: 497–503, 1977.
18. Carrier, G. O. and V. S. Bishop, The interaction of acetylcholine and norepinephrine on heart rate. *J. Pharmacol. Exp. Ther.* *180*: 31–37, 1972.
19. Cavey, D., J. P. Vincent, M. Lazdunski, The muscarinic receptor of heart cell membranes. *FEBS Lett.* *84(1)*: 110–114, 1977.
20. Chamales, M. H., R. D. Gourley, B. J. Williams, Effect of acetylcholine on changes in contractility, heart rate and phosphorylase activity produced by isoprenaline, salbutamol and aminophylline in the perfused guinea pig heart. *Br. J. Pharmacol.* *53*: 531–538, 1975.
21. Davis, L. D., Effects of autonomic neurohumors on transmembrane potentials of atrial plateau fibers. *Am. J. Physiol.* *229*: 1351–1364, 1975.
22. Dempsey, P. J. and T. Cooper, Ventricular cholinergic receptor systems: interaction with adrenergic systems. *J. Pharmacol. Exp. Ther.* *167*: 282–290, 1969.
23. De Palma, J. R., The role of acetylcholine in hydrocarbon-epinephrine arrhythmias. *J. Pharmacol. Exp. Ther.* *116*: 255–261, 1956.
24. Diamond, J., R. E. Ten Eick, A. J. Trapani, Are increases in cyclic GMP levels responsible for the negative inotropic effects of acetylcholine in the heart? *Biochem. Biophys. Res. Commun.* *79(3)*: 912–918, 1977.
25. Dresel, P. E. and M. C. Sutter, Factors modifying cyclopropane-epinephrine cardiac arrhythmias. *Circ. Res.* *9*: 1284–1290, 1961.
26. Ehlert, F. J., Y. Dumont, W. R. Roeske, H. I. Yamamura, Muscarinic receptor binding in rat brain using the agonist, [^{3}H]cis methyldioxolane. *Life Sci.* *26*: 961–967, 1980.
27. Ehlert, F. J., W. R. Roeske, H. I. Yamamura, The nature of muscarinic receptor binding. In *Handbook of Pharmacology*. eds. Iversen, Iversen, and Snyder, Plenum Press, 1981.
28. England, P. J., Correlation between contraction and phosphorylation of the inhibitory subunit of troponin in perfused rat heart. *FEBS Lett.* *50*: 57–60, 1975.
29. Fields, J. Z., W. R. Roeske, E. Morkin, H. I. Yamamura, Cardiac muscarinic cholinergic receptors: biochemical identification and characterization. *J. Biol. Chem.* *253(9)*: 3251–3258, 1978.

30. Galper, J. B., W. Klein, W. A. Catterall, Muscarinic acetylcholine receptors in developing chick heart. *J. Biol. Chem. 252(23)*: 8692–8699, 1977.
31. Galper, J. B. and T. W. Smith, Agonist and guanine nucleotide modulation of muscarinic cholinergic receptors in cultured heart cells. *J. Biol. Chem. 255(20)*: 9571–9579, 1980.
32. Galper, J. B. and T. W. Smith, Properties of muscarinic acetylcholine receptors in heart cell cultures. *Proc. Natl. Acad. Sci. USA 75(12)*: 5831–5835, 1978.
33. Gardner, R. M. and D. O. Allen, The relationship between cyclic nucleotide levels and glycogen phosphorylase activity in isolated rat hearts perfused with epinephrine and acetylcholine. *J. Pharmacol. Exp. Ther. 202*: 346–353, 1977.
34. George, W. J., L. J. Ignarro, R. J. Paddock, L. White, P. J. Kadowitz, Oppositional effects of acetylcholine and isoproterenol on isometric tension and cyclic nucleotide concentrations in rabbit atria. *J. Cyclic Nucleotide Res. 1*: 339–347, 1975.
35. George, W. J., L. J. Ignarro, and L. E. White, Muscarinic stimulation of cardiac guanylate cyclase. In *Recent Advances in Studies on Cardiac Structure and Metabolism,* Vol. 7. eds. P. Harris, R. J. Bing, and A. Fleckenstein, University Park Press, Baltimore, pp. 381–390, 1976.
36. George, W. J., J. B. Polson, A. G. O'Toole, N. D. Goldberg, Elevation of guanosine 3′,5′-cyclic phosphate in rat heart after perfusion with acetylcholine. *Proc. Natl. Acad. Sci. USA 66 (2)*: 398–403, 1970.
37. George, W. J., R.D. Wilkerson, P. J. Kadowitz, Influence of acetylcholine on contractile force and cyclic nucleotide levels in the isolated perfused rat heart. *J. Pharmacol. Exp. Ther. 184(1)*: 228–235, 1973.
38. Giles, W. and R. W. Tsien, Effects of acetylocholine on membrane currents in frog atrial muscle. *J. Physiol. (Lond) 246:* 64P-66p, 1975.
39. Glaviano, V. V., J. Goldberg, M. T. Pindok, Acetylcholine and norepinephrine interactions on cardiac lipids and hemodynamics. *Am. J. Physiol. 228(6):* 1678–1684, 1975.
40. Goldberg, N.D. and M. K. Haddok, Cyclic GMP metabolism and involvement in biological regulation. *Ann. Rev. Biochem. 46:* 823–896, 1977.
41. Goldstein, A., L. Aronow, S. M. Kalman, *Principles of Drug Action: The Basis of Pharmacology,* Wiley, New York, pp. 27–47, 1974.
42. Grodner, A. S., H. G. Lahrtz, P. E. Pool, E. Braunwald, Neurotransmitter control of sinoatrial pacemaker frequency in isolated rat atria and in intact rabbits. *Circ. Res. 27*: 867–873, 1970.
43. Halvorsen, S. W. and N. M. Nathanson, In vivo regulation of muscarinic acetylcholine receptor number and function in embryonic chick heart. *J. Biol. Chem. 256(15)*: 7941–7948, 1981.
44. Hartzell, H. C., Distribution of muscarinic acetylcholine receptors and presynaptic nerve terminals in amphibian heart. *J. Cell. Biol. 86*: 6–20, 1980.
45. Hayes, J. S., L. L. Brunton, S. E. Mayer, Selective activation of particulate cAMP-dependent protein kinase by isoproterenol and prostaglandin E_1. *J. Biol. Chem. 255(11)*: 5113–5119, 1980.
46. Higgins, C. B., S. F. Vatner, E. Braunwald, Parasympathetic control of the heart. *Pharmacol. Rev. 25(1)*: 119–155, 1973.
47. Hoffman, B. B. and R. J. Lefkowitz, Radioligand binding studies of adrenergic receptors: new insights into molecular and physiological regulation. *Ann. Rev. Pharmacol. Toxicol. 20*: 581–608, 1980.
48. Hoffman, B. F. and P. F. Cranefield, *Electrophysiology of the Heart.* McGraw Hill, New York, 1960.

49. Hoffman, B. F., A. A. Siebens, C. M. Brooks, Effect of vagal stimulation on cardiac excitability. *Am. J. Physiol. 169*: 377–383, 1952.
50. Hollenberg, M., S. Carriere, A. C. Barger, Biphasic action of acetylcholine on ventricular myocardium. *Circ. Res. 26*: 527–536, 1965.
51. Ingebretsen, C. G., Interaction between alpha and beta adrenergic receptors and cholinergic receptors in isolated perfused rat heart: effects on cAMP-protein kinase and phosphorylase. *J. Cyclic Nucleotide Res. 6(2)*: 121–132, 1980.
52. Inui, J. and H. Imamura, Effects of acetylcholine on calcium-dependent electrical and mechanical responses in the guinea-pig papillary muscle partially depolarized by potassium. *Naunyn Schmiedebergs Arch. Pharmacol. 299*: 1–7, 1977.
53. Jacob, R., D. T. Miller, J. P. Gilmore, Significance of antiadrenergic effects of acetylcholine for contractility and action potential of the mammalian ventricular myocardium. *Artziche Forschung 25*: 141–153, 1971.
54. Jakobs, K. H., K. Aktories, G. Schultz, GTp-dependent inhibition of cardiac adenylate cyclase by muscarinic cholinergic agonists. *Naunyn Schmiedebergs Arch. Pharmacol. 310*: 113–119, 1979.
55. Jones, L. R., H. R. Besch, Jr., J. W. Fleming, M. M. McConnaughey, A. M. Watanabe, Separation of vesicles of cardiac sarcolemma from vesicles of cardiac sarcoplasmic reticulum. *J. Biol. Chem. 254*: 530–539, 1979.
56. Katsuki, S., W. Arnold, C. Mittal, F. Murad, Stimulation of guanylate cyclase by sodium nitroprusside, nitroglycerin and nitric oxide in various tissue preparations and comparison to the effects of sodium azide and hydroxylamine. *J. Cyclic Nucleotide Res. 3*: 23–35, 1977.
57. Keely, S. L., Jr. and T. M. Lincoln, On the question of cyclic GMP as the mediator of the effects of acetylcholine on the heart. *Biochim. Biophys. Acta 543*: 251–257, 1978.
58. Keely, S. L., Jr., T. M. Lincoln, J. C. Corbin, Interaction of acetylcholine and epinephrine on heart cyclic AMP-dependent protein kinase. *Am. J. Physiol. 234(4)*: H432–H438, 1978.
59. Kent, R. S., A. DeLean, R. J. Lefkowitz, A quantitative analysis of beta-adrenergic receptor interactions: resolution of high and low affinity states of the receptor by computer modeling of ligand binding data. *Mol. Pharmacol. 17*: 14–23, 1980.
60. Kohlhardt, M. and K. Haap, 8-bromo-guanosine-3′,5′-monophosphate mimics the effect of acetylcholine on slow response action potential and contractile force in mammalian atrial myocardium. *J. Mol. Cell. Cardiol. 10*: 573–586, 1978.
61. Koski, G. and W. A. Klee, Opiates inhibit adenylate cyclase by stimulating GTP hydrolysis. *Proc. Natl. Acad. Sci. USA 78*: 4185–4189, 1981.
62. Kuo, J. F., T. P. Lee, P. L. Reyes, K. G. Walton, T. E. Donnelly, Jr., P. Greengard. Cyclic nucleotide-dependent protein kinases. *J. Biol. Chem. 247(1)*: 16–22, 1972.
63. Krause, E. G., W. Halle, A. Wollenberger, Effect of dibutyryl cyclic GMP on cultured beating rat heart cells. In *Advances in Cyclic Nucleotide Research*, Vol. 1. Raven Press, New York, pp. 301–305, 1972.
64. Laduron, P. M. and P. F. M. Janssen, Characterization and subcellular localization of brain muscarinic receptors labelled in vivo by [^{3}H]dexetimide. *J. Neurochem. 33*: 1223–1231, 1979.
65. Lane, M. A., A. Sastre, M. Law, M. M. Salpeter, Cholinergic and adrenergic receptors on mouse cardiocytes in vitro. *Dev. Biol. 57*: 254–269, 1977.
66. LaRaia, P. J. and E. H. Sonnenblick, Autonomic control of cardiac cAMP. *Circ. Res. 28*: 377–384, 1971.

67. Lavellee, M., J. deChamplain, R. A. Nadeau, N. Yamaguchi, Muscarinic inhibition of endogenous myocardial catecholamine liberation in the dog. *Can. J. Physiol. Pharmacol. 56*: 642–649, 1978.
68. Lee, T. P., J. F. Kuo, P. Greengard. Regulation of myocardial cyclic AMP by isoproterenol, glucagon and acetylcholine. *Biochem. Biophys. Res. Commun. 45*: 991–997, 1971.
69. Lee, T. P., J. F. Kuo, P. Greengard, Role of muscarinic cholinergic receptors in regulation of guanosine 3′5′-cyclic monophosphate content in mammalian brain, heart muscle, and intestinal smooth muscle. *Proc. Natl. Acad. Sci. USA 69(1)*: 3287–3291, 1972.
70. Levy, M. N. and B. Blattberg, Effect of vagal stimulation on the overflow of norepinephrine into the coronary sinus during cardiac sympathetic nerve stimulation in the dog. *Circ. Res. 38*: 81–85, 1976.
71. Levy, M. N. and P. J. Martin. Neural control of the heart. In *Handbook of Physiology. The Cardiovascular System I.* American Physiological Society, Bethesda, Maryland, pp. 581–620, 1979.
72. Lincoln, T. M. and S. L. Keely, Effects of acetylcholine and nitroprusside on cGMP-dependent protein kinase in the perfused rat heart. *J. Cyclic Nucleotide Res. 6(2)*: 83–91, 1980.
73. Lincoln, T. M. and S. L. Keely, Regulation of the cardiac cyclic GMP-dependent protein kinase. *Biochim. Biophys. Acta 676*: 230–244, 1981.
74. Lindemann, J. P., H. R. Besch, Jr., A. M. Watanabe, Indirect and direct effects of the divalent cation ionophore A23187 on guinea pig and rat ventricular myocardium. *Circ. Res. 44*: 472–482, 1979.
75. Lindemann, J. P., L. R. Jones, D. R. Hathaway, B. G. Henry, A. M. Watanabe, Beta-adrenergic stimulation of phospholamban phosphorylation and Ca^{2+}-ATPase activity in guinea pig ventricles. *J. Biol Chem., 258*: 464–471, 1983.
76. Linden, J. and G. Brooker, The questionable role of cyclic guanosine 3′5′-monophosphate in heart. *Biochem. Pharmacol. 28*: 3351–3360, 1979.
77. Loffelholz, K. and E. Muscholl, A muscarinic inhibition of the noradrenaline release evoked by postganglionic sympathetic nerve stimulation. *Naunyn Schmiedebergs Arch. Pharmacol. 265*: 1–15, 1969.
78. Loffelholz, K. and E. Muscholl, Inhibition by parasympathetic nerve stimulation of the release of the adrenergic transmitter. *Naunyn Schmiedebergs Arch. Pharmacol. 267*: 181–184, 1970.
79. Manalan, A. S. and L. R. Jones, Characterization of the intrinsic cAMP-dependent protein kinase activity and endogenous substrates in highly purified cardiac sarcolemmal vesicles. *J. Biol. Chem. 257(17)*: 10052–10062, 1982.
80. McAfee, D. A., G. J. Whiting, B. Siegel, Neurotransmitter and cyclic nucleotide modulation of frog cardiac contractility. *J. Mol. Cell. Cardiol. 10*: 705–716, 1978.
81. McConnaughey, M. M., L. R. Jones, A. M. Watanabe, H. R. Besch, Jr., L. T. Williams, R. J. Lefkowitz, Thyroxine and propylthiouracil effects on alpha- and beta-adrenergic receptor number, ATPase activities, and sialic acid content of rat cardiac membrane vesicles. *J. Cardiovasc. Pharmacol. 1*: 609–623, 1979.
82. McCullough, T. E. and D. A. Walsh, Phosphorylation and dephosphorylation of phosphorylase kinase in the perfused rat heart. *J. Biol. Chem. 254(15)*: 7345–7352, 1979.
83. Meester, W. D. and H. F. Hardman, Blockade of the positive inotropic actions of epinephrine and theophylline by acetylcholine. *J. Pharmacol. Exp. Ther. 158*: 241–247, 1967.

84. Michell, R. H., Inositol phospholipids and cell surface receptor function. *Biochim. Biophys. Acta 415*: 81–147, 1975.
85. Mirro, M. J., J. C. Bailey, and A. M. Watanabe, Dissociation between the electrophysiological properties and total tissue cyclic guanosine monophosphate content of guinea pig atria. *Circ. Res. 45*: 225–233, 1979.
86. Mirro, M. J., J. C. Bailey, A. M. Watanabe, The role of cyclic AMP in regulation of the slow inward current. In *The Slow Inward Current and Cardiac Arrhythmias*, eds. D. P. Zipes, J. C. Bailey, and V. Elharrar, Martinus Nijhoff. The Hague/Boston/London, pp. 111–126, 1980.
87. Mirro, M. J., J. F. Harper, A. L. Steiner, Compartmentation of the cGMP in sinus node: subcellular localization by immunocytochemistry. *Circulation 62*: III–239, 1980.
88. Mirro, M. J., A. S. Manalan, J. C. Bailey, A. M. Watanabe, Anticholinergic effects of disopyramide and quinidine on guinea pig myocardium: mediation by direct muscarinic receptor blockade. *Circ. Res. 47*: 855–865, 1980.
89. Murad, F., Y. M. Chi, T. W. Rall, E. W. Sutherland, Adenyl cyclase. *J. Biol. Chem. 237(4)*: 1233–1238, 1962.
90. Nawrath, H., Does cyclic GMP mediate the negative inotropic effect of acetylcholine in the heart? *Nature 267*: 72–74, 1977.
91. Noble, D. *The Initiation of the Heart Beat*. Oxford, Clarendon Press, 1975.
92. Olson, D. R., C. Kon, B. M. Breckenridge, Calcium ion effects on guanylate cyclase of brain. *Life Sci. 18*: 935–940, 1976.
93. Ong, S. H. and A. L. Steiner, Localization of cyclic GMP and cyclic AMP in cardiac and skeletal muscle: immunocytochemical demonstration. *Science 195*: 183–185, 1977.
94. Pappano, A. J., P. M. Hartigan, M. D. Coutu, Acetylcholine inhibits the positive inotropic effect of cholera toxin in ventricular muscle. *Am. J. Physiol. 243*: H434–H441, 1982.
95. Paton, W. D. and H. P. Rang, The uptake of atropine and related drugs by intestinal smooth muscle of the guinea pig in relation to acetylcholine receptors. *Proc. Roy. Soc. (Lond.) (Biol.) 163B*: 1–44, 1965.
96. Quist, E. E., Evidence for a carbachol stimulated phosphotidylinositol effect in heart. *Biochem. Pharmacol. 31*: 3130–3132, 1982.
97. Robison, G. A., R. W. Butcher, E. W. Sutherland. *Cyclic AMP*. Academic Press, New York and London, 1971.
98. Rosenberger, L. B., H. I. Yamamura, W. R. Roeske, Cardiac muscarinic cholinergic receptor binding is regulated by Na^+ and guanyl nucleotides. *J. Biol. Chem. 255*: 820–823, 1980.
99. Ross, E. M. and A. F. Gilman, Biochemical properties of hormone-sensitive adenylate cyclase. *Ann. Rev. Biochem. 49*: 533–564, 1980.
100. Sadavongvivad, C., P. Sanvarinda, J. Satayavivad, Mechanism of catecholamine antagonism in rat heart produced by pilocarpine and related drugs. *Br. J. Pharmacol. 52*: 97–100, 1974.
101. Sarnoff, S. J., S. K. Brockman, J. P. Gilmore, R. J. Linden, J. H. Mitchell, Regulation of ventricular contraction: influence of cardiac sympathetic and vagal nerve stimulation on atrial and ventricular dynamics. *Circ. Res. 8*: 1108–1122, 1960.
102. Schultz, G., J. G. Hardman, K. Schultz, C. E. Baird, E. W. Sutherland, The importance of calcium ions for the regulation of guanosine 3′5′-cyclic monophosphate levels. *Proc. Natl. Acad. Sci. USA 70(12)*: 3889–3893, 1973.

103. Schwegler, M. and R. Jacob, Catecholamine antagonism of acetylcholine and dibutyryl guanosine 3′,5′-monophosphate in the mammalian ventricular myocardium. In *Recent Advances in Studies on Cardiac Structure and Metabolism,* Vol. 7, eds. P. Harris, R. J. Bing, and A. Fleckenstein. University Park Press, Baltimore, pp. 391–399, 1976.
104. Sharma, V. K. and S. P. Banerjee, Muscarinic cholinergic receptors in rat heart: effects of thyroidectomy. *J. Biol. Chem. 252(21)*: 7444–7446, 1977.
105. Sharma, V. K. and S. P. Banerjee, Presynaptic muscarinic cholinergic receptors. *Nature 272*: 276–278, 1978.
106. Snyder, S. H., K. J. Chang, M. J. Kuhar, H. I. Yamamura, Biochemical identification of the mammalian muscarinic cholinergic receptor. *Fed. Proc. 34*: 1915–1921, 1975.
107. Sperelakis, N. and J. A. Schneider, A metabolic control mechanism for calcium influx which may protect the ventricular myocardial cell. *Am. J. Cardiol. 37*: 1079–1085, 1976.
108. Strawbridge, R. A., K. W. O'Connor, A. M. Watanabe, Depression of canine cardiac adenylate cyclase activity by muscarinic cholinergic agonists: evidence that the effect is mediated by acceleration of the rate of decay of enzyme activity. *Clin. Res. 29:* 244A, 1981.
109. Story, D. D., M. S. Briley, S. Z. Langer, The effects of chemical sympathectomy with 6-hydroxydopamine on alpha-adrenoceptor and muscarinic cholinoceptor binding in rat heart ventricle. *Eur. J. Pharmacol. 57*: 423–426, 1979.
110. Stull, J. T. and S. E. Mayer, Biochemical mechanisms of adrenergic and cholinergic regulation of myocardial contractility. In *Handbook of Physiology. The Cardiovascular System*. American Physiological Society, Bethesda, Maryland, pp. 741–774, 1979.
111. Taniguchi, T., M. Fujiwara, J. J. Lee, H. Hidaka, Effect of acetylcholine on the norepinephrine-induced positive chronotropy and increase in cyclic nucleotides of isolated rabbit sinoatrial node. *Circ. Res. 45*: 493–504, 1979.
112. Ten Eick, R., H. Nawrath, T. F. McDonald, W. Trautwein, On the mechanism of the negative inotropic effect of acetylcholine. *Pflugers Arch. 361*: 207–213, 1976.
113. Tuganowski, W., P. Kopec, M. Kopyta, J. Wezowska, Iontophoretic application of autonomic mediators and cyclic nucleotides in sinus node cells. *Naunyn Schmiedebergs Arch. Pharmacol. 299*: 65–67, 1977.
114. Trautwein, W., Generation and conduction of impulses in the heart as affected by drugs. *Pharmacol. Rev. 15*: 277–332, 1963.
115. Trautwein, W. and G. Trube, Negative inotropic effect of cyclic GMP in cardiac fiber fragments. *Pflugers Arch. 366*: 293–295, 1976.
116. Vatner, S. F., J. D. Rutherford, H. R. Ochs, Baroreflex and vagal mechanisms modulating left ventricular contractile responses to sympathomimetic amines in conscious dogs. *Circ. Res. 44*: 195–207, 1979.
117. Vincent, N. H. and S. Ellis, Inhibitory effect of acetylcholine on glycogenolysis in the isolated guinea pig heart. *J. Pharmacol. Exp. Ther. 139*: 60–68, 1963.
118. Wallach, D. and I. Pastan, Stimulation of membranous guanylate cyclase by concentrations of calcium that are in the physiological range. *Biochem. Biophys. Res. Commun. 72(3)*: 859–865, 1976.
119. Watanabe, A. M. and H. R. Besch, Jr., Cyclic adenosine monophosphate modulation of slow calcium influx channels in guinea pig hearts. *Circ. Res. 35*: 316–324, 1974.

120. Watanabe, A. M. and H. R. Besch, Jr., Interaction between cyclic adenosine monophosphate and cyclic guanosine monophosphate in guinea pig ventricular myocardium. *Circ. Res.* *37*: 309–317, 1975.
121. Watanabe, A. M., D. R. Hathaway, H. R. Besch, Jr., Mechanism of cholinergic antagonism of the effects of isoproterenol on hearts from hyperthyroid rats. In *Recent Advances in Studies on Cardiac Structure and Metabolism,* eds. T. Kobayashi, T. Sano, and N. S. Dhalla, University Park Press, Baltimore, pp. 423–429, 1978.
122. Watanabe, A. M., L. R. Jones, A. S. Manalan, H. R. Besch, Jr., Cardiac autonomic receptors: recent concepts from radiolabelled ligand binding studies. *Circ. Res.* *50*: 161–174, 1982.
123. Watanabe, A. M., J. P. Lindemann, L. R. Jones, H. R. Besch, Jr., J. C. Bailey. Biochemical mechanisms mediating neural control of the heart. In *Disturbances in Neurogenic Control of the Circulation,* eds. F. M. Abboud, H. A. Fozzard, J. P. Gilmore, and J. P. Reis, Waverly Press, Baltimore, pp. 180–203, 1981.
124. Watanabe, A. M., M. M. McConnaughey, R. A. Strawbridge, J. W. Fleming, L. R. Jones, H. R. Besch, Jr., Muscarinic cholinergic receptor modulation of beta-adrenergic receptor affinity for catecholamines. *J. Biol. Chem.* *253(14)*: 4833–4836, 1978.
125. Wei, J. W. and P. V. Sulakhe, Regional and subcellular distribution of myocardial muscarinic cholinergic receptors. *Eur. J. Pharmacol.* *52*: 235–238, 1978.
126. Wei, J. W. and P. V. Sulakhe, Cardiac muscarinic cholinergic receptor sites: opposing regulation by divalent cations and guanine nucleotides of receptor-agonist interaction. *Eur. J. Pharmacol.* *62*: 345–347, 1980.
127. Wei, J. W. and P. V. Sulakhe, Requirement for sulfhydryl groups in differential effects of magnesium ion and GTP on agonist binding of muscarinic cholinergic receptor sites in rat atrial membrane fraction. *Naunyn Schmiedebergs Arch. Pharmacol.* *314*: 51–59, 1980.
128. Wilkerson, R. D., R. J. Paddock, W. J. George, Effects of derivatives of cyclic AMP and cyclic GMP on contraction force of cat papillary muscles. *Eur. J. Pharmacol.* *36*: 247–251, 1976.
129. Williams, L. T., R. J. Lefkowitz, A. M. Watanabe, D. R. Hathaway, H. R. Besch, Jr. Thyroid hormone regulation of beta-adrenergic receptor number. *J. Biol. Chem.* *252*: 2787–2789, 1977.
130. Yamada, S., H. I. Yamamura, W. R. Roeske, Alterations in cardiac autonomic receptors following 6-hydroxydopamine treatment in rats. *Mol. Pharmacol.* *18*: 185–192, 1980.
131. Yamamura, H. R. and S. H. Snyder, Muscarinic cholinergic binding in rat brain. *Proc. Natl. Acad. Sci. USA* *71*: 1725–1729, 1974.

7

Neural Modulation of Cardiac Metabolism

STEPHEN B. JONES and JOHN X. THOMAS, JR.

A review of myocardial metabolic processes is warranted not only to give a more complete physiological picture of neural control, but also to shed light on the role of cardiac nerves in response to ischemia (see chapter 10) and the potential importance of cardiac denervation to the human patient (see chapter 18). This chapter will focus mainly on myocardial oxygen consumption, with special reference to selected aspects of intermediary metabolism and substrate utilization that impact on important questions of neural control. For a more complete discussion of the effects of catecholamines on intermediary myocardial metabolism, the reader is referred to several reviews [4,9,12,15,26,28,33].

ACUTE EFFECTS OF CATECHOLAMINES

It is generally accepted that acute exposure of the working myocardium to catecholamines results in an increase in oxygen consumption that is disproportionately greater than the resultant increase in cardiac work performed. The monograph of Wilhelm Raab [27] provides an excellent review of both European and American literature prior to the 1960's concerning this efficiency relationship. Rabb however, appears to be the first to speculate about the inefficiency that catecholamines create in the working heart and initiated the concept of "oxygen wasting" effects of catecholamines in the myocardium. Evidence in support of Rabb's concept has accumulated since 1970 and is derived from a variery of physiological studies.

Oxygen wasting by catecholamines implies excessive oxygen consumption and might involve elevated oxygen consumption under all conditions. However, catecholamine-induced increases in basal myocardial metabolism in the non-beating heart are not impressive. In studies using polarographic measurements, resting oxygen consumption was not altered by norepinephrine or epinephrine exposure in isolated cat papillary muscle [6,24]. This conclusion can also be drawn from the myothermic studies by Gibbs and Gibson [16] where rabbit papillary muscle preparations were used. Resting metabolic demand was also not altered in cat papillary muscle preparations by exposure to norepinephrine where muscle metabolism was determined by quantitating the rate of fall of high-energy phosphates following anoxia [3]. In whole-heart preparations subjected to potassium-induced arrest, high doses of norepinephrine, epinephrine, and isoproterenol produced only small increments in oxygen consumption [23]. Thus, myocardial muscle metabolism (exclusive of contractile activity) does not appear to be influenced by catecholamines.

In contrast to oxygen consumption in the absence of contractile activity, there is substantial evidence that catecholamines contribute to excessive oxygen consumption with reduced efficiency in the working myocardial muscle. Sonnenblick et al. [30] conducted a series of experiments with anesthetized dogs on right heart bypass. In this preparation, stroke volume, heart rate, and aortic pressure were kept constant while the velocity of contraction was increased either by paired pacing, norepinephrine, or calcium infusion. Myocardial oxygen consumption increased dramatically in response to all three experimental conditions and was closely correlated with increases in the velocity of contraction. Calculated tension-time index decreased with all three forcings and was not considered to be as important a determinant of oxygen consumption. These authors concluded that the "oxygen wasting" effect of norepinephrine is related to the increase in the velocity of contraction. An additional study by this group [17] involved the isovolumic left ventricle preparation in which wall tension was held constant while contractility was increased. In this way myocardial oxygen consumption could be determined while contractility was increased and all other variables which influence metabolic demand were held constant. These results clearly show that myocardial oxygen consumption correlated well with increases in contractility.

The relationship of increased contractility and elevated oxygen consumption was examined further using isolated cat papillary muscle with tension generated both isotonically and isometrically [6]. Isometric contractions were examined under conditions of constant developed tension by decreasing initial muscle length after the contractile state was augmented by exogenous norepinephrine. With constant developed tension, the velocity of shortening was linearly related to myocardial oxygen consumption. These results suggest that developed tension may be constant but metabolic rate may increase with increased rate of shortening. Thus, the oxygen wasting effect involves the increase in speed of tension development during exposure to catecholamines. In the case where increased rate of tension development did not result in increased total tension, more oxygen would be required to produce the same work and thus energy efficiency would be decreased.

Additional evidence of the inefficient effect of catecholamines on myocardial metabolism via the contractile apparatus is presented in a metabolic study by Chandler et al. [3]. These experiments involved isolated papillary muscle preparations which were subjected to different levels of work and contractile states. Just prior to the experimental work load, the tissues were perfused with iodoacetic acid and rendered anoxic to inhibit adenosine triphosphate (ATP) production. After a defined period of work with such metabolic inhibition, tissues were frozen and analyzed for creatine phosphate and ATP content. During isometric work, muscle preparations exposed to norepinephrine used 115% as much high-energy phosphates as nontreated muscle; they also underwent 59% as many contractions and performed 87% as much work. These results suggest that increased contractility with exogenous norepinephrine results in a disporportionate amount of chemical energy released in relation to the amount of work performed. It is assumed that substrate utilization with reduction in tissue high-energy phosphates, with glycolytic inhibition and anoxia, is an accurate reflection of energy utilization.

In considering decreased metabolic efficiency with increased catecholamines it could be argued that reduced catecholamines should result in increased efficiency, i.e. greater myocardial performance for the same level of oxygen utilization. The possibility that the oxygen wasting effect of norepinephrine is reversed when catecholamines are reduced from a control level must be answered using preparations which have catecholamines present under "control" conditions, i.e. intact innervated hearts. To address this question of the absence of the effect of norepinephrine, the experimental situation of exposure to blocking dosages of propranolol or related compounds with simultaneous measurements of myocardial oxygen consumption and the rate of tension development would be useful.

McKenna et al. [25] measured myocardial oxygen consumption (MVO_2) in anesthetized dogs (both during rest and simulated exercise), left ventricular (LV) work, developed left ventricular pressure, and an index of efficiency (LV work/MVO_2). At rest or during exercise propranolol did not change efficiency to any significant extent but there were decreases in both cardiac output and MVO_2.

Warltier et al. [31] substantiated these findings but in the isolated, blood-perfused dog heart model. Several variables were compared under control conditions where coronary blood flow was set to produce a perfusion pressure of 85 to 90 mm Hg. Delivery of 0.5 mg/kg propranolol to two groups of control hearts was followed by 15 minutes of stabilization, after which the same variables as in control conditions were measured. Some variations in the magnitude of the responses between the two control groups are evident, but the directional changes in the mean values following propranolol are the same for both groups. Heart rate decreased as did LV dP/dt, contractile force, epicardial/endocardial blood flow ratio, and A-V O_2 content. Coronary artery perfusion pressure increased, as did coronary artery vascular resistance. Myocardial oxygen consumption was reduced by 29 and 19% in the two groups. Stroke work was not calculated since these were isovolumic preparations with intraventricular balloons. However, considering the decreases in heart rate, LV dP/dt, contractile force, and myocardial oxygen consumption, with constant coronary flow, it does not appear that oxygen consumption fell disproportionately compared to performance. Since these preparations had no neural connections, it can be concluded that acute propranolol administrations block the effect of circulating catecholamines (if any) or any effect due to the presence of sympathetic innervation. In any event, these data suggest that acute beta blockade does not alter the basic efficiency of energy utilization involved in the contracting myocardium.

In summary, the experimental data from a variety of preparations and laboratories over the past 15 to 20 years suggest that increasing catecholamines acutely in the working myocardium results in a decrease in efficiency of energy utilization, or "oxygen wasting." In contrast, the acute removal of catecholamines from the immediate environment of the working myocardial muscle is difficult to achieve. In vitro preparations have already been removed from neural connections and sympathetic tone is not easily mimicked. Attempts to address this question have involved beta blockade as a means of acute removal of catecholamines. Results of beta-blockade experiments have failed to demonstrate the opposite effect to that of acute catecholamine elevation, i.e. increased efficiency.

CHRONIC EFFECTS OF CATECHOLAMINES

The chronic influence of autonomic nerves on myocardial metabolism and coronary blood flow was examined in the conscious dog by Gregg et al. [18]. They emphasized cardiac performance and coronary hemodynamics in response to exercise and excitement in animals that had undergone cardiac denervation. Protocols in conscious dogs were conducted 2 to 4 weeks following surgical denervation and implantation of electromagnetic flow probes. Circumflex artery blood flow, measured with an electromagnetic flow probe, was 50% lower in denervated hearts compared to controls, during resting conditions. With exercise or excitement, this flow increased in denervated hearts, but again only reached 50% of the maximal increase observed in the controls. Myocardial oxygen utilization was estimated by combining coronary blood flow measurements with monitoring of O_2 content in coronary sinus blood with an oximeter technique. There were no differences in coronary sinus O_2 content between control and denervated hearts at rest. However, at the time of maximum coronary flow with exercise, denervated hearts had greater reductions in coronary sinus O_2 content than controls. Nevertheless, oxygen utilization during exercise was still greater in control dogs due to the greater increase in coronary flow. Cardiac output, measured with aortic (electromagnetic) flow probes, did not differ in amount of increase during exercise or excitement in the two groups. Calculated cardiac work (kg/min) also increased similarly in both groups in response to exercise and/or excitement. Thus, denervation of the myocardium resulted in a reduced requirement for coronary blood flow and oxygen delivery, both at rest and during increased work (in exercise and excitement).

Questions of the completeness of denervation seem resolved by evidence of depletion of myocardial catecholamines, and lack of responsiveness to tyramine and atropine throughout the periods that the studies were conducted. More specific variables that influence oxygen consumption such as myocardial contractility, wall tension, and the degree of pressure-work versus volume-work cannot be precisely determined from the results. However, the major finding of this work is that in the conscious dog, chronic cardiac denervation appears to significantly reduce coronary blood flow and myocardial oxygen demand. Considering the review of the in vitro studies, it can be speculated that these changes involve the absence of an oxygen wasting effect of the catecholamines. Such extrapolation of results from the conscious dog should be made with reservation until more careful examination of the actual determinants of myocardial oxygen consumption is achieved. That type of evidence has been reported by Jones et al. [21].

In contrast to the work of Gregg et al. [18] Jones et al. [21] utilized an anesthetized open-chest dog that had undergone selective surgical ventricular sympathectomy or sham treatment 3 weeks prior to the experimental protocol. This surgical procedure [22] results in nearly complete depletion of ventricular catecholamines and loss of inotropic and chronotropic responses to nerve stimulation. Coronary blood flow was determined with an electromagentic flow probe positioned near the origin of the circumflex artery, and values were corrected for ventricular weight by determining the distribution of the dye perfusion after each experiment. Oxygen extraction was determined using an on-line oximeter technique and intraventricular pressures were measured directly. Aortic pressure could be varied using a hydraulic balloon occluder and thus afterload could be manipulated. With this instrumentation, tension-time index was obtained by planimetry of the area under the systolic portion of the left ventricular pressure curve. In addition, left ventricular dP/dt was obtained from the pressure wave, and myocardial oxygen consumption per 100 g of tissue was determined using the A-V O_2 difference, and coronary flow was corrected for ventricular weight.

The experimental protocol was designed to examine oxygen demand and coronary blood flow at different levels of left ventricular performance which were achieved by changing aortic pressure over the range from 50 to 150 mm Hg. Comparison of the chronic sympathectomized animal was made with time-matched, sham-operated controls. The relationship of increases in mean arterial pressure and resultant increases in tension-time index were the same for both groups. However, at each level of tension-time index, the resultant increase in MVO_2 was much less in the sympathectomized than in the sham-operated heart. Similarly, increases in coronary blood flow resulting from increased tension-time index were much lower in sympathectomized than in sham-treated hearts. Changes in oxygen extraction, A-V O_2 (ml/100 ml), as a function of increased tension-time index were not different between the two groups, nor were increases in coronary blood flow as MVO_2 became elevated. These results mean that at constant heart rate and given level of ventricular pressure load, the requirement of the sympathectomized heart for oxygen (and thus blood flow) is 50% lower than that of the sham-operated group. The reduced oxygen demand was accompanied by a reduction in blood flow. Estimates of contractility using left ventricular dP/dt show the same magnitude of change as tension-time index is increased. However, regression analysis of increasing left ventricular dP/dt as a function of increased tension-time index indicated a significant difference in slope of sympathectomized and sham-operated regression lines. Functional significance of these differences is difficult to assess, due to a large overlap in data points. Lack of clear differences in contractility suggests that basic changes in contractility do not occur in this model of denervation. Maximum left ventricular dP/dt is influenced by factors other than contractility, namely afterload, pressure, and end-diastolic fiber length. Wall distensibility and ventricular end-diastolic volume, in turn, influence these variables but were not examined. One final consideration is that the reduced demand for oxygen led to a reduced flow demand, and coronary blood flow was decreased at all levels of performance in the sympathectomized hearts. This is supported by the finding of constant level of A-V O_2 differences in both groups at the different work levels. A widening of A-V O_2 differences with increased work would suggest additional oxygen extraction stimulated by O_2 demand that could not be met by coronary flow. Thus, the absence of response in sympathectomized animals suggests that O_2 demand is met by existing flow and that reduced coronary flow is a consequence of reduced O_2 demand. This study [21] implicates the sympathetic nerves in significant levels of oxygen utilization during both basal and elevated levels of myocardial performance. This alteration may not involve changes in left ventricular dP/dt.

Other contemporary studies of neural influences on myocardial metabolism have not presented the same clear changes as those of Gregg et al. [18] or Jones et al. [21]. In fact, some contend that opposite effects occur. Daggett et al. [7] examined the effects of autotransplantation of the canine heart on cardiac performance and oxygen consumption. Six to 12 weeks after denervation, animals were subjected to a terminal experiment under anesthesia to examine myocardial function, coronary vascular dynamics, and myocardial oxygen utilization. Invasive procedures included right heart bypass with controlled heart rate and aortic pressure while measuring aortic and left ventricular pressure and dP/dt. Measurement of blood gases across the heart permitted calculation of oxygen consumption using coronary flow. By varying the bypass pump speed, cardiac output could be increased stepwise at constant heart rate and aortic pressure. In this way, ventricular function curves were generated by plotting stroke work against left ventricular end-diastolic pressure. Furthermore, coronary vascular resistance was calculated. Data from this work indicate very little difference between autotransplanted and control animals. There were no differences in coronary vascular resistance, or myocardial oxygen consumption per gram of tissue. Although the major emphasis of the authors was that autotransplantation did not impair cardiac performance, these results are in conflict with the work of Gregg and Jones. Potential experimental differences which could contribute to the variant results include the use of bypass procedures and pump perfusion of the heart, although Jones' study involved open-chest preparations.

In contrast to the study of Daggett et al. [7], Barta et al. [1] suggested increases in oxygen requirements for the denervated heart with significant reductions in cardiac performance. These conclusions are also in contrast to those of Gregg et al. [18], and Jones et al. [21], and careful examination of the experimental methods is warranted. These experiments were conducted on closed-chest anesthetized dogs with cannulation of the coronary sinus via the jugular vein, and with assessment of coronary blood flow using the nitrous oxide washout technique. Denervation was accomplished by removal of cardiac nerves from the stellate ganglia, vagosympathetic trunk, and pretracheal plexus. Completeness of the denervation was assessed by stimulation of nerves and atropine administration. Experiments were conducted 14 to 18 days after denervation. The most striking results relate to marked decreases in cardiac work performed and decreased efficiency of the left ventricle in terms of work and oxygen consumption. Coronary flow and coronary vascular resistance measurements indicate reduced flow and/or increased vascular resistance. Decreases in cardiac work in the denervated heart are related to the observed 50% decrease in cardiac output and 25% reduction in arterial blood pressure. Heart rates were also reduced by 30% in denervated hearts, which most likely reflects vagolytic action of the anesthetic in predenervated animals. It would be more meaningful to compare cardiac output and mean arterial pressure at the same heart rate, both before and after denervation. These measurements impact directly on cardiac work and efficiency. That is, to accurately assess left ventricular work and efficiency both before and after denervation, heart rate and arterial blood pressure should be the same in both groups. Since these variables were not controlled, it is difficult to interpret these results.

Additional data from this study suggest that the denervated heart may have been hypoxic, in that coronary sinus blood showed greater lactate content than arterial blood, suggesting a net myocardial output of lactate. The presence of hypoxic conditions appears contrary to reduced levels of coronary blood flow and elevated coronary vascular resistance. If the denervated myocardium were truly hypoxic, one would predict that coronary vascular resistance would decrease, in an attempt to supply metabolic substrates to meet the demands of mechanical performance. It would be more reasonable to suggest hypoxic conditions with net lactate production and elevated coronary blood flow and resultant decreased coronary vascular resistance. Oxygen consumption in tissue slices of control (innervated) and denervated myocardium demonstrated a significant decrease in basal metabolism of the denervated tissue. Although these in vitro measurements do not consider muscle contraction, they are supportive of the work of Gregg et al. [18] and Jones et al. [21] indicating reduced oxygen requirements of the denervated myocardium.

An additional major study concerning the innervation of the heart in intact animals has been reported by Drake et al. [13]. The findings of these investigators are contrary to that of the above studies in that at 2–3 weeks following cardiac denervation, myocardial blood flow and oxygen consumption (corrected for external work) were significantly elevated. Left ventricular lactate consumption, also corrected for external work, was significantly elevated. Drake et al. [13] concluded that under basal conditions, the cardiac nerves restrict coronary blood flow and myocardial oxygen consumption. Data were based on paired animal experiments where control measurements made before denervation and subsequently compared with similar measurements on the same animals made 2–3 weeks after denervation. Appropriate measures were taken to ensure complete denervation, techniques seem adequately described, and the experimental design appears to be sound. Measurements of heart rate, arterial pressure, and determinations of oxygen content and metabolic substrates in coronary sinus blood samples appear adequate. Determinations of cardiac output and coronary blood flow were based on single-point determinations involving the microsphere principle. Cardiac output was determined by infusion of technetium-99 human albumin microspheres. Unfortunately, only a single determination of cardiac output was made for each animal during control and following denervation, rather than continuous measurements with flow probes or multiple measurements with thermodilution procedures. In addition, coronary blood flow was measured using radiolabeled microspheres (15 μ size) both under control conditions (prior to denervation) and 2–3 weeks following denervation. Both sets of measurements were made under anesthesia. These single determinations of coronary flow are very important because they were used to calculate left ventricular oxygen and lactate consumption based on arterial and venous blood samples. Thus, the accuracy of oxygen and lactate consumption values are directly proportional to the measured values of coronary flow. Drake et al. [13] also corrected the values of coronary flow, oxygen, and lactate consumption for differences in external cardiac work which is the product of arterial pressure and cardiac output. Thus, such values, corrected for external work, depend on a single measurement of cardiac output. There is no question that the microsphere method for the determination of peripheral organ blood flow, and in particular coronary blood flow, provides accurate and reliable values under appropriate experimental conditions. However, whether all microspheres, trapped within the myocardium during control measurements, remained within the myocardium during the 2–3 week period following denervation is not certain. Loss of microspheres from ischemic myocardium has been shown to occur by Capurro et al. [2]. If there were significant loss of microspheres from normal myocardial tissue, this would result in erroneously low values of coronary blood flow, and thus falsely high values of coronary blood flow following denervation. Furthermore, correcting these values for external cardiac work involves the use of mean arterial pressure and cardiac output measurements. Although the latter measurement was not complicated by tissue microsphere movement, as was coronary flow, there is a greater possibility of error in single measurements of cardiac output in contrast to multiple measurements with thermodilution or continuous measurements with a flowmeter. Both of these possibilities, inaccurate assessment of cardiac output (either high or low), and falsely low control values of coronary flow could explain the apparent differences between the results of Drake et al. [13] and those of Gregg et al. [18] and Jones et al. [21]. Furthermore, other studies assessing coronary blood flow present evidence that sympathectomy reduces blood flow or oxygen concentration [5,29]. In contrast, Holtz et al. [19] reported an increase in coronary flow in regions of the myocardium subjected to sympathectomy with 6-hydroxydopamine. Such increases in blood flow, however, were reported within 3 days after the sympathectomy and may represent acute changes in coronary flow which are quite different from those occurring 2–3 weeks after removal of sympathetic nerves. Thus, data relating the influences of the cardiac innervation on myocardial oxygen consumption are presently inconsistent, and firm resolution of this important question remains impossible.

POTENTIAL MECHANISMS RELATED TO NEURAL CONTROL OF CARDIAC METABOLISM

Mechanisms responsible for the acute "oxygen wasting" observed with increases in catecholamine exposure are not clear. Since the decrease in energy efficiency in the presence of elevated catechols appears to depend on muscle contraction and occurs with increased rate of tension development, there is probably an important link with ionic mechanisms involved with contraction and energy transduction. In the process of excitation–contraction coupling, the intracellular reuptake of Ca^{2+} released with excitation is an energy-dependent process in the sarcoplasmic reticulum. With catecholamines, the rates of contraction and relaxation are increased. It is possible that increased energy utilization required to meet the demands of increased rate of relaxation compounds the energy used for work performed. A disproportionate amount of energy may also be involved in increasing the rate of contraction with catecholamines. Cellular processes involved in regulation of intracellular calcium appear to be the most likely site of metabolic–mechanical changes observed with catecholamines.

Trophic influences of nerves on myocardial metabolism may contribute to the observed decreases in oxygen consumption. Oxygen wasting may in part be due to altered enzyme activity involved with energy transduction. Dowell [10] has demonstrated in rats subjected to 3 weeks of peripheral sympathectomy with 6-hydroxydopamine, that myofibrillar ATPase activity was significantly reduced in comparison to control animals. 6-Hydroxydopamine was administered at weekly intervals to assure depression of peripheral catecholamines exclusive of the adrenal medulla. The possible acute toxic effect of 6-hydroxydopamine on ATPase activity was probably not a factor since no ATPase changes were observed 16–18 hrs following sympathectomy. This suggests that the myocardial myofibrillar ATPase changes following chronic sympathectomy are related to trophic actions of the local sympathetic nerve terminal. Since the adrenal medulla is known to compensate for reduced sympathetic tone, with sympathectomy increasing its output of epinephrine, adrenalectomized animals were also examined. No further alterations in myofibrillar ATPase were observed following adrenalectomy in a sympathectomized animal. These results imply that stimulation of cardiac receptors alone (as with increasing circulating epinephrine) cannot replace the action of local nerve-stimulated release of neurotransmitters on ATPase enzymes. It is also important that sympathectomized animals have reduced mean arterial blood pressure (95 vs. 123 mm Hg in control rats). Thus, the possibility exists that reduced afterload in the sympathectomized group resulted in reduced myofibrillar ATPase activity. Additional experiments are required to rule out the effect of reduced afterload in Dowell's experiments. Such information would provide more details about the relationship between myofibrillar ATPase activity and intact sympathetic nerves in the myocardium.

An interesting follow-up study by Dowell [11] contrasted the previous chronic sympathectomy with chronic beta-receptor blockade on myocardial myofibrillar ATPase activity. Rats were given blocking doses of propranolol twice daily for 2 weeks. Completeness of beta blockade was confirmed with isoproterenol challenge. No alterations in myofibrillar ATPase activity were observed following this regimen of propranolol, indicating that reduced beta-receptor stimulation does not mediate the reduced myofibrillar ATPase activity following chemical sympathectomy. Dowell [11] hypothesized that some constitutent of nerve-stimulated norepinephrine release, which has trophic action on the myocardial muscle, may be involved in determining the metabolic demand capacity of the heart. Interesting comparisons are made with skeletal muscle, in which the neural innervation plays an important role in determining the metabolic characteristics of different fiber types. Such trophic input may also be important in the myocardium, although related more to the absolute degree of sympathetic innervation than to innervation by different nerve types. Additional experiments of this type with particular reference to chronically denervated dog models would be interesting and may offer important explanations for the observed metabolic characteristics of the denervated heart.

Alterations in intermediary metabolism of the myocardium by norepinephrine have been proposed by Drake et al. [14]. Such changes are based on observations involving the chronic sympathectomized dog heart. Glucose utilization and the examination of key intermediates in glycolysis were used to assess the activity of regulatory enzymes on glucose metabolism in myocardial muscle. Glucose utilization across the heart was examined using ^{14}C labeled glucose. Small ventricular biopsy samples were taken under control (predenervated) conditions and after 3 weeks of cardiac denervation involving the mediastinal neural ablation technique. All dogs served as their own controls. Myocardial tissues were assayed for adenosine triphosphate, creatine phosphate, glucose-6-phosphate, and fructose-6-phosphate, as well as enzyme activity of phosphofructokinase and glycerolphosphate dehydrogenase. Blood lactate, glucose, and free fatty acids were also determined.

These experiments show that 3 weeks following denervation there was a decrease in A-V difference for $^{14}CO_2$ and a decrease in $^{14}CO_2$ production as a percent of total CO_2 production during the infusion of radiolabeled glucose. In denervated dog hearts, fructose-6-phosphate levels were increased but there was no increase in glucose-6-phosphate. All other measured metabolites were not altered by the denervation procedure. These findings suggest that myocardial glucose metabolism is reduced in the chronic absence of neural innervation. Drake et al. suggested that the increased level of fructose-6-phosphate, with little alteration in glucose-6-phosphate, is due to a reduced level of phosphofructokinase activity, although in vitro activity of phosphofructokinase is not altered under optimal conditions. Regulation and control of phosphofructokinase is well known and widely studied. However, results of this study do not suggest any alterations in metabolites which might mediate the reduced activity in situ. Whether the observed changes are mediated directly by norepinephrine, or (more likely) through some intermediate which was not measured, cannot be determined from the data. This most interesting finding of altered intermediary metabolism resulting from chronic cardiac denervation has important implications. Potential differences in myocardial metabolism as a result of denervation could be important in reducing oxygen demand and increasing metabolic efficiency. Although this notion is still speculative, the hypothesis that cardiac denervation can result in more efficient utilization of fuel for contraction and that this condition is mediated by alterations in intermediary metabolism is worth pursuing.

An additional characteristic of chronic denervation of the heart is the increase in myocardial glycogen. This has been reported by Jellinek et al. [20] and by Willman et al. [32]. Daw and Berne [8] examined glycogen levels as well as enzymes of synthesis and degradation to focus on the possible mechanism of altered glycogen storage. Using cats 4 to 5 weeks after sympathectomy, Daw and Berne were unable to demonstrate increased enzyme activity of glycogen synthesis or decreased enzymes of glycogen mobilization. To our knowledge, no other reports examining the mechanism involved in increased glycogen stores with chronic denervation have been reported.

CONCLUSIONS

The most well-defined aspect of the action of catecholamines on myocardial metabolism is the acute "oxygen wasting" effect. This excessive energy utilization for a given work load is associated with increased rate of tension development. Specific information involving ionic mechanisms or changes in contractile elements that could account for the decrease in energy efficiency are simply not available. In light of the compromising action that nerve-stimulated release of norepinephrine or circulating catecholamines displays in heart patients, understanding the mechanism of acute oxygen wasting would be of great clinical value.

Chronic effects of catecholamines are less clear than the acute effects, although the best experimental evidence suggests that prolonged absence of catecholamines in the heart improves the efficiency of energy utilization. In contrast to the denervated heart, there are no good models of chronically increased sympathetic nerve activity. Aortic banding, hypertension, or other situations of increased sympathetic nerve activity are also complicated by increased afterload and other alterations which prevent the singular examination of increased nerve activity.

Alterations in cellular metabolism at best have only begun to characterize the phenomenon of altered metabolism resulting from cardiac denervation. In light of the proposed application of denervation in the human patient in this monograph and the experimental evidence suggesting significant reductions in ischemic damage when hearts are chronically sympathectomized, characterization of the denervated heart metabolism will be essential. Certainly the influence of sympathetic nerves on substrate utilization, hormonal control of intermediary metabolism, and intracellular mechanisms will be essential to extend the application of the denervation concept and to understand the physiological role of the cardiac nerves.

REFERENCES

1. Barta E., E. Breuer, E. Pappova, L. Zlatos, Influence of surgical denervation on the heart on the energetic metabolism and cardiac efficiency. *Exp. Med. Surg. 24*:319–333, 1966.
2. Capurro, N. L., R. E. Goldstein, R. Aamodt, H. J. Smith, S. E. Epstein, Loss of microspheres from ischemic canine cardiac tissue. *Circ. Res. 44*:223–227, 1979.
3. Chandler, B. M., E. H. Sonnenblick, P. E. Pool, Mechanochemistry of cardiac muscle III. Effects of norepinephrine on the utilization of high-energy phosphates. *Circ. Res. 22*:729–735, 1968.
4. Clark, M. G., G. S. Patten, O. H. Filsell, Evidence for an alpha-adrenergic receptor-mediated control of energy production in heart. *J. Mol. Cell. Cardiol. 14*:313–321, 1982.
5. Cobb, F. R., R. J. Bache, C. L. Curry, P. A. Ebert, P. A. McHale, J. C. Greenfield Jr. Sympathetic influences on coronary and aortic flow responses to increasing heart rate. *Am. J. Physiol. 255*:538–545, 1973.
6. Coleman, H. N., E. H. Sonnenblick, and E. Braunwald, Mechanism of norepinephrine-induced stimulation of myocardial oxygen consumption. *Am. J. Physiol. 221*:778–783, 1971.
7. Daggett, W. M., V. L. Willman, T. Cooper, C. R. Hanlon, Work capacity and efficiency of the autotransplanted heart. *Circ. Res.* Suppl. 1 to 35 and 36:I96–I104, 1967.
8. Daw, J. C. and R. M. Berne, Effect of sympathectomy on cardiac UDPG-glycogen transferase activity in the cat. *Am. J. Physiol. 213*:1480–1484, 1967.
9. Donald, D. E., Myocardial performance after excision of the extrinsic cardiac nerves in the dog. *Circ. Res. 34*:417–424, 1974.
10. Dowell, R. T., Myocardial contractile function and myofibrillar adenosine triphosphatase activity in chemically sympathectomized rats. *Circ. Res. 39*:683–689, 1976.
11. Dowell, R. T., Myofibrillar ATPase activity in rat heart after chronic propranolol administration. *Am. J. Physiol. 237 (Cell Physiol. 6)*: C195–C199, 1979.
12. Drake, A., Substrate utilization in the myocardium. *Bas. Res. Cardiol. 77*:1–11, 1982.
13. Drake, A. J., J. Stubbs, M. I. M. Noble, Dependence of myocardial blood flow and metabolism on cardiac innervation. *Cardiovas. Res. 12*:69–80, 1978.
14. Drake, A. J., D. E. Papadoyannis, R. G. Butcher, J. Stubbs, M. I. M. Noble, Inhibition of glycolysis in the denervated dog heart. *Circ. Res. 47*:338–345, 1980.
15. Gibbs, C. L., Cardiac energetics. *Physiol. Rev. 58*:174–254, 1978.
16. Gibbs, C. L. and W. R. Gibson, Isoprenaline, propranolol and the energy output of rabbit cardiac muscle. *Cardiovas. Res. 6*: 508–515, 1972.
17. Graham, T. P. Jr., J. W. Covell, E. H. Sonnenblick, J. Ross Jr., E. Braunwald, Control of myocardial oxygen consumption: relative influence of contractile state and tension development. *J. Clin. Inves. 47*:375–385, 1968.
18. Gregg, D. E., E. M. Khouri, D. E. Donald, H. S. Lowensohn, S. Pasyk, Coronary circulation in the conscious dog with cardiac neural ablation. *Circ. Res. 31(2)*:129–144, 1972.

19. Holtz, J., E. Mayer, E. Bassenge, Demonstration of alpha-adrenergic coronary control in different layers of canine myocardium by regional myocardial sympathectomy. *Pflugers Arch. 372*:187–194, 1977.
20. Jellinek, M., M. P. Kaye, C. A. Nigh, T. Cooper, Alterations in chemical composition of canine heart after sympathetic denervation. *Am. J. Physiol. 206*:971–974, 1964.
21. Jones, C. E., T. W. Hurst, J. R. Randall, Reduced oxygen and blood flow demands in the chronically sympathectomized heart. *Circ. Shock 9*:469–480, 1982.
22. Kaye, M. P., D. V. Priola, J. Coyle, Depletion of ventricular catecholamine levels following peripulmonary neurectomy. *Proc. Soc. Exp. Biol. Med. 135*:844–848, 1970.
23. Klocke, F. J., G. A. Kaiser, J. Ross Jr., E. Braunwald, Mechanism of increase of myocardial oxygen uptake produced by catecholamines. *Am J. Physiol. 209*:913–918, 1965.
24. Lee, K. S. and D. H. Yu, Effects of epinephrine on metabolism and contraction of cat papillary muscle. *Am. J. Physiol. 206*:525–530, 1964.
25. McKenna, D. H., R. J. Corliss, S. Sialer, W. C. Zarnstorff, C. W. Crumpton, G. G. Rowe, Effect of propranolol on systemic and coronary hemodynamics at rest and during simulated exercise. *Cir. Res. 19*:520–527, 1966.
26. Opie, L. H., Role of cyclic nucleotides in heart metabolism. *Cardiovas. Res. 16*:483–507, 1982.
27. Raab, W., *Preventive Myocardiology—Fundamentals And Targets*, C. C. Thomas, Springfield, Ill., 1970.
28. Randle, P. J. and P. K. Tubbs, Carbohydrate and fatty acid metabolism. In *Handbook of Physiology*, Sec. 2, *The Cardiovascular System*, Vol. 1, *The Heart*, eds. R. M. Berne, N. Sperelakis, and S. Geiger. Baltimore, Williams and Wilkins, pp. 805–844, 1979.
29. Scott, J. C. and T. A. Balourdas, An analysis of coronary flow and related factors following vagotomy, atropine and sympathectomy. *Circ. Res. 31*:129–144, 1972.
30. Sonnenblick, E. H., J. Ross Jr., J. W. Covell, G. A. Kaiser, E. Braunwald, Velocity of contraction as a determinant of myocardial oxygen consumption. *Am. J. Physiol. 209*:919–927, 1965.
31. Warltier, D. C., G. J. Gross, H. F. Hardman, Effect of propranolol on regional myocardial blood flow and oxygen consumption. *J. Pharmacol. Exp. Ther. 198*:435–443, 1976.
32. Willman, V. L., M. Jellinek, T. Cooper, T. Tsunekawa, G. C. Kaiser, C. R. Hanlon. Metabolism of the transplanted heart: effect of excision and reimplantation on myocardial glycogen, hexokinase and acetylcholine esterase. *Surgery 56*: 266–269, 1964.
33. Will-Sahab, L. and E. G. Krause, Effect on myocardial metabolism. In *Handbook of Experimental Pharmacology* 54/I adrenergic activators and inhibitors, Part 1, Ed. L. Szekeres. New York, Springer-Verlag, pp. 135–223, 1980.

8

Neural Modulation of Coronary Blood Flow

JOHN X. THOMAS, JR., CARL E. JONES, and WALTER C. RANDALL

In general, sympathetic outflows are thought to be widely divergent, and to activate simultaneously organ systems throughout the body. However, the concept of selective excitation of sympathetic nerves to highly restricted regions of the body, and even within individual organs, has gradually emerged. Restricted activation of chronotropic, inotropic, dromotropic, or vasomotor influences in the heart has been demonstrated. Recent experiments have convincingly demonstrated the existence of an alpha-adrenergic vasoconstrictor mechanism in the coronary circulation, but its specific distribution and its functional implications in the physiological regulation of coronary blood flow remain unclear. The specific locations of vascular receptors along the coronary blood vessels, i.e. whether the receptors are confined to the larger conduit arteries, whether they extend to the arterioles, or whether they may reach the venous side remain controversial questions. There are investigators who advocate each of these locations, but the facts are still emerging. It is also not known whether the vasomotor fibers are present only in selected nerve pathways or equally distributed throughout all the cardiac nerves. To date, there have been no demonstrations of their restricted presence in different portions of the coronary vascular system supplying the ventricles or any preferential portion of the ventricles. Still, intense coronary arterial vasospasm is frequently demonstrated angiographically to be highly localized within sharply defined segments of coronary arteries. It may develop spontaneously, in association with emotional disturbances or cold reflex stimulation; or it may be induced by ergot derivatives. Such vascular spasm may often (but not invariably) be relieved by dilator drugs, relief from emotional tension, or alpha-adrenergic blockade.

Original data reported in this chapter were derived from work supported by a Grant-in-Aid from the Chicago Heart Association, by the Bane Charitable Trust Fund, by NIH grants HL-20286 and HL-29243, and by a Grant-in-Aid from the American Heart Association with funds contributed in part by the Texas Affiliate. The authors are indebted to Mr. David DeFily for his assistance in the preparation of this chapter.

Is there a basal underlying vasoconstrictor tone in coronary blood vessels which limits flow? A recent question has surfaced from observations that perhaps a vessel sustaining partial organic obstruction is more sensitive to adrenergic vasoconstriction, or what would normally be an inconsequential constriction may become catastrophic when superimposed upon existing occlusive disease [6]. These are just a few of the current questions. We will discuss some of them in this chapter. There are many significant areas and associated articles which would be appropriate to discuss here but which have not been included; we regret these exclusions. However, our goal has been to introduce the reader to the area and provide some sense of the flavor of the current issues. We will not provide a comprehensive review. For a comprehensive treatment the reader should refer to two recent reviews of the coronary circulation by Berne and Rubio [4] and by Feigl [21]. Finally, there are many excellent articles which have not been cited due to space limitations; for this we sincerely apologize.

During the recording of contractile force from multiple isometric gauges located at different regions of the ventricles, hypothalamic or stellate ganglion stimulation will elicit generalized, positive inotropic responses from nearly all surfaces of the heart. However, as smaller individual cardiac nerves are excited, such responses become more localized. That is, as the electrodes are progressively shifted more distally along a given cardiac nerve, local test regions are successively deleted from the overall response, and relatively independent regulation of small epicardial segments of the myocardium is revealed. Comparable patterns of selective endocardial innervation have also been demonstrated in such localized segments as the anterior and posterior papillary muscles within a single ventricle [54]. Equally clear distinctions between cardioaccelerator and augmentor responses have been demonstrated by electrically stimulating individual cardiac nerves. While considerable overlap in innervation of particular muscle segments exists, such highly selective distributions are of great interest and potential importance. From these observations it is clear that comparable vasomotor responsiveness of individual coronary blood vessels would be of even greater significance. These have been studied in several laboratories [3,16,22,42,57].

MICROSCOPIC STUDIES

The heart receives innervation from both divisions of the autonomic nervous system with the major nerve trunks traveling with the large central arteries to the myocardium. Indeed, Woolard concluded from light microscopy that the coronary arteries received the richest innervation of any arterial system in the body [68]. Using methylene blue stains, he described nerve fibers coursing along the main coronary artery branches, some (thick fibers) being restricted to the outer adventitial layer and not penetrating the smooth muscle; these could be traced distally to the arteriolar and precapillary levels. Thinner, nonmyelinated fibers gave off branches to smooth muscle cells in the arterial wall. Woolard thought the larger fibers were parasympathetic since they persisted while the thin fibers decreased in density after stellectomy. Thus, the thinner fibers were interpreted to be sympathetic in origin, and the large arteries were said to be supplied by both sympathetic and parasympathetic nerves. In Woolard's view, the smaller vessels were innervated only by sympathetic fibers. Nonidez drew similar conclusions, again from light microscopic studies [50]. This important question has been reexamined by many anatomists [1,30,43] and there is general agreement that both small and large coronary arteries are supplied by both sympathetic and parasympathetic nerves [5,30]. In an extensive literature review, Feigl [21] found that alpha-receptor mediated vasoconstriction is more prominent in large coronary vessels than in small epicardial arteries and arterioles, but such observations have not yet been confirmed in the in vivo, beating heart. Clinical angiography has revealed large epicardial constrictions of magnitude similar to, or even greater than, those in smaller vessels even though anatomical descriptions describe markedly fewer nerve terminations within appropriate distances from smooth muscle components [11].

Development of the fluorescent antibody technique by Falck and Owman [15] permitted more precise differentiation of adrenergic nerves than did silver or methylene blue staining techniques. Dahlstrom [8] suggested that in the canine heart, sympathetic fibers form a matrix loosely associated with myocardial muscle cells, small arterioles, and venules [8]. Plexuses were found close to the outer layer of smooth muscle. The muscular arteries have a compact sheath of adrenergic fibers just inside the media, but they extend only a very short distance into the muscular media [13]. The number of fibers decreases with the size of the artery, and the smallest arterioles have only one or two fibers, often at opposite poles of the vessel. Thus, adrenergic fibers run down to the smallest precapillary arterioles, perhaps over to postcapillary venules, but generally without evidence of innervation of capillaries. Unfortunately, fluorescence technology lacks the resolution necessary for certainty in determining termination sites. Suehiro and Ninomiya [63] recently described differential reflex participation of pericoronary nerves coursing along the main conduit arteries and Shimizu et al. [62] provided a schematic drawing of these nerves. Dolezel et al. [11] also described the distribution of fluorescent fibers only at opposite poles of small coronary arteries. These investigators found very scanty innervation of small veins, and concluded it to be much more sparse than that of comparable size arteries.

The cholinergic innervation of the coronary arteries has been demonstrated by acetylcholinesterase staining techniques [10,48,58] with delineation of relatively large fibers coursing in the adventitia and fine fibers at the outer (adventitial) border of the media. The latter fibers presumably serve as the parasympathetic efferent supply to the vascular smooth muscle. They originate from ganglion cells within the heart itself since vagal transection does not ablate the acetylcholinesterase activity [10,47].

Identification of nerve endings by electron microscopy also remains incomplete. At the arteriolar level, nerve bundles are reduced to fibers 1.0 μ in diameter, with separation of 0.3–0.7 μ from the coronary arteriolar wall. Nerve endings, as indicated by loss of Schwann cell investment and appearance of light (parasympathetic) and dense (sympathetic) core vesicles, together with small mitochondria, approach smooth muscle to within 0.2 μ, but specialized neuromuscular junctions have not been clearly identified [37]. There is a surprising paucity of nerve terminals closely associated with the muscle cells in the walls of large arteries of the guinea pig atrium. Many nerves were found in the adventitia of large arteries, but they were clearly preterminal. Arterioles (60–25 μ) showed many more nerve terminals, separated by distances of 0.08–0.15 μ. The terminals were not evenly distributed, but were grouped into discrete areas around a given vessel. In this study, terminals were found to be common around both arterioles and true capillaries, but it could not be ascertained whether they subserve efferent or afferent function.

Both light and electron microscopic studies fail to find many nerve terminals in the media of large coronary arteries; only the outer smooth muscle cells are innervated [4]. This introduces a confusing note in view of profound spasm frequently observed during coronary angiography, or in association with neural stimulation. As one proceeds distally, frequency of nerve terminals associated with smooth muscle increases. Proximity of terminals to smooth muscle also increases toward the periphery. Hence, the major anatomic substrate for effective neural control lies at the level of smaller arteries and precapillary resistance vessels, as in other systemic beds. During nerve activation, transmitter is presumably released close to vascular smooth muscle, but due to diffusion distance, the transmitter may influence only the smooth muscle in the outer portion of the vessel wall.

Thus, while electrical activation of sympathetic nerves to the heart characteristically elicits positive inotropic, chronotropic, dromotropic, and metabolic effects in the myocardium, the net change is usually augmentation in coronary blood flow. Any alpha-receptor mediated vasoconstriction is generally masked by multiple dilator influences; these responses obscured the true constrictor effect until the advent of well defined adrenergic blocking agents. Many earlier workers concluded, therefore, that vasoconstrictor responses did not occur. However, given the anatomical substrate for such tonic and reflex implications of vasomotor pathways to the coronary vasculature, there remain interesting and potentially important questions concerning their physiological involvement. Since the pathways exist, their participation (independent of inotropic, chronotropic, dromotropic reflex limbs of any outflow from vasomotor control centers) must be taken into account.

BLOOD FLOW STUDIES

Parasympathetic Effects

Historically, the effects of parasympathetic activation on coronary blood flow have been controversial due to technical limitations and nonuniform experimental designs. Katz and Jochim [33] first presented convincing functional evidence of vagal innervation of the canine coronary circulation. In an isolated, perfused, fibrillating heart preparation, vagal stimulation caused increased coronary flow which was abolished by atropine. Also, bilateral vagotomy produced coronary vasoconstriction. Since that time, other experiments using flowmeter measurements of coronary blood flow have failed to detect significant changes in systolic or diastolic coronary resistance during vagal stimulation [9,59]. However, in these experiments, some important variables affecting coronary blood flow were not carefully controlled. More recently, Feigl [18] illustrated functional innervation of the canine coronary vessels. With an intact, paced dog heart preparation, vagal stimulation reduced arterial pressure (presumably due to vagal depression of ventricular contractile force) with a concurrent increase in mean circumflex flow. Calculations of late diastolic coronary resistance revealed a 58% decrease during vagal stimulation. The vasodilator effect was transient, lasting only 20 seconds from the onset of stimulation, and was abolished by atropine. Anatomical evidence supporting cholinergic innervation of the coronary arteries has been reported in some species. Recently, Pillay and Reid [51] reported cholinesterase reacting fibers converging on the outer muscular layers of canine coronary arteries with outside diameters between 0.6 and 1.0 mm. They also described arterial branches with diameters less than 0.3 mm with extensive cholinergic innervation, sometimes terminating in the media in acetylcholinesterase rich terminals. In dogs pretreated with guanethidine, the innervation pattern was not significantly different, indicating that the fibers were probably not of the sympathetic cholinergic type. In contrast, comparable size arteries in the baboon did not appear to be innervated by cholinergic fibers. Thus, species variability must also be considered. Gross et al. [23] have reported that activation of the canine coronary muscarinic receptors with a submaximal vasodilator dose of acetylcholine produced a redistribution of coronary blood flow favoring the subendocardium which was independent of mechanical influences. This vasodilation was blocked with atropine. Hackett et al. [27] found that chemoreceptor stimulation resulted in activation of a coronary vasodilator pathway which was blocked by atropine or bilateral vagotomy. Also, the coronary vasodilation that resulted from carotid sinus nerve stimulation was due, in part, to parasympathetic activation, though the major component of the vasodilation was due to withdrawal of alpha-adrenergic tone. Others have reported reflex parasympathetic activation in response to chemoreceptor stimulation [29,66]. Reflex coronary vasodilation (which was abolished by atropine or vagotomy) following intracoronary administration of veratrum alkaloids has also been described [20]. Although these investigators have made a strong case for the presence of parasympathetic innervation of the coronaries and the ability to activate these nerves under experimental conditions, their precise role in the intact human has not been established.

Sympathetic Effects

Resolution of the question of sympathetic regulation of coronary blood flow has been even more complex than for parasympathetic, because of its profound influence on the heart as a whole. The effects of the adrenergic nerves and their agonists have been reviewed [56]. Increases in heart rate and myocardial contractility are associated with production of metabolites capable of directly altering coronary resistance independent of neural mechanisms. Early on, this led to conclusions that sympathetic activation primarily resulted in coronary vasodilation. Alpha-receptor mediated vasoconstriction has been described, although the physiological role of such sympathetics is not yet thoroughly understood. Further complications have arisen due to the teleologic supposition that neurally mediated vasoconstriction would be "deleterious" for cardiac performance.

Sympathetic Cholinergic. Feigl [16] reported that stimulation of cardiac and lumbar sympathetics produced alterations in coronary and hind-limb blood flow in anesthetized dogs. Both the stellate and lumbar sympathetic trunks were stimulated by two electrodes in parallel. There was a marked increase in coronary flow, and sharp constriction in femoral flow, consequent to simultaneous left stellate stimulation and lumbar sympathetic chain stimulation. These were accompanied by increased pulse pressure and heart rate. After beta blockade with propranolol, left stellate stimulation produced little change in pulse pressure and heart rate but produced coronary vasoconstriction due to concurrent excitation of alpha receptors. When the alpha receptors were blocked by dibenzyline (in addition to beta blockade), the coronary bed became unresponsive to left stellate stimulation, and there was no increase in flow, even though cholinergic mechanisms remained intact. Since pharmacological blockade of adrenergic receptors eliminated all changes in coronary flow, there do not appear to be sympathetic cholinergic dilator fibers in the coronary circulation comparable to those known to exist in skeletal muscle in some species. Using the same preparation, Feigl demonstrated coronary dilatation during defense area stimulation. Stimulation in the supraoptic region of the anterior hypothalamus (adrenalectomized dog) elicited increases in coronary flow, pulse pressure, heart rate, and blood pressure simultaneously with skeletal muscle vasodilation. The cardiac effects were blocked with propranolol while the cholinergic dilator response remained in the skeletal muscle. Subsequent studies have documented increases in coronary vascular resistance attending cardiac nerve stimulation after beta adrenergic blockade [49].

Sympathetic Adrenergic: Beta Receptors. Activation of cardiac beta receptors can dilate coronary resistance vessels directly by activation of vascular receptors (beta-2), or indirectly by metabolic vasodilation secondary to increased myocardial oxygen requirements resulting from positive inotropic and chronotropic effects of the agonist (beta-1). Direct vascular effects have been observed in arrested hearts or in hearts which have received blocking doses of beta-1 receptors to minimize metabolic effects of sympathetic stimulation or agonist administration. Klocke et al. [36] reported that isoproterenol reduced coronary vascular resistance in the beating as well as the potassium-arrested canine heart. Since vasodilation occurred in the arrested heart, Klocke concluded that one component of this response was due to a direct vascular action and a mechanism was present for direct sympathetic vasodilation. Immediately thereafter, Zuberbuhler and Bohr [71] reported that isoproterenol caused relaxation of isolated coronary arterial helical strips both from large (1.5–2.4 mm) and small (250–500 μ) coronary arteries. Pitt et al. [52] reported the presence of both alpha and beta adrenergic receptors in the coronary arteries of unanesthetized dogs, independent of adrenergic receptors located in the myocardium. Intravenous or intracoronary catecholamines elicited beta-adrenergic receptor activity which was characterized by an early initial vasodilation occurring prior to any myocardial or systemic hemodynamic changes. Gross and Feigl [24] also found evidence of coronary beta-2 vasodilation following beta-1 blockade with practolol in a potassium-arrested canine heart. Thus, although the presence of coronary vascular beta receptors has been documented by several investigators, their physiological significance has not been established. When an in situ modified Langendorf preparation was used isoproterenol induced a dose-dependent coronary vasodilation after beta-1 blockade with practolol [28] in anesthetized dogs. Stellate stimulation following beta-1 blockade resulted in coronary vasoconstriction. After alpha blockade (Dibozane), stellate stimulation resulted in a small transient vasodilation which was still present after treatment with propranolol. The persistent vasodilation during stellate stimulation was unexplained. Hamilton and Feigl concluded that although there were beta-2 receptors present in the coronary circulation, the physiological effect of neural activation of these receptors was relatively minor. Domenech and MacLellan [12] recently reported that activation of the beta-2 receptors resulted in coronary vasodilation and redistributed myocardial blood flow toward the subepicardium. This phenomenon also was present in the empty beating heart, but was enhanced in the intact beating heart by the transmural resistance gradient to flow imparted by normal cardiac contraction. These results suggest a progressive decrease in beta-2 receptor density from subepicardium to subendocardium. Activation of these receptors during physiological stress, such as ischemia, may tend to exaggerate shifts in the endo/epi blood flow ratio. Most of the studies cited thus far have been from anesthetized, open-chest preparations or isolated vessel studies.

Vatner et al. [65] recently studied the effects of beta-adrenergic activation of large and small coronary arteries in conscious dogs. In these studies, large coronary artery cross sectional area (CSA) was calculated from dimensions measured by sonomicrometry and small-vessel caliber was assessed by calculating late diastolic coronary resistance (LDCR). Intravenous isoproterenol caused significant increases in both CSA and LDCR. However, the peak effect on LDCR preceded that on CSA. The reason for the different time courses was not determined, but the peak CSA occurred at a time when arterial pressure was still below control levels. Following beta-1 blockade with atenolol, isoproterenol still produced significant increases in both CSA and LDCR, although significantly less than before blockade. Surprisingly, beta-1 blockade attenuated the vasodilation of large coronary vessels more than in small coronary vessels. Pirbuterol, a selective beta-2 agonist, produced similar effects to isoproterenol after beta-1 blockade. Vatner et al. suggested that coronary vasodilation in responce to beta activation in the conscious dog results from (1) beta-1 stimulated increases in metabolism followed by metabolic vasodilation; (2) direct stimulation of coronary vascular beta-2 receptors; and (3) direct stimulation of vascular beta-1 receptors. However, the issue is far from settled since pharmacological activation of receptors and physiological activation of neural vasodilator pathways might represent totally different situations.

Sympathetic Adrenergic: Alpha Receptors. Sympathetic mediated coronary vasoconstriction has been demonstrated by several different investigators. Transient decreases in coronary blood flow following administration of catecholamines to in situ fibrillating dog hearts have been reported [3]. Feigl [16] found coronary vasoconstriction in anesthetized dogs during stellate ganglion stimulation following beta-receptor blockade with propranolol. This vasoconstriction was eliminated with phenoxybenzamine. Granata et al. [22] reported a small decrease in coronary blood flow at the onset of stellate ganglion stimulation in the unanesthetized dog. Zuberbuhler and Bohr [71] reported that helical strips taken from large coronary arteries occasionally contracted following exposure to catecholamines. These contractions were blocked by dibenzyline. Recently, it has been demonstrated that alpha-receptor stimulation increases coronary vascular resistance, but the large vessels account for only 60% of the increased resistance for the whole vascular bed [34]. Thus, constriction of the large coronary vessels contributes to the increased resistance following alpha-receptor activation, but is not the "dominant site" of vasoconstriction. Sympathetic vasoconstriction has been shown to influence myocardial oxygen tension [19] and limit metabolic vasodilation [44] and even limit the increase in coronary blood flow during exercise [25,46,61]. Reflex activation of the sympathetics via the carotid sinus has been shown to increase resistance in the left [17] coronary circulation of the dog and the right coronary circulation of both the dog and pig [14]. Whether coronary arterial resistance is under a continuous tone (vasoconstrictor) from the sympathetics remains a controversial question, although it has received considerable attention in both anesthetized and conscious dog preparations. In addition, Klassen and Armour [35], have recently raised the question as to whether autonomic innervation of the coronary veins might participate in the regulation of coronary blood flow and ventricular function by affecting the rate of venous outflow. This requires further investigation.

The interpretation of increases in coronary blood flow following alpha-receptor blockade is more complex and has recently been demonstrated in one of our laboratories (C. Jones, unpublished results). Pentobarbital anesthetized dogs were acutely prepared with an extracorporeal shunt to the left coronary arteries with perfusion pressure held constant by a servo pump. Left ventricular contractile force was monitored with a Walton-Brodie strain gauge arch. Myocardial arterial–venous oxygen differences were monitored on line with an Avox oximeter. Phenoxybenzamine (0.37 mg/min) for a total dose of (0.5 mg/kg), which blocks all alpha receptors and prazosin (0.15 mg/min), for a total dose of 2 mg, which blocks primarily alpha-1 receptors were administered to the heart through the shunt. Total left coronary stenosis was simulated by lowering the perfusion pressure from 90 to 50 mm Hg. Figure 8-1 shows the results from a typical experiment using phenoxybenzamine. In A, the perfusion pressure was

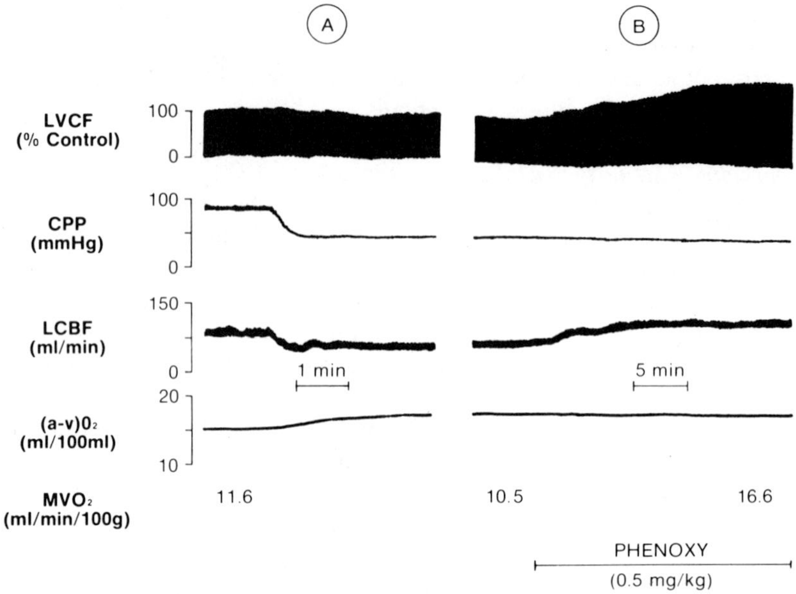

Fig. 8-1. Tracing of left ventricular contractile force (LVCF), coronary perfusion pressure (CPP), left coronary blood flow (LCBF), and arteriovenous oxygen differences before (A) and following (B) intracoronary administration of phenoxybenzamine. Calculated values for myocardial oxygen consumption are shown below.

lowered. Note the decrease in coronary blood flow and increase in oxygen extraction. The calculated value for myocardial oxygen consumption is shown at the bottom prior to the change in coronary perfusion pressure. After stabilization (B), phenoxybenzamine was slowly infused. It is clear that phenoxybenzamine resulted in a large increase in flow during coronary stenosis. However, the increase in flow was accompanied by large increases in contractile force and left ventricular oxygen consumption. Therefore it is difficult to discern whether the increase in flow resulted primarily from blockade of an alpha-constrictor tone or from the metabolic effects of the increase in cardiac performance. In this regard, the positive inotropic action of phenoxybenzamine may result in blockade of presynaptic alpha-2 receptors with an increased release of norepinephrine.

In order to address this question, the selective alpha-1 block of prazosin was employed and typical results are shown in Fig. 8-2. Note that prazosin infusion also resulted in an increase in flow, although not as great as that seen with phenoxybenzamine. Also, with prazosin there was no increase in left ventricular contractile force (LVCF). The increase in myocardial oxygen consumption seen with prazosin may have resulted from the abolition of vasoconstrictor tone and an increase in oxygen delivery to the ischemic myocardium. These results suggest that a vasoconstrictor tone is indeed present in the coronary circulation during ischemia and may limit oxygen delivery. A large portion of the increase in flow seen with phenoxybenzamine may result from postsynaptic alpha-1

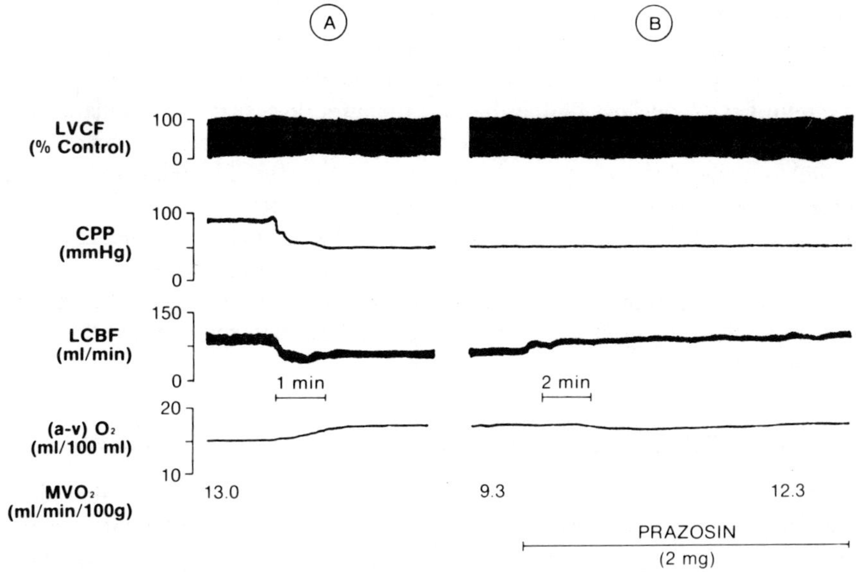

Fig. 8-2. Similar tracing to Fig. 8-1 (all abbreviations are the same) before (A) and following (B) the intracoronary administration of prazosin.

blockade, but a portion also seems to result from presynaptic alpha-2 blockade. This point becomes clearer if the ratio of the change in coronary flow to the change in myocardial oxygen consumption with phenoxybenzamine and prazosin are compared. Thus, with phenoxybenzamine (Fig. 8-1) this ratio was about 6 while with prazosin (Fig. 8-2) the ratio was about 10; this difference indicates that with phenoxybenzamine the change in flow was more closely associated with a change in myocardial oxygen consumption. With prazosin, the change in flow was more independent of the change in myocardial oxygen consumption, indicating a more direct vascular action of prazosin. The results shown in Figs. 8-1 and 8-2 typify those in four phenoxybenzamine experiments and five prazosin experiments. The mean results are summarized in the Table 8-1.

To summarize, total alpha blockade results in an increase in coronary blood flow which is due to (1) blockade of the alpha-1 receptor on the coronary vessel, and (2) blockade of the presynaptic alpha-2 receptor which results in increased norepinephrine release from the terminal which leads to an increase in contractile force and myocardial oxygen consumption.

The interpretation of increases in coronary blood flow following alpha-recep-

Table 8-1. Mean results

	LCBF	(A-V)O_2	LVCF	MVO_2
Phenoxy	+65%	−5%	+64%	+57%
Prazosin	+25%	−12%	+23%	+24%

tor blockade has been complicated by the recent report of Holtz et al. [32]. They found that alpha-2 blockade was more effective in blocking norepinephrine-induced contractions than alpha-1 receptor blockade. They analyzed changes in circumflex blood flow in anesthetized mongrel dogs that were spinalized at C-2, vagotomized, and had received beta blockers. The circumflex artery was cannulated and perfused at constant pressure with arterial blood. Alterations in coronary blood flow in response to adrenergic agonists were analyzed before and after selective alpha-1 or alpha-2 blockade. Holtz et al. concluded that norepinephrine contractions were mediated mainly through activation of postsynaptic alpha-2 receptors. Thus, considerable controversy exists as to the nature and physiological significance of the alpha adrenergic tone in the coronary arteries.

Adrenergic Influence on the Coronary Circulation of Conscious Animals

Several recent investigations have focused on alpha-adrenergic mediated alterations in coronary blood flow without the complicating factors of anesthesia and acute surgical trauma. In anesthetized, open-chest preparations, experiments have been designed to (1) accentuate adrenergic activity by physiological means (i.e. reflexes) or by administration of the neurotransmitter or some sympathomimetic agent; (2) eliminate the neural pathway; (3) eliminate the neurotransmitter by depletion or by blocking the appropriate receptor type. Vatner et al. [64] reported that intravenous norepinephrine resulted in a biphasic response in the coronary circulation of conscious dogs. Initially, there was vasodilation which was blocked by beta-adrenergic blocking agents, followed by vasoconstriction which was antagonized by phentolamine. Later, Vatner et al. [67] demonstrated in conscious dogs that large vessel coronary diameter (as measured with an ultrasonic dimension gauge) constricted below control levels and coronary vascular resistance increased by 92% following intravenous methoxamine. These changes were not attributable to alterations in myocardial metabolic demand or direct effects or arterial pressure on large coronary vessels. Vasoconstriction following an intracoronary injection of phenylephrine and norepinephrine (after beta blockade) has also been reported in conscious dogs [26]. Schwartz and Stone [60] have reported that the hyperemic response to a brief coronary occlusion was potentiated after removing the left stellate ganglion, suggesting a sympathetic mediated vasoconstrictor tone.

Holtz et al. [31] have reported substantial alpha-adrenergic coronary artery activity in the resting, conscious dog. Regional myocardial sympathectomy was accomplished by intracoronary administration of 6-hydroxydopamine directly into the circumflex artery. Mean myocardial blood flow was measured using radioactive microspheres and was found to be lower in normally innervated ventricular muscle supplied by left anterior descendens artery than in the center of the 6-hydroxydopamine-treated area. Subendocardial flow was substantially higher than that to subepicardial segments. These results demonstrated substantial alpha-receptor constrictor coronary tone operative in conscious dogs at rest, with similar magnitude in different layers of the ventricular wall. Following chemical sympathectomy of a restricted portion of the coronary vasculature, blood flow to the sympathectomized segments was 80% greater when compared with innervated segments of the same heart. Alpha blockade abolished the difference. Holtz et al. proposed that this sympathetic tone was required to maintain relatively low myocardial perfusion under steady-state conditons. This level of difference was surprising, but confirmed a similar finding of high constrictor tone by Vatner and McRitchie [66], who compared interactions between a chemoreflex and pulmonary inflation reflex controls of coronary circulation in conscious dogs. Nicotine stimulation of carotid chemoreceptors induced striking coronary dilatation with two components: (1) a minor component involving chemoreflex with efferent pathways in the vagi, and (2) a major component following increased depth in respiration, and its efferent pathway involved withdrawal of alpha-receptor constrictor tone.

These conclusions that resting coronary blood flow is under tonic restraint due to sympathetic vasoconstrictor activity in the conscious, resting dog have been strongly challenged [7]. Regional sympathectomy was produced by local epicardial application of phenol, and regional myocardial blood flow was measured in the conscious state under normal resting conditions, both before and after administration of adrenergic blocking agents. The findings extend the observations of Martins and Zipes [38] that cardiac sympathetic nerves traverse and penetrate the myocardium via the epicardial surface. Left sympathetic stimulation caused increased myocardial extraction ratios for oxygen and lactate in the normally innervated regions of the ventricle. This reduction in myocardial oxygen tension is not accompanied by development of myocardial anaerobic metabolism. Myocardial blood flow and its transmural distribution were not significantly different in normally innervated and sympathectomized regions of the ventricle under conscious, resting conditions. Blood flow was not altered in either region following adrenergic blockade. Thus, these data do not support the accumulating evidence for resting sympathetic coronary vasoconstrictor tone in the conscious animal.

CLINICAL EVIDENCE FOR CORONARY VASOSPASM

The hypothesis that coronary vasospasm causes angina was advanced by clinicians many years ago, most clearly in the recognition of angina of vasospastic origin by Prinzmetal [53]. The idea has reappeared recently in interpretations of "variant" angina [69,70]. Coronary angiography during attacks demonstrates severe spasm of one or more major coronary vessels that involves long conduit artery segments in a given patient during angina at rest [39]. These observations require revision of the traditional notion that angina ensues only when myocardial metabolic demand increases beyond the capability of coronary vessels to deliver oxygen. Maseri et al. [41] proved that there might not be an increase in myocardial metabolic demand before the episode of pain, and concluded that recurrent coronary arterial spasm appears to be the most likely mechanism.

Also, severe reductions in myocardial perfusion have been demonstrated during angina induced by rapid pacing [40]. At least some patients with "variant" angina respond favorably to treatment with alpha blockade [69].

Thus evidence is strong that sympathetic vasoconstrictor fibers have alpha-receptor characteristics, but virtually nothing is known about their patterns of distribution to the coronary vessels. The practical question of the exact stimulus that results in coronary arterial spasm also remains unanswered. The spasm has been described as (1) highly localized, (2) widely diffuse, (3) close to the catheter tip, (4) induced by ergot alkloids, and (5) present with or without localized sclerosis. Some workers have reported induction of coronary spasm with methacholine or epinephrine; many have assumed the autonomic nervous system is involved. Others have been unable to induce spasm in similar patients with pharmacological agents. In fact, there is no really good evidence that pharmacologically induced spasm is comparable to spontaneously occurring spasm.

To date, the crucial role of spasm in production of myocardial ischemia or infarction has not been established unequivocally [2]. However, in response to a cold stimulus, coronary vascular resistance increases more in patients with obstructive coronary artery disease than in those with radiographically normal coronary arteries; the constriction can be abolished by phentolamine [45].

Thus, the presence of alpha-adrenergic coronary vasoconstriction has been well demonstrated in recent years both in the experimental animal and in human patients, yet its role in coronary blood flow regulation has not been firmly established. Sympathetic coronary alpha-receptor vasoconstriction is effectively unmasked by beta-receptor blockade of metabolic regulation, and is a functional component of baro- and chemoreceptor reflexes. Substantial alpha-adrenergic activity may exist to maintain relatively low myocardial perfusion in the resting heart.

DIFFERENTIAL DISTRIBUTION OF CORONARY VASOCONSTRICTOR PATHWAYS; REGIONAL CORONARY ALPHA CONSTRICTION

Finally, we wished to determine how the alpha-adrenergic constrictor system is distributed to the heart. Are the nerves evenly distributed? Are they intermingled with those sympathetic nerves that have been shown to regulate highly localized inotropic, chronotropic, and dromotropic functions? To address these questions, a series of experiments was designed by Rinkema et al. [55] to determine the magnitude of coronary flow reduction which could be induced by strong stimulation of the vasoconstrictor nerves, and whether consistent patterns of constriction could be found in ventricular muscle. Since right and left stellate stimulation have different chronotropic and inotropic effects, it seemed logical to test whether different vasomotor controls exist.

Dogs anesthetized with pentobarbital, paced atrium, and decentralized cardiac innervation, were given a challenge dose of isoproterenol, followed by propranolol (1 mg/kg), with a second isoproterenol injection to test for beta-adrenergic blockade. When beta block was complete, radiolabeled microspheres (15

μ) were injected into the left atrium, to assess regional blood flow. Two to five minutes later, a second species of microsphere was injected during either right or left stellate ganglion stimulation. Microspheres were injected over a 20-second period, beginning 3–5 seconds after onset of nerve stimulation. Measurements of blood flow were made in eleven dogs during left stellate stimulation and in eleven dogs during right stellate stimulation. The heart was then fibrillated, excised, and the ventricles cut into 20 pieces, the latter further sectioned into smaller pieces for counting. The pieces were also cut into epi- and endocardial halves. The tissues were weighed and counted with reference to blood samples for radioactivity; blood flow was calculated from standard equations. A paired t-test was used to compare control and stimulation values for a single area. For tests among areas, an analysis of variance was employed.

Blood flows for right and left ventricles (ml/min/100 g) are shown in Table 8-2.

The first control data were collected 15 minutes after beta block. Mean right ventricular flow was 50 ± 4.7, while mean left ventricular flow was 82 ± 4.7. Right ventricular flow significantly decreased during left but not during right stellate stimulation. In the left ventricle, significant constriction followed both right and left stellate stimulation. Overall, this decrease averaged 17% of control during left and 10% during right stellate stimulation. The changes were not due to altered perfusion pressure or heart rate. LV oxygen extraction was measured using an A-VOX on-line oximeter, and LV oxygen consumption did not change. Figure 8-3 illustrates the manner in which the ventricles were divided in order

Table 8-2. Left and right ventricular blood flow

	Right stellate (n = 11)		Left stellate (n = 11)	
	Control	Stimul.	Control	Stimul.
Mean myocardial blood flow (ml/min/100 g)				
Right ventricle	45.9	43.8	55.0	44.1
(SEM)	±4.7	±4.4	±4.9	±6.4
Left ventricular base				
Endocardial	92.3	82.8	99.2	82.2
(SEM)	±7.6	±6.2	±7.8	±10.2
Epicardial	72.6	66.0	80.4	63.9
(SEM)	±6.6	±5.9	±6.9	±8.2
Left ventricular apex				
Endocardial	86.2	76.0	91.1	76.0
(SEM)	±7.4	±6.5	±8.1	±10.2
Epicardial	72.1	64.3	78.3	63.5
(SEM)	±6.2	±5.6	±6.4	±7.8
Mean arterial pressure, mm Hg	106.0	104.0	100.0	102.0
(SEM)	±7.0	±7.0	±7.0	±8.0
Left ventricular oxygen consumption	13.26	12.33	12.07	12.76
(ml/min/100 ±g)	±1.3	±0.96	±1.93	±2.34

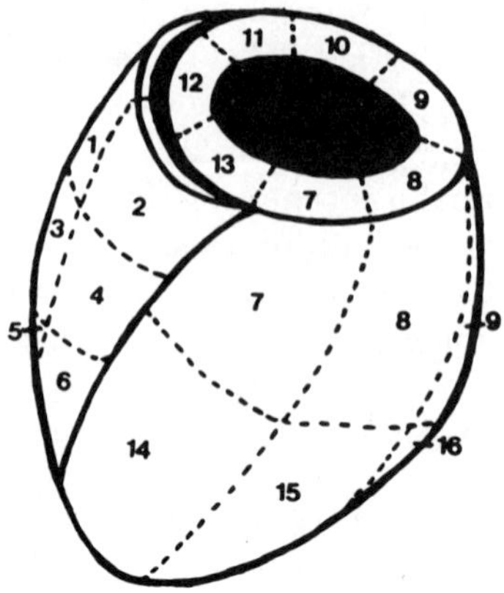

AREA	LOCATION
1 - 6	RIGHT VENTRICLE
1	Conus - Posterior
2	Conus - Anterior
3	Mid - Posterior
4	Mid - Anterior
5	Apex - Posterior
6	Apex - Anterior

AREA	LOCATION	AREA
BASE	LEFT VENTRICLE	APEX
7	Anterior Free Wall	14
8	Anterior-Lateral Free Wall	15
9	Posterior-Lateral Free Wall	16
10	Posterior Free Wall	17
11	Posterior Septum	18
12	Mid Septum	19
13	Anterior Septum	20

Fig. 8-3. Schematic drawing of the heart showing the way it was sectioned for radioactive counting. Right ventricular samples were transmural; left ventricular pieces were divided into endocardial and epicardial portions.

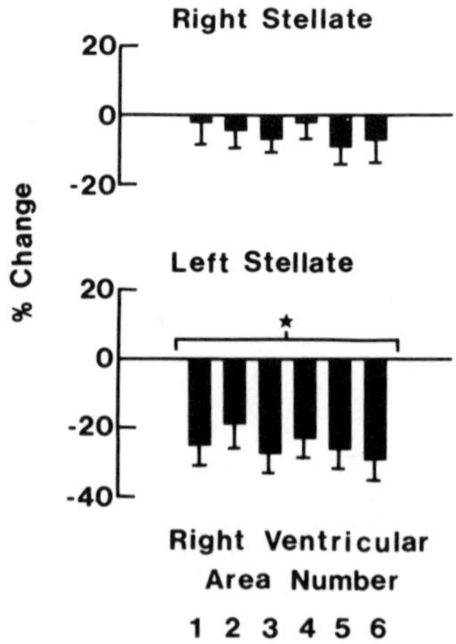

Fig. 8-4. Changes in blood flow elicited by right (RSS) and left (LSS) stellate stimulation in the right ventricular areas indicated in Fig. 8-3. No significant differences were found with RSS, but LSS caused a significant decrease (*$p < 0.05$) in blood flow to all areas of the right ventricle.

to achieve consistent comparisons and label counts from animal to animal. It also identifies each of the small ventricular segments in which separate blood flows were determined.

Figure 8-4 shows right ventricular areas 1–6, with transmural tissue segment blood flow changes during right stellate stimulation (above) and left stellate stimulation (below). During right stellate stimulation (at stimulation intensities previously shown to induce profound tachycardia), right ventricular blood flow changed only slightly, while left stellate stimulation elicited an average of 26% reduction in flow. There was little regional variation.

Figures 8-5 and 8-6 show similar data for the left ventricular areas 7–20 (from Fig. 8-4). Figure 8-5 shows the changes in flow in the left ventricular basal areas (7–13) during nerve stimulation. Right stellate stimulation induced a 7% change in epicardial segments. Left stellate stimulation produced nonuniform changes, 28% posteriorly and 16% anteriorly, all changes being significantly different from controls. The posterior wall constrictions were significantly greater than the anterior wall constrictions, suggesting a differential distribution of constrictor nerves along the circumflex and LAD arteries. Statistically significant changes were observed in endocardial flows during left stellate stimulation, but only in a few endocardial areas during right stellate stimulation. These results were essentially characteristic of the apical surfaces (areas 14–20), although the magnitude of the changes was somewhat less (13% during right and 23% during left stellate stimulation).

In summary, right and left stellate stimulation produced markedly different coronary artery vasoconstrictor responses, both in magnitude and in regional distribution within the ventricles. Right stellate stimulation produced little constriction except along the distribution of the LAD. In contrast, left stellate stim-

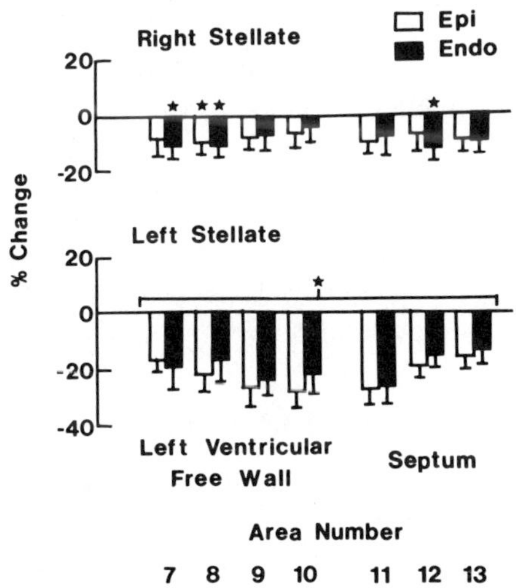

Fig. 8-5. Changes in blood flow elicited by RSS and LSS in the left ventricular base. Epicardial (open bars) and endocardial (solid bars) are shown. °$p < 0.05$.

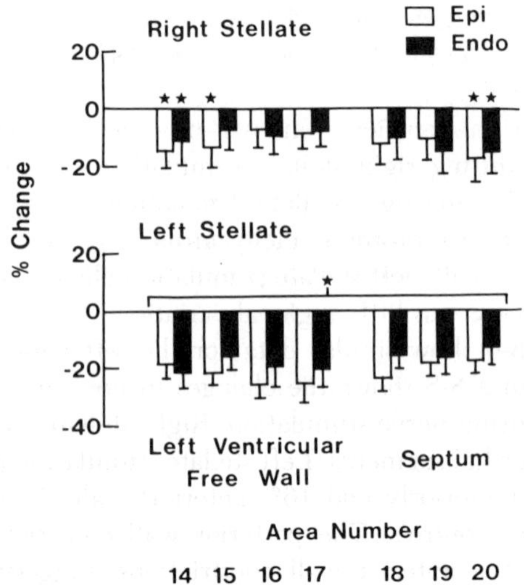

Fig. 8-6. Changes in blood flow in the left ventricular apex. During RSS, significant changes were observed only in the anterior left ventricle. Significant changes were seen in all areas following LSS. °$p < 0.05$.

ulation produced significant constrictions in all of the areas studied. The flow decrease was uniformly distributed across the endocardial surfaces, but in the epicardium, the decreases were more pronounced in the posterior regions, and greater in the circumflex than in the LAD distribution.

CONCLUSIONS

There is a great deal of experimental evidence indicating the presence of sympathetic and parasympathetic innervation in various segments of the coronary vasculature. A growing body of evidence supports the alpha-receptor innervation of arterioles. However, much work remains before the precise function of the innervation, in both normal and abnormal physiology, is understood. At present, there is little convincing evidence for a direct coronary sympathetic vasodilator system, although there have been several reports regarding the activation of a parasympathetic vasodilator system.

REFERENCES

1. Abraham, A. Die mikroskopische innervation des herzens und der blutgefasse von vertebraten, Budapest: Akademiai Kiado, Verlog der Ungarischen Akademie der Wissenschaften, 1964.
2. Arnett, E. N. and W. C. Roberts, Acute myocardial infarction and angiographically normal coronary arteries. An unproven combination. *Circ.* 53: 395–400, 1976.
3. Berne, R. M., H. DeGeest, M. N. Levy, Influence of the cardiac nerves on coronary

resistance. *Am. J. Physiol. 208*: 763–769, 1965.

4. Berne, R. M. and R. Rubio, Coronary Circulation. In *Handbook of Physiology. The Cardiovascular System,* eds. R. M. Berne and N. Speralakis. American Physiology Society, Washington, D.C., 1979 Sec. 2, vol. 1, Chap. 25, p. 873–952.
5. Boucek, R. J., R. Takshita, R. Fojaco, Relation between microanatomy and functional properties of the coronary arteries (dog). *Anat. Rec. 147*: 199–207, 1963.
6. Buffington, C. W. and E. O. Feigl, Adrenergic coronary vasoconstriction in the presence of coronary stenosis in the dog. *Circ. Res. 48*: 416–423, 1981.
7. Chilian, W. M., R. B. Boatwright, T. Shoji, D. M. Griggs, Jr., Evidence against significant resting sympathetic coronary vasoconstrictor tone in the conscious dog. *Circ. Res. 49*: 866–876, 1981.
8. Dahlstrom, A., K. Fuxe, M. Mya-tu, E. M. Zetterstrom, Observations on adrenergic innervation of the dog heart. *Am. J. Physiol. 209*: 689–692, 1965.
9. Denison, A. B., Jr. and H. D. Green, Effects of autonomic nerves and their mediators on the coronary circulation and myocardial contraction. *Circ. Res. 6*: 633–643, 1958.
10. Denn, M. J. and H. L. Stone, Autonomic innervation of dog coronary arteries. *J. Appl. Physiol. 41*: 30–35, 1976.
11. Dolezel, S., M. Gerova, J. Gero, T. Sladek, J. Vasku, Adrenergic innervation of the coronary arteries and the myocardium. *Acta Anat. 100*: 306–316, 1978.
12. Domenech, R. J. and P. R. MacLellan, Transmural ventricular distribution of coronary blood flow during coronary B-2 adrenergic-receptor activation in dogs. *Circ. Res. 46*: 29–36, 1980.
13. Ehinger, B., B. Falck, H. Persson, B. Sporrong, Adrenergic and cholinesterase containing neurones of the heart. *Histochemie 16*: 197–205, 1968.
14. Ely, S. W., D. C. Sawyer, D. L. Anderson, J. B. Scott, Carotid sinus reflex vasoconstriction in right coronary circulation of dog and pig. *Am. J. Physiol. 241 (Heart Circ. Physiol. 10)*: H149–H154, 1981.
15. Falck, B. and C. Owman, A detailed methodological description of the fluroscence method for the cellular demonstration of biogenic monoamines. *Acta Univ. Lund. II,* No. 7, 1–25, 1965.
16. Feigl, E. O., Sympathetic control of coronary circulation. *Circ. Res. 20*: 262–271, 1967.
17. Feigl, E. O., Carotid sinus reflex control of coronary blood flow. *Circ. Res. 23*: 223–237, 1968.
18. Feigl, E. O. Parasympathetic control of coronary blood flow in dogs. *Circ. Res. 25*: 509–519, 1969.
19. Feigl, E. O., Control of myocardial oxygen tension by sympathetic coronary vasoconstriction in the dog. *Circ. Res. 37*: 88–95, 1975.
20. Feigl, E. O., Reflex parasympathetic coronary vasodilation elicited from cardiac receptors in the dog. *Circ. Res. 37*: 175–182, 1975.
21. Feigl, E. O., Coronary physiology. *Physiol. Rev. 63*: 1–205, 1983.
22. Granata, L., R. A. Olsson, A. Huvos, D. E. Gregg, Coronary inflow and oxygen usage following cardiac sympathetic nerve stimulation in unanesthetized dogs. *Circ. Res. .6*: 114–120, 1965.
23. Gross, G. J., J. D. Buck, D. C. Warltier. Transmural distribution of blood flow during activation of coronary muscarinic receptors. *Am. J. Physiol. 240 (Heart Circ. Physiol. 9)*: H941–H946, 1981.
24. Gross, G. J. and E. O. Feigl, Analysis of coronary vascular beta receptors in situ. *Am. J. Physiol. 228*: 1909–1913, 1975.

25. Gwirtz, P. A. and H. L. Stone, Coronary blood flow and myocardial oxygen consumption after a-adrenergic blockade during submaximal exercise. *J. Pharmacol. Exp. Ther. 217*: 92–98, 1981.
26. Gwirtz, P. A. and H. L. Stone, Coronary blood flow changes following activation of adrenergic receptors in the conscious dog. *Am. J. Physiol. 243 (Heart Circ. Physiol. 12)*: H13–H19, 1982.
27. Hackett, J. G., F. M. Abboud, A. L. Mark, P. G. Schmid, D. D. Heistad, Coronary vascular responses to stimulation of chemoreceptors and baroreceptors. Evidence for reflex activation of vagal cholinergic innervation. *Circ. Res. 31*: 8–17, 1972.
28. Hamilton, F. N. and E. O. Feigl, Coronary vascular sympathetic beta-receptor innervation. *Am. J. Physiol. 230*: 1569–1576, 1976.
29. Hashimoto, K., S. Igarashi, I. Uei, S. Kumakura, Carotid chemoreceptor reflex effects on coronary flow and heart rate. *Am. J. Physiol. 206*: 536–540, 1964.
30. Hirsch, E. F. and A. M. Borghard-Erdle, The innervation of the human heart. I. The coronary arteries and the myocardium. *Arch. Pathol. 71*: 384–407, 1961.
31. Holtz, J., E. Mayer, E. Bassenge, Demonstration of alpha-adrenergic coronary control in different layers of canine myocardium by regional myocardial sympathectomy. *Pfluegers Arch. 372*: 187–194, 1977.
32. Holtz, J., M. Saeed, O. Sommer, E. Bassenge, Norepinephrine constricts the canine coronary bed via postsynaptic a2-adrenoceptors. *European J. Pharmacol. 82*: 199–202, 1982.
33. Katz, L. N. and K. Jochim, Observations on the innervation of the coronary vessels of the dog. *Am. J. Physiol. 126*: 395–401, 1939.
34. Kelley, K. O. and E. O. Feigl, Segmental a-receptor-mediated vasoconstriction in the canine coronary circulation. *Circ. Res. 43*: 908–917, 1978.
35. Klassen, G. A. and J. A. Armour, Epicardial coronary venous pressures: autonomic responses. *Can. J. Physiol. Pharmacol. 60*: 698–706, 1982.
36. Klocke, F. J., G. A. Kaiser, J. Ross Jr., E. Braunwald, An intrinsic adrenergic vasodilator mechanism in the coronary vascular bed of the dog. *Circ. Res. 16*: 376–382, 1965.
37. Malor, R., C. J. Griffin, S. Taylor, Innervation of the blood vessels in guinea-pig atria. *Cardiovasc. Res. 7*: 95–104, 1973.
38. Martins, J. B. and D. P. Zipes, Epicardial phenol interrupts refractory period responses to sympathetic but not vagal stimulation in canine left ventricular epicardium and endocardium. *Circ. Res. 47*: 33–40, 1980.
39. Maseri, A., A. L' Abbate, S. Chierchia, O. Parodi, Coronary artery spasm—diagnostic and therapeutic implications. *Am. Heart J. 96*: 554–555, 1978.
40. Maseri, A., A. L' Abbate, A. Pesola, C. Michelassi, M. Marzilli, M. De Nes. Regional myocardial perfusion in patients with atheroschlerotic coronary artery disease, at rest and during angina pectoris induced by tachycardia. *Circ. 55*: 423–433, 1977.
41. Maseri, A., R. Mimmo, S. Chierchia, C. Marchesi, A. Pesola, A. L' Abbate, Coronary artery spasm as a cause of acute myocardial ischemia in man. *Chest 68:* 625–633, 1975.
42. McRaven, D. R., A. L. Mark, F. M. Abboud, H. E. Mayer, Responses of coronary vessels to adrenergic stimuli. *J. Clin. Invest. 50*: 773–778, 1971.
43. Mitchell, G. A. G. and J. Learmouth, Anatomy of the autonomic nervous system. E. and S. Livingstone, Edinburgh, 1953.
44. Mohrman, D. E. and E. O. Feigl, Competition between sympathetic vasoconstriction and metabolic vasodilation in the canine coronary circulation. *Circ. Res. 42*: 79–86, 1978.

45. Mudge, G. H., Jr., W. Grossman, R. M. Mills, Jr., M. Lesch, E. Braunwald. Reflex increase in coronary vascular resistance in patients with ischemic heart disease. *N. Engl. J. Med. 295*: 1333–1337, 1976.
46. Murray, P. A. and S. F. Vatner, a-Adrenoceptor attenuation of the coronary vascular response to severe exercise in the conscious dog. *Circ. Res. 45*: 654–660, 1979.
47. Navaratnam, V., P. R. Lewis, C. C. D. Schute, Effects of vagotomy on the cholinesterase content of the preganglionic innervation of the rat heart. *J. Anat. 103*: 225–232, 1968.
48. Navaratnam, V. and A. Palkama, Cholinesterases in the walls of the great arterial trunks and coronary arteries. *Acta Anat. 60*: 445–448, 1965.
49. Nayler, W. G. and V. Carson, Effect of stellate ganglion stimulation on myocardial blood flow, oxygen consumption, and cardiac efficiency during beta- adrenoceptor blockade. *Cardiovasc. Res. 7*: 22–29, 1973.
50. Nonidez, J. F., Studies on the innervation of the heart. I. Distribution of the cardiac nerves, with special reference to the identification of the sympathetic and parasympathetic postganglionics. *Am. J. Anat. 65*: 361–413, 1939.
51. Pillay, C. V. and J. V. O. Reid, Histochemical localization of acetylcholinesterase in the wall of cardiac blood vessels in the baboon, dog, and vervet monkey. *Bas. Res. Cardiol. 77*: 213–219, 1982.
52. Pitt, B., E. C. Elliot, D. E. Gregg, Adrenergic receptor activity in the coronary arteries of the unanesthetized dog. *Circ. Res. 21*: 75–84, 1967.
53. Prinzmetal, M., R. Kennamer, R. Kerliss, T. Wada, R. Bor, Angina pectoris: 1. A variant form of angina pectoris. *Am. J. Med. 27*: 375–388, 1959.
54. Randall, W. C., J. A. Armour, W. P. Geis, D. B. Lippincott, Regional cardiac distribution of the sympathetic nerves. *Fed. Proc. 31:* 1199–1208, 1972.
55. Rinkema, L. E., J. X. Thomas, Jr., W. C. Randall, Regional coronary vasoconstriction in response to stimulation of stellate ganglia. *Am. J. Physiol. 243 (Heart Circ. Physiol. 12)*: H410–H415, 1982.
56. Ross, G., Adrenergic responses of the coronary vessels. *Circ. Res. 39*: 461–465, 1976.
57. Ross, G. and D. G. Mulder, Effect of right and left cardiosympathetic nerve stimulation on blood flow in the major coronary arteries of the anesthetized dog. *Cardiovasc. Res. 3*: 22–29, 1969.
58. Schenk, E. A. and A. E. Badawi, Dual innervation of the arteries and arterioles. A histochemical study, *Z. Zellforsch, Mikrosk. Anat. 91*: 170–177, 1968.
59. Schreiner, G. L., E. Berglund, H. G. Borst, R. G. Monroe, Effects of vagus stimulation and of acetylcholine on myocardial contractility, O_2 consumption, and coronary flow in dogs. *Circ. Res. 5*: 562–567, 1957.
60. Schwartz, P.J. and H. L. Stone, Tonic influence of the sympathetic nervous system on myocardial reactive hyperemia and on coronary blood flow distribution in dogs. *Circ. Res. 41*: 51–58, 1977.
61. Schwartz, P. J. and H. L. Stone, Effects of unilateral stellectomy upon cardiac performance during exercise in dogs. *Circ. Res. 44*: 637–645, 1979.
62. Shimizu, T., D. F. Peterson, V. S. Bishop, Reflex circulatory changes due to the afferent stimulation of the cat pericoronary nerve. *Am. J. Physiol. 235 (Heart Circ. Physiol. 4)*: H759–H766, 1978.
63. Suehiro, S. and I. Ninomiya, Pericoronary nerve mediates inhibitory sympathetic response to coronary occlusion. *Am. J. Physiol. 243 (Heart Circ. Physiol. 12)*: H170–H174, 1982.

64. Vatner, S. F., C. B. Higgins, E. Braunwald, Effects of norepinephrine on coronary circulation and left ventricular dynamics in the conscious dog. *Circ. Res. 34*: 812–823, 1974.
65. Vatner, S. F., T. H. Hintze, P. Macho, Regulation of large coronary arteries by B-adrenergic mechanisms in the conscious dog. *Circ. Res. 51*: 56–66, 1982.
66. Vatner, S. F. and R. J. McRitchie, Interaction of the chemoreflex and the pulmonary inflation reflex in the regulation of coronary circulation of conscious dogs. *Circ. Res. 37*: 664–673, 1975.
67. Vatner, S. F., M. Pagani, W. T. Manders, A. D. Pasipoularides, Alpha adrenergic vasoconstriction and nitroglycerin vasodilation of large coronary arteries in the conscious dog. *J. Clin. Invest. 65*: 5–14, 1980.
68. Woolard, H. H., The innervation of the heart. *J. Anat. Physiol. 60*: 345–373, 1926.
69. Yasue, H., M. Touyama, H. Kato, S. Tanaka, F. Akiyama, Prinzmetal's variant form of angina as a manifestation of alpha- adrenergic receptor-mediated coronary artery spasm: documentation by coronary arteriography. *Am. Heart J. 91*: 148–155, 1976.
70. Yasue, H., M. Touyama, M. Shimamoto, H. Kato, S. Tanaka, F. Akiyama, Role of autonomic nervous system in the pathogenesis of Prinzmetal's variant form of angina. *Circ. 50*: 534–539, 1974.
71. Zuberbuhler, R. C. and D. F. Bohr, Responses of coronary smooth muscle to catecholamines. *Circ. Res. 16*: 431–440, 1965.

9

Subsidiary Atrial Pacemakers and Their Neural Control

WALTER C. RANDALL, STEPHEN B. JONES,
STEPHEN L. LIPSIUS, and GEORGE J. ROZANSKI

In 1907, Keith and Flack reported a group of "primitive fibers" at the junction of the superior vena cava and the right atrium which they believed to be responsible for the origin of the mammalian heart beat [25]. In the same year, Erlanger and Blackman found that the right auricle, in the vicinity of the mouth of the great veins, possessed the highest degree of automaticity of any cells within the heart [9]. Martin Flack, a student of Keith, published additional details in 1910 and concluded that this area was, in fact, the pacemaker region of the heart [15]. He also noted that the vagus and sympathetic nerves exerted their main influences on this region of the heart. In commenting on an anatomical description of the nodal region by Davies [7] several years later, Keith reaffirmed this localization and told how

> One very hot day in 1906, my wife and I, returning from a bicycle ride, were bade by Martin Flack to look through the microscope at a very strange structure he had found at the junction of the superior vena cava and the right auricle. The structure was muscular but quite different from the musculature round about . . . we set to work and found it at the same site in all the mammalian hearts at our disposal. In structure it resembled the node of Tawara; hence we inferred it to be the site at which the cardiac rhythm was normally initiated. (ref. 26)

Electrophysiological identification of the region is traced primarily to Lewis, who stimulated this region at the base of the superior vena cava to yield a complex closely resembling that of a normal beat [28]. He further reported "the point of primary negativity" to be directly superficial to the Keith-Flack node [29]. These results were confirmed by Eyster and Meek who also observed shifts

Experimental data derived from research grants HLO8682, HL28205, HL27652, Chicago Heart Assoc. grants C80-12, C81-12, The Bane Charitable Trust Fund, Chicago, Ill., and the James DePauw Fund of Chicago, Ill.

within the nodal region during vagal stimulation, during KCl injection, or during local applications of cold [11,12].

Brooks and Lu [4] observed that the innovative microelectrode and intracellular recording techniques of Gerard et al. [17,30] marked the beginning of a new era in studies of cardiac pacemakers [1946–49]. It became possible to differentiate pacemaker cells from other myocardial cells as well as to localize more precisely the functional pacemakers. Cells with spontaneous diastolic depolarization were found first in the false tendon of the dog and kid hearts by Coraboeuf and Weidmann in 1949 [6] and later by Draper and Weidmann [8]; still later in the frog sinus by Trautwein and Zink [52], and finally in the rabbit S-A node by West in 1955 [62]. Primary pacemaker function was found still later to be confined to specific types of nodal cells [53] and intracellular recordings have since demonstrated shifts in dominant pacemaker sites within the node [33,34,51].

SUBSIDIARY PACEMAKER IDENTIFICATION

Early observations demonstrated the ability of A-V node or even ventricular tissue to initiate the heart beat when S-A node tissues were blocked or damaged [34], and it has been shown that such lower pacemakers are actually suppressed by normal S-A node driving rates [27,32]. Thus, while the heart beat normally originates in the S-A node of mammalian hearts, there are subsidiary cells that can effectively generate a heart beat. These classical teachings [9,11–13,28–29,36,54], together with the clinical impression that the A-V node assumes the role of pacemaker when the sinus node stops functioning or fails to transmit impulses [46], have received recent experimental support [54–55, 58–60]. Within the A-V node there are cells designated as P cells which are thought to be comparable to those in the sinus node [20,24]; these conceivably could serve as substitute pacemakers [61]. This view is highlighted in most cardiac electrophysiology chapters in modern physiology texts. However, the concept must now be revised to allow for the functional performance of well-documented auxiliary pacemakers available within restricted portions of the right atrium [39]. This is not to say that all atrial cells are capable of generating pacemaker potentials for, clearly, they are not. However, specific cells within the atrium but outside the S-A node are fully capable of rescuing the heart from standstill or the relatively slow rates of junctional or idioventricular escape rhythms. Sealy et al. clearly demonstrated the functional dominance of a permanent, low, right atrial pacemaker site in dog hearts in which the S-A node had been surgically excluded from the remaining atrium [48–50].

Clear understanding of the hierarchy of supraventricular pacemakers is of more than academic interest and importance. Since Ferrar [14] emphasized the so-called sick sinus syndrome in 1973, much attention has been directed to sinus dysfunction and the sick sinus (escape) syndrome [35]. Cardiac surgeons need to recognize the sites of secondary pacemakers as they plan their incisions for correction of structural defects or for interruption of pathways involved in rhythm disturbances. Corrections of transposition of the great vessels, following the general design of the Mustard procedure, may be complicated by serious dysrhythmias. The latter could be prevented or greatly attenuated by careful placement of incisions so as to avoid critical areas harboring subsidiary pacemaker cells [5]. Finally, interaction and competition among subsidiary atrial pacemakers (SAPs) deserve special attention in considering degrees of overdrive suppression, and in marked variability in ultimate achievement of stable pacemaker function.

IN VIVO EXPERIMENTS

In 1970 our laboratory reported that excision of the S-A node released residual pacemaker activity arising within the right atrium [16]. Discrete excision of only the S-A node, verified histologically, is followed by a supraventricular (atrial) rhythm in both resting and exercising dog models. The ECG is characterized by a definite P-wave, normal P-R interval, and is associated in time with the atrial electrogram. Waxing and waning in heart rate, generally referred to as sinus arrhythmia, continues in the awake animal after complete excision of the S-A node. This arrhythmia is responsive to both adrenergic and cholinergic interventions, thus indicating the presence of both sympathetic and parasympathetic regulation of the functionally dominant subsidiary atrial pacemaking tissues [38]. More recently an additional study was conducted, in which a longer segment of atrial tissue along the sulcus terminalis (3–4 cm), including the S-A node, was excised in a group of dogs that was studied chronically in the conscious state. After a brief interval in which the cardiac rhythm alternately shifted from an inferior atrial site to one in the junctional zone, a stabilized P-wave with a P-R interval of 80 to 100 msec became established. The period of relative instability lasted from only a few moments or hours to a few days. Maximum heart rates in this group of awake animals demonstrated the following comparisons:

Functional comparisons of S-A node and SAP

	Maximum Heart Rate		
	SAN	SAP	p value
Nembutal	133	97	0.005
Exercise	276	219	0.001
Isoproterenol	272	226	0.001
Stellate stim.	273	197	0.001

In these comparisons, a clear hierarchy of functional performance appeared in which the intact S-A node pacemakers possessed predominance, followed by the subsidiary atrial, the A-V junctional, and finally by ventricular pacemakers. Once S-A node primacy was destroyed, however, the subsidiary atrial pacemakers demonstrated capacity to successfully control cardiac performance, and they were immediately and effectively responsive to neurohumoral regulation

[22]. Employing an epicardial suction electrode in reference to plunge electrodes in fixed positions within the atrium, the SAP was definitively localized just superior to the inferior vena cava–inferior right atrial junction in 80% of the test animals. In a related study, a group of animals was maintained for 3–10 months after excision of the S-A node together with the sulcus (crista) terminalis. A junctional rhythm appeared immediately after surgery, followed by an unstable ectopic atrial rhythm which persisted at varying times during the first postoperative week in 94% of the dogs. Pacemaker instability was characterized by spontaneous pacemaker shifts and periodic episodes of asystole. The latter persisted for several weeks or months in some of the dogs. In contrast to the sinus arrhythmia which characterized all of the dogs before surgery, the ectopic atrial arrhythmias were not related to respiration, but promptly disappeared after atropine or during treadmill exercise.

In a recent series of experiments described by Boineau, Schuessler et al. [1–3,47], multiple epicardial electrode pickups suggested a multicentric origin of right atrial pacemakers. These locations were generally situated within or close to the classical Keith-Flack region (point B), at a superior right atrial-posterior SVC location (point A), or several millimeters caudal to the Keith-Flack region (point C). While these specific locations do not correspond to those detected by an exploring electrode used to map the SAPs in our chronic animal models [22,23], they do reinforce our contention that viable auxiliary pacemakers exist within the right atrium, and that they are capable of assuming functional control in the event the S-A node ceases to operate.

Thus, the electrophysiological data of Boineau et al., the surgical experiences of Sealy et al., and our prolonged studies in conscious animals in which the S-A node has been totally ablated, are clearly incompatible with the concept that when the sinus node defaults, the major subsidiary pacemaker is confined to the A-V junctional region [61].

Thus, after surgical ablation of the S-A node as histologically [11–12,13,36] and electrophysiologically [28,29] identified in the classical literature, follow-up ECG and atrial electrograms in the conscious, normally performing animal, reveal consistent patterns of pacemaker location, progressing from temporary focus in the A-V junction to permanent location in the inferior right atrium. To examine more precisely the emergence of SAPs under acute conditions, a protocol was designed in which the S-A node and adjacent tissue along the sulcus terminalis were surgically excised in sequential but multiple segments. Under chloralose anesthetic and prior to the initial excision, the focus of initial activation was found in all animals to be in the classical area of the S-A node, and discharging regularly at a rate of 130/min (Fig. 9-1). Four successive excisions were made and four different foci of excitation origin were localized by the exploring electrode following the excisions. There was stepwise reduction in rate with each successive excision until the final rate of 60/min was reached. The electrogram sequences at the bottom of the figure compare activation at the exploring suction electrode located within the proximal but intact segment of the sulcus with that at each of the stationary electrodes. The figure depicts the sites of each successive excision with a solid dot representing location of the

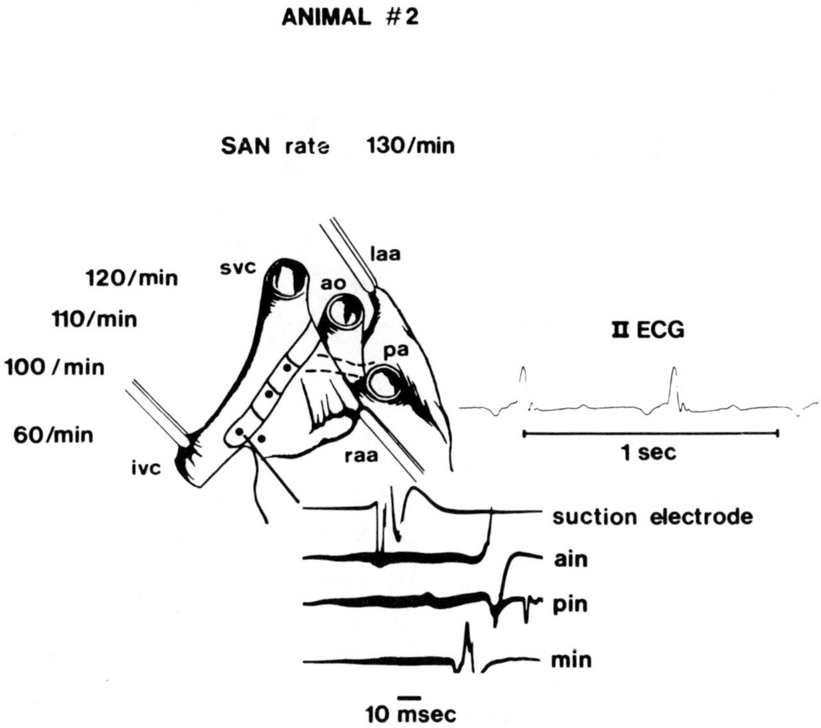

Fig. 9-1. Schematic diagram of exposed myocardium indicating epicardial foci of initial electrical activation following sequential excisions of the SAN (S-A node) and adjacent sulcus terminalis in the dog. ivc, inferior vena cava; svc, superior vena cava; ao, aorta; laa, left atrial appendage; pa, pulmonary artery; raa, right atrial appendage (retracted). ECG and electrical activation sequences are illustrated for the third focus (arrow). Fixed bipolar plunge electrodes were located in the regions of the anterior (ain), posterior (pin), and middle (min) internodal pathways which were in Bachman's bundle, Eustachean ridge, and limbus of the fossa ovalis, respectively. (From ref. 23, with permission of the authors and the American Physiological Society)

residual focus after each excision. Lead II of the ECG was recorded simultaneously with the electrogram sequence and is characterized by an inverted P-wave and normal (115 msec) P–R interval. The P-wave was concurrent with the stationary electrograms. The time interval between suction electrode and (min) electrograms was consistently attenuated by moving the suction electrode in any direction away from the anatomic position indicated by the solid circle. After the fourth excision, the focus was not at the A-V junction, but an inverted P-wave persisted and the initial area of activation was close to the suture line but still in atrial tissue. Note also the retrograde activation of the superior (ain) electrogram. These locations and rates of atrial ectopic firing support the concept that the A-V junctional region is not the fastest pacemaker in the absence of the S-A node and indicate that the atrial ectopic pacemakers are intermediate in the hierarchy of cardiac pacemakers in the dog [23].

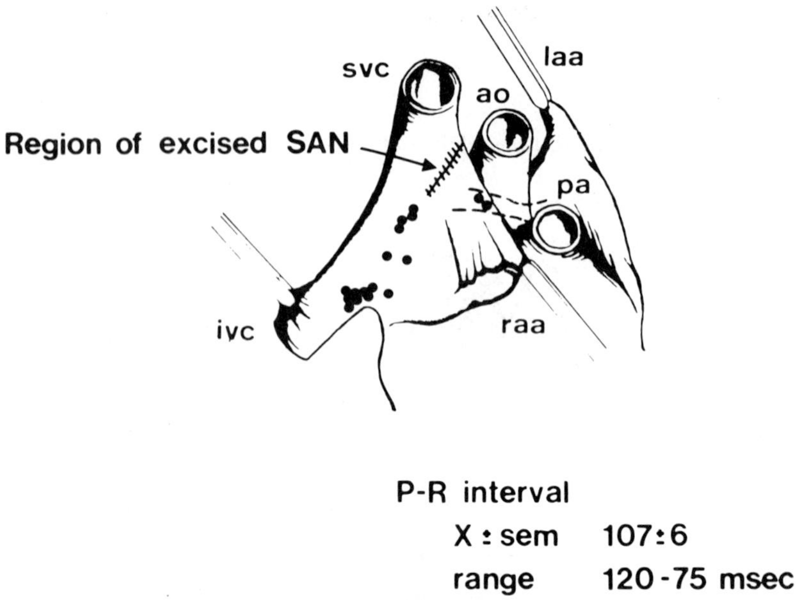

Fig. 9-2. Composite representation of atrial ectopic pacemaker locations and P–R intervals from a series of 12 canine experiments in which the SAN (S-A node) region had been removed (cross-hatched). Labels as in Fig. 9-1. Solid circles show locations of initial activation, mapped electrophysiologically, as the SAPs emerged following successive, acute, small segmental excisions along the sulcus terminalis. (From ref. 23, with permission of the authors and the American Physiological Society)

Figure 9-2 is a composite of atrial ectopic pacemaker locations and P–R intervals summarizing this series of acute animal experiments [23] in which the classical S-A node region and adjoining sulcus terminalis were surgically removed and in which the right atrium was electrophysiologically mapped subsequent to SAP stabilization. All of the pacemaker locations were along the sulcus terminalis, or in the atrial free wall just superior to the junction of the inferior vena cava and the right atrium.

"Selective perfusion" of the S-A node region as originally described by James and Nadeau [19] and more recently elaborated [56,59–60] to allow mathematical comparison of S-A node and A-V junctional pacemaker discharge rates, is thought by some to involve exclusive distribution to the S-A node by way of the node artery. However, injection of contrast media [37], radioactive microspheres [63], or vitally staining dyes [18] directly into the S-A node artery clearly demonstrates explicit atrial vascular distribution to much of the free wall of the right atrium as well as to portions of the interatrial septum. The distribution areas clearly include SAP sites along the crista terminalis and inferior right atrium [18].

Well documented studies using the technique of cannulation and perfusion of the sinus node artery with cholinergic drugs provide strong evidence for the existence of A-V junctional pacemakers [21,54,57,58,60]. Although the validity of the experimental results are not challenged, the notion that these data secure the argument that the A-V junction is the site of the next fastest cardiac pacemaker in the absence of the S-A node [60] seemed untenable. Accordingly, a concentrated solution of highly visible dye was injected directly into the S-A node artery, permitting visualization of dye distribution patterns from both epicardial and endocardial surfaces of the open atrium [18]. Figure 9-3 illustrates a typical distribution of indocyanine green following injection into the S-A node artery near its origin from the right coronary artery. On the epicardial surface (Fig. 9-3A & B), dye extended well beyond the S-A node region to include nearly the entire posterior atrial wall, as well as the atrial sections of the superior and inferior vena cava and even the azygos vein. Dye is visible also in part of

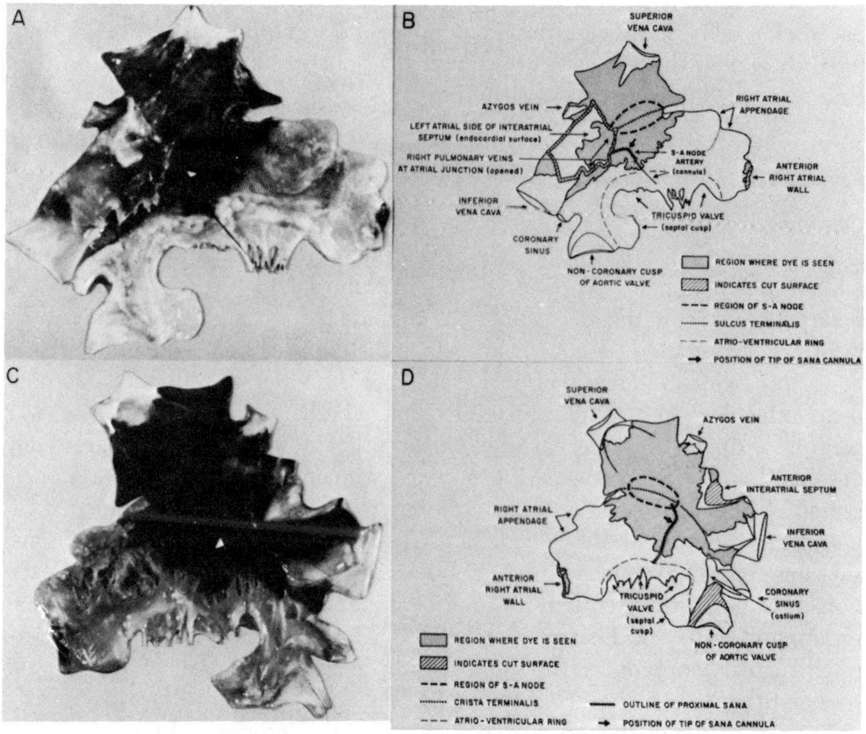

Fig. 9-3. Right atrium of dog heart displayed for visualization of dye (indocyanine green) distribution after its injection into the SANA (S-A node artery). (A) Epicardial surface showing location of SANA cannula tip (white arrow). (B) Identification of anatomic structures in A. Cannula tip (arrow) was about 1.5 cm from SANA origin. Note dye distribution to region of the SAN, but also to inferior atrium, portions of interatrial septum, and junctions with large veins. (C) Endocardial surface, and (D) anatomical correlates of C. Note wide distribution area for dye to the SAN, surrounding region, crista terminalis, atrial septum, and inferior atrium. Dye extended up to, but not beyond, coronary sinus ostium. (From ref. 18, with permission of authors and the American Physiological Society)

the interatrial septum (left side) and in the atriopulmonary venous junction. The anterior atrial wall and most of the atrial appendage were free of dye.

The endocardial distribution (Fig. 9-3 C & D) included much the same areas as shown in the epicardium. In addition, however, dye extended beyond the septal border of the posterior atrial wall into the interatrial septum (right side), up to, but not beyond, the ostium of the coronary sinus. The dye was more concentrated on the endocardial surface.

These dye distribution patterns clearly show that S-A node artery distribution is not exclusively to the S-A node but is widespread to much of the right atrium, including the sulcus terminalis and a large portion of the free wall. These regions incorporate the tissue immediately rostral to the junction of the inferior vena cava and the right atrium, precisely the location of subsidiary pacemakers following destruction or removal of the S-A node. Thus, cholinergic drugs infused via the S-A node artery would suppress the SAP as well as the S-A node pacemaker cells. So much atrial tissue is exposed to suppressive drugs administered by way of the S-A node artery that A-V junctional pacemakers must then emerge to dictate the dominant rhythm.

HOLTER MONITORING STUDIES

Our experiments have documented the functional existence, and even the probable anatomical localization of the SAPs in the dog right atrium. We next wished to functionally characterize the SAP and compare them with the S-A node pacemakers in the alert, conscious animal model. Employing Holter monitoring, we compared 24-hour heart rate and rhythm traces in intact, conscious dogs, both before and after surgical excision of the S-A node [40]. Mean 24-hour heart rates were not significantly different, whether under S-A node or SAP control for the first few days or weeks after surgery, although they progressively decreased with time in the SAP group and remained significantly lower for a period of months. Under resting conditions, propranolol failed to influence 24-hour heart rates in either S-A node or SAP-controlled animals. While junctional rhythms commonly (but not invariably) occurred immediately after SAN excision, P-waves with essentially normal configuration reappeared within a few minutes or hours and became stabilized within a few days or weeks. Electrophysiological mapping of the right atrium after stabilization of the P-wave revealed the earliest site of activation to be along the sulcus (crista) terminalis or at the junction of the inferior vena cava and the inferior right atrium.

Figure 9-4 illustrates the heart rate and rhythms recorded by Holter monitoring or cardiac electrograms in the conscious dog before (A–D), at the time of S-A node excision (E–F), and immediately after S-A node excision (G–L), including tracings during sympathetic and parasympathetic blockade. Panel A represents the normal resting rhythm, and is marked by clear, well-formed complexes and normal intervals. A respiratory arrhythmia of sinus origin is apparent with asystoles of 1.22 second duration and average heart rate of 75/minute. Neither heart rate nor duration of asystole were noticeably altered by a blocking dose of propranolol during quiet rest (B). Atropine (intramuscular,

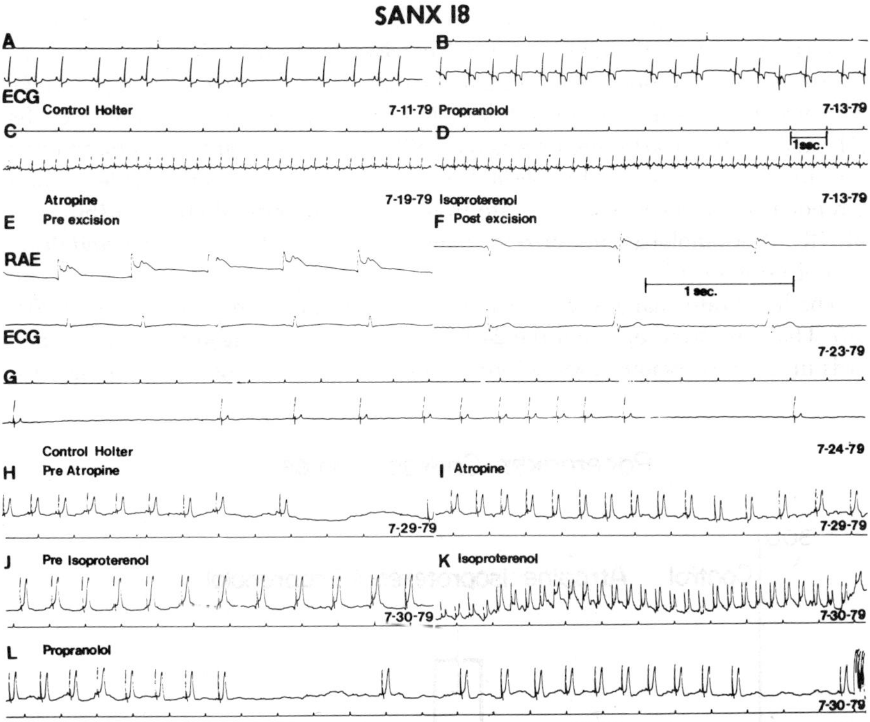

Fig. 9-4. Separate ECG strips from Holter monitor during preoperative control, quiet rest (A), after propranolol (B), atropine (C), and isoproterenol (D). Note different dates, reflecting different 24-hour series for each tracing. E shows simultaneous ECG and right atrial electrogram (RAE) during pentobarbital anesthesia, immediately before excision of the SAN. F was recorded immediately after excision; note shifting pacemaker. G was from Holter monitor on day after excision—note "wandering pacemaker" and prolonged asystoles. H is pre- and I post-atropine; J is pre- and K is post-isoproterenol injection. L shows response to large oral dose of propranolol. (From ref. 40, with permission of authors and the American Physiological Society)

2.0 mg/kg) induced an elevation in heart rate, achieving a maximum of 180/minute during the third half-hour (C), with total abolition of the respiratory arrhythmia. Isoproterenol was injected intravenously (2.0 μg/kg) to elicit a maximum heart rate of 180/minute (D). All of these interventions were made on different days in the trained, unanesthetized dog; isoproterenol was recorded before administration of propranolol. The chest was then opened, and a bipolar electrode was sutured to the right atrial appendage, with a preexcision record illustrated (E). Note that the P-wave in the ECG and the initial fast component of the right atrial electrogram (RAE) occurred simultaneously. Immediately after surgical excision of the S-A node region, a junctional rhythm occurred. Panel F shows a shift in pacemaker as the RAE complex appeared concurrently with the QRS during the first two cycles, but preceded it and became simultaneous with the P-wave on the next sequential beat.

The day following operation (Fig. 9-4G), the P-wave was markedly unstable and wandered in and out of the QRS. Note also the profound periods of asystole (5–10 sec in some dogs) that occurred spontaneously in the conscious animal. This instability lasted for several days, but a P-wave characterized most cycles (H), and resting heart rates averaged 50–60/minute. Atropine accelerated heart rate to 90/minute (I) and abolished the prolonged periods of asystole. Isoproterenol again accelerated heart rate from the control rate of 60 (J) to 150/minute (K). Propranolol again failed to change the resting, slow heart rate and duration of asystole (L).

The heart rate changes observed in these experiments are summarized in Fig. 9-5. The open bars represent the 24-hour heart rates averaged from Holter records in seven conscious dogs before excision of the S-A nodes, and the hatched

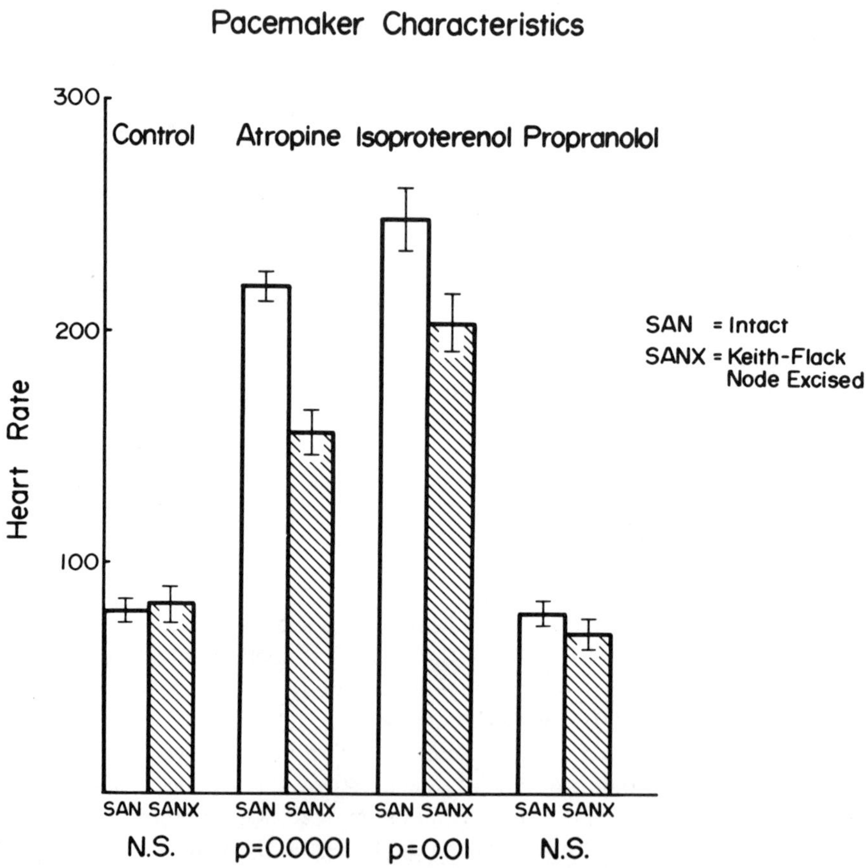

Fig. 9-5. Graphic representation of 24-hour heart rates (Holter monitor) in seven dogs before (SAN) and after (SANX) surgical excision of the sinoatrial region of right atrium. All rates were compared in all seven animals after atropine, isoproterenol, and propranolol, within 1–2 weeks before and after SAN excision. (From ref. 40, with permission of authors and the American Physiological Society)

bars are entirely comparable averages from the same animals after S-A node excision. The control observations indicate no significant differences in quietly resting heart rates as a result of extirpation of the Keith-Flack nodal region. Atropine consistently blocked vagal tone resulting in acceleration in heart rates of sinus origin to an average of 230/minute. A comparable average in the same animals after excision of the Keith-Flack node (S-A node excision) was significantly lower, 160/minute ($p < 0.0001$). This indicates that the SAPs within the first 1–2 weeks after destruction of S-A node are capable of driving the heart, but at a rate considerable slower during parasympathetic blockade.

Isoproterenol induced maximal heart rates (250–260/min), a value slightly higher than that induced by parasympathetic blockade (atropine), in the con-

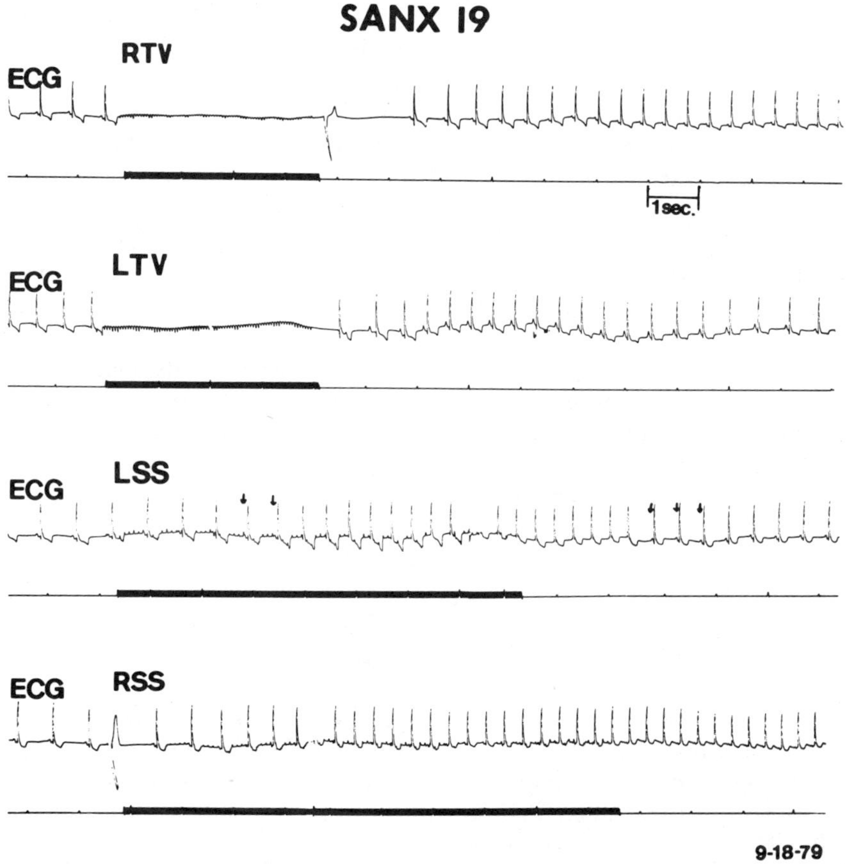

Fig. 9-6. Electrocardiographic (ECG) responses to direct electrical excitation (10–20 Hz, 5.0 msec, 4–6 volts) of right (RTV) and left (LTV) thoracic vagus, and left (LSS) and right (RSS) sympathetic (combined ansae subclavia) stimulations in dog sustaining histologically verified SAN excision 5 weeks previously. Arrows emphasize presence and reappearance of P-waves during LSS. (From ref. 40 with permission of authors and the American Physiological Society)

trol, conscious animals with S-A node intact. However, subsidiary atrial pacemakers (in the same animals after S-A node excision) responded to isoproterenol with significantly lower ($p < 0.01$) heart rates. Thus, within the first two weeks after S-A node excision, subsidiary pacemakers of atrial origin assume control of heart rate and rhythm, but they are not capable of comparably high maximum rates of acceleration during either parasympathetic blockade or direct beta-adrenergic drive by isoproterenol.

These experiments demonstrated the functional presence of direct autonomic innervation of the SAP with varying levels of both sympathetic and parasympathetic regulation in the alert, conscious animal. Figure 9-6 illustrates the direct responses of the SAP to electrical excitation of the right and left vagi, as well as the left and right sympathetics (both anterior and posterior ansae) in an animal in which the chest was reopened (under pentobarbital) in order to replace the atrial electrode. Vagal stimulation (RTV,LTV) elicited cardiac standstill without escape, with relatively prolonged recovery periods immediately following cessation of stimulation. P-waves were present in all control traces, although of low, biphasic amplitude in channel 2 (LTV), with P–R intervals between 95 and 100 milliseconds. Nonatrial beats marked the initial recovery cycles following vagal stimulation, but atrial beats were restored during the second recovery cycle. Both left and right sympathetic stimulation (LSS and RSS) elicited prominent acceleration in heart rate, right more so than left, with a prominent shift in P-wave during LSS (at arrows during stimulation period). Arrows also mark the reappearance of P-waves during the recovery phase. Left sympathetic stimulation consistently shifted the pacemaker away from its normal S-A node location to a junctional focus. These experiments demonstrate that comparable LSS also shifted the pacemaker away from SAP locations, presumably into similar junctional sites. Right Sympathetic Stimulation accelerated SAP rates directly, without pacemaker shifts, although to a lesser maximum than comparable stimulation in the presence of intact S-A node pacemakers.

OVERDRIVE SUPPRESSION

To further distinguish pacemakers in the canine right atrium, cardiac cycle lengths after rapid atrial pacing were measured in the alert, conscious dog. With implanted bipolar electrodes on the atrial appendage, pacing was established at a rate 100% above spontaneous heart rate, and was continued for periods of 30, 60, 120, or 180 seconds. The average control cycle length subtracted from the first recovery cycle after cessation of pacing was termed the corrected recovery time (CRT). In order to compare responses of the S-A node with those of the SAP, CRT was measured before and at intervals after excision of the S-A node. Figure 9-7 illustrates typical alterations in magnitude of overdrive suppression in the conscious dog on the first day following excision of the S-A node as compared with the degree of suppression in the same animal before S-A node excision [41]. The figure also reveals progressive changes in magnitude of overdrive suppression in the conscious animal in the days and weeks following S-A node excision. Panel A shows control tracings of lead II of the ECG and a simulta-

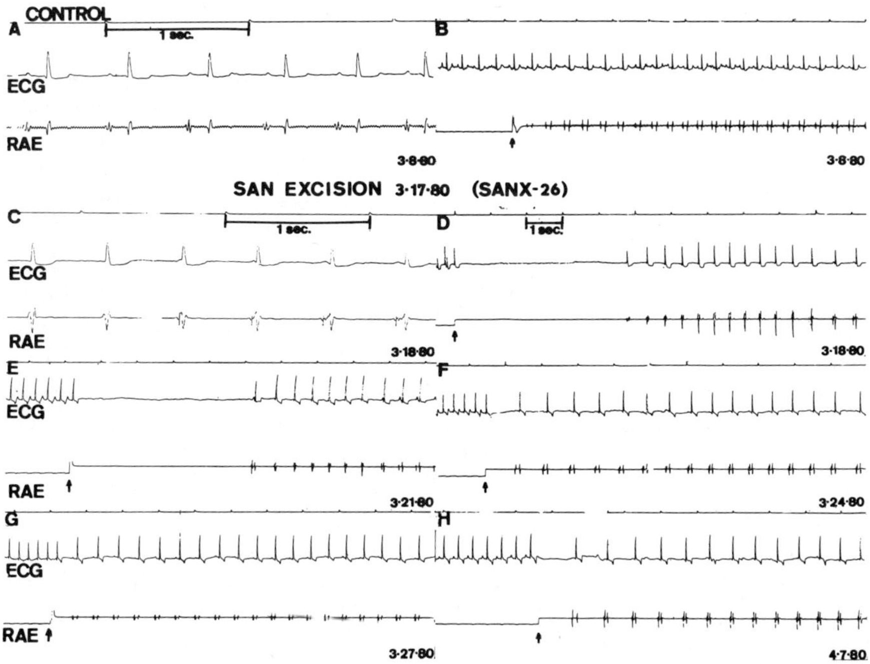

Fig. 9-7. Electrocardiographic (ECG) and right atrial electrograms (RAE) from the conscious, alert dog before (A and B) and after (C–H) surgical excision of the SAN (excision date was 3-17-80). Individual records were made while animal stood quietly in laboratory (dates indicate relationship to excision) and show progressive alterations in duration of overdrive suppression. Arrow indicates exact time of cessation of atrial pacing which was double the spontaneous heart rate. (From ref. 41 with permission from authors and the American College of Cardiology)

neous trace from the right atrial electrogram (RAE), recorded during a control (preoperative) period in the conscious, alert animal. Observe the simultaneous onset of atrial activation (RAE) and the upstroke of the P-wave. Panel B illustrates the cessation of rapid atrial pacing (225/min) at a rate 100% above control, spontaneous heart rate. Frequently this rate of atrial pacing induced atrioventricular block. The corrected recovery time in this experiment was only 25 milliseconds, and in repeated trials in this same animal, averaged less than 100 milliseconds. The first recovery beat was marked by a clear P-wave associated with activation in the RAE. Heart rate gradually accelerated during the following 8–10 seconds. Panel C was recorded on the day following surgical excision of the S-A node and shows a progressive shift from junctional rhythm (first two cycles) to an atrial rhythm characterized by a P-wave and associated precedence in RAE. Note the emergence of an early potential wave (third cycle, RAE) and a very short P–R interval. The latter progressively lengthened during subsequent cycles, thus providing evidence for a "wandering P-wave" as was common during the first few days after operation. Still, a P-wave was present most of the time. Panel D illustrates an enormously lengthened period of overdrive suppression following cessation of atrial pacing on the first day after S-A node excision. Again, the pacing rate was 100% above the spontaneous heart rate, and was marked by a CRT of 4.8 seconds. A minimal oscillation appeared in the position of the P-wave (both ECG and RAE) of the first recovery beat, but a junctional rhythm marked the next 11 cycles. A clear P-wave then emerged and remained throughout the recovery period. Panel E was recorded, again in the conscious animal, three days later to reveal a similarly prolonged CRT (5.0 sec). The initial recovery beat showed a vestigial P-wave with a very short P–R interval and a junctional rhythm for the next six cycles. A P-wave then emerged and progressed into a normally appearing atrial excitation pattern. Three days later (panel F) rapid atrial pacing induced a significantly shorter CRT (350 msec) and the initial recovery beat was associated with a clear P-wave. Thus, a dramatic prolongation in overdrive suppression was observed immediately following excision of the S-A node, and this was repeatedly observed over the next several postoperative days in the conscious animal model. However, within one week, there occurred an equally dramatic reduction in CRT, generally associated with reappearance of a stable, functional P-wave and an atrial pacemaker. Two subsequent determinations (panels G and H) confirmed these findings, with evidence for continuing instability of the atrial pacemaker and relatively prolonged CRTs following overdrive stimulation. The CRT in panel H, made approximately 3 weeks after surgery, was slightly more than 400 milliseconds, a value significantly greater than that found in the same control, unoperated animal, but dramatically shorter than that immediately following S-A node excision.

Four animals in this series of 15 dogs continued to show prolonged periods of asystole during Holter monitoring, particularly during quiet resting hours. Figure 9-8 illustrates the course of change in CRT in one of these animals. Panel A shows the normal association between P-wave and atrial electrogram (RAE) before excision of the node, and panel B shows a normal overdrive suppression immediately following cessation of pacing. Both records were made while the S-A node remained intact with the animal standing quietly in the laboratory. Panels C and D were made on the day following S-A node excision, again in the awake animal. Panel C reveals a "wandering" pacemaker, with P-waves appearing and disappearing in successive ECG tracings. Each P-wave is associated with an appropriate atrial activation spike in RAE. Note also the prolonged period of asystole (2.5 sec) which occurred during the control tracing. A prominent P-wave was associated with the recovery beat following the asystole. Overdrive pacing (panel D) was followed by prolonged suppression (6.3 sec) and syncope (note motion artifacts in the ECG). None of the recovery beats shown were atrial in origin. Two days later (panel E), control tracings revealed the regular presence of a P-wave and spontaneously prolonged asystole (3.7 sec), with supraventricular activation in the recovery cycle. Subsequent beats were junctional in origin. Rapid pacing (panel F) again resulted in prolonged suppression (7.9 sec) followed by junctional beats. One week after S-A node excision, rapid pacing was associated with A-V block and prolonged suppression following cessation of pacing. Junctional beats were apparent early in recovery,

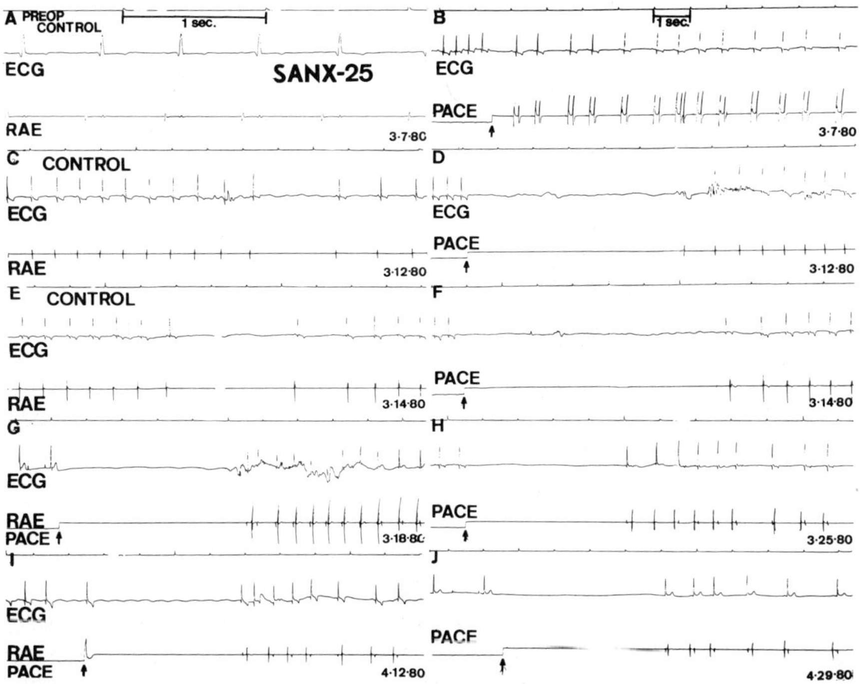

Fig. 9-8. Segments from pre- (A and B) and post-excision (3-11-80 was excision date) electrocardiographic (ECG) and RAE traces in a dog showing relatively slow recovery of an inferior atrial pacemaker. Labels as in Fig. 9-7. Note prolonged duration of exaggerated CRT and asystolic periods following SAN excision. Even in these animals, however, stable SAPs became firmly established. (From ref. 41, with permission of authors and the American College of Cardiology)

but a P-wave persisted after the last cycle shown (panel G). After a second week passed, CRT was still prolonged (4.8 sec) and the first two recovery cycles were junctional in origin (panel H). The third cycle, however, was atrial in origin and a "wandering" pacemaker marked the remainder of the recovery period. Similar periods of exaggerated CRT remained after an additional 18 (panel I) and 35 (panel J) days. While a P-wave was clearly present during much of the dogs waking hours, it failed to become permanently stabilized for several weeks. Thus, in contrast to the animal illustrated in Fig. 9-7, this animal (S-A node excision number 25) was characterized by a markedly unstable pacemaker following excision of the sinoatrial node, and this instability persisted for a period of seven weeks. Thereafter the P-wave became stable, asystolic periods became progressively attenuated during quietly resting (Holter) control circumstances, and the duration of overdrive suppression was markedly reduced.

Figures 9-7 and 9-8 therefore illustrate two different time sequences in recovery from SAN excision, one representing a majority of animals (Fig. 9-7) who responded with greatly exaggerated CRT lasting for 1 to 5 days with progressive return toward much shorter periods of overdrive suppression. The other (Fig.

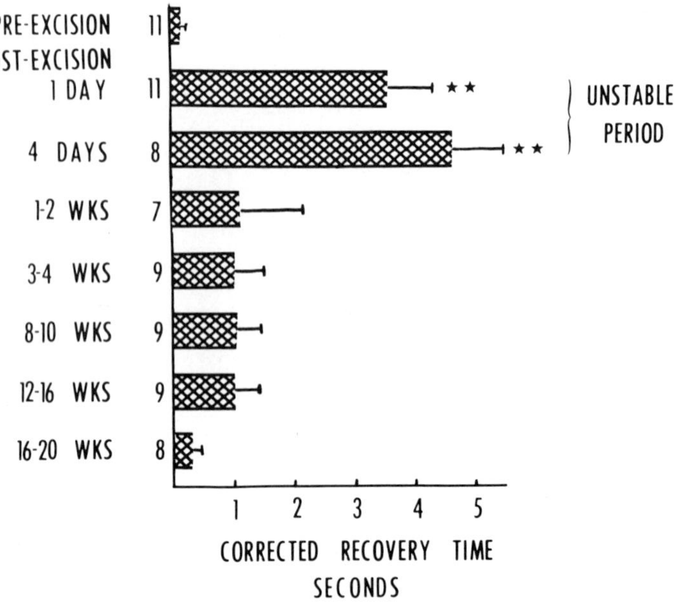

Fig. 9-9. Graphic representation of changes in corrected recovery times (CRT) before (pre-excision) and at regular intervals after SAN excision. Number of animals tested at each interval shown at base of each bar. CRT was significantly prolonged ($p < 0.001$) over control values immediately after excision, and P-wave became most unstable at this time. Relative instability and changing CRTs are revealed in large standard errors during recovery period. (From ref. 41, with permission of authors and the American College of Cardiology)

9-8) represents four dogs in which the recovery in CRT was much more prolonged.

Figure 9-9 summarizes the successive alterations in CRT in the entire series of chronic, conscious dogs in which comparisons were made between responses of the S-A node and SAP pacemakers to overdrive atrial pacing. The average CRT before S-A node excision was 267 milliseconds. Immediately after excision and after recovery from the barbiturate anesthesia, CRT was consistently and significantly ($p < 0.001$) prolonged; this interval was characteristically extended over a period of 3 days to 1 week. This period also incorporated the time of greatest pacemaker instability following S-A node surgery. Thereafter the P-wave became more stable, and assumed essentially normal configuration with P–R interval between 80 and 100 msec, while CRT progressively shortened. The latter continued to average considerably longer than the control, preoperative value, even in the presence of stable P-waves. While CRTs progressively returned toward those characterizing the intact S-A node, they remained slightly exaggerated even after 16 to 20 weeks. P-waves were generally stable at this time, and Holter monitoring revealed essentially normal, quietly resting cardiac rhythms.

After recovery periods of 3 to 10 months, all of these animals were anesthetized and the atrium mapped electrophysiologically. Once again, all of the sites of earliest activation were along the sulcus terminalis, and within approximately 2 mm of either its atrial or caval borders.

IN VITRO PREPARATIONS

While the in vivo demonstrations of subsidiary atrial pacemaker function were in process, a search for cardiac cells possessing appropriate cellular and transmembrane characteristics was also under way. This required development of an in vitro model of subsidiary atrial pacemaker activity that would avoid the limitations inherent to in vivo preparations. Employing the technique originally described by James and Nadeau [19], the S-A node artery of an adult mongrel dog was cannulated via the right coronary artery and perfused with warm Tyrode's solution in situ. The heart, with at least 2 cm of vena cava attached, was quickly excised, and immersed in Tyrode's solution. The in vitro preparation was then modified with the technique of Woods et al. [64]. The right atrium was separated from the rest of the heart, while it was continuously perfused through the S-A node artery. After the right atrium was opened, the entire free wall including portions of both venae cavae, but excluding the coronary sinus and interatrial septum, was transferred to a large (200 ml capacity) tissue bath and pinned endocardial side up. A perfusion pump delivered warmed (36°) oxygenated Tyrode's solution, adjusted to a constant perfusion pressure that yielded a flow of 4.7 ml/minute. The preparation was also superfused with warmed oxygenated Tyrode's solution at 10–12 ml/minute. Three stationary and one mobile extracellular bipolar electrodes were used to locate the site of earliest activation (SEA) and to study changes in spontaneous rate under various conditions. In 93% of the atria studied, the control SEA was located within the S-A node region (shaded area, Fig. 9-10) [42,44]. The trace at the left demonstrates that the SEA beneath the mobile electrode (filled circle) depolarized before the three stationary electrodes, located along the crista terminalis (positions 1,2,3).

In order to elicit spontaneous subsidiary pacemaker activity in this preparation, S-A node pacemaker activity was suppressed by ligating the S-A node artery just caudal to the S-A node region, as illustrated in Fig. 9-11 [42,44]. Following suppression of S-A node activity, subsidiary pacemaker activity was found invariably within the crista terminalis, primarily at the junction of the inferior right atrium and the inferior vena cava. Note the position of the SEA (solid circle) and the retrograde conduction recorded by electrodes 3-2-1. The appearance of this pacemaker activity depended on the presence of a background level of norepinephrine (10^{-8}M) in the perfusing solution [43,44].

Experiments were done to compare the responses of this isolated right atrial preparation when activated by the S-A node and when activated by SAPs, under similar conditions [44]. In the presence of background norepinephrine, the average spontaneous rate of SAP activity was significantly less (78 ± 1.2) than S-A node activity (105 ± 5.3) ($p < 0.005$). Perfusion on the preparation

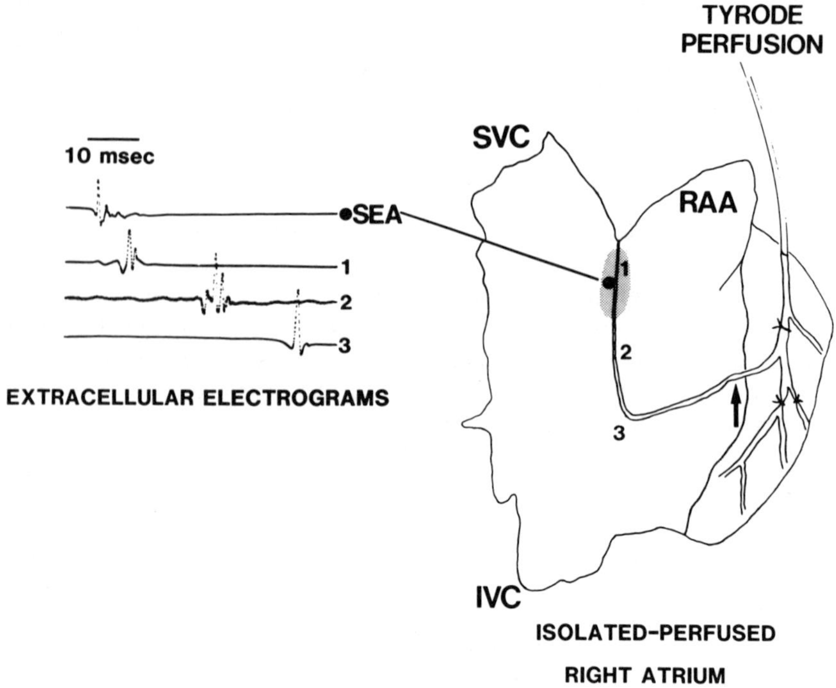

Fig. 9-10. Schematic diagram of the perfused atrial free wall preparation as it appears in the tissue bath, epicardial side up. The stippled area represents the SAN region and the arrow locates the tip of the perfusion cannula in the SAN artery. The three reference electrodes are in position 1, 2, and 3 and each of their recordings are shown in the left-hand panel. Under control conditions the site of earliest activation (SEA) was located within the SAN region. SVC = superior vena cava; IVC = inferior vena cava; RAA = right atrial appendage. (From ref. 44, with permission of the authors and the American Heart Association)

with propranolol or norepinephrine-free Tyrode's solution reduced the spontaneous rate of S-A node activity. However, the same interventions completely abolished SAP activity, rendering the preparation quiescent. The response to neuromediators was tested by introducing ACh or NE into the perfusate and constructing concentration-response curves. These experiments showed that SAP activity is more sensitive to the chronotropic effects of ACh than are S-A node pacemakers. The concentration-response curve for SAP activity was shifted far to the left of the S-A node curve. When NE sensitivity was tested, S-A node activity always had a greater maximal chronotropic response than SAP activity. These differences were small and nearly parallel at lower NE concentrations ($<10^{-7}$M) but became highly significant and diverged at higher concentration ($>10^{-7}$M). The larger differences resulted from abrupt increases in SAN activity that were associated with transient shifts in activation sequence, suggesting shifts in pacemaker location within the S-A node. In contrast, shifts

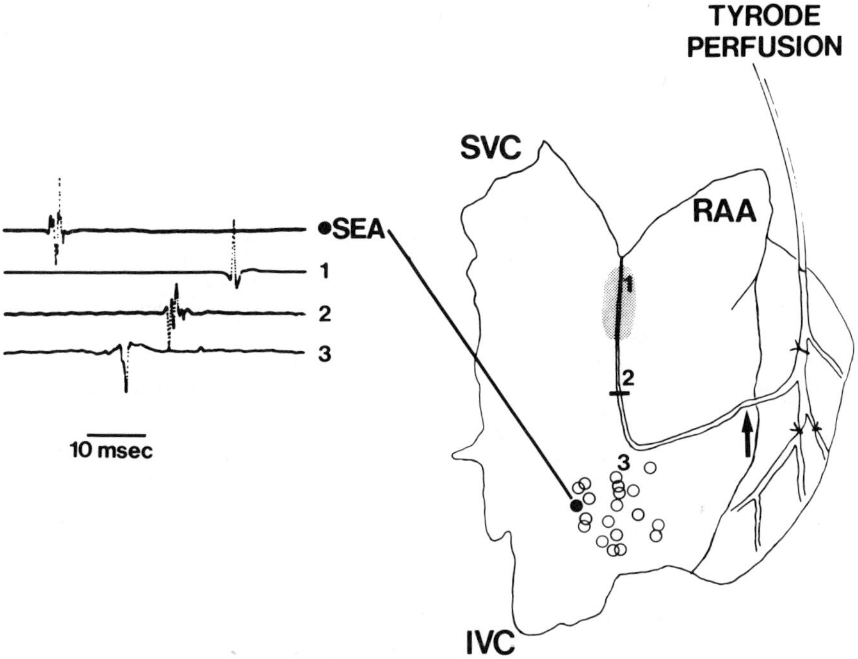

Fig. 9-11. Subsidiary SEA located following ligation of the SAN artery in 20 perfused right atrial preparations. The solid horizontal bar indicates the approximate site of ligation. The solid circle represents the subsidiary SEA located with the recordings shown in the left panel and the open circles represent the other 19 preparations. Note that the mobile electrogram precedes the reference electrograms and that the activation sequence of the reference electrograms is reversed from control (see Fig. 9-10)

were not observed with the positive chronotropic response of SAP activity to NE. Another important characteristic distinguishing SAP from S-A node activity was the response to overdrive pacing. With comparable rates and periods of overdrive pacing, SAP activity had significantly longer periods of overdrive suppression than S-A node activity. The suppression for S-A node activity was measured in milliseconds, in contrast to SAP suppression measured in seconds.

In order to gain insight into the cellular electrophysiological mechanisms responsible for SAP activity, intracellular microelectrode techniques were used to record transmembrane potentials from tissues excised from right atrial preparations exhibiting SAP activity [31,42]. As described earlier, SAP activity in this preparation was found primarily in a distinct region of the inferior right atrium–inferior vena cava. When perfused in the tissue bath, this region was pale in color and therefore easily distinguished from the surrounding atrial tissue. This pale region is illustrated, in Fig. 9-12, in relation to the sulcus terminalis and other epicardial structures of the right atrium. It was found approximately 2–3 cm caudal from the S-A node and ranged in dimensions from 2 × 4 mm to 7 × 12 mm. Once the earliest site of SAP activity was located in the

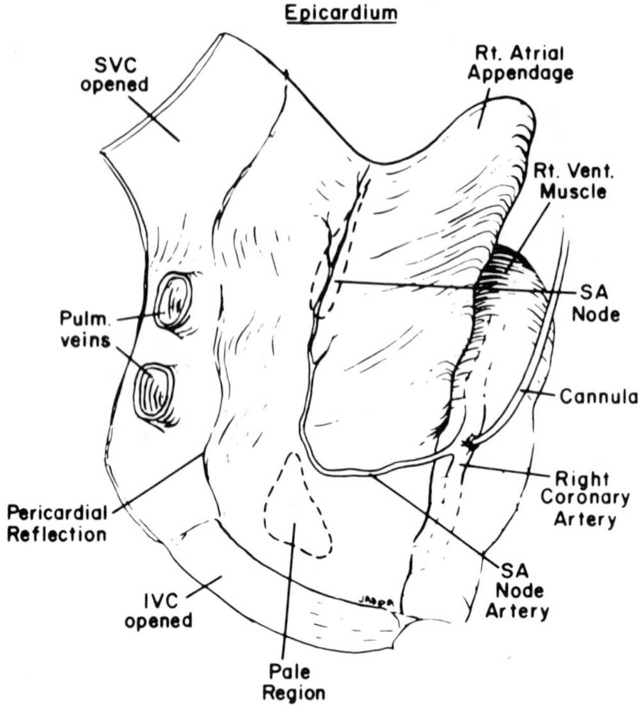

Fig. 9-12. Epicardial view of canine right atrium, revealing the relationship between SAN, SAN artery, and the "pale region" located immediately rostral to the junction of the inferior vena cava and the right atrium.

perfused right atrial preparation with the extracellular electrodes, this region, with at least 5 mm of surrounding atrial muscle, was excised and superfused with Tyrode's solution in a smaller tissue bath, endocardial side up. In the presence of background NE, all of these isolated tissues beat spontaneously. In addition, the spontaneous rate of the isolated preparations (74.9 $\pm$ 7.0) was not significantly different from the subsidiary spontaneous rate of the perfused right atria from which they were excised (75.7 $\pm$ 8.3). Pacemaker cells generating the earliest activity in this preparation were located by placing one extracellular bipolar electrode on the periphery of the tissue and one intracellular microelectrode to record from individual cells. Invariably, the pacemaker cells with the earliest activation were found within the pale region and corresponded closely with the site of earliest activation found with extracellular mapping of the right atrium.

The most frequent type of action potentials recorded from this preparation were typical fast responses, characteristic of plateau fiber action potentials. However, the cells generating the earliest activity displayed action potentials more typical of slow responses, possessing primary pacemaker features [42]. This is shown in Fig. 9-13, where action potentials were recorded from the pale region. Although these pacemaker action potentials appear to be slow response,

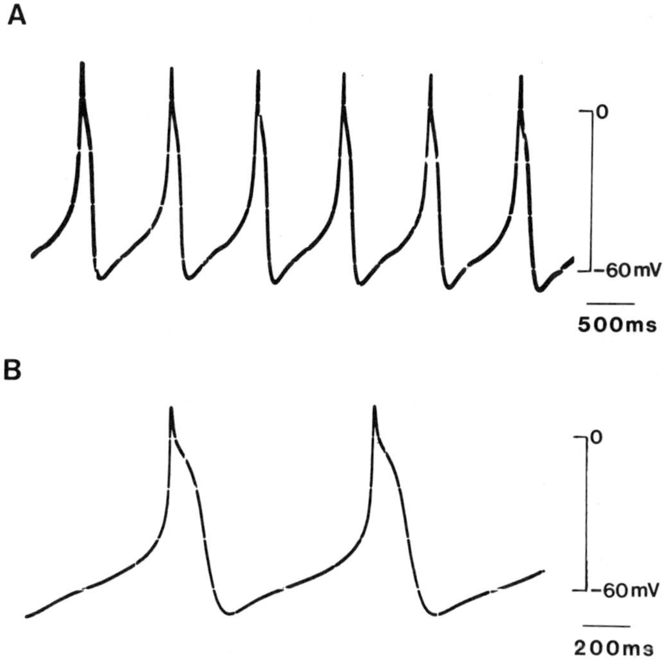

Fig. 9-13. Spontaneous pacemaker action potentials recorded from the endocardial surface of a tissue excised from the "pale region" of the inferior right atrium. A and B are the same recordings taken at two different sweep speeds to show the smooth transition of diastolic depolarization (phase 4) into the upstroke (phase 0).

preliminary experiments suggest that a partially inactivated sodium channel may contribute to the automaticity of these fibers.

The requirement of NE for the appearance of SAP activity was investigated by recording action potentials from a pacemaker cell and extracellular electrograms from the surrounding tissue [31]. With this technique it was possible to monitor changes in both impulse formation and impulse conduction of SAP activity. When the background NE was reduced below 10^{-8}M or removed from the perfusate, conduction of SAP activity to the surrounding tissue was partially or completely blocked. However, SAP impulse formation continued, although at a slower rate. Restoring NE to the perfusate restored control activity. Similarly, adding low concentrations of ACh (5×10^{-8}M) to the superfusate resulted in partial or complete exit block, with little or no direct effect on SAP automaticity.

In some experiments on the perfused right atrial preparation it was not possible to elicit subsidiary pacemaker activity following ligation of the S-A node artery, even in the presence of higher concentrations of NE. From these quiescent tissues, the pale region along with some surrounding tissue was excised for transmembrane recordings. These studies revealed that fibers within the pale region possess a unique sensitivity to NE, which is not displayed by the surrounding atrial tissue. In the presence of NE (10^{-6}M), electrical stimulation at

60 beats/minute generated action potentials from the pale region that displayed prominent afterhyperpolarizations and what appeared to be steep diastolic depolarizations. This was not observed in action potentials from surrounding tissue. Upon stopping the stimulation, action potentials from the pale region were followed by prominent, late afterdepolarizations not generated by the surrounding fibers. In some preparations, late afterdepolarizations reached threshold and generated nondriven action potentials and in some cases sustained repetitive activity [43]. This triggered activity was abolished by removing NE or by administering verapamil.

These results support the idea that subsidiary pacemakers exist in the canine right atrium. In the atrial model used here, we have found a high concentration of subsidiary sites in a distinct pale region of tissue, at the junction of the inferior right atrium–inferior vena cava. This is essentially the same location in which subsidiary atrial pacemakers were found following excision of the S-A node, in vivo. These subsidiary pacemakers generate action potentials more typical of slow responses. Appearance of SAP activity may critically depend on the level of autonomic tone at any time. Withdrawal of beta adrenergic activity or enhanced cholinergic activity may result in block of SAP propagation and possible shift in pacemaker site to another region of the atrium or the heart. Due to inherent membrane characteristics, these subsidiary pacemakers may respond to higher concentrations of adrenergic stimulation with dysrhythmias in the form of triggered activity. The cellular properties and responses of these subsidiary atrial pacemakers in vitro, are consistent with the autonomically mediated dysrhythmias recorded with subsidiary atrial pacemaker activity following excision of the SAN in vivo.

CONCLUSIONS

There is an important hierarchial organization of pacemaker function in the canine heart, with the sinoatrial node exerting dominance under normal, resting conditions. Damage to this region however, results in assumption of dominance by subsidiary cells located in the inferior right atrial free wall (subsidiary atrial pacemakers or SAP), followed by atrioventricular junctional, and finally by ventricular foci. The hierarchy is characterized by progressively decreasing spontaneous discharge rates, achievement of lower heart rate maxima under direct beta-adrenergic stimulation (isoproterenol), and release from parasympathetic tone (atropine) during exercise or during electrical excitation of the stellate ganglia.

Excision of the S-A node may be followed instantaneously by an A-V junctional rhythm, but within minutes or hours, the SAPs assume dominance. The SAP may be situated within or close to the intact crista terminalis, or if this region is also damaged, in a "pale region" in the inferior right atrium immediately rostral to the junction of the inferior right vena cava and the atrium. The primary arterial supply to the SAPs is via the sinoatrial nodal artery which also supplies the S-A node in the dog heart. The SAPs are under comprehensive autonomic control and function promptly and effectively in the alert, conscious animal sustaining chronic excision of the S-A node. While the SAPs are marked by greatly prolonged periods of overdrive suppression immediately following destruction of the S-A node, the CRT progressively shortens with time (days or weeks), the level of performance coinciding with P-wave stability. The SAPs eventually assume stable pacemaker function with relatively short overdrive suppression characteristics approximating those of the S-A node pacemaker cells.

In animals in which activity from the classical S-A node region has been excluded, subsidiary pacemaker location has been identified in both in vivo and in vitro experiments. Surgical isolation of the cannulated, perfused-superfused right atrial free wall consistently results in dominant pacemaker location in the S-A node region. Ligation of the SAN artery however, promptly results in shift of the pacemaker to a relatively thin, pale region in the inferior right atrium. This region is identical to that identified in the chronic animal model in which the S-A node has been previously removed. Transmembrane potential recordings consistently reveal spontaneous slow response activity from cells within the "pale region" but fast responses from the surrounding "pink" atrial tissues. It appears likely that these cells are responsible for the establishment of stable P-waves and normal P–R intervals in alert, awake animals sustaining chronic damage to, or removal of, the classical Keith-Flack S-A node region.

REFERENCES

1. Boineau, J. P., R. B. Schuessler, C. R. Mooney, A. C. Wylds, C. B. Miller, R. D. Hudson, J. M. Burroughs, C. W. Brockus, Multicentric origin of atrial depolarization wave. The pacemaker complex. *Circulation 58*: 1036–1048, 1978.
2. Boineau, J. P., R. B. Schuessler, D. B. Hackel, C. B. Miller, C. W. Brockus, A. C. Wylds, Widespread distribution and rate differentiation of the atrial pacemaker complex, *Am. J. Physiol. 239*: H406–H415, 1980.
3. Boineau, J. P., R. B. Schuessler, D. B. Henkel, A. C. Wylds, C. B. Miller, C. W. Brockus, Multicentric distribution and rate differentiation of the atrial pacemaker system, In *The Physiology of Atrial Pacemakers and Conductive Tissues*, ed. R. C. Little. Futura, Mt. Kisco, N.Y., pp. 221–260, 1980.
4. Brooks, C. M. and H. H. Lu, *The Sinoatrial Pacemaker of the Heart*. C. C. Thomas, Springfield, Ill., 1972, pp. 68–124.
5. Clarkson, P. M., B. G. Barratt-Boyes, J. M. Neutze, Late dysrhythmias and disturbed conduction following Mustard operation for complete transposition of the great arteries, *Circulation 53*: 519–524, 1976.
6. Coraboeuf, E. and S. Weidmann, Potentiel de repos et potentiels d' action du muscle cardioque mesures a l'aide d'electrodes internes, *C. R. Soc. Biol. 143*: 1329–1331, 1949.
7. Davies, F. The conducting system of the vertebrate heart, *Br. Heart J. 4*: 66–76, 1942.
8. Draper, M. H. and S. Weidmann, Cardiac resting and action potentials recorded with an intracellular electrode, *J. Physiol. 115*: 74–94, 1951.
9. Erlanger, J. and J. R. Blackman, A study of relative rhythmicity and conductivity in various regions of the auricles of the mammalian heart, *Am. J. Physiol. 19*: 125–174, 1907.

10. Euler, D. E., S. B. Jones, W. P. Gunnar, J. M. Loeb, D. K. Murdock, W. C. Randall, Cardiac arrhythmias in the conscious dog after excision of the sinoatrial node and crista terminalis, *Circulation 59*: 468–475, 1979.
11. Eyster, J. A. E. and W. J. Meek, Experiments on the origin and propagation of the impulse in the heart, *Heart 5*: 137–140, 1914.
12. Eyster, J. A. E. and W. J. Meek, Experiments on the origin and conduction of the cardiac impulse. VI. Conduction of the excitation from sinoauricular node, *Arch. Intern. Med. 18*: 775–799, 1916.
13. Eyster, J. A. E. and W. J. Meek, The origin and conduction of the heart beat, *Physiol. Rev. 1*: 1–43, 1921.
14. Ferrar, M. I. The sick sinus syndrome, *Circulation 47*: 635–641, 1973.
15. Flack, M. An investigation of the sino-auricular node of the mammalian heart, *J. Physiol. (Lond.) 41*: 64–77, 1910–11.
16. Geesbreght, J. M., W. C. Randall, G. Brynjolfsson, Area localization of supraventricular pacemaker activity before and after SA node excision, *The Physiologist 13*: 202, 1970.
17. Graham, J. and R. W. Gerard, Membrane potential and excitation of impaled single muscle fibers, *J. Cell. Comp. Physiol. 28*: 99–117, 1946.
18. Hardie, E. L., S. B. Jones, D. E. Euler, D. L. Fishman, W. C. Randall, Sinoatrial node artery distribution and its relation to hierarchy of cardiac automaticity, *Am. J. Physiol. 241*: H45–H53, 1981.
19. James, T. N., R. A. Nadeau, Direct perfusion of the sinus node. An experimental model for pharmacologic and electrophysiologic studies of the heart, *Henry Ford Hosp. Med. Bull. 10*: 21–25, 1962.
20. James, T. N. and L. Sherf, Ultrastructure of the human AV node, *Circulation 37*: 1049–1070, 1968.
21. James, T. N. The sinus node as a servo-mechanism, *Circ. Res. 32*: 307–313, 1973.
22. Jones, S. B., D. E. Euler, E. L. Hardie, W. C. Randall, G. Brynjolfsson, Comparison of SA nodal and subsidiary atrial pacemaker function and location in the dog, *Am. J. Physiol. 234*: H471–H476, 1978.
23. Jones, S. B., D. E. Euler, W. C. Randall, G. Brynjolfsson, E. L. Hardie, Atrial ectopic foci in the canine heart. Hierarchy of pacemaker automaticity, *Am. J. Physiol. 238*: H788–H793, 1980.
24. Kawamura, K., Electron microscopic studies on the cardiac conduction system of the dog. II. The sinoatrial and atrioventricular nodes, *Jap. Circ. J. 25*: 973–1013, 1961.
25. Keith, A. and M. Flack, The form and nature of the muscular connections between the primary divisions of the vertebrate heart, *J. Anat. Physiol. 41*: 172–189, 1906–07.
26. Keith, A., The sino-auricular node: a historical note, *Br. Heart J. 4*: 77–79, 1942.
27. Lange, G., Action of driving stimuli from intrinsic and extrinsic sources on in situ cardiac pacemaker tissue, *Circ. Res. 17*: 449–459, 1965.
28. Lewis, T., Galvanometric curves yielded by cardiac beats generated in various areas of the auricular musculature. The pacemaker of the heart, *Heart 2*: 23–40, 1910.
29. Lewis, T., B. X. Oppenheimer, A. Oppenheimer, The site of origin of the mammalian heart beat—the pacemaker in the dog, *Heart 2*: 147–196, 1910.
30. Ling, G. and R. W. Gerard, The normal membrane potential of frog sartorius fibers, *J. Cell. Comp. Physiol. 34*: 383–396, 1949.
31. Lipsius, S. L., G. J. Rozanski, W. C. Randall, Autonomic modulation of subsidiary atrial pacemaker impulse propagation, *Fed. Proc. 41*: 1505, 1982.

32. Lu, H. H., G. Lange, C. M. Brooks, Factors controlling pacemaker action in cells of the sinoatrial node, *Circ. Res. 17*: 460–471, 1965.
33. Lu, H. H. and C. M. Brooks, Intranodal shifts of pacemaker action, *Circulation 40, Suppl. III*: 136, 1969.
34. Lu, H. H., Shifts in pacemaker dominance within the sinoatrial region of cat and rabbit hearts resulting from increase of extracellular potassium, *Circ. Res. 26*: 339–346, 1970.
35. Mandel, W. T., M. M. Laks, K. Obagaski, Sinus node function. Evaluation in patients with and without sinus node disease, *Arch. Intern. Med. 135*: 388–394, 1975.
36. Meek, W. J. and J. A. E. Eyster, Experiments on the origin and propagation of the impulse in the heart, *Heart 5*: 227–244, 1916.
37. Meek, W. F., M. Keenan, H. J. Theisen, The auricular blood supply in the dog. I. General auricular supply with special reference to the sino-auricular node, *Am. Heart J. 4*: 591–599, 1929.
38. Randall, W. C., J. Talano, M. P. Kaye, D. E. Euler, S. B. Jones, G. Brynjolfsson, Cardiac pacemakers in the absence of the SA node. The response to exercise and autonomic blockade. *Am. J. Physiol. 234*: H465–470, 1978.
39. Randall, W. C., W. H. Wehrmacher, S. B. Jones, Hierarchy of supraventricular pacemakers, *J. Thor. Cardiovasc. Surg. 82*: 797–800, 1981.
40. Randall, W. C., L. E. Rinkema, S. B. Jones, J. F. Moran, G. Brynjolfsson, Functional characterization of atrial pacemaker activity, *Am. J. Physiol. 242*: H98–H106, 1982.
41. Randall, W. C., L. E. Rinkema, S. B. Jones, J. F. Moran, G. Brynjolfsson, Overdrive suppression of atrial pacemaker tissues in the alert, awake dog before and chronically after excision of the sinoatrial node, *Am. J. Cardiol. 49*: 1166–1175, 1982.
42. Rozanski, G. J., S. L. Lipsius, W. C. Randall, Electrophysiology of pacemaker activity in the isolated canine right atrium, *Fed. Proc. 39*: 816, 1980.
43. Rozanski, G. J., S. L. Lipsius, W. C. Randall, The dependence of right atrial subsidiary pacemaker activity on norepinephrine, *The Physiologist 23*: 160, 1980.
44. Rozanski, G. J., S. L. Lipsius, W. C. Randall, Functional characteristics of sinoatrial and subsidiary pacemaker activity in the canine right atrium, *Circulation, 67*: 1378–1387, 1983.
45. Rozanski, G. J., S. L. Lipsius, S. B. Jones, W. C. Randall, Neuromediator regulation of chronic vs. acute subsidiary pacemaker activity in the canine right atrium, *Fed. Proc. 40*: 414, 1981.
46. Scherf, D., S. Blumenfeld, M. Yildiz, Experimental studies on A-V nodal rhythm following suppression of activity of the sinus node, *Am. J. Cardiol. 10*: 234–238, 1962.
47. Schuessler, R. B., J. P. Boineau, A. C. Wylds, C. B. Miller, C. W. Brockus, Dynamics of atrial activation, In *The Physiology of Atrial Pacemaker and Conductive Tissue*, ed. R. C. Little. Futura, Mt. Kisco, N. Y. pp. 182–206, 1980.
48. Sealy, W. C., R. J. Bache, A. V. Seaber, S. K. Bhattacharga, The atrial pacemaker site after surgical exclusion of the sinoatrial node, *J. Thor. Cardiovasc. Surg. 65*: 841–850, 1973.
49. Sealy, W. C. and A. Seaber, Cardiac rhythm following exclusion of the sinoatrial node and most of the right atrium from the remainder of the heart, *J. Thor. Cardiovasc. Surg. 77*: 436–447, 1979.
50. Sealy, W. C. and A. V. Seaber, Surgical isolation of the atrial septum from the atria, *J. Thor. Cardiovasc. Surg. 80*: 742–749, 1980.

51. Toda, N. and K. Shimamoto, The influence of sympathetic stimulation on transmembrane potentials in the S-A node, *J. Pharmacol. Exp. Ther. 159*: 298–305, 1968.
52. Trautwein, W. and K. Zink, Ueber membran und aktion potentiale einzelner myokardfasern des kat-und warmbluterherzens, *Pflugers Arch. ges. Physiol. 256*: 68–84, 1952.
53. Trautwein, W. and K. Uchizono, Electron microscopic and electrophysiologic study of the pacemaker in the sinoatrial node of the rabbit heart, *Zeit. fur Zell. 61*: 96–109, 1963.
54. Urthaler, F., C. R. Katholi, J. Macy, T. N. James, Mathematical relationship between automaticity of the sinus node and the A-V junction, *Am. Heart J. 86*: 189–195, 1973.
55. Urthaler, F. and T. N. James, Effects of tetrodotoxin on A-V conduction and the junctional rhythm, *Am. J. Physiol. 224*: 1155–1161, 1973.
56. Urthaler, F., C. R. Katholi, J. Macy, T. N. James, Mathematical relationship between automaticity of the sinus node and the AV junction, *Am. Heart J. 86*: 189–195, 1973.
57. Urthaler, F., K. Millar, M. J. Burgess, J. A. Abildskov, T. N. James, Comparative dependence on adrenergic neural tone by automaticity in the sinus node and in the atrioventricular junction, *J. Pharmacol. Exp. Ther. 187*: 269–279, 1973.
58. Urthaler, F., J. H. Isobe, T. N. James, Comparative effects of glucagon on automaticity of the sinus node and the atrioventricular junction, *Am. J. Physiol. 227*: 1415–1421, 1974.
59. Urthaler, F., C. R. Katholi, J. Macy, T. N. James, Electrophysiological and mathematical characterization of the escape rhythm during complete AV block, *Cardiovasc. Res. 8*: 173–186, 1974.
60. Urthaler, F. and T. N. James, Cholinergic and adrenergic control of the sinus node and AV junction, In *Neural Regulation of the Heart*, ed. W. C. Randall. Oxford Univ. Press, New York, pp. 247–288, 1977.
61. Urthaler, F. and T. N. James, Hierarchy of supraventricular pacemakers, *J. Thor. Cardiovasc. Surg. 80*: 750–753, 1980.
62. West, T. C., Effects of chronotropic influences on subthreshold oscillations in the sino-atrial node, In *The Specialized Tissues of the Heart*, eds. A. Paes De Carvalho, W. C. DeMello, B. F. Hoffman. Elsevier, New York, 1961, pp. 81–94.
63. White, C. W., M. L. Marcus, F. M. Abboud, Distribution of coronary artery flow to the canine right atrium and sinoatrial node, *Circ. Res. 40*: 342–347, 1977.
64. Woods, W. T., F. Urthaler, T. N. James, Spontaneous action potentials of cells in the canine sinus node, *Circ. Res. 39*: 76–82, 1979.
65. Woods, W. T., R. E. Katholi, F. Urthaler, T. N. James, Electrophysiological effects of magnesium on cells in the canine sinus node and false tendon, *Circ. Res. 44*: 182–188, 1979.

10

Sympathetic Imbalance and Cardiac Arrhythmias

PETER J. SCHWARTZ

The importance of the autonomic nervous system, particularly its sympathetic limb, in the genesis of cardiac arrhythmias has become progressively more evident [39,43,62,76,86]. Extensive research has brought new insights into the genesis of arrhythmias and new strategies for the prevention and management of the more serious, and often life-threatening, cardiac arrhythmias. Activation of localized nerve pathways or unilateral sympathetic discharges may be even more arrhythmogenic than massive but homogeneous activation of the sympathetic nervous system. With regard to the susceptibility to cardiac arrhythmias, these findings have led to the concept of "sympathetic imbalance" which is the subject of this chapter. The realization that there are clinical conditions characterized by life-threatening arrhythmias and dependent, or likely to depend, on sympathetic imbalance has greatly increased interest in this topic.

This chapter will not deal with the problems of "autonomic imbalance" [85], sympathetically mediated shifts in pacemaker origin [17,19], or supraventricular arrhythmias. Because of the greater clinical implications and larger number of detailed studies, the relationship between sympathetic imbalance and ventricular arrhythmias will be stressed.

HISTORICAL NOTE

What follows is a brief chronological review of some of the studies that are most relevant, directly or indirectly, to the concept of sympathetic imbalance.

In 1892 Langley [37], confirming an observation made by Boehm and Nuss-

I am grateful to Drs. A. M. Brown, E. Feigl, and A. Malliani for reviewing the manuscript and for helpful criticism. I wish to express deepest gratitude to my friend and partner Dr. H. L. Stone without whose continuing cooperation this work on sympathetic imbalance would not have been possible.

baum in 1875, reported that "the accelerator nerves in the thorax have much less effect on the left side than on the right."

In 1899 Hunt observed in cats and in dogs "irregularities of the heart" [26] after removal of the right stellate ganglion. Figure 10-1 shows the effects on blood pressure of right stellectomy in a vagotomized dog: the sudden drops are clearly the hemodynamic counterpart of premature ventricular contractions. While the electrocardiogram was not yet available, left ventricular pressure was recorded and Hunt noted that during what he called "long beats" there were often brief rises of left ventricular pressure, obviously produced by premature ventricular beats. These changes were never observed following left stellectomy.

In 1946 Pannier [52] extended the earlier work by Langley and demonstrated that electrical stimulation of right rami communicantes produced much larger increases in heart rate than stimulation of left rami communicantes.

In 1956 [55], thanks in part to an accidental delay in the delivery of some equipment necessary to perform studies on sweating and temperature regulation [53], Randall and Rohse completed a preliminary and serendipitous observation made by Randall in 1952 and started the first comprehensive analysis of

THE

American Journal of Physiology.

VOL. II. JULY 1, 1899. NO. V.

DIRECT AND REFLEX ACCELERATION OF THE MAMMALIAN HEART WITH SOME OBSERVATIONS ON THE RELATIONS OF THE INHIBITORY AND ACCELERATOR NERVES.[1]

BY REID HUNT.

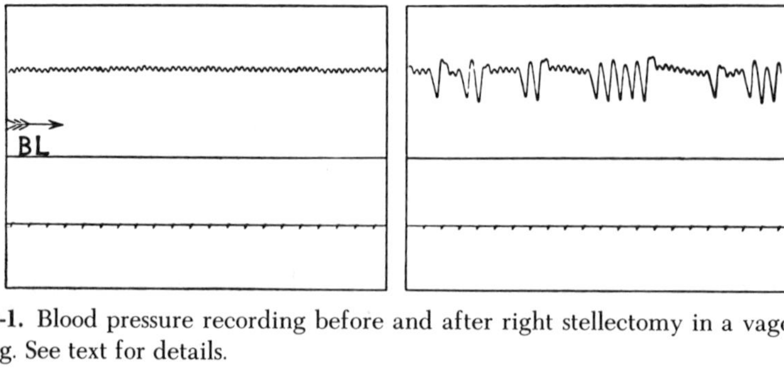

Fig. 10-1. Blood pressure recording before and after right stellectomy in a vagotomized dog. See text for details.

different effects produced by stimulation of right and left cardiac sympathetic nerves. They initially showed that acceleration of heart rate always accompanies elevation of blood pressure when the right stellate ganglion is stimulated, but only occasionally and much less following left stellate ganglion stimulation [55].

In 1966 a medical student, Frank Yanowitz, found that unilateral stimulation and removal of the stellate ganglia produced QT interval lengthening after either right stellectomy or left stellate ganglion stimulation [90]. In both conditions there was dominance of left-sided sympathetic nerves. This observation led Abildskov's group to extensive studies of relationships between the individual sympathetic nerves, their distribution, and some electrophysiologic effects. Mechanisms which may increase the QT interval are subjects of interest because of the tight association between QT prolongation and propensity to reentrant arrhythmias and sudden death [48,67].

In 1972 Armour et al. [3], using electrical stimulation of various local cardiac nerves, found that ventricular arrhythmias could be more easily elicited by stimulation of a large branch originating from the left stellate ganglion, the ventrolateral cardiac nerve.

In 1974 Schwartz et al. [77] found that blockade by cold of the left stellate ganglion during acute myocardial ischemia had an antiarrhythmic effect, while blockade of the right stellate ganglion surprisingly had the opposite effect, namely arrhythmias were increased and ventricular fibrillation more frequent. This observation led to the first study in which a "sympathetic imbalance" created by leaving the heart exposed to reflex sympathetic discharges mediated through only part of cardiac sympathetic innervation, was investigated in specific relationship to cardiac arrhythmias [78].

In 1976 Randall et al. [54] employed a total denervation of the canine heart, but spared the ventrolateral cardiac nerve, to create the first conscious animal model of autonomic imbalance. When these dogs were subjected to strenuous exercise a variety of arrhythmias, including ventricular tachycardia, were produced in the majority of animals.

In 1979 Austoni et al. [5] showed that sympathetic imbalance with left dominance is also arrhythmogenic in humans. This investigation involved patients with Raynaud's syndrome treated with right or left stellectomy and evaluated with an exercise stress test.

DEFINITIONS

Some confusion has arisen from indiscriminate use of the following expressions: autonomic imbalance, vagosympathetic or parasympathetic imbalance, and sympathetic imbalance. Actually, the first three are synonyms and only indicate a "disturbance" in cardiac homeostasis; this depends indeed on a balance of the usually antagonistic influences of the inhibitory parasympathetic nervous system and of the excitatory sympathetic nervous system. A classic example of autonomic imbalance is the situation during the first few hours of an acute myocardial infarction where, depending on the site of the infarct, excessive vagal or sympathetic activity may be present; both may even occur simultaneously, as manifested by concomitant bradycardia and hypertension [88]. Autonomic imbalance, if temporary, is not necessarily pathological since it may occur during normal physiological activity, e.g. exercise. In the latter case it seems that the autonomic balance is altered to actually allow a better cardiac performance; likewise it may allow better adaptation to unusual circumstances, e.g. the diving reflex.

Sympathetic imbalance is a term properly used for conditions in which sympathetic activity is altered or absent in some cardiac nerves but not in others, and typically identifies states in which the heart receives neural impulses in quantities or ratios different from normal from the right and left components of cardiac sympathetic innervation. An early example of sympathetic imbalance was reported by Jonnesco in 1921 [29]. This patient underwent ablation of the left stellate ganglion in the successful and pioneering attempt to interrupt anginal pain; after surgery the heart was exposed only to sympathetic discharges originated through the right cardiac nerves and a state of sympathetic imbalance thus was created.

CARDIAC ARRHYTHMIAS

Two concepts have emerged during the last decade: the left cardiac sympathetic nerves have a prominent arrhythmogenic potential and right stellectomy may produce detrimental effects.

Stimulation Experiments

Armour et al. in 1972 and Hageman et al. in 1973 [3,21] have indicated that while right-sided stimulation induces only sinus tachycardia, stimulation of nerves originating from the left stellate ganglion results in a variety of rhythm disturbances. Most of these arrhythmias are supraventricular [3,21,36]. Stimulation of the left stellate ganglion of an intact heart, may induce reentrant ventricular tachyarrhythmias, e.g. ventricular tachycardia (Fig. 10-2) [78]. This

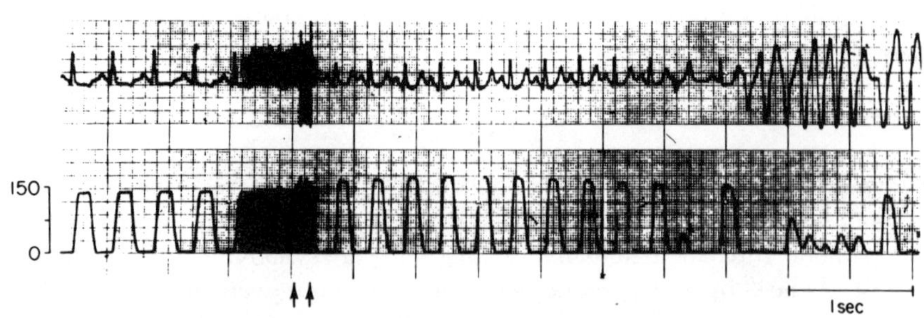

Fig. 10-2. Electrocardiogram and left ventricular pressure in an anesthetized dog. The arrows indicate the electrical stimulation of the left stellate ganglion, which lengthens the QT interval and results in an episode of ventricular tachycardia with significant hemodynamic consequences. (From Schwartz et al., ref. 78)

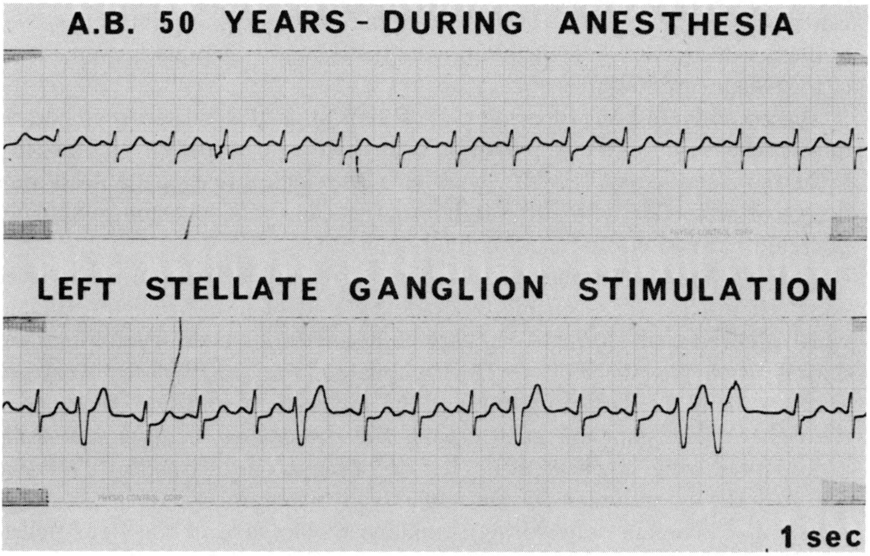

Fig. 10-3. Electrocardiographic tracing in an anesthetized man 50 days after occurrence of an anterior myocardial infarction complicated by ventricular fibrillation. The patient was in sinus rhythm until the left stellate ganglion was mechanically stimulated, leading to frequent premature ventricular beats and couplets. This patient is participating in a multicenter clinical trial in which survivors of an anterior myocardial infarction complicated by ventricular fibrillation are randomly allocated to treatment with either placebo, beta-adrenergic blockade with oxprenolol, or left stellectomy (high thoracic left sympathectomy). (From Schwartz and Stone, ref. 76)

arrhythmogenic potential of left sympathetic stimulation becomes manifest in the presence of myocardial infarction or of acute myocardial ischemia [23,79]. When the left stellate ganglion is briefly stimulated during a short-lasting coronary artery occlusion, ventricular tachycardia and fibrillation are consistently elicited and constitute a reliable and meaningful model for the evaluation of antiarrhythmic interventions [79,80]. Also, when the heart is sensitized to catecholamines by probucol, ventricular fibrillation almost always follows left stellate ganglion stimulation but seldom results from right stellate ganglion stimulation [91].

The arrhythmogenic potential of left-sided cardiac nerves can be observed in humans (idiopathic long QT syndrome) [58] and we have now observed it in patients with ischemic heart disease (Fig. 10-3).

Denervation Experiments

These experiments, to be meaningful, have to be performed in association with cardiac arrhythmias largely dependent on sympathetic activity. A classic example of such a condition is coronary artery occlusion. Acute myocardial ischemia excites sympathetic afferent fibers [41] and elicits an excitatory cardiocardiac sympathetic reflex [42]. This reflex plays a critical role in the arrhythmias associated with acute artery occlusion with significant reduction following section of the dorsal roots C1–T8 which represent the sympathetic input from the heart to the spinal cord [63].

There is a large body of evidence [74] indicating that bilateral sympathectomy protects against these arrhythmias; the most popular study is probably that by Harris et al. in 1951 [22]. It would have been logical to expect at least some degree of protection with either right or left stellate ganglionectomy. Actually, the reality turned out to be quite different.

To avoid the shortcomings associated with irreversible procedures, we developed the method of reversible blockade by cold of either stellate ganglion, which allowed us to alternate coronary occlusion during control conditions and during stellate ganglia blockade. During unilateral blockade the heart is exposed to sympathetic discharge only through the contralateral ganglion. Blockade of the right stellate ganglion greatly enhanced the development of ventricular arrhythmias, while blockade of the left had a major protective effect [78]. Figure 10-4 shows examples of ventricular tachyarrhythmias induced by acute myocardial ischemia only during simultaneous blockade of the right stellate ganglion but not when both ganglia were normally functioning. Thus, despite the fact that the heart was exposed to less sympathetic discharge, the incidence of life-threatening arrhythmias was higher. Similarly, the incidence of ventricular fibrillation was much higher during coronary occlusion performed during right stellate ganglion blockade than during control occlusions.

This was the first evidence for a paradoxical arrhythmogenic effect of right stellectomy and was subsequently confirmed under a variety of experimental conditions. Noteworthy are those of Pandey et al. [51] who have almost exactly duplicated our experimental protocol [78] to obtain exactly the same results.

Did these surprising observations depend on the model used, which involved anesthetized open-chest animals subjected to acute myocardial ischemia? This possibility was disproved in four separate studies in conscious dogs and humans.

Randall and associates [54], pursuing their finding of arrhythmias induced by electrical stimulation of the ventrolateral cardiac nerve (which originates from the left stellate ganglion), evaluated the effect of exercise stress in dogs after cardiac denervation which spared only this nerve. Ventricular arrhythmias were elicited in five of six animals, while no arrhythmias were observed in four dogs with total denervation. These dogs were stressed with maximal exercise beginning on the first day postsurgery; on the other hand, these arrhythmogenic responses were present for prolonged periods of time, although they were more difficult to induce 2 to 5 months after operation.

Schwartz and Stone tested the arrhythmogenic effect of right stellectomy in dogs subjected to submaximal exercises 2–3 weeks after surgery [73]. The incidence of ventricular arrhythmias during exercise was 8% in control dogs (2 of 25) 11% in dogs with left stellectomy (1 of 9), and 86% in dogs with right stellectomy (6 of 7). This result confirmed that susceptibility to ventricular arrhythmias could be enormously increased by simply removing the right stellate ganglion in an otherwise normally innervated heart.

The same type of sympathetic imbalance was found, in a different study [57],

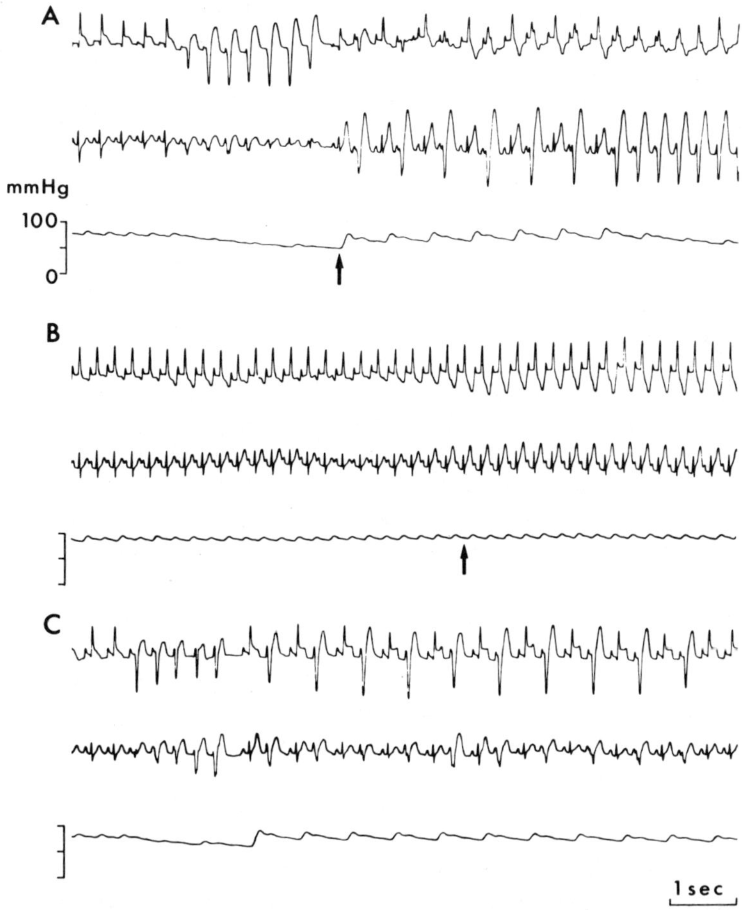

Fig. 10-4. Tracings, from top to bottom, are: ECG (D_1 and D_2), aortic blood pressure. Paper speed 25 mm/sec. Effect of a 20-sec occlusion of both circumflex and left descending coronary artery during the right stellate ganglion blockade and in control. The arrows indicate the release of the occlusion; in C the occlusion was released 2 sec after the end of the strip. A. Coronary artery occlusion during right stellate ganglion blockade: an episode of ventricular tachycardia followed by ventricular bigeminy is evident. B. Coronary artery occlusion under control conditions. No arrhythmias. C. Coronary artery occlusion during right stellate ganglion blockade. Again, ventricular tachycardia and ventricular arrhythmias. These occlusions were consecutive. The control occlusions preceding A and following C produced only a few ectopic beats. (Modified from Schwartz et al., ref. 78)

to facilitate the development of life-threatening arrhythmias in conscious cats exposed to a psychological stress.

Furthermore, the arrhythmogenic effect of right stellectomy was confirmed in man [5]. Seventy-one patients affected by Raynaud's syndrome, without cardiac involvement, and treated with unilateral and bilateral stellectomy were studied with a submaximal exercise stress test and compared to a group of healthy controls. Exercise-induced ventricular arrhythmias appeared in 6 of 34 patients with right stellectomy (18%) in significant contrast with 1 of 32 controls (3%), 1 of 19 patients with left stellectomy (5%), and none of 18 patients with bilateral stellectomy. Stellectomy in man produces less complete denervation than in animals and therefore these findings are likely to underestimate the true effect of unilateral denervation. As discussed below, in order to achieve a degree of denervation in man comparable to that obtained with stellate ganglionectomy in animals, it is necessary to remove the first 4–5 thoracic ganglia.

VULNERABILITY TO VENTRICULAR FIBRILLATION

Electrical stimulation of sympathetic nerves lowers the ventricular fibrillation threshold, i.e. increases vulnerability to fibrillation [87]. As to denervation, only left stellectomy has been evaluated, probably on the assumption that right or bilateral stellectomy would have not added much. Left stellectomy was found to increase ventricular fibrillation threshold by 31% above control values [33].

Unexpected results with right stellectomy prompted us to investigate the specific effect of unilateral stellectomy, or cold block, on ventricular fibrillation threshold in dogs. While ablation or cooling of the left stellate ganglion increased the threshold by 72%, ablation or cooling of the right stellate ganglion reduced ventricular fibrillation threshold by 48% (Fig. 10-5) [70]. These findings have clinical implications, as discussed later, relevant to both the pathogenesis of the long QT syndrome and to the prevention of sudden death in high-risk patients.

During the data analysis one consideration was made which is methodologically important. In 5 out of 25 dogs no change in ventricular fibrillation threshold was observed following ablation of one stellate ganglion and even after bilateral stellectomy. When this group of animals was compared with the group which showed major changes, it became evident that while the level of blood pressure was similar (136 ± 25 vs. 123 ± 9 mm Hg) a large (40 beats/min) and significant difference was present in heart rate (197 ± 19 vs. 157 ± 21 beats/min). This simply indicates, keeping in mind that all animals were vagotomized, that these five animals had low sympathetic activity. It should be obvious that if sympathetic activity is low, no change can be expected by removal of sympathetic nerves.

The effect of unilateral stellectomy on ventricular vulnerability as evidenced by the repetitive extrasystole threshold [44], was subsequently studied by Brooks et al. [11]. A clear difference was found between left stellectomy, which raised the threshold by 27%, and right stellectomy which did not modify (1% difference from control) the threshold for repetitive extrasystole in six dogs. Their conclusion, although in agreement for the protective effect of left stellectomy, did not support the paradoxical effect of right stellectomy. Analysis of the data suggests an explanation for this discrepancy. Despite a blood pressure significantly lower compared to our dogs (117 ± 24 vs. 136 ± 26 mm Hg), the heart rate after vagotomy was considerably lower (176 ± 31 beats/min) in the 12 ani-

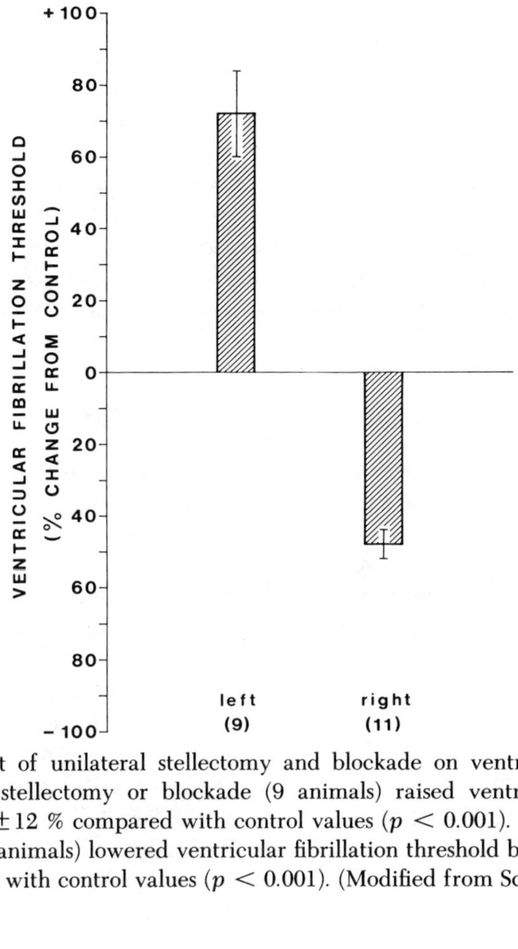

Fig. 10-5. Effect of unilateral stellectomy and blockade on ventricular fibrillation threshold. Left stellectomy or blockade (9 animals) raised ventricular fibrillation threshold by 72±12 % compared with control values ($p < 0.001$). Right stellectomy or blockade (11 animals) lowered ventricular fibrillation threshold by 48±3 % (mean ±SE) compared with control values ($p < 0.001$). (Modified from Schwartz et al., ref. 70)

mals to be studied with either right or left stellectomy. This strongly suggests that many of their animals had a very low resting sympathetic activity, and if the majority were studied with right stellectomy the lack of difference from controls could be easily explained. At any rate, mixing animals with low and normal sympathetic activity certainly blunts the effects of denervation and this may well explain the quantitative differences in our findings with left stellectomy (+72%) and those of Kliks et al. [33] (+31%) and of Brooks et al. [11] (+ 27%).

Studies of ventricular vulnerability to electrical stimuli always require confirmation with life-threatening arrhythmias occurring spontaneously. A clinical example may be represented by amiodarone; its efficacy in protecting patients susceptible to ventricular tachycardia is not predicted by the results with electrophysiologic studies involving programmed electrical stimulation [92].

Significant evidence on the antifibrillatory effect of left stellectomy has been established in a recent study in conscious animals [74]. Thirty-two dogs had an anterior myocardial infarction produced by ligation of the left anterior descending coronary artery. One week later they were randomly allocated to a control or to an experimental group that underwent left stellectomy. One month after ligation while the dogs were conscious, a balloon occluder previously positioned around the circumflex coronary artery was inflated and the ensuing coronary occlusion was maintained for 10 minutes. Ventricular fibrillation occurred in 11 of 17 (65%) control dogs, compared with 5 of 15 (33%) in the experimental group. This study indicated that left stellectomy exerts a major protective effect in reducing the incidence of ventricular fibrillation when conscious dogs with a previous anterior myocardial infarction are exposed to an episode of acute myocardial ischemia.

INSIGHTS ON MECHANISMS

Two aspects of the relationship between sympathetic imbalance and cardiac arrhythmias brought out in experiments detailed above require further clarification: the protective effect of left stellectomy and the paradoxical arrhythmogenic effect of right stellectomy.

Using the coronary flow response to 10-second occlusions in conscious dogs, we found that removal of the left stellate ganglion greatly increased reactive hyperemia, and this result could be mimicked by alpha-adrenergic blockade [72]. Thus, the ability of the coronary bed to dilate increases after left stellectomy. This study indicated that in conscious dogs there is a tonic vasoconstrictor tone dependent on the sympathetic nerves; these results extended the pioneering study by Feigl in 1967 [15] who showed that in anesthetized dogs pretreated with beta blockers, electrical stimulation of the left stellate ganglion induced coronary vasoconstriction. Furthermore, sympathetically mediated vasoconstriction could be demonstrated even when the metabolic demand was elevated in the anesthetized dog [46]. In a further attempt to characterize the role of the sympathetic nervous system in controlling coronary flow in physiologic and clinically relevant conditions, we found that coronary flow was increased by left stellectomy, even during exercise [73].

Concordant evidence on the beneficial effects of left sympathectomy on coronary flow comes from two recent studies employing quite different techniques. In a collaborative study with Janse, DC extracellular electrograms were simultaneously recorded from 60 left ventricular epicardial sites in anesthetized dogs during repeated 5-minute coronary occlusions performed under control conditions and after left or right stellectomy [28]. The degree of TQ segment depression, interpreted as depolarization of resting membrane potential of ischemic cells and thus serving as a quantitative marker of ischemia, was decreased by left stellectomy and, once more paradoxically, augmented by right stellectomy. Also, the electrophysiological border zone, defined as the area where TQ potentials began to become negative, was markedly shifted in opposite directions by left and right unilateral stellectomy.

The effect of left stellectomy on infarct size produced by an 8-hour occlusion of the left anterior descending coronary artery was evaluated in anesthetized cats [83]. Left stellectomy significantly reduced, by approximately 25%, the infarcted area. These data are relevant not only to the neural control of coronary circulation but also to the relationship between sympathetic imbalance and cardiac arrhythmias. It seems that the direct electrophysiologic actions discussed earlier act synergistically with the effects on coronary flow to explain the protective effect of left stellectomy, at least in the setting of acute myocardial ischemia. Conversely, the observed worsening in degree and extension of ischemia produced by right stellectomy at the time of a coronary occlusion [28] certainly helps in understanding how this maneuver may increase the incidence of ventricular arrhythmias during acute myocardial ischemia [78].

However, the overall problem of the paradoxical effect of right stellectomy requires a more comprehensive explanation. A critical piece of information was provided by a study with Verrier and Lown [81] which evaluated sympathetic and vagal influences on ventricular refractoriness using the strength–interval curve [49], which is commonly used as an index of ventricular excitability. Left stellectomy shifted the strength–interval curve later in diastole, indicating

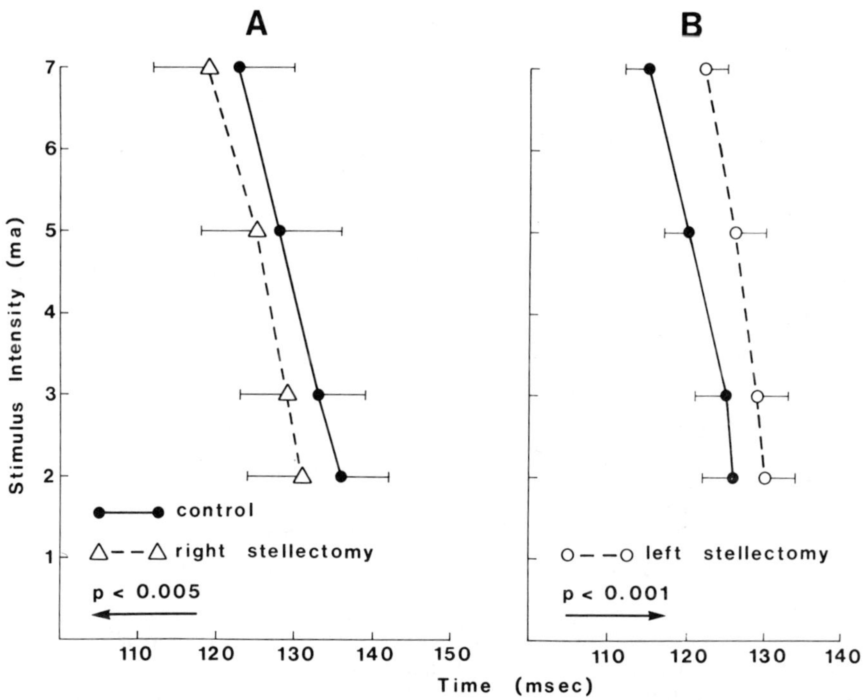

Fig. 10-6. Effect of unilateral stellectomy on the endocardial strength-interval curve in vagotomized dogs. Right stellectomy in six dogs (panel A) shifted the strength-interval curve 3–5 msec earlier; left stellectomy in five dogs (panel B) produced an opposite effect of moving the strength–interval curve 4–7 msec later. Values are expressed as mean ±SE. (From Schwartz et al., ref. 81)

decreased excitability, while right stellectomy had the opposite effect, namely the refractory period was shortened (Fig. 10-6). The effects of bilateral stellectomy were then evaluated by removing the intact ganglion. While the effect of left stellectomy was undeniably greater from a quantitative point of view, right stellectomy—when performed *after* left stellectomy—increased refractoriness (Fig. 10-7). This study indicated that the paradoxical effects of unilateral right stellectomy are dependent on the presence of an intact left stellate ganglion.

Shortly afterwards Haws and Burgess [24] provided important evidence on the quantitative dominance of left-sided nerves. While evaluating the effects of unilateral right, unilateral left, and bilateral stellate stimulation on ventricular refractory periods at sites of overlapping cardiac sympathetic innervation [34], they found that the influences of increased left sympathetic tone exceeded that exerted by right sympathetic nerves. Furthermore, a bilateral increase in cardiac sympathetic tone had no greater effect on recovery properties than the effects of stimulating the left stellate ganglion alone.

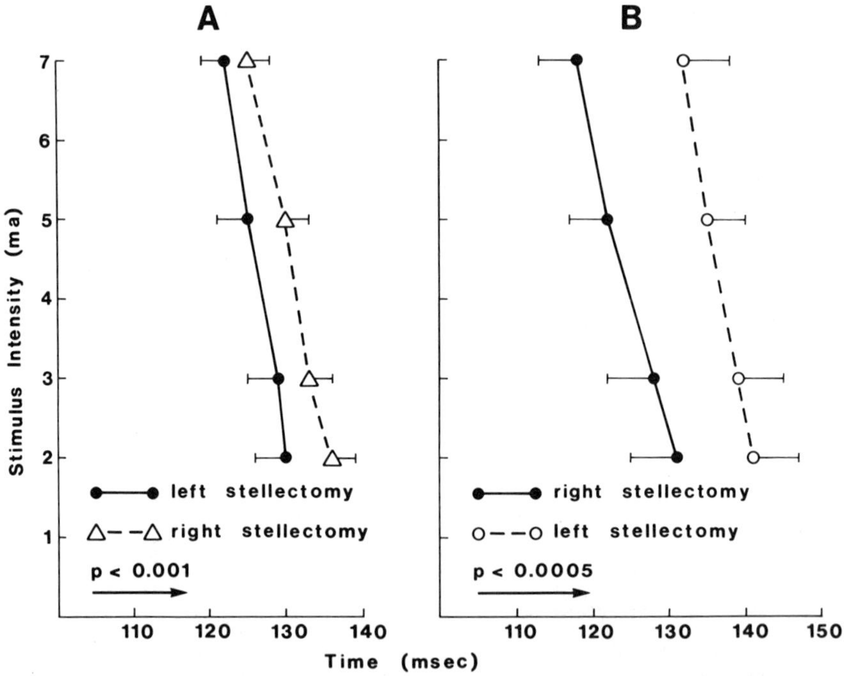

Fig. 10-7. Effect of right and left stellectomy after contralateral stellate ganglion removal. In five dogs in which the left stellate ganglion had been previously removed, right stellectomy shifted the strength–interval curve 3–6 msec later (A). The direction of this shift was opposite to that observed in dogs with an intact left stellate ganglion (Fig. 10-6). Left stellectomy in six dogs with ablated right stellate ganglia shifted the strength–interval curve 10–14 msec later. This effect was qualitatively similar to that observed in dogs with intact right stellate ganglia. (From Schwartz et al., ref. 81)

These findings and a study by McCall et al. [45] (see below) suggested two possible explanations for the effect of right stellectomy [73,81]: (1) when one stellate ganglion is ablated, consequent reduction in systemic arterial pressure and/or in heart rate decreases carotid sinus baroreceptor activity which results in increased sympathetic activity through the contralateral stellate ganglion. Thus, unilateral stellectomy, while suppressing sympathetic activity in the ipsilateral side, may reflexly increase it in the contralateral side. The net change in electrophysiological properties of the ventricles will depend on the net difference between the two opposite influences. In this regard, a crucial role is played by the quantitatively dominant left stellate ganglion; (2) another mechanism is suggested by the work of McCall et al. [45]. Spinal interneurons located in the vicinity of the intermediomedial nucleus directly inhibit part of the sympathoexcitatory pathways located in the intermediolateral spinal nucleus. These inhibitory interneurons receive part of their input from sympathetic afferents in the inferior cardiac nerve. Thus, removal of these afferents—as with unilateral stellectomy—would interrupt the inhibitory pathway and result in increased sympathetic activity through the contralateral stellate ganglion.

These mechanisms, which may provide a working hypothesis to explain the strikingly different effects of unilateral right and left stellectomy, are exemplified in Fig. 10-8. In normal conditions cardiac afferent sympathetic fibers exert reciprocal inhibitory influences on the contralateral stellate ganglion and the heart receives influences which are quantitatively larger from the left side. For simplicity, the diagrams do not show that, under special circumstances, there is also a potential for excitatory influences of a stellate ganglion on its contralateral counterpart through the central nervous system [68].

With left stellectomy, the right stellate ganglion is no longer under inhibitory control and its efferent activity increases; however, because of the lack of dominant tonic activity through the left stellate ganglion, the net result is a decrease in the sympathetic effects on the heart. With right stellectomy, the left stellate ganglion is no longer under inhibitory control and its efferent activity increases; however, the absence of right-sided efferent activity does not compensate for the increase in the already dominant activity of left sympathetic nerves and the net result is now an increase in the sympathetic effects on the heart.

Experimental right stellectomy has provided results consistent with this hypothesis. It is more difficult to evaluate the effects of left stellectomy because of the overall dominance of left-sided nerves. One exception is the sympathetic control of heart rate. This is primarily exerted through the right-sided nerves which, at level of the sinus node, are dominant [55,71]. According to Figure 10-8, one would expect a higher heart rate or enhanced heart rate response after left stellectomy. Indeed, this is the case. After left stellectomy compared to control conditions, heart rate increases more in dogs exercising on a treadmill [73] and in response to a blood pressure reduction induced by nitroprusside (Schwartz and Stone, in preparation). Thus, data available on changes of responses after unilateral stellectomy seem to fit the sequence of events expressed schematically in Fig. 10-8.

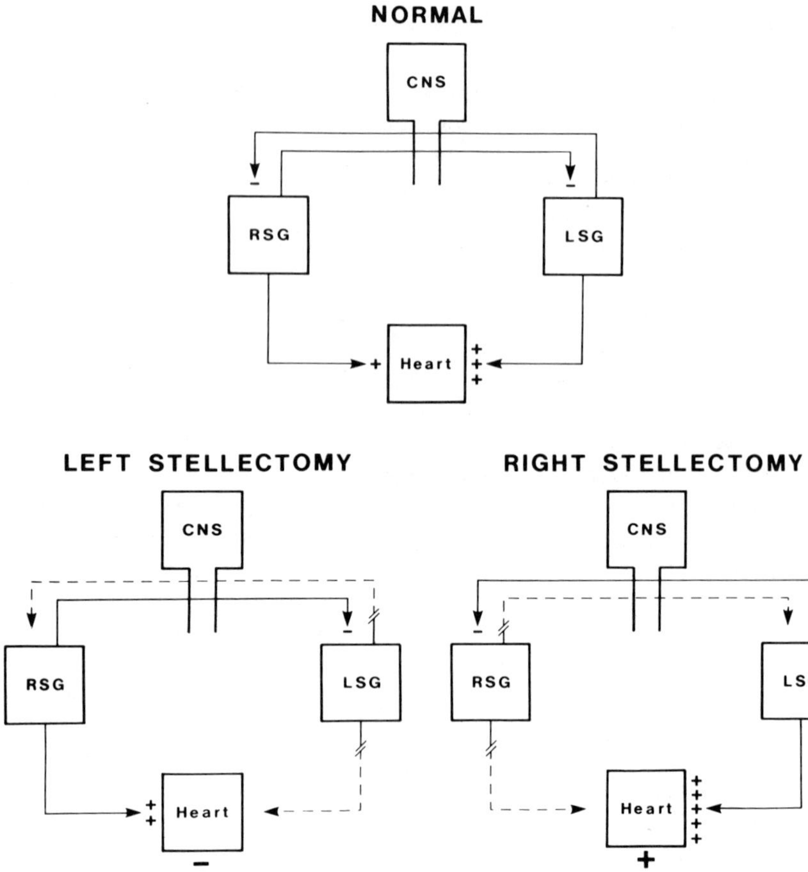

Fig. 10-8. Diagram representing a working hypothesis to explain the effects of unilateral stellectomy. CNS: central nervous system; RSG: right stellate ganglion; LSG: left stellate ganglion. For details see text.

CLINICAL IMPLICATIONS

Sympathetic imbalance has far reaching clinical implications. They are particularly evident in idiopathic long QT syndrome which is a paradigmatic example. Cardiac sympathetic imbalance may provide the key to pathogenetic mechanisms of the long QT syndrome and possibly part of the Sudden Infant Death Syndrome; its analysis has indeed demonstrated the high protective effect of left stellectomy. This latter aspect is currently under extensive investigation because its relevance seems also to extend to the prevention of life-threatening arrhythmias in ischemic heart disease.

The Idiopathic Long QT Syndrome

The long QT syndrome (LQTS) seems to provide a mechanistic link between neural and cardiac factors in the genesis of sudden death and represents the most provocative example of neurally mediated, noncoronary sudden cardiac death [48,58, 67,69].

The affected patients have syncopal attacks in conditions such as violent emotions or physical stresses, associated with sudden increases in sympathetic activity. The syncopal episodes are due to "torsades de pointe," a severe type of ventricular tachycardia which often degenerates into ventricular fibrillation. Typically, these patients have several attacks which frequently are self-terminating but eventually prove fatal. The mortality in untreated patients is 77% [58,69]. An hereditary pattern is relatively common but there are also many sporadic cases.

The only evident abnormalities are in the electrocardiogram which presents a marked prolongation of the QT interval and, usually in coincidence with emotional or physical stresses, episodes of alternation of the T wave [65]. It has been suggested that the same disease may be present even with a normal QT interval in the surface ECG [58].

A critical role for the autonomic nervous system in the pathogenesis of LQTS was suggested by the association of syncopal episodes with increases in sympathetic activity, as produced by vigorous physical activity or by emotional stresses. However, it was necessary to find a unitarian interpretation for the peculiar ECG abnormalities. This was provided by the experimental results of Yanowitz et al. [90], Schwartz and Malliani [65], and by the clinical studies of Moss and Mc Donald [47] and Crampton [13]. Basically, QT prolongation and alternation of the T wave were obtained by either stimulation of the left stellate ganglion or by blockade of the right stellate ganglion. These observations suggested that the LQTS patients may have a congenital imbalance between right and left cardiac sympathetic innervation with left dominance.

An imbalance with left dominance may depend either on primary hyperactivity of left sympathetic nerves or primary hypoactivity of right-sided nerves. The sympathetic control of heart rate is almost exclusively exerted through the right stellate ganglion [55]. This notion, added to the observation that most LQTS patients have unusually low heart rates and that many of them have a diminished heart rate response to exercise, led Schwartz et al. [69] to suggest that a lower than normal right cardiac sympathetic activity might be the basic defect for LQTS. This concept became the useful working hypothesis which has generated a number of experimental studies relevant to both the LQTS and to the understanding of sympathetic imbalance.

The main question was how a lower-than-normal cardiac sympathetic activity could favor arrhythmias and sudden death. Within a few years the following observations were made using right stellectomy or right stellate ganglion blockade as a tool to mimic sympathetic imbalance with left dominance due to reduced right cardiac sympathetic activity. This maneuver increased ventricular arrhythmias during acute myocardial ischemia [78], during exercise in dogs [73] and in man [5], and during emotional stress [57]; it also lowered the threshold for ventricular fibrillation [70] and shortened the ventricular refractory period [81]. Manipulation of the sympathetic nervous system has produced concordant results in patients with LQTS [13,47].

Important support for this hypothesis comes from a recent study by Abildskov et al. [1]. They determined the body surface distribution of ECG potentials in 11 patients with LQTS and compared them to 200 normal adults. Their findings showed prolonged repolarization in anterior and lateral ventricular walls which are predominantly innervated by right-sided sympathetic fibers and, therefore, are entirely consistent with deficient right cardiac sympathetic activity in LQTS patients. Thus, the available experimental and clinical data support the hypothesis of sympathetic imbalance characterized by a lower-than-normal right cardiac sympathetic activity in patients with LQTS. However, the possibility of an unknown intracardiac abnormality which decreases electrical stability and sensitizes the heart to sympathetic discharges mostly mediated through the particularly arrhythmogenic left-sided nerves cannot be excluded.

The rational choice of an adequate therapy merely reflects the degree of understanding of mechanisms of a given disease. The previous analysis clearly indicates that the syncopal episodes of the LQTS depend on sympathetic discharges mostly mediated through left-sided cardiac nerves. Favorable results may thus be expected with either beta-adrenergic blocking agents or left stellectomy.

The first surgical interventions for LQTS were successfully performed by Moss and Mc Donald in 1970 [47] and later on, in 1973, by Schwartz and Malliani [65].

The evaluation of therapeutic efficacy in an uncommon disease presents difficulties. The great sense of cooperation of physicians around the world has allowed, mostly through personal contacts, an analysis based on 576 patients [67] which extends and confirms an earlier survey made in 1975 [69]. The main points are the following: the mortality for untreated patients is extremely high (77%); with miscellaneous treatment, which does not include beta blockers, it remains high (50%); with beta blockers it is markedly decreased (7%); 14 patients all refractory to beta blockers at full dose underwent left stellectomy and their mortality was 7%. It is quite obvious that both antiadrenergic interventions are very effective; however it has to be noted that if the 14 patients who continue having syncopal attacks despite beta blockers did not have the chance of sympathetic denervation the mortality figure for beta blockers would certainly be higher. These patients clearly represented the subgroup at highest risk. Keeping this fact in mind, we realize that the results obtained with left stellectomy are extremely rewarding. The significance and implications of these data have been extensively discussed elsewhere [58,69].

The original rationale of left stellectomy was to shorten the QT interval; however, the experience with 14 patients indicates that QT interval shortened significantly, after left stellectomy, in only half of them despite protection from malignant arrhythmias. The experimental studies listed above have indicated that the main goal now is to afford protection against ventricular fibrillation independently of changes in QT interval. In the last few years left sympathectomy has become the treatment of choice for those patients who, despite beta blockade, continue to have syncopal episodes.

Sudden Infant Death Syndrome (SIDS)

With the exception of the first week postnatally, the leading cause of death in the first year of life is the Sudden Infant Death Syndrome (SIDS). In the U.S. it claims 8,000–10,000 victims annually. The typical clinical story is that an apparently healthy infant, age two to four months, routinely put to sleep for a nap or for the night, is found dead sometime shortly thereafter or the next morning. A thorough postmortem examination fails to demonstrate an adequate cause of death.

There is almost a consensus that SIDS depends on a respiratory defect; nonetheless, the possibility of a primary cardiac death in SIDS was proposed in 1968 [27] and is logically tenable [16]. The cardiac theory proposed that at least some cases of SIDS might depend on sudden sympathetic discharges taking place through an asymmetrically developed cardiac sympathetic innervation with left dominance [56,59], similar to that congenitally present in the idiopathic long QT syndrome.

This developmental imbalance would manifest itself with a temporary prolongation of the QT interval, evident either at birth or during the first few months of life, thus allowing early identification of the "at risk" babies.

A prospective study specifically designed to test this hypothesis, referred to as the QT hypothesis, is currently ongoing and has already provided some interesting information. Over 4200 newborns have been enrolled, and it has been found that QTc (QT interval corrected for heart rate) lengthens during the second month of life, remains prolonged during the fourth month, and by the sixth month returns to baseline values [66]. This curve matches that of the incidence of SIDS and indicates that during development there is a tendency toward a *temporary* decrease in cardiac electrical stability as manifest by the increase in the QT interval. Three SIDS cases have already occurred and their QTc exceeded the mean by more than 2, 3, and 9 standard deviations respectively. These findings are too limited numerically to draw any conclusion, but are consistent with the QT hypothesis.

Evidence for developmental imbalance in the cardiac sympathetic innervation comes from a study by Kralios and Millar [35]. They found evidence in puppies for a nonuniform maturation of cardiac nerves and, more specifically, observed that at third week of life there is a predominance of left-sided nerves. This may represent the explanation for the temporary prolongation of QT interval observed in normal babies [66] and may provide the physiological substrate for a time-limited decrease in electrical stability of the heart which favors life-threatening arrhythmias, as previously postulated [56].

It is entirely possible that other types of developmental abnormalities in cardiac innervation may occur in some infants predisposing to ventricular fibrillation. They may involve, among others, an insufficient vagal activity with lack of its protective effect [86] and may become manifest by specific alterations, e.g. higher than normal heart rate or abnormally low heart rate variability.

The "QT hypothesis" has generated a controversy which has been discussed in detail elsewhere [59,60].

Ischemic Heart Disease

The relationship between sympathetic imbalance and ischemic heart disease is primarily based on the protective effects of left stellectomy; however, recent data may extend this relationship.

Zipes' group has found that experimental transmural infarction produces a sympathetic denervation even in the noninfarcted area below the infarct site, probably dependent on destruction of the nerve fibers passing through the infarcted area [6,7].

Myocardial infarction involving the anterior ventricular surface would result in greater destruction of right-sided sympathetic nerves than of left-sided nerves, thus reproducing the arrhythmogenic condition of sympathetic imbalance with left dominance. This may contribute to the well-known propensity of anterior wall myocardial infarctions to ventricular tachyarrhythmias. Also, since this denervation is postganglionic, a functionally effective and complete reinnervation would be expected within 9–12 months [30]. This may contribute to the fact that cardiac electrical instability is particularly high in the first year after myocardial infarction and then gradually returns to normal. Finally, this observation may help in understanding the mechanism underlying QT prolongation, and susceptibility to sudden death, in patients with myocardial infarction. In 1976, and more extensively in 1978, Schwartz and Wolf demonstrated that prolongation of the QT interval in patients with a previous myocardial infarction is an important predictor of subsequent sudden death [82]. This finding has been confirmed [2,25] and QT interval prolongation has been found to have a strong association with life-threatening arrhythmias even in the acute stage of myocardial infarction [83]. Also in dogs with one-month old anterior myocardial infarction, QT prolongation identifies a subgroup at higher risk of sudden death [74]. This electrocardiographic change may partially depend on the extent of the infarcted area but, as we have speculated [74], it may also reflect damage of adrenergic terminals mostly innervated by right-sided nerves, thus mimicking effects of right stellectomy, which are associated with prolongation of the QT interval [90] and ventricular arrhythmias [78]. This view is now supported by the studies of Zipes' group [6,7].

The high arrhythmogenic potential of left-sided cardiac sympathetic nerves, discussed earlier, has unavoidably led to the realization of the antiarrhythmic effect of their removal. Left stellectomy, directly or indirectly, increases electrical stability of the heart. It reduces ventricular arrhythmias associated with acute myocardial ischemia [78] and increases the threshold for ventricular fibrillation [70]. It lengthens the ventricular refractory period, thus decreasing cardiac excitability [81]. It halves the incidence of ventricular fibrillation in conscious dogs undergoing acute myocardial ischemia one month after an anterior myocardial infarction [74]. It reduces to zero (0 out of 14) from 66% (6 out of 35) the incidence of ventricular fibrillation in dogs subjected to a brief episode of acute myocardial ischemia superimposed at the end of an exercise stress test, also in this case one month after an anterior myocardial infarction [61]. Also, left stellectomy, by increasing the capability of coronary bed to dilate, both at rest and during exercise [72,73], may limit the ischemic area by improving the perfusion of the border zone [28,84] and contribute to the preservation of ventricular function.

It is noteworthy that left stellectomy, unlike most antiarrhythmic drugs, is not accompanied by a negative inotropic effect. Thus, myocardial contractility is not reduced by left stellectomy either at rest or during exercise stress testing [73]. Of particular clinical relevance is the fact that this lack of negative effects on the contractility of the left ventricle is present in dogs with a prior myocardial infarction performing an exercise stress test [64]. Also in humans, left stellectomy does not induce the appearance of dyspnea during exertion in an exercise stress test, in contrast with what happens with bilateral stellectomy [4].

These data have led to a clinical trial in which a subgroup of patients with anterior myocardial infarction at high risk for sudden death is randomized between placebo, the beta blocker oxprenolol, and high thoracic left stellectomy. Whatever its outcome, this trial, ongoing in Northern Italy since 1979, is evidence of the tight relationship between experimental and clinical cardiology.

The utilization of coronary bypass surgery has focused new interest on the possibility of performing surgical denervation at the same time. Since the first formal proposal by Kaye and Randall in 1974 [31], several reports have appeared on various interventions in patients with Prinzemetal's angina [8–10,12,20]. Since this issue is specifically dealt with in chapter 13, only a few considerations seem appropriate, particularly on some of the limitations of these procedures, be they plexectomy, ventricular denervation, or autotransplantation.

The first limitation concerns the complexity, the magnitude, and the high potential for incompleteness of these interventions, the simpler one being a ventricular sympathetic denervation as discussed by Kaye and Randall [32]. This means that the surgery requires considerable expertise and carries a degree of risk for the patients.

Second, total ventricular denervation leaves the heart completely without adrenergic support which, in ischemic hearts with an already reduced left ventricular function, may be detrimental.

The third and main limitation of all of these interventions is that they produce a postganglionic denervation. This implies that within a variable amount of time, most likely less than a year [30], neural regeneration will occur, thus minimizing potential benefits. Admittedly, this regeneration may not be complete; however, in the possible case of an earlier or greater reinnervation from the left-sided nerves, the most dangerous type of sympathetic imbalance may occur and predispose to life-threatening arrhythmias. Also, since a postganglionic denervation depletes myocardial catecholamines, denervation supersensitivity has to be expected with many potential ill effects. These two latter points represent, in my opinion, a major limitation for the long-term clinical validity and for the physiological significance of this group of surgical interventions.

These limitations may be contrasted with left stellectomy (high thoracic left sympathectomy), which constitutes minor surgery, being performed extrapleurally without entering the chest. After left stellectomy the heart still receives adrenergic support from the right-sided cardiac sympathetic nerves; thus, the heart rate control remains intact and, together with partial innervation of the ventricles, allows the maintenance of a normal ventricular performance. This is documented by the enormous difference in myocardial contractility between dogs with left stellectomy and dogs with bilateral stellectomy [73].

Furthermore, because in humans the stellate ganglion is the fusion between the inferior (or caudal) cervical ganglion and the first thoracic ganglion [38], this surgery not only is preganglionic but removes also most cardiac sympathetic synaptic connections located in these two ganglia [89]. As a result. significant reinnervation does not occur. This is confirmed by almost ten years' experience with left stellectomy in patients with idiopathic long QT syndrome [58,67]. Finally, left stellectomy does not induce denervation supersensitivity [75].

METHODS OF STUDY AND LIMITATIONS

Sympathetic imbalance may be studied in two ways. The first involves augmentation in the activity of some cardiac sympathetic nerves, mostly by the use of electrical stimulation. The second involves section, or blockage, of cardiac sympathetic branches innervating the heart. With the latter procedure the heart remains exposed to the neural discharges originating from one side or from part of one side only.

Electrical stimulation of cardiac nerves is a seemingly simple maneuver in widespread use. It is certainly useful in identifying neural circuits, areas of innervation, and in suggesting neurally mediated effects on cardiac functions and parameters. However, it has both serious limitations and pitfalls.

Results obtained with this technique should be interpreted with caution, considering the artificial nature of the stimulus. First of all, it shows the effect of massive activation of all nerve fibers present in the stimulated nerves, an unlikely event in a system characterized by a very high degree of specificity [50] (Fig. 10-9). Also, the rate of firing of sympathetic neurons, even during reflex excitation, is much lower than that usually produced by electrical stimulation [40,42,50]. In addition, many postganglionic nerves contain vagal efferent fibers, so that adrenergic and cholinergic effects are simultaneously produced, but the results are frequently interpreted as "pure" sympathetic effects. Extreme examples of these diffculties are those experiments [18] in which cardiac arrhythmias resistant to any pharmacologicel intervention had been produced because, as shown later by Randall's group [14], the electrical simulation had been performed so distally that a column of cardiac muscle fibers is included.

Another major set of problems exists. In most cases when the stellate ganglia are stimulated they are not decentralized and this, in addition to the stimulation of efferent fibers, results in the simultaneous reflex activation of the contralateral stellate ganglion concurrently with an inhibition of the cardiac vagal efferent activity [68]. Thus, once more, what is claimed to be the result of a purely unilateral sympathetic stimulation is instead the algebraic summation of several individual effects. On the other hand, if the more correct stimulation of a decen-

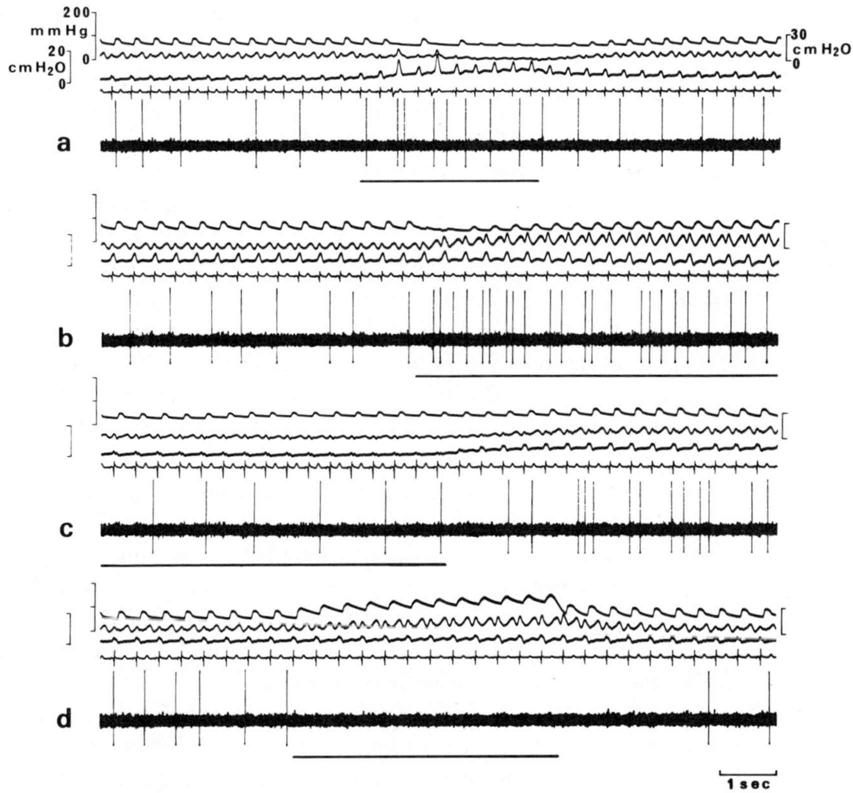

Fig. 10-9. Anesthetized cat, with spinal section at C1, bilateral vagotomy, and bilateral carotid sinus denervation. Increases or decreases in the discharge of the same sympathetic preganglionic neuron obtained with different stimuli. Tracings represent, from top to bottom, the carotid arterial blood pressure, the left atrial pressure, the right atrial pressure, the ECG, and the nervous recording. (a) Stenosis of the pulmonary artery by a snare; (b) obstruction of the left ventricular outflow by inflating a balloon in the root of the aorta; (c) release of a transient occlusion of the inferior vena cava; (d) obstruction of the midthoracic aorta by a snare. The first three maneuvers activate cardiac receptors and elicit a reflex increase in sympathetic efferent activity, while the latter also activates aortic receptors and induces an inhibition of the sympathetic outflow. (From Pagani, et al., ref. 50)

tralized stellate ganglion is performed, other problems are encountered. Namely, the "control" condition, just before stimulation, is artificial. A unilaterally or bilaterally sympathetically denervated heart is suddenly exposed to the major and unrealistic shift from no sympathetic activity to a massive neural discharge.

The second approach studies the effects of selective denervation and explores the importance of the tonic sympathetic activity present in the nerves under investigation. In addition, it allows observation, in a physiological context, of the manifestations and consequences of sympathetic imbalance.

One requirement is essential for drawing valid conclusions from the results of denervation studies and constitutes a prerequisite for meaningful experiments: a high resting level in sympathetic activity. Since these studies are based on evaluation of the effects of unilaterally withdrawing the resting level of sympathetic activity, it is quite evident that should this level be low, very minor changes could be expected. Therefore, denervation experiments are properly conducted: (1) using room air for respiration and avoiding the chemoceptive inhibition of sympathetic outflow induced by high oxygen; (2) using bilateral vagotomy in order to eliminate the inhibitory vagal afferent control on sympathetic efferent activity; (3) performing the experiments under conditions of naturally increased sympathetic activity, such as exercise, psychologic stress or, to a lesser extent, acute myocardial ischemia. Another related and important factor is individual variability and it is known that some animals, for unknown reasons, have a low sympathetic activity. They are readily identified by a relatively low heart rate for a given level of blood pressure [70]. Failure to account for these variables predisposes to misleading results and faulty conclusions.

Another cause of error is traumatic damage in the preparation of the nerves to be stimulated, blocked, or sectioned. Sympathetic nerves are quite sensitive to stretch, and to exposure to heat or to dry environment, and while apparently intact, their function and activity is easily and irreversibly damaged. Electrophysiological recording of single sympathetic fibers is extremely useful for realizing what really goes on in the cardiac nerves, and to learn that even minor mismanagement of sympathetic nerves annuls or greatly reduces this activity. Unfortunately, in most experiments the surgical technique used, while adequate for dissecting muscles and vessels, may severely damage sympathetic nerves.

Sympathetic imbalance, in relation to cardiac arrhythmias or to other functions, may also be studied in humans. When a study is performed before and after unilateral sympathectomy [4,5], there are no major problems. However, most commonly a pharmacological blockade is attempted. This procedure, although potentially very useful, is liable to misinterpretations [69]. The main difficulty is represented by the unavoidable uncertainty of the effectiveness of the blockade. A persistent misconception is that the appearance of a Horner syndrome is a marker of an effective blockade of the stellate ganglion. Actually, since the fibers going to the eye traverse the upper part of the stellate ganglion, the Horner syndrome indicates only that the local anesthetic used for the block has reached the cephalic pole of the stellate ganglion; it provides no clue whatsoever to the simultaneous blockade of the fibers directed to the heart which are located more caudally. A somewhat greater likelihood of a correct interpretation may be achieved by observing a simultaneous rise of temperature of the thumb or fingers, augmented pulse in the forefingers by plethysmograph, and changes of galvanic skin resistance [13]. However, a pharmacological blockade of the cardiac sympathetic fibers running through one stellate ganglion may only be estimated. This means that only if a *change* in a cardiovascular parameter occurs is this assumption legitimate; if no changes are observed it is almost impossible to discriminate between a lack of effective procedure and failure to achieve complete blockade of the cardiac sympathetic fibers. An exception is the blockade of the right stellate ganglion after atropinization; this maneuver produces a substantial fall in heart rate which may serve as a guide throughout the procedure [78].

Reversible blockade of one stellate ganglion may conveniently be achieved in experimental animals by cold [70,78]. The advantage of a cold blockade is that it allows rapid shifts between control conditions and unilateral blockade and this may be done several times during one experiment. In this way effects due to unilateral blockade of one stellate ganglion may be clearly and convincingly demonstrated.

REFERENCES

1. Abildskov, J. A., G. M. Vincent, A. K. Evans, M. J. Burgess, Distribution of body surface ECG potentials in familial QT interval prolongation, *Am. J. Cardiol. 47*: 480, 1981.
2. Ahnve, S., C. Helmers, T. Lundman, N. Rehnqvist, A. Sjogren, QTc interval in acute myocardial infarction: first year prognostic implications. *Clin. Cardiol. 3*: 303–308, 1980.
3. Armour, J. A., G. R. Hageman, W. C. Randall, Arrhythmias induced by local cardiac nerve stimulation. *Am. J. Physiol. 223*: 1068–1075, 1972.
4. Austoni, P., R. Rosati, L. Gregorini, E. Bianchi, E. Bortolani, U. Fox, P. J. Schwartz, Effects of stellectomy on exercise-induced QT changes in man. *Circulation 56, Suppl. III*: 184, 1977.
5. Austoni, P., R. Rosati, L. Gregorini, E. Bianchi, E. Bortolani, P. J. Schwartz, Stellectomy and exercise in man. *Am. J. Cardiol. 43*: 399, 1979.
6. Barber, M. J., T. M. Mueller, D. P. Zipes, Evidence that transmural infarct ablates electrophysiologic responses to sympathetic nerve stimulation outside the infarct. *Clin. Res. 29*: 749A, 1981.
7. Barber, M. J., T. M. Mueller, J. P. Phillips, D. P. Zipes, Chronic transmural infarction prevents refractory period shortening by sympathetic nerve stimulation in noninfarcted areas apical to infarct. *Am. J. Cardiol. 49*: 899, 1982.
8. Bertrand, M. E., J. M. Lablanche, M. F. Rousseau, H. H. Jr. Warembourg, C. Stankowiak, G. Soots, Surgical treatment of variant angina: use of plexectomy with aortocoronary bypass. *Circulation 61*: 877–882, 1980.
9. Bertrand, M. E., J. M. Lablanche, P. Y. Tilmant, Treatment of Prinzmetal's variant angina. Role of medical treatment with nifedipine and surgical coronary revascularization combined with plexectomy. *Am. J. Cardiol. 47*: 174–178, 1981.
10. Bertrand, M. E., J. M. Lablanche, P. Y. Tilmant, C. Ducloux, H. Jr. Warembourg, G. Soots, Complete denervation of the heart (autotransplantation) for treatment of severe, refractory coronary spasm. *Am. J. Cardiol. 47*: 1375–1378, 1981.
11. Brooks, W. W., R. L. Verrier, B. Lown, Influence of vagal tone on stellectomy-induced changes in ventricular electrical stability. *Am. J. Physiol. 234*: H503–H507, 1978.
12. Clark, D. A., R. A. Quint, R. L. Mitchell, W. W. Angell, Coronary artery spasm. Medical management, surgical denervation and autotransplantation. *J. Thorac. Cardiovasc. Surg. 73*: 332–339, 1977.
13. Crampton, R. S., Preeminence of the left stellate ganglion in the long Q-T syndrome. *Circulation 59*: 769–778, 1979.

14. Euler, D. E., H. K. Jacobs, E. R. Hageman, W. C. Randall, An explanation for the pharmacological resistance of arrhythmias induced by sympathetic nerve stimulation. *Fed. Proc. 34*: 375, 1975.
15. Feigl, E. O., Sympathetic control of coronary circulation. *Circ. Res. 20*: 262–271, 1967.
16. Froggatt, P. and T. N. James, Sudden unexpected death in infants. Evidence on a lethal cardiac arrhythmia. *Ulster Med. J. 52*: 136–152, 1973.
17. Geesbreght, J. M. and W. C. Randall, Area localization of shifting pace-makers during sympathetic stimulation. *Am. J. Physiol. 220*: 1522–1527, 1971.
18. Gillis, R. A., O. L. Pearle, T. Hoekman, Failure of beta-adrenergic receptor blockade to prevent arrhythmias induced by sympathetic nerve stimulation. *Science 185*: 70–72, 1974.
19. Goldberg, J. M., J. M. Geesbreght, W. C. Randall, G. Brynjolfsson, Sympathetically induced pacemaker shifts following sinus node excision. *Am. J. Physiol. 224*: 1468–1474, 1973.
20. Grondin, C. M. and R. Limet, Sympathetic denervation in association with coronary artery grafting in patients with Prinzmetal's variant angina. *Ann. Thorac. Surg. 23*: 111–117, 1977.
21. Hageman, G. R., J. M. Goldberg, J. A. Armour, W. C. Randall, Cardiac dysrhythmias induced by autonomic nerve stimulation. *Am. J. Cardiol. 32*: 823–830, 1973.
22. Harris, S. A., A. Estandia, R. F. Tillotson, Ventricular ectopic rhythms and ventricular fibrillation following cardiac sympathectomy and coronary occlusion. *Am. J. Physiol. 165*: 505–512, 1951.
23. Harris, A. S., H. Otero, A. J. Bocage, The induction of arrhythmias by sympathetic activity before and after occlusion of a coronary artery in the canine heart. *J. Electrocardiol. 4*: 34–43, 1971.
24. Haws, C. W. and M. J. Burgess, Effects of bilateral and unilateral stellate stimulation on canine ventricular refractory period. *Circ. Res. 42*: 195–198, 1978.
25. Haynes, R. E., A. P. Hallstrom, and L. A. Cobb, Repolarization abnormalities in survivors of out-of-hospital ventricular fibrillation. *Circulation 57*: 654–658, 1978.
26. Hunt, R., Direct and reflex acceleration of the mammalian heart with some observation on the relations of the inhibitory and accelerator nerves. *Am. J. Physiol. 2*: 395–470, 1899.
27. James, T. N. Sudden death in babies. *Am. J. Cardiol. 22*: 479–506, 1968.
28. Janse, M. J., P. J. Schwartz, Effect of cardiac sympathetic nerves on electrophysiologic changes induced by acute myocardial ischemia in dogs, *Europ. Heart J. 4*: Supp E, 38, 1983.
29. Jonnesco, T., Traitement chirurgical de l'angine de poitrine par la resection du sympathetic cervico-thoracique. *Presse Med. 20*: 193–194, 1921.
30. Kaye, M. P., W. C. Randall, G. R. Hageman, W. P. Geis, D. V. Priola, Chronology and mode of reinnervation of the surgically denervated canine heart: functional and chemical correlates. *Am. J. Physiol. 233*: 431–437, 1977.
31. Kaye, M. P. and W. C. Randall, Coronary artery surgery. Could it be better? *Curr. Med. Dialog. 41*: 531–532, 1974.
32. Kaye, M. P. and W. C. Randall, Cardiac denervation with aortocoronary bypass. *Circulation 62*: 1389, 1980.
33. Kliks, B. R., M. J. Burgess, J. A. Abildskov, Influence of sympathetic tone on ventricular fibrillation threshold during experimental coronary occlusion. *Am. J. Cardiol. 36*: 45–49, 1975.

34. Kralios, F. A., L. Martin, M. J. Burgess, C. K. Millar, Local ventricular repolarization changes due to sympathetic nerve branch stimulation. *Am. J. Physiol. 228*: 1621–1626, 1975.
35. Kralios, F. A. and C. K. Millar, Functional development of cardiac sympathetic nerves in newborn dogs: evidence for asymmetrical development. *Cardiovasc. Res. 12*: 547–554, 1978.
36. Kralios, F. A. and C. K. Millar, Sympathetic neural effects on regional atrial recovery properties and cardiac rhythm. *Am. J. Physiol. 240*: H590–H596, 1981.
37. Langley, J. N., On the origin from the spinal cord of the cervical and upper thoracic sympathetic fibres, with some observations on white and grey rami communicantes. *Phil. Trans. Roy. Soc. London 183 B, 107*: 85–124, 1892.
38. Leriche, R. and R. Fontaine, The surgical treatment of angina pectoris: what it is and what it should be. *Am. Heart J. 3*: 649–671, 1927/28.
39. Lown, B. Sudden cardiac death: the major challenge confronting contemporary cardiology. *Am. J. Cardiol. 43*: 313–328, 1979.
40. Malliani, A., M. Pagani, G. Recordati, P. J. Schwartz, Spinal sympathetic reflexes elicited by increases in arterial blood pressure. *Am. J. Physiol. 220*: 128–134, 1971.
41. Malliani, A., G. Recordati, P. J. Schwartz, Nervous activity of afferent cardiac sympathetic fibres with atrial and ventricular endings. *J. Physiol. 229*: 457–469, 1973.
42. Malliani, A., P. J. Schwartz, A. Zanchetti, A sympathetic reflex elicited by experimental coronary occlusion. *Am. J. Physiol. 217*: 703–709, 1969.
43. Malliani, A., P. J. Schwartz, A. Zanchetti, Neural mechanisms in life-threatening arrhythmias. *Am. Heart J. 100*: 705–715, 1980.
44. Matta, R. J., J. E. Lawler, B. Lown, Ventricular electrical instability in the conscious dog. Effects of psychologic stress and beta-adrenergic blockade. *Am. J. Cardiol. 38*: 594–598, 1976.
45. R. B. McCall, G. L. Gebber, S. M. Barman, Spinal interneurons in the baroreceptor reflex arc. *Am. J. Physiol. 232*: 657–665, 1977.
46. Mohrman, D. E. and E. O. Feigl, Competition between sympathetic vasoconstriction and metabolic vasodilatation in the coronary circulation. *Circ. Res. 42*: 79-86, 1978.
47. Moss, A. J. and J. McDonald, Unilateral cervicothoracic sympathetic ganglionectomy for the treatment of long QT interval syndrome. *N. Eng. J. Med. 285*: 903–904, 1971.
48. Moss, A. J. and P. J. Schwartz, Delayed repolarization (QT or QT prolongation) and malignant arrhythmias. *Mod. Conc. Cardiovasc. Med. 51*: 85–90, 1982.
49. Orias, O., C. McC. Brooks, E. E. Suckling, Excitability of the mammalian ventricle throughout the cardiac cycle. *Am. J. Physiol. 163*: 272–282, 1951.
50. Pagani, M., P. J. Schwartz, R. Banks, F. Lombardi, A. Malliani, Reflex responses of sympathetic preganglionic neurones initiated by different cardiovascular receptors in spinal animals. *Brain Res. 68*: 215–225, 1974.
51. Pandey, R. C., R. D. Srivastava, V. N. Bathnagar, Effect of unilateral stellate ganglion blockade and stimulation on experimental arrhythmias. *Ind. J. Physiol. Pharmacol. 23*: 305–314, 1979.
52. Pannier, R., Contribution à l'innervation sympatique du coeur. Les nerfs cardioaccélérateurs, *Arch. Int. Pharmacodyn. 73*: 193–259, 1946.
53. Randall, W. C. *Neural Regulation of the Heart.* Oxford University Press, New York, 1977.

54. Randall, W. C., M. P. Kaye, G. R. Hageman, H. K. Jacobs, D. E. Euler, W. H. Wehrmacher, Cardiac dysrhythmias in the conscious dog following surgically induced autonomic imbalance. *Am J. Cardiol.* *38*: 178–183, 1976.
55. Randall, W. C. and W. G. Rohse, The augmenter action of the sympathetic cardiac nerves. *Circ. Res.* *4*: 470–475, 1956.
56. Schwartz, P. J., Cardiac sympathetic innervation and the sudden infant death syndrome. A possible pathogenetic link. *Am. J. Med.* *60*: 167–172, 1976.
57. Schwartz, P. J., Experimental reproduction of the long QT syndrome. *Am. J. Cardiol.* *41*: 374, 1978.
58. Schwartz, P. J., The long Q-T syndrome. In *Sudden Death*, ed. H. E. Kulbertus and H. J. J. Wellens, M. Nijhoff, The Hague, 1980, pp. 358–378.
59. Schwartz, P. J. The sudden infant death syndrome. In *Reviews in Perinatal Medicine*, Vol. 4, ed. E. M. Scarpelli and E. V. Cosmi. Raven Press, New York, 1981, pp. 475–524.
60. Schwartz, P. J., Autonomic nervous system, ventricular fibrillation and SIDS. In *Sudden Infant Death Syndrome*, Eds. J.T. Tildan, L.M. Roeder, A. Steinschneider, Academic Press, New York, 1983, p. 319–340.
61. Schwartz, P. J., G. E. Billman, H. L. Stone, Autonomic interventions in a new animal model for sudden death. *Circulation 64, Suppl 4*: 289, 1981.
62. Schwartz, P. J., A. M. Brown, A. Malliani, A. Zanchetti, eds., Neural *Mechanisms in Cardiac Arrhythmias*. Raven Press, New York, 1978.
63. Schwartz, P. J., R. D. Foreman, H. L. Stone, A. M. Brown, Effect of dorsal root section on the arrhythmias associated with coronary occlusion. *Am. J. Physiol.* *231*: 923–928, 1976.
64. Schwartz, P. J., P. A. Gwirtz, H. L. Stone, Cardiac performance before and after left stellectomy in dogs with an anterior myocardial infarction. *Proc. 8th Europ. Congr. Cardiol.*, Paris, 1980, pp. 121.
65. Schwartz, P. J. and A. Malliani, Electrical alternation of the T wave: clinical and experimental evidence of its relationship with the sympathetic nervous system and with the long QT syndrome. *Am. Heart J.* *89*: 45–50, 1975.
66. Schwartz, P. J., M. Montemerlo, M. Facchini, P. Salice, D. Rosti, G. Poggio, R. Giorgetti, The Q-T interval throughout the first six months of life: a prospective study. *Circulation* *66*: 496–501, 1982.
67. Schwartz, P. J. and A. J. Moss, QT interval prolongation. What does it mean? *J. Cardiovasc. Med.*, *7*: 1317–1330, 1982.
68. Schwartz, P. J., M. Pagani, F. Lombardi, A. Malliani, A. M. Brown, A cardiocardiac sympathovagal reflex in the cat. *Circ. Res.* *32*: 215–220, 1973.
69. Schwartz, P. J., M. Periti, A. Malliani, The long Q-T syndrome. *Am. Heart J.* *89*: 378–390, 1975.
70. Schwartz, P. J., N. G. Snebold, and A. M. Brown, Effects of unilateral cardiac sympathetic denervation on the ventricular fibrillation threshold. *Am. J. Cardiol.* *37*: 1034–1040, 1976.
71. Schwartz, P. J. and H. L. Stone., Role of right stellate ganglion during exercise. *Europ. J. Clin. Invest.* *6*: 328, 1976.
72. Schwartz, P. J. and H. L. Stone, Tonic influence of the sympathetic nervous system on myocardial reactive hyperemia and on coronary blood flow distribution. *Circ. Res.* *41*: 51–58, 1977.
73. Schwartz, P. J. and H. L. Stone, Effects of unilateral stellectomy upon cardiac performance during exercise in dogs. *Circ. Res.* *44*: 637–645, 1979.

74. Schwartz, P. J. and H. L. Stone, Left stellectomy in the prevention of ventricular fibrillation caused by acute myocardial ischemia in conscious dogs with anterior myocardial infarction. *Circulation 62*: 1256–1265, 1980.
75. Schwartz, P. J. and H. L. Stone, Left stellectomy and denervation supersensitivity in conscious dogs. *Am. J. Cardiol. 49*: 1185–1190, 1982.
76. Schwartz, P. J. and H. L. Stone, The role of the autonomic nervous system in sudden coronary death. *Ann. N.Y. Acad. Sci. 382*: 162–181, 1982.
77. Schwartz, P. J., H. L. Stone, and A. M. Brown, Effect of unilateral cardiac sympathetic denervation on arrhythmias induced by coronary occlusion. *Circulation 50*: 204, 1974.
78. Schwartz, P. J., H. L. Stone, A. M. Brown, Effects of unilateral stellate ganglion blockade on the arrhythmias associated with coronary occlusion. *Am. Heart J. 92*: 589–599, 1976.
79. Schwartz, P. J. and E. Vanoli, Cardiac arrhythmias elicited by interaction between acute myocardial ischemia and sympathetic hyperactivity: a new experimental model for the study of antiarrhythmic drugs. *J. Cardiovasc. Pharmacol. 3*: 1251–1259, 1981.
80. Schwartz, P. J., E. Vanoli, A Zaza, The prevention of cardiac arrhythmias associated with myocardial ischemia and dependent upon increases in sympathetic activity. In *Calcium Antagonism in Cardiovascular Therapy (Experience with Verapamil)* Eds. A. Zanchetti and D. M. Krikler. Excerpta Medica, Amsterdam, 1981, pp. 314–325.
81. Schwartz, P. J., R. L. Verrier, B. Lown, Effect of stellectomy and vagotomy on ventricular refractoriness in dogs, *Circ. Res. 40*: 536–540, 1977.
82. Schwartz, P. J. and S. Wolf, QT interval prolongation as predictor of sudden death in patients with myocardial infarction. *Circulation 57*: 1074–1077, 1978.
83. Taylor, G. J., R. S. Crampton, R. S. Gibson, P. T. Stebbins, M. T. G. Waldman, G. A. Beller, Prolonged Q-T interval at onset of acute myocardial infarction in predicting early phase ventricular tachycardia. *Am. Heart J. 102*: 16–24, 1981.
84. Vanoli, E., A. Zaza, G. Zuanetti, M. Pappalettera, P. J. Schwartz, Reduction in infarct size produced by left stellectomy. *IX World Congr. Cardiol.*, Moscow, 2:1312, 1982.
85. Verrier, R. L. and B. Lown, Sympathetic-parasympathetic interactions and ventricular electrical stability. In *Neural Mechanisms in Cardiac Arrhythmias*, Eds. P. J. Schwartz, A. M. Brown, A. Malliani, A. Zanchetti. Raven Press, New York, 1978, pp. 75–86.
86. Verrier, R. L. and B. Lown, Autonomic nervous system and malignant cardiac arrhythmias. In *Brain Behaviour and Bodily Disease*, eds. H. Wiener, M. A. Hofer, A. J. Stunkard. Raven Press, New York, 1981, pp. 273–291.
87. Verrier, R. L., P. L. Thompson, B. Lown, Ventricular vulnerability during sympathetic stimulation: role of heart rate and blood pressure. *Cardiovasc. Res. 8*: 602–610, 1974.
88. Webb, S. W., A. A. J. Adgey, J. F. Pantridge, Autonomic disturbance at onset of acute myocardial infarction. *Br. Med. J. 3*: 89–92, 1972.
89. Wechsler, J. S., J. B. Pace, J. M. Goldberg, W. C. Randall, Location of synaptic connections in canine sympathetic cardiac innervation. *Am. J. Physiol. 217*: 1789–1794, 1969.
90. Yanowitz, R., J. B. Preston, J. A. Abildskov, Functional distribution of right and left stellate innervation to the ventricles: production of neurogenic electrocardio-

graphic changes by unilateral alteration of sympathetic tone. *Circ. Res. 18*: 416–428, 1966.

91. Zipes, D., V. Elharrar, A. M. Watanabe, W. E. Gaum, H. R. Besch, Induction of ventricular fibrillation in probucol treated dogs. *Clin. Res. 25*: 459A, 1977.
92. Hamer, A. W., W. B. Finerman Jr., T. Peter, W. J. Mandel, Disparity between the clinical and electrophysiologic effects of amiodarone in the treatment of recurrent ventricular tachyarrhythmias. *Am. Heart J. 102*: 992–1000, 1981.

11

Neural Influences in Myocardial Ischemia: Effects of Neural Ablation

CARL. E. JONES and JOHN X. THOMAS, JR.

The physiological roles of the autonomic nervous system in the regulation of cardiac function and coronary blood flow have been discussed in previous chapters. This chapter concerns the effects of neural stimulation of the heart during a pathological condition, myocardial ischemia. Sympathetic influences will be emphasized since sympathetic stimulation of the heart during ischemia has been especially implicated as a factor contributing to decreased myocardial viability. The chapter will be largely devoted to a discussion of relatively new results from our two laboratories which suggest that chronic cardiac denervation or sympathectomy exerts a substantial protective effect on myocardial performance and viability following acute coronary artery occlusion.

Sympathetic Stimulation of the Heart During Myocardial Ischemia

During myocardial ischemia, sympathetic stimulation of the heart and its vasculature may increase subtantially. Thus, Webb et al. [48] reported that of 74 patients monitored within 30 minutes after acute myocardial infarction, 36% showed evidence of increased sympathetic discharge, including sinus tachycardia. The incidence of increased sympathetic discharge was more prevalent following anterior than following posterior infarction. While these observations suggest an enhanced sympathetic stimulation of the heart during myocardial ischemia in humans, they do not provide information regarding the basis of the response.

An increased sympathetic discharge to the heart during myocardial ischemia may partially be due to reductions in cardiac output and systemic arterial pressure with activation of the baroreceptor reflex. In examining this phenomenon,

Data reported in this chapter were derived from work supported by NIH grants HL-20286 and HL-22243, by a Grant-in-Aid from the American Heart Association with the funds contributed in part by the Texas Affiliate, and by the Bane Charitable Trust Fund. Dr. Thomas is a recipient of a Career Development Award from the Schweppe Foundation of Chicago.

Karlsberg et al. [24] studied the relationships between plasma catecholamines and both cardiac output and arterial pressure following acute coronary occlusion in conscious dogs. Throughout 1 hour of observation, the levels of both norepinephrine and epinephrine were directly related to the magnitude of the decreases in cardiac output and arterial pressure. These data suggest that both adrenal secretory activity and sympathetic neural activity are increased during myocardial ischemia and that the fall in cardiac output and arterial pressure may be major factors causing these increases.

The cardiac sympathetic response in ischemia is partly, but not fully, accounted for by the baroreceptor reflex. Thus, in many patients, Webb et al. [48] noted a sinus tachycardia with no change or with an increase in arterial pressure. Similar observations have been made by others in humans and experimental animals. This increase in sympathetic discharge to the heart in the absence of the baroreceptor reflex may be attributable to stimulation of neural receptors within the ischemic heart itself and to activation of an exitatory cardiocardiac reflex as described by Malliani et al. [28,29]. Basically, the reflex may be initiated by abnormal mechanical or chemical events in the ischemic heart. Stimulation of the cardiac receptors increases sympathetic afferent nerve traffic from the heart to the thoracic spinal cord and, thereby, elicits an increased discharge from the cord through cardiac sympathetic efferent nerves. Several investigators have observed that the net effects of ischemic, chemical or, electrical stimulation of afferent sympathetic cardiac nerves in experimental animals are positive chronotropic and inotropic responses in the heart [30,31,36]. However, it should be noted that stimulation of certain cardiac receptors following coronary occlusion may induce a powerful depressor reflex [4,45]. Nerve traffic from these receptors is carried by vagal afferent fibers, and stimulation of these fibers leads to bradycardia. Thus, during myocardial ischemia, the ultimate responses of the heart may depend on an interaction between vagal inhibitory and sympathetic excitatory afferent signals as well as signals generated by the baroreceptor reflex. In this regard, it should be noted that inhibitory cardiac receptors may be preferentially located in the posterior wall of the left ventricle [43]. Such a distribution would explain the excitatory response seen primarily with anterior wall infarction in man [48] and experimental animals [36].

One final mechanism of increased cardiac sympathetic stimulation during myocardial ischemia should be noted. Following coronary occlusion, an ischemia-induced release of norepinephrine from sympathetic nerve terminals may occur even in the absence of an increased efferent nerve discharge [17,50]. Such an increased release of norepinephrine into a localized ischemic region may not exert effects on the entire heart, but could influence the viability of the local ischemic region through effects on myocardial oxygen demand or on perfusion.

Sympathetic Influences on Myocardial Oxygen Demand and Viability During Ischemia

The viability of the flow-compromised heart largely depends on the blood flow requirement, or the oxygen demand, of the myocardium. Factors that increase the oxygen demand of the ischemic heart also increase the severity of myocardial damage; factors that reduce the oxygen demand reduce the myocardial injury [15]. The following discussion is an overview of the effects of sympathetic stimulation on the oxygen demand of the heart and, therefore, on myocardial viability during ischemia.

The major determinants of myocardial oxygen demand include heart rate, contractile state of the heart, and systolic wall tension as set by chamber diameter and developed pressure [49]. Oxygen demand increases when any of these factors increase, but these determinants do not operate independently. Thus, a change in heart rate or a global change in contractile state will affect oxygen demand both directly and indirectly through an accompanying change in wall tension. Indeed, in the dilated, failing heart, catecholamines may cause an actual decline in oxygen consumption. This effect is due to the reduction in systolic wall tension resulting from an increase in contractility and a consequent reduction in end-diastolic diameter [3]. However, it is crucial to recognize that myocardial oxygen demand during adrenergic stimulation always increases unless myocardial damage is associated with global ventricular failure and dilation [3]. When localized ischemic injury is not accompanied by global failure, myocardial oxygen demand is increased by catecholamines, or sympathetic stimulation, and ischemic injury is exacerbated.

The influence of sympathetic stimulation on ischemic injury has been shown by studying either the effects of increased sympathetic nerve discharge or sympathomimetic agents. Davidson et al. [7] studied the effects of the beta-adrenergic agonist isoproterenol on contractile function in the nonischemic and ischemic rat heart. In the nonischemic heart, continuous isoproterenol infusion elicited a sustained increase in left ventricular systolic pressure. However, in the ischemic heart isoproterenol elicited only a transient increase in systolic pressure followed by a rapid decline to a value less than control. Similar effects of sympathomimetic agents during ischemia have been reported by others [46,47]. In addition, Giudicelli et al. [11] noted that after coronary artery occlusion in dogs, stimulation of the left stellate ganglion increased S–T segment elevation in ischemic myocardium. The enhancement of ischemic injury and the decline in performance of ischemic myocardium during sympathetic stimulation have been largely attributed to the increase in oxygen demand with an exaggeration of the imbalance between oxygen demand and supply.

The deleterious effect of sympathetic stimulation on ischemic myocardium is also evident from the effects of sympathetic inhibition. Thus, it is well known that beta-adrenergic antagonists may relieve anginal pain and reduce ischemic injury in humans [15]. In animal studies, beta blockade, particularly with propranolol, has been reported to reduce infarct size after coronary occlusion. Although the precise mechanism behind this protective effect is still unclear, it is at least in part attributed to a reduction in heart rate, contractility, and, consequently, in myocardial oxygen demand [26].

Sympathetic Influences on the Coronary Circulation During Ischemia

The direct effect of sympathetic stimulation on the coronary circulation is vasoconstriction, and evidence suggests that during ischemia, a sympathetic vasoconstrictor influence on the coronary circulation may be an important factor limiting perfusion of the myocardium. As early as 1939, the studies of Manning et al. [32] in dogs suggested that following mechanical occlusion of a major coronary artery, the vessels distal to the primary occlusion underwent a neurally mediated spasm which further opposed perfusion of the ischemic myocardium. Prinzmetal et al. [34] later applied this concept to human ischemic heart disease when they described a variant angina. They proposed that this syndrome was due to coronary artery spasm superimposed on a partial atheromatous stenosis. A multitude of studies have now been directed toward the role of vasospasm in ischemic heart disease, and it is generally accepted that coronary artery spasm in either normal coronary arteries or in arteries with hemodynamically insignificant lesions causes myocardial ischemia in humans and gives rise to variant angina [16,42]. For example, it has been convincingly demonstrated using myocardial scintigraphic techniques that in patients with little or no atheromatous coronary artery disease, myocardial perfusion is drastically reduced during episodes of variant angina and returns to normal, or to hyperemic levels, after disappearance of angina. Although less conclusive, recent evidence also suggests that coronary artery spasm may produce actual myocardial infarction in patients with normal coronary arteries [16] or with severe coronary stenotic lesions [16,14].

The precise cause of coronary artery spasm is uncertain. However, it appears that whenever spasm occurs, an altered sympathetic influence on the coronary vasculature is involved. Thus, Mudge et al. [33] observed that in response to a cold pressor test, coronary resistance increased more in patients with preexisting coronary lesions than in patients with normal coronary arteries. This reflex coronary vasoconstriction could be blocked by the alpha-adrenergic antagonist phentolamine. Although these results suggest that spasm is due to a pathologic increase in alpha-adrenergic constrictor tone in the coronary vessel, the increased constrictor tone may not be due to an actual increase in sympathetic nerve discharge. For example, Robertson et al. [38] found no increase in plasma or urinary levels of catecholamines during episodes of variant angina. Thus, the apparent increased sympathetic influences on the coronary artery during spasm may be due to some local change in the vessel wall itself, leading to an increased alpha-adrenergic responsiveness to catecholamines.

While much attention has focused on alpha-adrenergic mediated vasospasm, relatively little has been directed toward the possibility that, even in the absence of a net increase in coronary resistance, an alpha-adrenergic constrictor tone may limit the extent of metabolically coupled vasodilation and, thereby, oppose myocardial oxygenation under certain conditions. It is now clear that an alpha-adrenergic tone may oppose metabolic dilation under physiological conditions. However, the consequent limitation in coronary flow is balanced by an increased oxygen extraction from blood such that myocardial oxygen delivery is not compromised. On the other hand, with substantial reductions in coronary perfusion pressure, like that caused by partial coronary stenosis or systemic hypotension, the metabolic coronary vasodilation is insufficient to maintain adequate myocardial oxygenation, and oxygen extraction may increase to a near maximal value. Under these conditions, an alpha-adrenergic constrictor tone in the coronary vasculature powerful enough to limit metabolic dilation may effectively form a barrier to myocardial oxygenation. In this regard, Buffington and Feigl [5] examined the possible presence of an alpha-adrenergic constrictor tone in the coronary circulation of the dog during partial coronary stenosis, a condition in which the metabolic vasodilatory signal would be high and might mask the constrictor signal. They observed that following a 70% coronary stenosis, a constrictor tone was still demonstrated and could be blocked with phenoxybenzamine.

One author of this chapter has studied the role of coronary alpha-adrenergic constrictor tone in limiting myocardial oxygenation during severe coronary stenosis (Jones, unpublished results). In alpha-chloralose anesthetized dogs, left coronary blood flow (LCBF) was monitored with a flow probe in line with a Gregg cannula inserted into the left coronary ostium. Left ventricular oxygen extraction [(a–v)O_2] was continuously monitored, and ventricular oxygen consumption (MVO_2) was calculated. Left ventricular contractile force (LVCF) was measured with a strain gauge attached to the ventricular surface. Coronary sinus and arterial blood samples were periodically withdrawn for determination of ventricular lactate extraction ratio (LER). Mean systemic arterial pressure

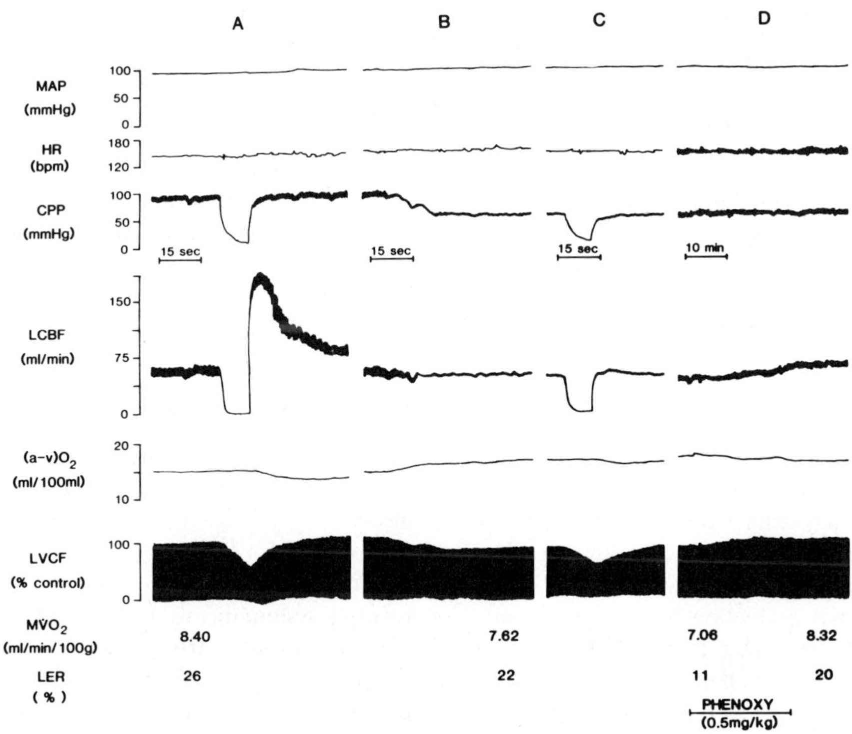

Fig. 11-1. Dog heart experiment showing the effects of coronary alpha-adrenergic blockade during severe coronary stenosis. See text for explanation and abbreviations. (Data from Jones, unpublished observations)

(MAP), coronary perfusion pressure (CPP) at the coronary cannula tip, and heart rate (HR) were also monitored. Figure 11-1 shows typical results. Panel A illustrates the various control values and shows a large coronary reactive hyperemic response following a 15-second total occlusion of coronary inflow. Panel B shows the drastic fall in CPP when the coronary inflow line was partially occluded. Note that the fall in LCBF was not nearly as great as the fall in CPP because of metabolic coronary vasodilation (autoregulation). However, because of the decline in LCBF, $(a-v)O_2$ increased substantially. Despite the metabolic and the increased $(a-v)O_2$, both MVO_2 and LER began to decline, indicating myocardial ischemia. The production of ischemia was accompanied by a slight reduction in LVCF. Panel C shows that during partial coronary stenosis, a 15-second coronary occlusion was not followed by reactive hyperemia, indicating that the coronary vasculature was "maximally" dilated. Panel D shows the effects of slow infusion of phenoxybenzamine into the left coronary bed during the partial stenosis. Note that coronary alpha-adrenergic blockade caused a further coronary dilation with an improvement in LCBF to a slightly hyperemic level. This increase in LCBF was associated with a near restoration of MVO_2, LER, and LVCF. Results similar to those shown in Figure 11-1 have also been observed during severe systemic hypotension (Jones, unpublished results) and suggest that during myocardial ischemia, an alpha-adrenergic constriction may oppose and limit metabolic vasodilation in the coronary circulation and, consequently, may limit myocardial oxygen delivery.

PROTECTIVE EFFECT OF CHRONIC CARDIAC DENERVATION

Both collaborative and independent studies from our two laboratories have shown that chronic cardiac denervation substantially protects the heart following acute coronary artery ligation. The studies have also examined the possible mechanisms underlying this effect. The following discussion is an integrated review of our experiments as well as pertinent work by others.

Effect of Chronic Cardiac Denervation on Myocardial Viability

Over 50 years ago, Leriche and Fontaine [27] noted that stellate ganglionectomy in the dog resulted in a reduced myocardial necrosis when a major coronary artery was ligated. Interestingly, they also noted that myocardial injury seemed less extensive in animals sympathectomized for longer periods of time prior to coronary occlusion. This apparent time-dependent nature of myocardial protection by cardiac denervation was not systematically described until Jones et al. [21] showed that infarct size following coronary artery occlusion was much smaller in chronically denervated than in control, sham-operated, or acutely denervated hearts. For chronic cardiac denervation, the intrapericardial denervation technique of Randall et al. [37] was employed; the infarct size experiments were performed 2 weeks after denervation. To ascertain whether any reduction in infarct size seen in the chronically denervated hearts was due to the surgical trauma, control animals subjected to a simultaneous sham denervation procedure were also studied. For acute cardiac denervation, the heart was decentralized, and both alpha and beta adrenergic blockades were produced pharmacologically; the infarct size experiments were performed immediately after completion of the preparation. In order to minimize variation in infarct size within each group, only animals showing the same epicardial distribution of the left anterior descending coronary artery (LAD) were used. The LAD was ligated immediately above its apical branch, and infarct size was determined 5 hours later using the nitro-blue tetrazolium (NBT) method. Table 11-1 compares infarct sizes in all four groups. Mean infarct size in sham-operated hearts was nearly identical to that in the control group in which no surgery had been performed prior to the experiment, implying that the trauma involved in the chronic denervation procedure did not affect infarct size. It may also be seen that the acutely denervated group showed approximately a 25% reduction in infarct size. Interestingly, this degree of reduction is very similar to that caused by propranolol alone when the NBT method is used for infarct size determination [41]. Thus, the reduction in infarct size caused by acute cardiac denervation in conjunction with alpha and beta adrenergic blocking agents may be primarily due to the pharmacological blockade of the beta receptor. As pointed out earlier, this protective effect may result from a reduction in heart rate, contractility, and myocardial oxygen demand. Indeed, in our experiments, the acutely denervated group showed significantly lower heart rates than either the sham-operated or control groups following coronary ligation. As also shown in Table 11-1, the most dramatic effect on infarct size was seen in the chronically denervated group. In these hearts infarct size was less than 20% of that in the control or sham-operated hearts and only 25% of that in acutely denervated hearts. These observations clearly imply that the protective effect of cardiac denervation is time-dependent and cannot be completely accounted for by acute abolition of sympathetic efferents to the heart or by removal of adrenergic function during ischemia.

This protective effect of chronic cardiac denervation has been confirmed by investigators using techniques other than the NBT method to assess infarct size. Barber et al. [1] used the radio-labeled microsphere technique to determine

Table 11-1. Mean infarct sizes

	Control (N = 10)	Sham-operated (N = 4)	Acute denervation (N = 6)	Chronic denervation (N = 7)
Left ventricular weight (g)	80.5	100.4	91.1	82.0
Infarct weight (g)	16.1	20.6	13.7	3.1
% Infarct	20.1	21.0	15.0°	3.8°,†

°P < 0.05 when compared to control.
†P < 0.05 when compared to acutely denervated group.
From Jones et al. [21].

local myocardial blood flow following acute coronary ligation and correlated blood flow changes with subepicardial and subendocardial ST-segment elevations in both 2-week denervated and sham-operated dog hearts. They observed that in severely ischemic myocardial regions (blood flow less than 30 ml/min/100 g), ST-segment elevation in chronically denervated hearts was less than half that in sham-operated controls. Since this reduced injury was seen in myocardial areas with an ischemic blood flow similar to that in sham-operated hearts, it was proposed that the protection afforded by chronic cardiac denervation is in large measure due to a reduction in myocardial metabolic demand. Later Barber et al. [2] also examined infarct sizes using the NBT technique in chronically denervated, acutely denervated, and control dog hearts. These experiments differed from those of Jones et al. [21] in two important ways. First, an increase in sympathetic stimulation of the heart following coronary ligation was prevented in nondenervated controls by section of the left and right cervical vagi and ansae subclavia in conjunction with a constant electrical stimulation of the peripheral end of the left ansae. Second, the LAD was ligated at a much higher level than in the experiments of Jones et al. It was observed that the acutely denervated group showed an approximately 25% and the chronically denervated group an approximately 53% smaller infarct size when compared to controls. Infarct size in chronically denervated hearts was significantly less than either the control or acutely denervated hearts. These results qualitatively agree with the earlier studies of Jones et al., although the reduction in infarct size seen in the chronically denervated hearts was quantitatively less in the experiments of Barber et al. This difference may be due to the prevention of an increase in sympathetic stimulation in the control hearts. In the study of Jones et al., such an increase in sympathetic stimulation may have caused a larger infarct size in the control group. Also, in the study of Barber et al., since the LAD was ligated at a much higher level, the area at risk was larger.

Recent collaborative studies from our two laboratories have employed analyses of myocardial creatine phosphokinase (CPK) activity and ST-segment changes to assess the effect of chronic cardiac denervation on ischemic myocardial injury (Jones and Thomas, unpublished results). In control dog hearts and in hearts denervated 2 weeks earlier by the method of Randall, the LAD was ligated immediately above its apical branch. Before and 15 minutes following coronary ligation, subepicardial and subendocardial ST-segment elevations were assessed in 10 control and 8 denervated hearts at 10 different sites within the center and the periphery of the ischemic region. In 9 control and 9 denervated hearts, the pericardium and chest were closed after coronary ligation. After 24 hours, the chest was reopened, and transmural myocardial samples were obtained from the same 10 sites within the ischemic area. One nonischemic myocardial sample was obtained from the perfusion territory of the circumflex artery. Subepicardial and subendocardial CPK activities were determined in each of these transmural samples. The results showed a dramatic difference in both ST-segment elevations and CPK activities between the chronically denervated and control hearts. In control hearts, mean ST-segment elevations in ischemic subepicardial and subendocardial regions were uniformly greater than 2 mV. However, in chronically denervated hearts, mean ischemic ST-segment elevations in both subepicardium and subendocardium were only approximately 1 mV. Only two central ischemic sites showed elevations greater than 2 mV. Also, in control hearts, subepicardial and subendocardial CPK activities were significantly reduced to less than 50% of those in nonischemic muscle. However, in the chronically denervated hearts, CPK activity was significantly reduced only in the subendocardium of the central ischemic area.

As an index of the severity of ischemia resulting from coronary occlusion in control and chronically denervated dog hearts, S. B. Jones and Thomas studied myocardial lactate production (unpublished results). They noted that following release of 5-minute LAD occlusion, coronary sinus lactate concentration increased 182% in controls but only 79% in denervated hearts. These data suggest that during LAD occlusion, the imbalance between oxygen demand and supply was substantially less in chronically denervated than in nondenervated control hearts.

Elson et al. [10] used a microelectrode technique to assess ischemic injury in the acutely and chronically denervated dog heart. At various times following circumflex artery ligation, the posterior papillary muscle was removed and assessed for cellular injury. Forty minutes after ligation, hearts denervated immediately before coronary occlusion showed a 40% reduction in the extent of papillary muscle injury; however, hearts denervated 2 weeks before circumflex ligation showed more than a 90% reduction. Interestingly, if cellular injury was assessed 80 minutes after circumflex ligation, there was no difference between chronically denervated and control hearts. This observation suggests that the protective effect of chronic cardiac denervation is a temporary one, simply delaying the onset of myocardial injury. Although the time course of the protection afforded by chronic cardiac denervation needs further exploration, it is felt that the transient nature of the protection observed in posterior papillary muscle may be unique. In this regard, it should be recalled that analysis of CPK activity showed a substantial preservation of myocardial viability in the chronically denervated heart 24 hours after coronary ligation.

Effect of Chronic and Selective Cardiac Sympathectomy on Myocardial Viability

All of the studies reviewed above used a chronically and totally denervated dog heart as a model. Because of the known sympathetic influences on viability of ischemic myocardium, it was thought that the protective effect observed with chronic denervation was due primarily to chronic ablation of sympathetic nerves. This hypothesis was verified in later experiments by Jones et al. [18] in which infarct sizes in control and sham-operated hearts were compared to those in hearts which had been sympathectomized 2 weeks before the experiments. The peripulmonary neurectomy method of Kaye [25] was used for selective sympathectomy. This technique produces a complete sympathectomy of both ventricles, as indicated by abolition of the ventricular inotropic response to stellate stimulation [18] and by a decline in ventricular catecholamines to a level comparable to that seen after cardiac autotransplantation [25]. The chronotropic responses to both stellate and vagal stimulation remain intact. Infarct sizes in the three groups of animals were assessed using the NBT method 5 hours after occlusion of the LAD. It was observed that arterial pressure and heart rate in the three groups of animals were not significantly different throughout the 5 hours following coronary ligation. However, mean infarct size in the chronically sympathectomized hearts was approximately 40% of that in sham-operated or control hearts. Similar findings have been observed by Barber et al. [2], who compared infarct sizes in 2-week denervated, 2-week sympathectomized, and control hearts. They observed that infarct sizes in both chronically denervated and chronically sympathectomized hearts were about 50% of those in control hearts.

Effect of Chronic Cardiac Denervation on Myocardial Contractile Function

The preservation of myocardial viability following coronary occlusion, as assessed by infarct size studies, implies that chronic cardiac denervation may also exert a substantial protective effect on myocardial contractile function during ischemia. However, relatively few studies have been directed to this question. Thomas et al. [44] examined contractile function in control, sham-operated, acutely denervated, and chronically denervated dog hearts following acute coronary occlusion. Chronic cardiac denervation was produced by the method of Randall 2 weeks prior to the experiments. For acute denervation, the heart was decentralized, and alpha and beta adrenergic blockade was produced pharmacologically. Sham-operated animals underwent a sham denervation procedure 2 weeks before experiment. To assess contractile function, two strain gauge arches were attached to the anterior left ventricular surface. Several small arterial branches supplying the muscle beneath one gauge were isolated and simultaneously ligated. This provides a measure of epicardial contractile force in the ischemic region following coronary occlusion. The remaining strain gauge provided a measure of nonischemic contractile force. Figure 11-2 shows typical recordings of arterial pressure and contractile forces in ischemic and nonischemic myocardium following coronary occlusion in both an acutely denervated (A) and chronically denervated (B) heart. Following coronary occlusion in the acutely denervated heart, contractile force in the ischemic region abruptly fell to an extremely low level. Compare this response to that seen in the chronically denervated heart where contractile force in the ischemic region was not affected by coronary ligation. In the control, sham-operated, and acutely denervated groups, mean reductions in contractile force 30 minutes after coronary ligation were 67–74%; there was no statistically significant difference between any of the groups. However, in the chronically denervated hearts, the mean reduction in ischemic myocardial contractile force was only 22%, which was significantly less than in any of the other groups.

These findings suggest that following acute coronary ligation in the chronically denervated heart, contractile function in the myocardium normally sup-

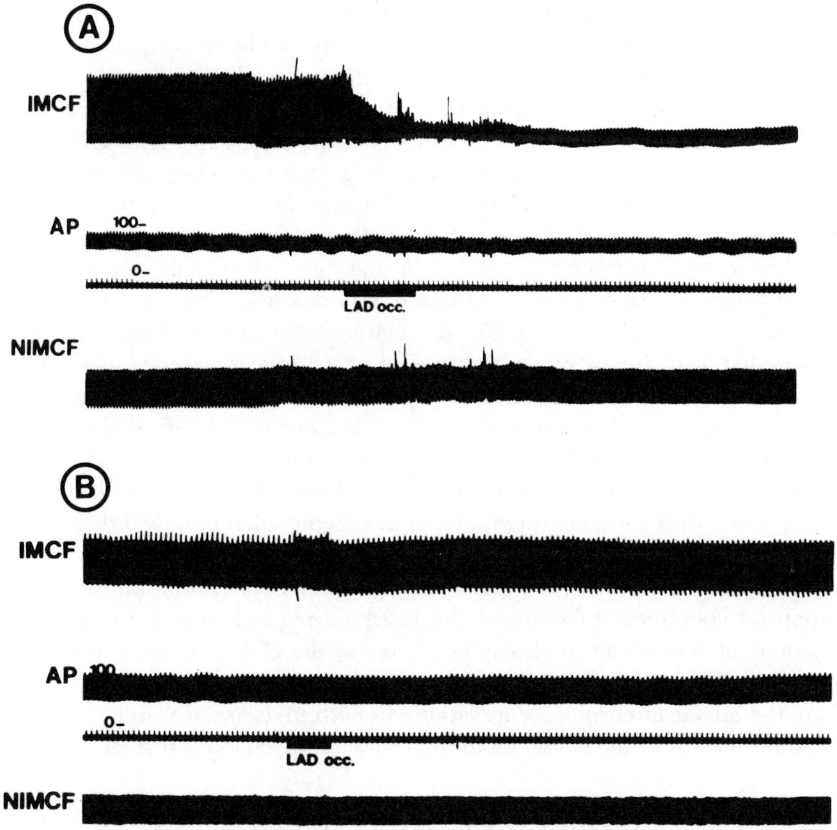

Fig. 11-2. The effect of acute coronary ligation on ischemic myocardial contractile force (IMCF) and nonischemic myocardial contractile force (NIMCF) in both an acutely denervated (A) and a chronically denervated (B) dog heart. AP = arterial pressure. Each small deflection on the time scale represents 5 seconds. (Data from Thomas et al. Part of this figure reproduced through courtesy of *Am. Heart J.*, ref. 42)

plied by the occluded vessel is largely preserved. However, studies by Randall et al. [35] suggested that following coronary occlusion, the decline in global left ventricular function is not prevented by chronic cardiac denervation. In these experiments, both nondenervated dogs and dogs which had been subjected to complete cardiac denervation 2 or more weeks before the experiment were chronically instrumented to permit recordings of left ventricular pressure, left ventricular dP/dt, mean arterial pressure, left ventricular stroke volume, and heart rate. In the conscious animal, the circumflex artery was abruptly occluded near its origin, and it was observed that the major difference between the cardiac response in the two groups was significantly greater increase in heart rate in the innervated animals. The responses of mean arterial pressure, stroke volume, and left ventricular diastolic pressure were similar in both groups. More importantly, there was a similar decline in ventricular dP/dt in both groups, suggesting a similar decline in global contractility.

Although the cause of the different results in two studies is at present unclear, certain factors must be considered. Thus, in the study of Thomas et al. [42], contractile function in a localized region of the myocardium following localized coronary occlusion in the anesthetized dog was assessed. By contrast, in the study of Randall et al. [35], an index of global contractile function was evaluated in the conscious dog following occlusion of a major coronary artery with the consequent production of ischemia in a major portion of the left ventricle. Nevertheless, in view of the magnitude of the protective effect on myocardial viability as seen in numerous studies in anesthetized animals, and the maintained contractile force seen the localized ischemia in anesthetized animals, the observation of no difference in global function between control and chronically denervated heart following an occlusion of even a major coronary artery in the conscious dog is somewhat unexpected. However, it should also be recognized that in the study of Thomas et al., contractile force in the very shallow subepicardial muscle was assessed. Since the deeper subendocardial muscle is more vulnerable to ischemic damage in the dog heart, it is conceivable that the absence of a decline in contractile force in subepicardial muscle did not reflect changes in the transmural contractile state.

It is apparent that the potentially important effect of chronic cardiac denervation on contractile function of the heart during ischemia must be further explored. It is essential to clearly characterize the effects on local, transmural contractile function and on global pump function following coronary occlusion. Also, the effects of chronic denervation, on both myocardial viability and contractile function in the conscious animal, should be explored further.

FACTORS INVOLVED IN THE PROTECTIVE EFFECT OF CHRONIC CARDIAC DENERVATION

After initially observing a dramatically reduced infarct size in the chronically denervated heart, we thought that this effect must be due to a reduced blood flow demand, an increased perfusion of myocardium distal to the coronary occlusion, or both. As pointed out earlier, sympathetic stimulation of the heart is known to increase myocardial oxygen and blood flow demands, and inhibition of sympathetic influences are known to reduce these demands. However, the magnitude of the reduction in infarct size in the chronically denervated heart led us to believe that this protective effect was not entirely due to a reduction in myocardial metabolic demand and that an increased perfusion of ischemic myocardium may also be involved.

Myocardial Oxygen Demand in the Chronically Denervated Heart

Many investigators have examined the effect of cardiac denervation on myocardial blood flow, myocardial oxygen consumption, and the efficiency of oxygen utilization. Donald [8] reviewed these studies and pointed out that the results have been extremely contradictory. He stated that the basis of the conflicting results may be differences in animal species employed or in the method and duration of cardiac denervation.

The first indication that myocardial oxygen and blood flow demands may be reduced in the dog heart following chronic cardiac sympathectomy by the peripulmonary neurectomy method of Kaye et al. [25], as used in our infarct size studies, came from experiments using the tracer microsphere technique. The results showed that subepicardial and subendocardial blood flows in the perfusion territory of the LAD in hearts which had been sympathectomized for 2 weeks were approximately 30–35% less than in control hearts [18]. Almost identical results were later observed in the perfusion territory of the circumflex coronary artery of the dog heart [9]. The reductions in resting myocardial blood flow were observed even though heart rate and arterial pressure were similar in the chronically sympathectomized and control hearts. These initial findings were recently supported by Barber et al. [2] who used the tracer microsphere technique to compare nonischemic blood flows in control hearts to those in hearts which had been totally denervated by the method of Randall et al. [36] or sympathectomized by the method of Kaye et al. [25] 2 weeks earlier. These workers noted that subepicardial and subendocardial flows in both denervated and sympathectomized hearts were approximately 20–25% less than those in control hearts. The substantial reduction in myocardial blood flow as observed in these studies implies a substantial reduction in myocardial oxygen demand following chronic cardiac denervation or sympathectomy. Such a reduction in oxygen demand may aid in preserving the viability of myocardium when coronary blood flow is compromised. This proposal is given credence by Barber et al. [1] who reported that following coronary ligation, selected regions of chronically denervated myocardium with the same ischemic blood flow level seen in selected areas of control myocardium showed less evidence of myocardial injury.

In the studies cited above, left ventricular oxygen consumption was not directly assessed. In the classic studies of Gregg et al. [13], however, the left ventricular blood flow and oxygen extraction were measured in control dog hearts and in hearts which had been totally denervated for 3–6 weeks. The results demonstrated that resting oxygen consumption and blood flow in denervated left ventricles were only about 50% of those in controls, although heart rate, arterial pressure, and ventricular pressure-volume work were no lower in the denervated hearts. They also observed that during treadmill exercise, the increases in oxygen consumption and coronary flow in the denervated heart were less than 50% of those in controls although the increases in pressure-volume work were nearly identical in both groups. These results strongly suggest that at any given level of cardiac output, the chronically denervated heart operated with reduced oxygen and blood flow demands.

Recently, the potentially important effects of chronic cardiac sympathectomy on left ventricular oxygen demand and blood flow were further explored by Jones et al. [22]. In these experiments, left ventricular oxygen consumption and blood flow were compared in chronically sympathectomized and sham-operated dog hearts over a wide range of afterload pressures. Afterload pressure is a major determinant of ventricular developed wall tension and, thereby, of ventricular oxygen demand. Therefore, greater efficiency of oxygen utilization by the chronically sympathectomized heart in performing external work should be reflected by a reduced left ventricular oxygen consumption at any given afterload pressure. In these experiments, 8 animals which had been sham-operated 3 weeks earlier and 7 animals which had undergone cardiac sympathectomy by the method of Kaye 3 weeks earlier were used. In each animal the heart was paced at 150 beats/minute. To estimate left ventricular oxygen extraction, the difference in oxygen concentration between arterial and coronary sinus blood was continuously monitored. Circumflex blood flow was measured using an electromagnetic flow probe placed around the circumflex artery at its origin. After each experiment, the heart was weighed, and the circumflex perfusion territory was calculated as 37% of the heart weight, a value found in a large number of dog hearts by Gregg et al. [13] and verified in this laboratory. Circumflex blood flow was normalized to a 100 g perfusion territory, and left ventricular oxygen consumption was calculated from normalized blood flow and oxygen extraction. To monitor left ventricular pressure and afterload pressure (aortic pressure), a dual-sensor catheter-tip pressure transducer was inserted into a femoral artery and advanced until the tip sensor was in the left ventricle, while the proximal sensor was in the ascending aorta. The tension-time-index per beat was obtained by planimetry of the area under the systolic portion of the recorded left ventricular pressure signal. Tension-time-index was measured since it is directly influenced by ventricular afterload pressure and is a primary correlate of oxygen consumed by the left ventricle to pump against a pressure load. After the preparation was complete, ventricular afterload pressure was varied either by aortic constriction or by hemorrhage. During aortic constriction, mean peripheral arterial pressure was maintained at 100 mm Hg using a blood-filled reservoir connected to a femoral artery. To reduce afterload pressure, the animal was bled into this reservoir. In each animal, values for ventricular oxygen extraction, circumflex blood flow, oxygen consumption, and tension-time-index were obtained at 3–5 levels of afterload pressure. Among both groups of animals, values for afterload pressure ranged from 60 to 150 mm Hg. and pressure maintained at each level for at least 5 min before data were obtained. In analyzing the data, the linear regressions of oxygen comsumption, coronary flow, and oxygen extraction on tension-time-index and of circumflex flow on oxygen consumption were obtained. For any relationship the statistical significance of the difference between the two groups of animals was assessed by calculating a probability using the F-test.

Figure 11-3 shows the relationship between ventricular oxygen consumption and tension-time-index in the two groups of animals. This figure clearly indicates that at any value of tension-time-index, oxygen consumption in the chronically sympathectomized left ventricle was dramatically less than that in the sham-operated ventricle. The regressions of coronary blood flow on tension-time-index showed an identical difference between the two groups of hearts,

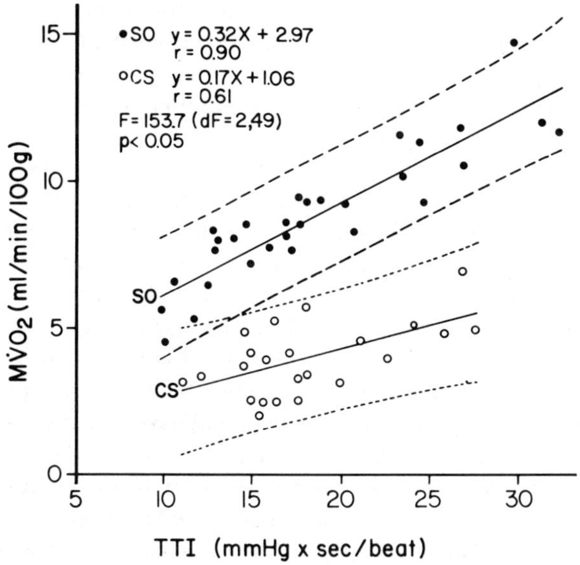

Fig. 11-3. Regression of left ventricular oxygen consumption (MVO_2) on tension-time-index (TTI) in sham-operated (SO) and chronically sympathectomized (CS) dog hearts. Indicated are the regression equations and the correlation coefficients found in each group of hearts. The calculated F value with degrees of freedom is also shown. The regressions in the two groups of hearts were significantly different. (Data from Jones et al. Reproduced through courtesy of *Circ. Shock*, ref. 22)

indicating that the reduction in oxygen consumption in the sympathectomized ventricles was completely paralleled by a reduction in coronary blood flow; there was no difference in the regressions of oxygen extraction on tension-time-index. The parallel reductions in oxygen consumption and coronary blood flow in the chronically sympathectomized heart were also demonstrated by the regressions of coronary flow on oxygen consumption in the two groups of hearts. Although mean coronary blood flow and oxygen consumption were substantially less in the chronically sympathectomized groups, the regression of flow on oxygen consumption in the chronically sympathectomized ventricle was nearly identical to that in the sham-operated control and to that reported under a variety of conditions by others [39]. Thus, these data again strongly suggest that following chronic cardiac sympathectomy, the oxygen required by the left ventricle to pump against a pressure load, a primary determinant of myocardial oxygen demand, is substantially reduced. This reduction in oxygen demand is accompanied by an equal reduction in coronary blood flow.

Similar results have also been observed by Thomas and Barber (unpublished results) who compared oxygen consumptions in sham-operated control and chronically sympathectomized dog ventricles. In these experiments, left ventricular perfusion was determined using the tracer microsphere technique, and simultaneous measurements of left ventricular oxygen extraction were made.

Measurements were made only under resting conditions. However, it was observed that although mean arterial pressure and heart rate were identical in the two groups of animals, both oxygen consumption and left ventricular perfusion in the chronically sympathectomized ventricle were only about 60% of those in controls.

It is noteworthy that the effect of chronic cardiac denervation on coronary blood flow, as illustrated in the studies above, differs from the effect of acute denervation or adrenergic blockade as reported by many others. Thus as pointed out in chapter 8, numerous investigators have reported that acute cardiac denervation or adrenergic blockade in the dog leads to a substantial increase in coronary blood flow, which is attributed to the removal of an alpha-adrenergic constrictor tone from the coronary circulation. Since oxygen consumption of the myocardium is not affected by this acute procedure, the increase in flow is accompanied by a reduction in oxygen extraction. Therefore, the overall results seem to indicate that the acute effect of denervation is coronary hyperemia, while several days to weeks following denervation, a reduced coronary flow is observed. This proposal may be questioned on the basis of recent studies by Chilian et al. [6] in the conscious dog. These researchers reported that 2 weeks following regional sympathectomy of the left ventricle by topical application of phenol, blood flow in sympathectomized myocardium was not different from that in innervated myocardium. They suggested that in the conscious, resting animal, there is only an insignificant sympathetic vasoconstrictor tone in the coronary circulation. The interpretation of and reasons for the discrepancy between these results and others is at present unclear.

Two weeks following surgical denervation of the heart, coronary flow is substantially reduced in the anesthetized dog. The precise basis of such an apparent time-dependent effect on coronary flow is at present uncertain. However, this reduction may partly depend on an increased tendency toward metabolically coupled vasoconstriction secondary to the substantial reduction in myocardial oxygen demand which accompanied chronic denervation. Indeed, the observation that the relationship between coronary flow and oxygen consumption in the chronically denervated heart was identical to that in control hearts at least suggests that the final level of coronary flow after chronic denervation was largely influenced by the level of myocardial oxygen demand.

The basis for the reduction in oxygen consumption following chronic cardiac sympathectomy or denervation has not been systematically defined. However, a possible explanation relates to the effect of chronic denervation on myocardial contractile state. Although the studies of Gregg et al. [13] and those from our two laboratories have related oxygen consumption in control and denervated hearts to either pressure-volume work, tension-time-index at constant heart rate, or to the heart rate-arterial pressure product, an additional major determinant is myocardial contractility. This parameter is much more difficult to evaluate accurately. Thus, it is possible that the reduced oxygen consumption was caused by a reduced contractile state of the chronically denervated heart or sympathectomized left ventricle. However, further studies are required to answer this question.

Perfusion of Ischemic Myocardium in the Chronically Denervated Heart

It was thought early in our studies that an improved perfusion of ischemic myocardium may also play a role in the protective effect of chronic cardiac denervation. The first support for this proposal came from semiquantitative experiments using the fluorescing dye thioflavin S to delineate areas of myocardium receiving very low flow following ligation of the LAD [21]. In both control and 2-week denervated dog hearts, the low flow area observed immediately after coronary ligation closely approximated the infarcted area determined in separate groups of animals 5 hours after the ligation. These observations imply that improved perfusion distal to the ligation may have caused the reduced infarct size.

Perfusion of ischemic myocardium in the chronically sympathectomized dog heart was quantitatively assessed using the radiolabeled tracer microsphere technique [18]. In these experiments, controls and 2-week ventricular sympa-

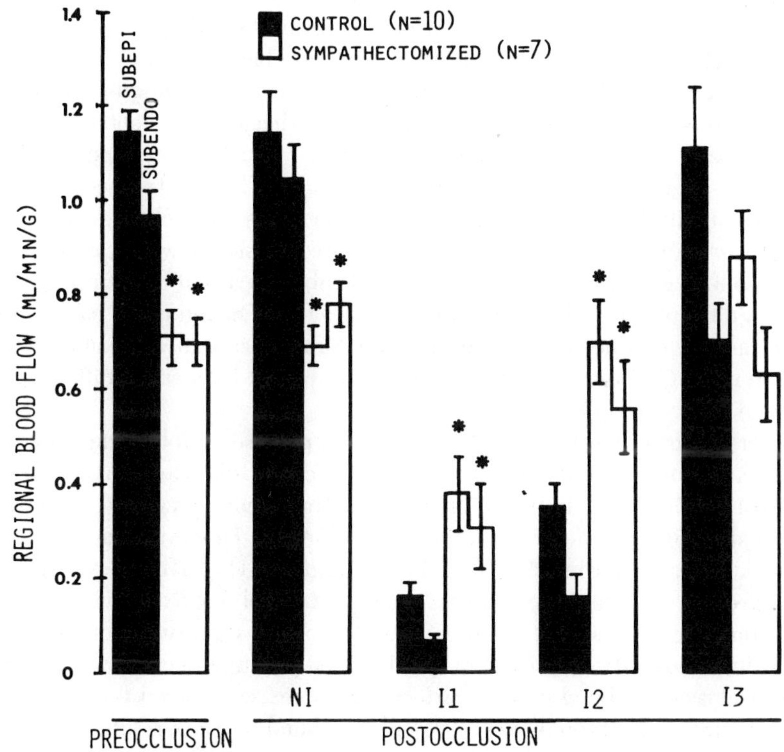

Fig. 11-4. Regional perfusions in control and chronically sympathectomized dog ventricles both before and after ligation of the left anterior descending coronary artery. Vertical bars are standard errors. An asterisk indicates that perfusion in a particular region in the sympathectomized heart was signficantly different from the corresponding perfusion in the control heart. ($P < 0.05$). (Data from Jones et al. Reproduced through courtesy of *Am. J. Physiol.*, ref. 18)

thectomized dog hearts were used. A first species of microspheres was injected to estimate preocclusion left ventricular blood flow, and a second species was injected 5 minutes after ligation of the LAD above its apical branch. Immediately after injection of the second microsphere species, the dye thioflavin S was injected to permit visual delineation of the myocardial region of very low flow. The animal was then killed, and the left ventricle was sliced into 7–9 sections. A section proximal to the ligation was used to obtain a sample of nonischemic muscle. To sample ischemic muscle, the second section distal to the occlusion was examined under ultraviolet light, and the center of the nonfluorescing zone was located. Samples were obtained (Fig. 11-4) from the center of the ischemic zone (sample I-1), 1.5 cm from the center (I-2), and 3 cm from the center (I-3). In all cases, transmural samples were obtained and divided into subepicardial and subendocardial halves. Radioactivity in all muscle aliquots was counted, and blood flow was estimated.

Figure 11-4 shows the results of the tracer microsphere experiments. The preocclusion flows from all four regions sampled were pooled to obtain the mean preocclusion blood flows shown. As mentioned, preocclusion perfusions in the chronically sympathectomized hearts were substantially less than those in controls. After coronary occlusion, there was no change in flow to the nonischemic muscle in either group of animals. However, even though flows in nonischemic muscle were substantially less in sympathectomized ventricles, perfusions in the two most central ischemic regions (I-1 and I-2) were approximately 100–300% greater in sympathectomized ventricles. These differences were statistically significant. Also, when postocclusion flows in each region of both groups were compared to the corresponding preocclusion flow, it was noted that in the control group both subepicardial and subendocardial flows in region I-3 were significantly less than the preocclusion value. On the other hand, in the chronically sympathectomized group, only subendocardial and subepicardial flows in region I-1 and subendocardial flows in region I-2 were significantly less than the preocclusion level.

Experiments similar to those above were also performed following circumflex artery occlusion in the dog [9]. In contrast to results following LAD occlusion, there was no difference in perfusion of the central ischemic region (I-1) between chronically sympathectomized and control hearts. However, in the region immediately surrounding this central zone (region I-1), perfusion was substantially greater in sympathectomized than in control hearts. Thus, following occlusion of either the LAD or the circumflex arteries, perfusion of the bed of the occluded artery is improved in the chronically sympathectomized ventricle. With occlusion of the circumflex artery, this increase in blood flow is not distributed uniformly throughout the vascular bed and does not result in increased perfusion of the central most ischemic region.

Several factors may explain the increase in perfusion of ischemic myocardium observed in the chronically sympathectomized heart. First, it may be postulated that this increased perfusion is due to the removal of alpha-adrenergic constrictor influences from the coronary bed. As pointed out earlier, such constrictor influences may oppose metabolic vasodilation and may in some cases lead to vasospasm. It can be seen that removal of these vasoconstrictor influences from ischemic myocardium distal to a coronary occlusion would permit improved perfusion of this myocardium through collateral vessels originating on nonoccluded coronary arteries. Second, the improved perfusion of ischemic myocardium may result from the removal of vasoconstrictor influences from the collateral vessels themselves. However, if either of the two mechanisms above were influential in reducing infarct size in the chronically denervated heart, it may be reasonable to expect a similar reduction in infarct size in the acutely denervated heart in conjunction with pharmacological alpha- and beta-adrenergic blockages. But the results clearly show that chronic denervation results in a much greater reduction in infarct size. Thus, these data suggest that the improved perfusion of ischemic myocardium following chronic cardiac denervation is not due only to the removal of vasconstrictor influences. Nevertheless, these data must be interpreted with some degree of caution. Thus, in our acutely denervated heart preparation, coronary ligation may have elicited a massive ischemia-induced release of norepinephrine from sympathetic nerve endings. If a complete pharmacological blockade of vascular alpha-adrenergic receptors was not produced, such a release of norepinephrine may still have caused a vasocontrictor effect in ischemic myocardium. In such a case, infarct size in the acutely denervated hearts may have been greater than that in chronically denervated hearts in which norepinephrine stores were depleted. An additional explanation may be that chronic ventricular sympathectomy causes an expansion of the perfusion territories of the coronary arteries. In this case the perfusion territories of nonoccluded vessels may substantially overlap those of the occluded vessel and cause a consequent increased perfusion distal to the coronary ligation. As a final possibility, the increased ischemic perfusion may be due to an active growth of collateral vessels following cardiac denervation similar to that which occurs during chronic or progressive coronary occlusion. With coronary occlusion in the chronically denervated heart, an increased ischemic perfusion then could occur through an enlarged collateral circulation.

Because of the magnitude of the increased ischemic perfusion in the chronically denervated heart, it is conceivable that a reduction in resistance to flow through collateral channels was involved, either by removal of vasoconstrictor influences from these channels or by active growth of these channels. Jones and Scheel [23] used an isolated dog heart preparation to estimate coronary collateral resistance in acutely denervated and 2-week sympathectomized hearts. In these experiments the major epicardial arteries (right, LAD, circumflex) were perfused separately but simultaneously under conditions of maximal dilation. The preparation permitted the collateral resistances in both directions between all three arteries to be estimated from measurements of retrograde flows. Furthermore, the minimum antegrade coronary resistances through the vascular beds of each of the three coronary arteries could be determined from pressure-flow relationships obtained in each artery. These measurements were made because it was hypothesized that if the increased ischemic perfusion in the chronically denervated heart was due to an enlargement of the perfusion territories of the coronary beds, such an enlargement would be reflected by a

Table 11-2. Coronary collateral resistances in acutely denervated control and chronically sympathectomized dog hearts

	R_{A-C}	R_{C-A}	R_{C-R}	R_{R-C}	R_{A-R}	R_{R-A}
Control (N = 12)	13.6	14.0	90.0	31.7	149.0	45.4
Sympathectomized (N = 8)	6.7	6.8	47.3	13.1	51.6	15.7
% Change	−51°	−52°	−47°	−59°	−64°	−65°

°$P < 0.05$. Mean resistance values are expressed as mm Hg/ml/min. R_{A-C} = resistance from left anterior descending to circumflex artery; R_{C-A} = resistance from circumflex to left anterior descending artery; R_{C-R} = resistance from circumflex to right artery; R_{R-C} = resistance to circumflex artery; R_{A-R} = resistance from left anterior descending to right artery; R_{R-A} = resistance from right to left anterior descending artery.

From Jones and Scheel [22].

reduction in the minimum resistances to flow through these beds. Table 11-2 compares coronary collateral resistances determined in acutely denervated control and chronically sympathectomized hearts. All six collateral resistances determined were substantially and significantly less in chronically sympathectomized hearts than in controls. This finding strongly supports the proposal that the increased perfusion of ischemic myocardium in the chronically sympathectomized heart is largely due to a reduction in the resistances of collateral channels supplying the occluded vascular bed. Indeed, the reductions in collateral resistances determined in the isolated heart were comparable to the increases in ischemic perfusions observed in the chronically sympathectomized in situ heart following ligation of either the LAD [18] or the circumflex [9] coronary arteries. As noted earlier, the increased collateral flow following circumflex ligation is apparently not distributed uniformly and does not increase perfusion of the most central ischemic region.

The results of the isolated heart experiments also showed that the antegrade resistances of the three coronary beds were not different in the control and sympathectomized hearts. These data imply that the increased ischemic perfusion noted in the chronically sympathectomized heart is not due to a structural enlargement of the coronary vascular beds. Histological evidence also indicates that myocardial capillary density in the two-week sympathectomized dog heart is not different from that in controls [20].

It is generally agreed that collateral channels connecting the right, circumflex, and LAD coronary arteries in the dog heart are largely located on the epicardial surface. By contrast, in the human heart, collateral vessels are thought to be distributed throughout the myocardial wall with only few at the epicardial surface. For this reason, we questioned whether chronic cardiac sympathectomy also leads to a reduction in the resistances of intramyocardial collateral channels. The septal artery in the dog heart is a deep intramyocardial vessel, and any collateral channels connecting it to the beds of the major epicardial arteries must be intramyocardial. Therefore, in subsequent isolated dog heart experiments, the resistances of collateral channels connecting the septal artery to the major epicardial arteries were determined in acutely denervated control and 2-week sympathectomized hearts [40] (Jones and Scheel, unpublished results). In these experiments, all three major epicardial arteries were occluded simultaneously, and retrograde flows were collected. Since the septal artery is the only vessel supporting myocardial perfusion, any retrograde flows collected on the three occluded vessels must reflect collateral flow from the septal artery. The results indicated that in the chronically sympathectomized heart, the resistances of these intramyocardial collateral channels were 40–60% less than in controls. These results are very similar to the reduction in epicardial collateral resistances shown in Table 11-2, and may be particularly relevant to the human heart since the septal artery collaterals are probably similar to those in the human.

The underlying cause of the reduced collateral resistances in the chronically sympathectomized heart is at present uncertain. If the effect resulted from an abolition of constrictor influences from collateral vessels, one would expect an equal reduction in infarct size in both acutely denervated, alpha-adrenergic blocked hearts and in chronically denervated hearts. But such was not the case. In addition, in the experiments of Jones and Scheel [23], collateral resistances determined 2 weeks after ventricular sympathectomy were compared to those determined immediately after cardiac denervation for the isolated heart procedure. The finding of reduced collateral resistances in the chronically sympathectomized heart supports the argument that the effect was not due to the simple removal of an autonomic constrictor tone from preexisting vessels. Furthermore, pilot studies performed during the experiments of Jones and Scheel showed that during isolated experiments on control hearts, injection of high doses of the alpha-adrenergic blockers phenotolamine and phenoxybenzamine into the blood perfusion system did not alter collateral resistances in these hearts. Thus, the evidence indicates that the reduction in collateral resistances after sympathectomy is time-dependent and is not fully manifest immediately after abolition of sympathetic inputs. This implies that the reduction in collateral resistances may be due to an active growth or development of collateral channels. This proposal has qualitative support from the studies of Jones and Cannon [19,20], in which histochemical techniques were used to assess the reactivities of selective enzymes and other metabolic components in coronary microvessels in control and 2-week sympathectomized dog hearts. They observed histochemical changes in sympathectomized hearts indicative of increased protein synthesis. Although the histochemical data are qualitative and subject to broad interpretation, they add evidence for structural development of the coronary collateral circulation following chronic cardiac sympathectomy.

A proposal that the reduced collateral resistances following chronic sympathectomy may be due to a structural development of the collateral circulation is hindered by a lack of understanding of the underlying mechanism. At present, major stimuli for enlargement of the collateral circulation are considered to be myocardial hypoxia and an alteration of physical forces within the coronary circulation consequent to stenosis [12]. Whether either of these stimuli elicits reduced collateral resistances observed after chronic sympathectomy is not clear. Furthermore, precisely how these factors trigger an enlargement of the collateral circulation is not well understood. Thus, although indirect evidence indicates that the reduced collateral resistances following chronic sympathectomy may be due to a structural development of the collateral circulation, a complete understanding of the phenomenon must await further investigation.

SUMMARY

Sympathetic stimulation of the heart may increase substantially in myocardial ischemia. This may increase the oxygen demand and further limit perfusion of ischemic myocardium; therefore, it is detrimental to the viability and contractile performance of the flow-compromised heart. Evidence indicates that acute abolition of sympathetic influences on ischemic myocardium may be beneficial in preserving viability. However, investigations from our two laboratories and by others indicate that chronic surgical denervation of the heart or, more specifically, chronic surgical sympathectomy of the ventricles exerts a far greater protective effect following coronary occlusion than does acute denervation or acute adrenergic blockade.

There seem to be two factors underlying the substantial protective effect of long-term removal of sympathetic influences. First, for any given level of cardiac work, the oxygen demand of the chronically sympathectomized myocardium may be reduced as much as 40–50%. The precise cause of this effect is at present unclear but may be related to a reduction in myocardial contractile state. Second, an improved perfusion of ischemic myocardium following coronary occlusion in the chronically sympathectomized ventricle may accompany the reductions in oxygen and blood flow requirements. The net effect of these two factors is an improvement in the imbalance between oxygen demand and supply. Factors underlying the increased ischemic perfusion in chronically sympathectomized myocardium are not well delineated. Evidence favors the time-dependent reduction in coronary collateral resistances following surgical ventricular sympathectomy, although an understanding of this phenomenon is currently incomplete.

REFERENCES

1. Barber, M. J., D. E. Euler, J. X. Thomas, Jr., W. C. Randall, Changes in blood flow and S-T segment during coronary arterial occlusion in denervated and nondenervated canine hearts. *Am. J. Cardiol. 45*: 973–978, 1980.
2. Barber, M. J., J. X. Thomas, Jr., S. B. Jones, W. C. Randall, Effect of sympathetic nerve stimulation and cardiac denervation on myocardial blood flow during coronary artery occlusion. *Am. J. Physiol. 243*: H566–H574, 1982.
3. Braunwald, E., J. W. Covell, P. R. Maroko, J. Ross, Jr., Effects of drugs and of counterpulsation on myocardial oxygen comsumption. Observations on the ischemic heart. *Circulation. 40*: 220–230, 1969.
4. Brown, A. M., Coronary pressor reflexes. *Am. J. Cardiol. 44*: 849–851, 1979.
5. Buffington, C. W. and E. O. Feigl, Adrenergic coronary vasoconstriction in the presence of coronary stenosis in the dog. *Circ. Res. 48*: 416–423, 1981.

6. Chilian, W. M., R. B. Boatwright, T. Shoji, D. M. Griggs, Jr., Evidence against significant resting sympathetic coronary vasoconstrictor tone in the conscious dog. *Circ. Res. 49*: 866–876, 1981.
7. Davidson, S., P. R. Maroko, E. Braunwald, Effects of isoproterenol on contractile function of the ischemic and anoxic heart. *Am. J. Physiol. 227*: 439–443, 1974.
8. Donald, D., Myocardial performance after excision of the extrinsic cardiac nerves in the dog. *Circ. Res. 34*: 417–424, 1974.
9. DuPont, E., C. E. Jones, R. A. Luedecke, E. E. Smith, Chronic ventricular sympathectomy: effect on myocardial perfusion after ligation of the circumflex artery in dogs. *Circ. Shock. 6*: 324–331, 1979.
10. Elson, J. L., R. E. Ten Eick, D.H. Singer Autonomic nervous system and cellular injury from circumflex ligation in dogs. *Am. J. Physiol.* (*Heart Cir. Physiol.* 9): H738-H745, 1981.
11. Giudicelli, J., A. Berdeaux, F. Tato, M. Garnier, Left stellate stimulation: regional myocardial flows and ischemic injury in dogs. *Am. J. Physiol. 239 (Heart Circ. Physiol. 8)*: H359–H354, 1980.
12. Gregg, D. E., The natural history of coronary collateral development. *Circ. Res. 35*: 335–344, 1974.
13. Gregg, D. E., E. M. Khouri, D. E. Donald, H. A. Lowensohn, S. Pasyk, Coronary circulation in the conscious dog with cardiac neural ablation. *Circ. Res. 31*: 129–144, 1972.
14. Hellstrom, H. R., Coronary artery vasospasm: the likely immediate cause of acute myocardial infarction. *Br. Heart J. 41*: 426–432, 1979.
15. Hillis, L. D. and E. Braunwald, Myocardial ischemia. *New Eng. J. Med. 296*: 971–978, 1977.
16. Hillis, L. D. and E. Braunwald, Coronary-artery spasm. *New Eng. J. Med. 299*: 695–702, 1978.
17. Hirche, H. J., C. H. R. Franz, L. Bos, R. Bissing, R. Lang, M. Schramm, Myocardial extracellular I^+ and H^+ increase and noradrenaline release as possible causes of early arrhythmias following acute coronary artery occlusion in pigs. *J. Mol. Cell. Cardiol. 12*: 579–593, 1980.
18. Jones, C. E., L. Y. Beck, E. DuPont, G. E. Barnes, Effects of coronary ligation on the chronically sympathectomized ventricle. *Am. J. Physiol. 235 (Heart Circ. Physiol. 4)* H429–H434, 1978.
19. Jones, C. E. and M. S. Cannon, The myocardium and its vasculature: a histochemical comparison of the normal and chronically sympathectomized dog heart. *Histochem. J. 12*: 9–22, 1980.
20. Jones, C. E. and M. S. Cannon, Evidence for increased protein synthesis in myocardial microvessels after chronic sympathectomy in the dog. *Acta Anat. 109*: 313–320, 1981.
21. Jones, C. E., M. D. Devous, J. X. Thomas, Jr., E. DuPont, The effect of chronic cardiac denervation on infarct size following acute coronary occlusion. *Am. Heart J. 95*: 738–746, 1978.
22. Jones, C.E., T.W. Hurst, and J.R. Randall. Reduced oxygen and blood flow demands in the chronically sympathectomized heart. *Circ. Shock 9*:469–480, 1982.
23. Jones, C. E. and K. W. Scheel, Reduced coronary collateral resistances after chronic ventricular sympathectomy. *Am. J. Physiol. 238 (Heart Circ. 7)*: H196–H201, 1980.
24. Karlsberg, R. P., P. A. Penkose, P. E. Cryer, P. B. Corr, R. Roberts, Rapid activation of the sympathetic nervous system following coronary artery occlusion: rela-

tionship to infarct size, site, and haemodynamic impact. *Cardiovas. Res. 13*: 523–531, 1979.
25. Kaye, M. P., D. V. Priola, J. Coyle, Depletion of ventricular catecholamine levels following peripulmonary neurectomy. *Proc. Soc. Exp. Biol. Med. 135*: 844–848, 1970.
26. Kloner, R. A. and E. Braunwald, Observations on experimental myocardial ischemia. *Cardiovasc. Res. 14*: 371–395, 1980.
27. Leriche, R. and R. Fontaine, Les resultats actuels du traitment chirurgical de l'angine de poitrine. *J. De Chir. 38*: 785–815, 1931.
28. Malliani, A., Afferent cardiovascular sympathetic nerve fibres and their function in the neural regulation of the circulation. In *Cardiac Receptors*, eds. R. Hainsworth, C. Kidd, and R. J. Linden. Cambridge University Press, Cambridge, 1979, pp. 319–338.
29. Malliani, A. and F. Lombardi, Neural reflexes associated with myocardial ischemia. In *Neural Mechanisms In Cardiac Arrhythmias*, eds. P. J. Schwartz and A. M. Brown. Raven Press, New York, 1978,p p. 209–219.
30. Malliani, A., M. Parks, R. P. Tuckett, A. M. Brown, Reflex increases in heart rate elicited by stimulation of afferent cardiac sympathetic nerve fibers in the cat. *Circ. Res. 32*: 9–14, 1973.
31. Malliani, A., D. G. Peterson, V. S. Bishop, A. M. Brown, Spinal sympathetic cardiocardiac reflexes. *Circ. Res. 30*: 158–166, 1972.
32. Manning, G. W., C. G. McEachern, G. E. Hall, Reflex coronary artery spasm following sudden occlusion of other coronary branches. *Arch. Int. Med. 64*: 661–674, 1939.
33. Mudge, G. H., Jr., W. Grossman, R. M. Mills, M. Lesch, E. Braunwald, Reflex increase in coronary vascular resistance in patients with ischemic heart disease. *New Eng. J. Med. 295*: 1333–1337, 1976.
34. Prinzmetal, M., R. Kennamer, R. Merliss, T. Wada, N. Bor, Angina Pectoris I. A variant form of angina pectoris. *Am. J. Med. 27*: 375–388, 1959.
35. Randall, D. C., J. M. Evans, G. E. Billman, G. A. Ordway, C. F. Knapp, Neural, hormonal and intrinsic mechanisms of cardiac control during acute coronary occlusion in the intact dog. *J. Autonomic Nerv. Syst. 3*: 87–99, 1981.
36. Randall, D. C., D. M. Hasson, V. J. Brady, Acute cardiovascular consequences of anterior descending coronary artery occlusion in unanesthetized monkey. *Proc. Soc. Exp. Biol. Med. 158*: 135–140, 1978.
37. Randall, W. C., M. P. Kaye, J. X. Thomas, M. J. Barber, Intrapericardial denervation of the heart. *J. Surg. Res. 29*: 101–109, 1980.
38. Robertson, D., R. M. Robertson, A. S. Nies, J. A. Oates, G. C. Friesinger. Variant angina pectoris: investigation of indexes of sympathetic nervous function. *Am. J. Cardiol. 43*: 1080–1085, 1979.
39. Rubio, R. and R. M. Berne, Regulation of coronary blood flow. *Prog. Cardiovasc. Diseases. 18*: 105–122, 1975.
40. Scheel, K.W. and C.E. Jones. Reduced resistances of septal artery collateral channels after cardiac sympathectomy. *Basic Res. Cardiol. 78*:373–383, 1983.
41. Shatney, C. H., D. J. MacCarter, R. C. Lillehei, Effects of allopurinol, propranolol, and methylprednisolone on infarct size in experimental myocardial infarction. *Am. J. Cardiol. 37*: 572–580, 1976.
42. Shubrooks, S. J., Variant angina: more variants of the variant. *Am. J. Cardiol. 43*: 1245–1247, 1979.

43. Thames, M. D., H. S. Klopfenstein, F. M. Abboud, A. L. Mark, J. L. Walker, Preferential distribution of inhibitory cardiac receptors with vagal afferents to the inferoposterior wall of the left ventricle activated during coronary occlusion in the dog. *Circ. Res.* *43*: 512–519, 1978.
44. Thomas, J. X., Jr., W. C. Randall, C. E. Jones, Protective effect of chronic versus acute cardiac denervation on contractile force during coronary occlusion. *Am. Heart J.* *102*: 157–161, 1981.
45. Thoren, P. Vagal depressor reflexes elited by left ventricular C-fibers during myocardial ischemia in cats. In *Neural Mechanisms in Cardiac Arrhythmias*, eds. P. J. Schwartz, A. M. Brown, A. Malliani, and A. Zanchelti. Raven Press, New York, 1978, pp. 179–190.
46. Vatner, S. F. and H. Baig, Comparison of the effects of ouabain and isoproterenol on ischemic myocardium of conscious dogs. *Circulation* *58*: 654–662, 1978.
47. Vatner, S. F., R. J. McRitchie, P. R. Maroko, T. A. Patrick, E. Braunwald, Effects of catecholamines, exercise, and nitroglycerin on the normal and ischemic myocardium in conscious dog. *J. Clin. Invest.* *54*: 563–575, 1974.
48. Webb, S. W., A. A. J. Adgey, J. F. Pantridge, Autonomic disturbance at onset of acute myocardial infarction. *Br. Med. J.* *3*: 89–92, 1972.
49. Weber, K. T. and J. S. Janicki, The metabolic demand and oxygen supply of the heart: physiologic and clinical considerations. *Am. J. Cardiol.* *44*: 722–729, 1979.
50. Wollenberger, A. and L. Shahab, Anoxia-induced release of noradrenaline from the isolated perfused heart. *Nature.* *207*: 88–89, 1965.

12

Denervation and Reinnervation of the Heart

MICHAEL P. KAYE

Techniques for acute and chronic studies of the partially and totally denervated heart are by no means of recent origin. Clinical and laboratory investigations of the denervated heart appeared often in the medical literature of the late 1800's. In an elegant article, Reid Hunt, in 1899 [58], reviewed the historical aspects of the neural control of the heart and presented data from a large series of acute denervation experiments dealing with the direct and reflex control of the mammalian heart. In the same year, Francois Franck [43] proposed that cardiac sympathectomy be considered in the surgical treatment of angina pectoris. Shortly thereafter, bilateral cervical ganglionectomy was performed for relief of angina pectoris by C. H. Mayo, although he did not report the successful relief of angina in this case until 1925 [82]. Even before Cannon's description of the effect of adrenal secretion on the denervated heart [14], Carrel and Guthrie reported the first attempts at cardiac transplantation in 1905 [15]. Gasser and Meek, in 1914 [44], described a technique for chronic cardiac denervation that is still, or was until very recently, in use. Such studies have continued through the years on both an experimental and a clinical basis. A review of these early studies was presented by Cutler and Fine in 1926 [26]. A more complete review of the current clinical utilization of selective cardiac denervation is included in this chapter in the section entitled "Partial Denervation."

Interest in cardiac transplantation seems to have been revived in the 1930's when Mann and associates [80] developed a technique of cervical transplantation that brought about the crucial factor of donor coronary perfusion more simply. Numerous investigators [3,9,10,16,18,29,39,81,100,101,119] have subsequently used the Mann technique or modifications of it in studying the problems of heart transplantation. Late in 1951, Demikhov, in the USSR, made the first attempt to perform orthotopic cardiac transplantation in experimental animals, and by January, 1955, he had been successful in obtaining good cardiac function in two animals for periods of 11½ and 15½ hours. The brilliance of these technical feats must be acknowledged because they were successfully accomplished without the use of hypothermia or cardiopulmonary bypass. With the advent of a means of supporting the recipient during the operative procedure, workers in this area become more ambitious and many described techniques and functional results of orthotopic cardiac transplantation. This work culminated in the major advances of Lower and Shumway, in 1960, when they reported a series of eight consecutive cardiac homotransplantations in which five of the recipient animals lived 6 to 21 days [77,78]. These authors and their colleagues have added considerable knowledge to the study of the function of the denervated (transplanted) heart in both experimental animals and humans [38,76]. Their clinical experience with 206 patients undergoing 227 cardiac transplantations has recently been reviewed [94].

Extensive studies of the autotransplanted heart have been carried out by Willman and colleagues, who analyzed the physiology [122], histology [21,86], metabolism [22], and pharmacology [23] in dogs and in primates [106]. Studies utilizing other techniques for cardiac denervation have also been carried out and have contributed significant knowledge to our understanding of the function of the partially or totally denervated heart. This work has been reviewed by Donald [30] and by Kent and Cooper [67].

TOTAL CARDIAC DENERVATION TECHNIQUES

There are numerous techniques for total cardiac denervation including those performed with and without extracorporeal circulation. The use of hypothermia or extracorporeal circulation (or both) has been described by Willman and associates [121] and by Lower and associates [78]. The latter group's technique is that currently used in human orthotopic cardiac transplantation.

Before the technique of regional neural ablation was published by Cooper and his colleagues in 1961 [20], many methods had been proposed for total cardiac denervation without transplantation. For the most part these various techniques consisted of a staged cervical or thoracic vagectomy and sympathetic ganglionectomy. Conflicting results were obtained in many of these studies because of varying degrees of cardiac denervation and variable destruction of autonomic nerves to other viscera and vascular beds. The procedure described by Cooper and associates was based on studies of the neuroanatomy of the dog, leading the authors to conclude that regional ablation of the autonomic structures in the mediastinum should result in an experimental preparation that would circumvent these objections.

This procedure was performed in dogs through a median sternotomy. The phrenic nerves were freed from the pericardium and pleura beginning at the thoracic inlet and continuing to the diaphragm. The pericardium was excised from the diaphragm to its reflection over the great vessels and the aorta, and the origins of the brachiocephalic and subclavian arteries were mobilized and stripped of adventitia. The superior vena cava was mobilized from the level of the innominate vein to the right atrium, and the azygos vein was divided. The right pulmonary artery was cleaned of adventitia from its origin to its main branches. Fat, lymphatics, and nervous tissue in the pretracheal plexus were excised to expose the dorsal wall of the left atrium. The trachea, from its bifurcation to the level of T-3, was cleaned by excising all remaining mediastinal elements between the aorta and the superior vena cava. On the left side, the pulmonary artery was cleaned of adventitia from its origin to its main branches. The ligamentum arteriosum, the vestigial fold of Marshall, and the pericardial attachments were all denuded. The left atrial wall was exposed in the region of the left superior pulmonary vein, and all adjacent mediastinal tissue was excised. The pericardial reflections about the left and right pulmonary veins were divided, and the interatrial groove was developed. The pericardium and pleura were excised from the supradiaphragmatic portion of the inferior vena cava, and the sulcus terminalis was dissected. All remaining pericardium was excised. The completeness of denervation was verified postoperatively by direct electrical stimulation of the main vagal and sympathetic trunks.

Because of the limited assurance of total denervation after regional neural ablation [93], and because of the demanding postoperative care and excessive mortality involved in denervation by autotransplantation [121], Geis and colleagues [46] proposed in 1971 an additional technique for total cardiac denervation. This technique involves two separate thoracotomies staged 3 to 12 days apart. During the first procedure, the adventitia of the main pulmonary artery and the aorta, along with intervening tissues, is transected. In addition, the free wall of the left atrium is transected and reanastomosed near the pericardial reflection. After recovery from this operative procedure, the animal is subjected to a right thoracotomy, at which time the medial protion of the superior vena cava is transected and reanastomosed from the margin of the previous superior left atriotomy incision to the anterior superior vena cava. The lateral superior vena cava is transected and reanastomosed from the anterior superior vena cava to the superior margin of the interatrial groove. The interatrial groove is dissected free of all fatty tissue and nerve fibers from the upper border of the right superior pulmonary vein to the lower border of the right inferior pulmonary vein. Through a right atriotomy performed during occlusion of the venae cavae, the interatrial septum is incised longitudinally from below the coronary sinus through the limbus of the fossa ovalis. This septal incision is then closed with a continuous suture. Extensive physiological studies performed 7 to 15 days postoperatively verified completeness of denervation.

Because of the "two-stage" nature of the Geis procedure, intraoperative documentation of total denervation by direct nerve stimulation is not possible. Consequently, we developed a one-stage technique that permits precise documentation of denervation during the surgical procedure [62]. This procedure, performed through a median sternotomy, was in most aspects similar to that described by Geis and associates [46]. However, two major differences between the procedures should be noted. First, in the one-stage procedure, careful attention was directed to transection of all connective tissue between the pulmonary arteries and the left atrium. Secondly, in contrast to the Geis technique, transection of the atrial septum was not carried out. Documentation of complete denervation was carried out at the time of surgery by direct electrical stimulation of the vagosympathetic trunks and stellate ganglia.

Because of the morbidity secondary to median sternotomy in dogs, we continued our studies to refine the technique of cardiac denervation without transplantation. Currently the denervation procedure is performed as follows. The chest is entered through a left thoracotomy in the fourth intercostal space, the lung is retracted, and the pericardium is incised longitudinally above and parallel to the phrenic nerve from the apex of the heart to its reflection over the pulmonary artery. At this point, the pericardial incision is directed toward the superior vena cava and continued to the point where it reflects onto the anterior aspect of this structure. Walton-Brodie strain gauge arches are sutured to the atria and ventricles to record myocardial contractile force, and systemic blood pressure and the electrocardiogram are recorded. Predenervation data are obtained by electrically stimulating the intrathoracic vagi and stellate ganglia and recording the responses.

The ventrolateral cardiac nerve is transected at the level of the left superior pulmonary vein. By dissecting in the transverse sinus, the pericardial attachments to the left atrium are severed from the left to the right superior pulmonary veins. Connective tissue between the right pulmonary artery and the atrium is also transected. Attention is now directed to the right-sided innervation. With the aorta retracted to the left and the right atrial appendage retracted caudally, the tissue between the aorta and the superior vena cava is transected at the level of the pericardial reflection onto the superior vena cava. The adventitia of the superior vena cava is sectioned circumferentially. The right pulmonary artery is freed of any residual connective tissue between it and the left atrium and superior vena cava. The azygos vein is ligated and divided. Finally, circumferential transection of the adventitia of the pulmonary artery and the adjacent aorta as well as interposed connective tissue is carried out to complete the denervation procedure. At this point, functional studies are repeated and compared with controls to confirm complete denervation.

In addition to the aforementioned surgical techniques, complete chemically induced cardiac denervation has been achieved after the administration of atropine with reserpine [89], 6-hydroxydopamine [59], and beta blockade and immunosympathectomy [112]. Although much information has been provided from such studies, the lack of specificity of chemical denervation for cardiac tissues prevents these techniques from providing specific information on the function of the totally denervated heart.

Finally, considering the clinical implications of complete or partial cardiac denervation, the autonomic neuropathies and consequent cardiac denervation which may accompany diabetes mellitus [74] and Chagas' heart disease [1] should be kept in mind when the results of these studies are analyzed.

FUNCTION OF THE DENERVATED HEART

Before the functional results of total cardiac denervation are discussed, it must be emphasized that any data presented on this subject must be evaluated in terms of the technique used to accomplish denervation, the time from denervation to the time of study, and the anesthetic agents employed. These factors are of extreme importance since it has been shown, for example, that as few as 15% of animals subjected to mediastinal neural ablation are totally denervated, that denervation of other viscera may result, that reinnervation may be found as early as 26 days in subhuman species, and that barbiturates, even in small doses, depress both peripheral and central nervous transmission of cardiovascular responses [93].

In 1963, Donald and Shepherd [34] reviewed the results of previous studies on the effect of exercise in animals after cardiac denervation and presented detailed data on the capacity for work in dogs subjected to regional neural ablation. The resting heart rate in awake dogs with cardiac denervation was between 90 and 120 beats/min. In all animals sinus arrhythmia was absent and the R-R interval remained almost constant for periods of 1 hour or more. Startle did not cause any immediate change in heart rate in contrast to the change that is seen in the normal animal. The heart response to mild exercise was a modest

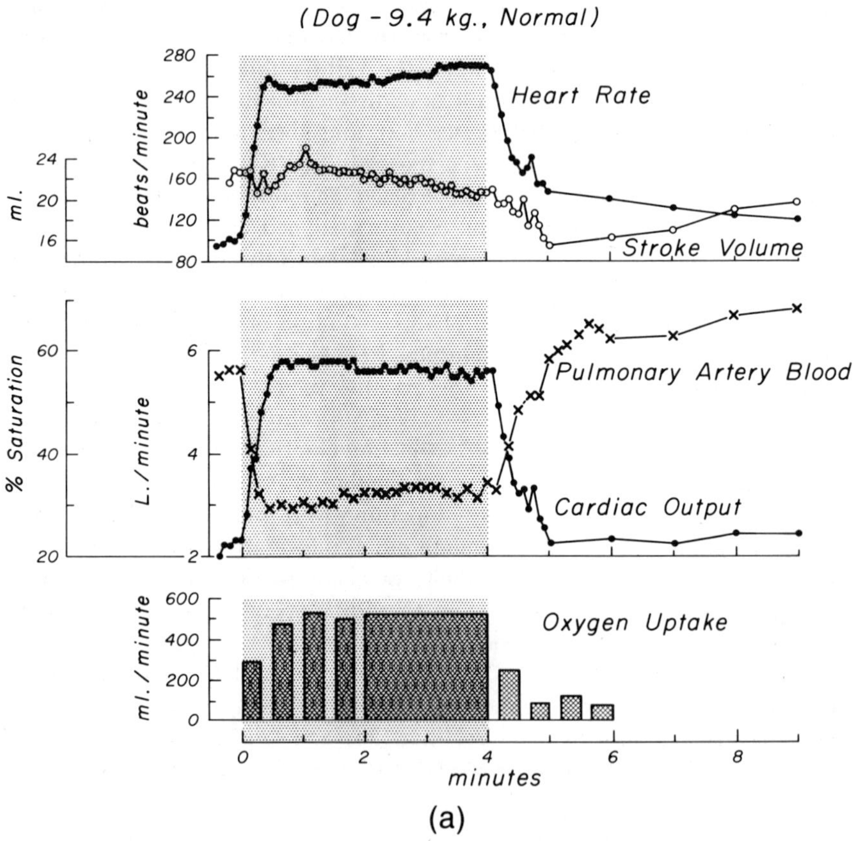

Fig. 12-1. Cardiorespiratory changes with exercise (5.5 km/hour, 21% grade). (A) Normal dog, 9.4 kg. (B) Dog with chronic cardiac denervation, 8.0 kg. (Reproduced through courtesy of Donald and Shepherd and *Am. J. Physiol.* 207: 1325, 1964)

increase in heart rate with an absence of any sudden changes as seen in control animals. With more severe levels of exercise, heart rate increased slowly to a peak value lower than that of controls and returned more slowly to control levels. When compared over equal increments in oxygen consumption, the increase in heart rate in cardiac-denervated dogs was approximately one-third that of controls.

In further studies relevant to the response of the dog with cardiac denervation to exercise, these authors demonstrated that the salient differences between normal and denervated dogs occur within the first minute of running [35]. With mild work, the increase in cardiac output in the denervated group was almost wholly due to an increase in stroke volume, whereas the increase in the normal group of dogs was entirely a result of increased rate (Fig. 12-1). The increase in left ventricular end-diastolic pressure and internal diameter suggests that the increased initial fiber length is the responsible mechanism for the increased stroke volume in these denervated hearts. Although this marked increase in stroke volume contributes extensively to the increase in cardiac output, the maximal stroke volume is not very different from that measured in conscious dogs at rest with heart rates of 50 to 70 beats/min. Similar compensatory mechanisms

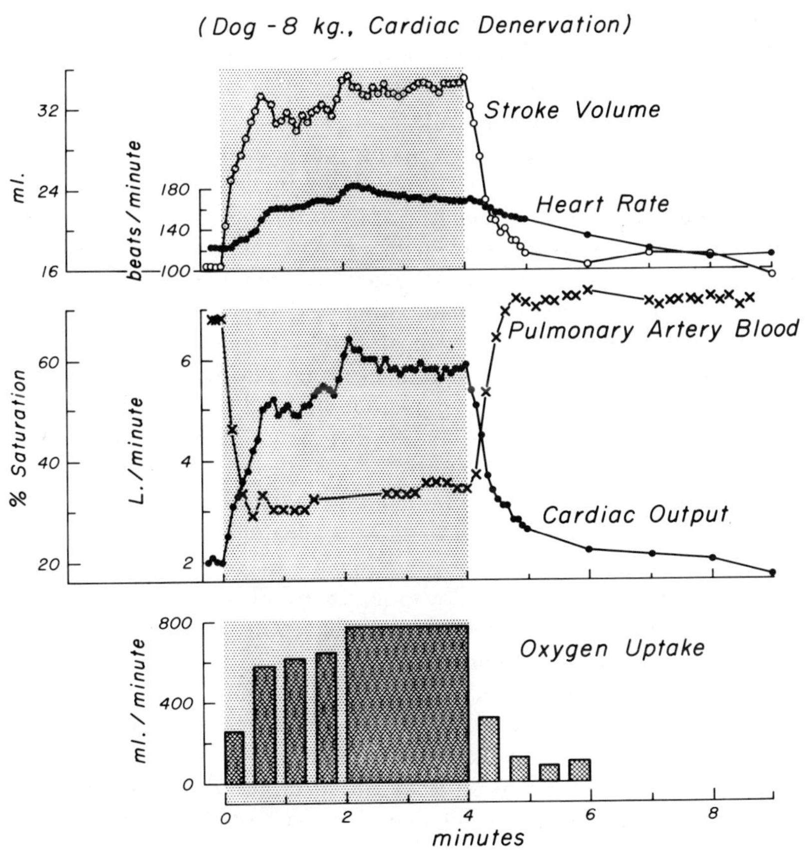

(b)

for increasing cardiac output in response to the stress of mild exercise have been reported in man after cardiac transplantation [102,108,113].

As levels of exercise are increased, cardiac output cannot be augmented by the Starling mechanism alone. As demonstrated by Bishop and Horwitz [11], stroke volume depends not only on initial fiber length but also on an increase in the velocity and extent of fiber shortening caused by sympathetic stimulation. Guyton and co-workers [55] have demonstrated that myocardial supersensitivity to circulating catecholamines is a quantitatively sufficient mechanism to account for the apparently normal augmentation of ventricular performance in the cardiac-denervated dog. This development of supersensitivity to circulating catecholamines appears to compensate fully for the loss of direct neural support of ventricular performance. These data are substantiated by those of Donald and colleagues [31,32], who have demonstrated that the racing times and maximal heart rates are only slightly less than controls in cardiac-denervated, trained racing greyhounds. These authors further demonstrated, however, that when the cardiac effects of circulating catecholamines are prevented by beta blockade, the greyhound with a denervated heart shows a marked reduction in racing performance and in heart rate [31]. Similarly in man, Shaver and associates [108] have reported that after cardiac transplantation beta blockade significantly decreases the donor heart rate response to exercise.

Additional studies on the response of the denervated heart in animal and in man to induced stress have demonstrated the effects of arterial hypertension and hypotension, hypoxia, and anemia [5,51,71,113,117]. In cardiac-denervated dogs subjected to hemorrhage, the response was similar to that of control animals except for the increases in heart rate shown by the control animals. Under the circumstances of the experiments, it appears that adjustments in the peripheral vasculature were adequate to maintain systemic arterial blood pressures [71]. If, however, hypotension was produced in anesthetized animals by acetylcholine infusion [117], then cardiac output and heart rate increased less in denervated dogs than in controls. If heart rate was controlled by pacing, both groups showed similar responses of cardiac output. The increase in arterial pressure load in response to arterial hypertension induced by angiotension infusion [117] or carotid occlusion [25] was sustained equally well by normal and denervated hearts.

Studies by Glick and colleagues [48] and by Greenfield and Ebert [52] demonstrated that the response of the denervated heart to hypoxia is similar but somewhat less pronounced than the response in control animals. Similar responses to acute anemia induced by exchange transfusions [49] were recorded. Mild hypoxia in patients studied after cardiac transplantation can cause an increase in the innervated recipient sinus node rate without causing changes in the denervated donor sinus node rate. Increases in donor sinus node rate during more severe degrees of hypoxia are probably due to the release of circulating catecholamines [51]. In all of these studies, data are presented to support the conclusion that a neurally induced tachycardia constitutes an important part of the cardiac response to stress and that the denervated (transplanted) heart response is less than normal in these situations.

Shaver and associates have suggested [108] that not only do circulating catecholamines play a role in increasing heart rate after cardiac transplantation, but that the transplanted human heart itself has the ability to increase its intrinsic rate after beta blockade. Similar observations were reported by Donald and Samueloff [33] in cardiac-denervated dogs after administration of propranolol, and Blinks [12] has described a positive chronotropic effect of increasing right atrial pressure in the isolated heart.

The dependence of the denervated heart on circulating catecholamines is enhanced to a great degree by the supersensitivity of the heart to these substances. Studies by Dempsey and Cooper [28], Ebert [40], and others [23,33,36,96] indicated that the heart follows Cannon's "Law of Denervation" and responds with increases of heart rate, contractile force, and cardiac output to infusions of minute quantities of norepinephrine. Dempsey and Cooper [28] have stated that this supersensitivity can be explained by a loss of intraneuronal binding loci for norepinephrine. Almost total depletion of myocardial catecholamines has been reported by various laboratories [20,24,50] after total sympathetic denervation or transplantation of the heart. Potter and associates [95] have reported on the ability of the transplanted heart to bind, store, and synthesize norepinephrine and dopamine, and they have suggested that these functions are almost completely dependent on its content of adrenergic nerves. Retention of administered dopamine was reduced to about 4% of normal. Uptake and retention of norepinephrine for 15 minutes was reduced to about 6% of normal in denervated hearts. Synthesis of norepinephrine from dopamine after perfusion with dopamine was only 2.8% of that found in normal hearts. Denervation produced little change in total in vitro activity of the enzymes that metabolize norepinephrine, monamine oxidase, and catechol-O-methyltransferase (COMT). In transplanted hearts, norepinephrine apparently does not enter neurons, with the result that it is largely degraded by COMT-like circulating catecholamines. The overall inactivation of administered norepinephrine by binding and metabolism was noted to be considerably less in the denervated heart than in the normal. The authors attributed part of the increased chronotropic and inotropic responsiveness of transplanted hearts to the fact that more free norepinephrine is present at the receptor cell. These studies demonstrate the importance of the adrenergic innervation of the heart for normal synthesis, storage, and inactivation of norepinephrine.

Recently Palmer and associates [91] presented data that argue strongly for the fact that some neuronal postjunctional alterations occur following cardiac denervation. Their results show that adenylate cyclase activities from the atria and ventricles of denervated hearts exhibit a twofold to threefold increase in response to norepinephrine as compared with control hearts. The possible involvement of the catalytic site of adenylate cyclase in mechanisms of supersensitivity is reflected by the enhanced response of the ventricular enzyme preparation to fluoride. The authors suggest that denervation supersensitivity therefore may involve changes in both the reuptake mechanism (prejunctional) and the adrenergic receptor itself (postjunctional).

The response of the denervated heart to other drugs has been studied in both animals and man after cardiac transplantation [23,72,88,113]. In cardiac-denervated dogs, administration of tyramine in doses of 60 μg/kg results in neither cardiac augmentation nor acceleration as seen in normal animals, although a modest pressor response remains [23]. In man, intravenous administration of tyramine produces an initial depression of the recipient atrial rate during the phase of rising atrial pressure, followed by a prolonged period of relative tachycardia. During this time the donor heart rate remains stable [113]. The responses to metaraminol, ephedrine, and mephentermine were attenuated in animals with denervated hearts. In contrast, the cardiac autotransplant responds to ouabain administration in an apparently normal manner. Similarly, the positive inotropic action of calcium chloride is apparently unaffected. The cryptenamine alkaloids, which induce bradycardia mediated by the Bezold-Jarisch reflex in control animals, are, as expected, without effect after transplantation. The potent inotropic and chronotropic effects of glucagon are apparently unaltered in the transplanted heart [72].

Other metabolic changes that may or may not occur in the transplanted or denervated heart have been reviewed by Donald [30], who supports the general impression that there are no major alterations in myocardial metabolism in the long-term surviving animal. The question is by no means settled. Gregg and associates [53] have suggested that the oxygen requirements and circumflex coronary artery flow in dogs with denervated hearts are less both at rest and during exercise and excitement than are those of dogs with intact cardiac nerves under similar conditions.

The effects of cardiac afferent fiber loss after transplantation are perhaps even more controversial than the metabolic effects of the procedure [75]. Disagreements arising in this area stem in large part from inadequate knowledge about the exact location and nature of afferent receptors and pathways and about the techniques for specific ablation of receptor response. For example, although an increase in blood volume has been noted after cardiac denervation, its mechanism is obscure. Mulcahy and associates [85] have demonstrated that in dogs with denervated hearts the elevation of blood volume results almost entirely from an increase in the plasma components. In addition, these animals demonstrated a large deficit in intracellular water. In the face of this elevated blood volume, the concentration of antidiuretic hormone in plasma was diminished and was associated with decreased urinary osmolality and increased urine volume after surgery.

Thames and associates [116] have demonstrated abnormal increases in peripheral plasma renin activity in response to bleeding in dogs after cardiac autotransplantation and have suggested that receptors in the heart other than those near the orifices of the great vein and posterior wall of the atria are involved in mediating these changes.

Some of the controversy about the effects of denervation of receptor function is no doubt a consequence of the denervation technique employed, as has been pointed out by Willman and associates [125] in comparing their results with those obtained by Gilmore and Daggett [47]. The latter authors studied animals with cardiac denervation produced by mediastinal neural ablation and found more striking alteration in urine production than was found in Willman and associates ' autotransplanted animals. Willman's group consistently reported troublesome fluid retention after transplantation, with generalized edema, pleural effusion, and ascites; these findings persisted despite therapy with digitalis and diuretics. In contrast, in animals undergoing cardiac autotransplantation according to the technique described by Shumway, this finding has not been reported [75]. It should be noted that, following the technique of Willman, the venae cavae are sectioned some distance from the heart, whereas in the Shumway technique the posterior right atrial wall remains intact and the cavae are not incised. Perhaps careful study of the receptor function of the venae cavae and other atrial tissues (as reviewed in chapter 5) will provide needed answers to some of the questions concerning cardiac afferent pathways.

REINNERVATION

It has been well established in experimental animals [37,41,69,70,87,93, 98,106,123] including primates, that reinnervation of the transplanted heart occurs. Such is not the case in humans subjected to cardiac transplantation and followed up to 9 years [4,102,114]. Evidence for reinnervation in animals has been confirmed not only after autotransplantation but also in allografted animals given immunosuppressive therapy [70]. Using techniques of direct electrical stimulation of the vagosympathetic trunks and stellate ganglia, Peiss and coworkers [93] were able to demonstrate vagal reinnervation occurring as early as 26 days, and both vagal and sympathetic reinnervation as early as 74 days after autotransplantation in dogs. After 1, 2, and 3 years, the functional responses to reflex and electrical activation of the nervous system were similar to those in normal dogs [93]. Other studies [66] have demonstrated even earlier sympathetic reinnervation when the cardiac denervated animals were treated with nerve growth factor. Norvell and Lower, using histochemical techniques, demonstrated regeneration of adrenergic fibers 1 year after cardiac autografting and confirmed that no changes in the quantity of cholinergic fibers were observed after transplantation [87]. We have correlated functional reinnervation of various segments of the heart with local catecholamine content and segmental supersensitivity and have also demonstrated return of the Bezold-Jarisch reflex 6 to 9 months after denervation.

Figure 12-2 illustrates a portion of the data obtained from an animal studied 3 months after denervation. Stimulation of the right stellate ganglion increased heart rate with a resultant atrial alternans and second-degree heart block. An increase in force of contraction was seen in both atria. Stimulation of the left stellate ganglion increased heart rate and force of contraction in the atria and in the left ventricular basal area. Stimulation of the distal end of the transected right cervical vagosympathetic trunk resulted in an increase in heart rate and atrial force rather than the expected slowing and depression of atrial contractile force. In contrast, stimulation of the distal left vagosympathetic trunk decreased

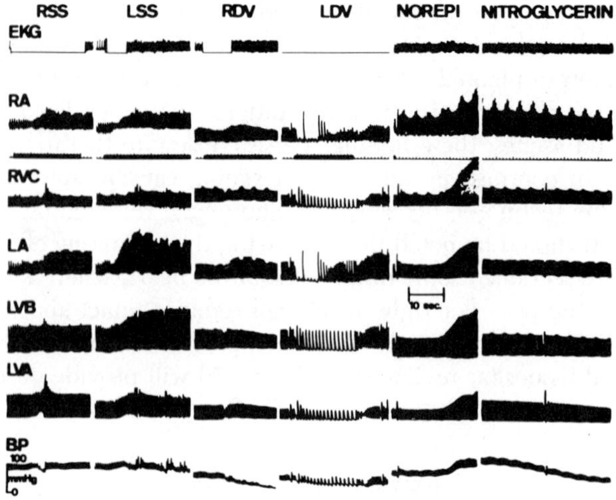

Fig. 12-2. Effects of nerve stimulation and drug administration 3 months after denervation. RSS = right stellate ganglion stimulation; LSS = left stellate ganglion stimulation; RDV and LDV = stimulation of right and left distal vagus; NOREPI = norepinephrine; RA = right atrial contractile force; RVC = right ventricular conus contractile force; LA = left atrial contractile force; LVB = left ventricular base contractile force; LVA = left ventricular apex contractile force; BP = systemic arterial blood pressure.

heart rate and force of atrial contraction. With cessation of stimulation, function of the vagosympathetic components in this nerve was manifest by the increase in heart rate. The presence of functional vagosympathetic fibers was verified in this animal after the administration of atropine. Norepinephrine (0.1 μg) infused into the superior vena cava resulted in a strong inotropic response in all gauges. Intravenous nitroglycerin caused hypotension but no reflex tachycardia. Infusion of cryptenamine was without effect.

In three animals studied at 4 months after denervation, stimulation of the stellate ganglia again gave evidence for inotropic and chronotropic reinnervation of the atria. Bradycardia with left distal vagosympathetic stimulation was noted in these animals, and right vagosympathetic stimulation resulted in small increases in heart rate.

Figure 12-3 illustrates data obtained from an animal studied 6 months after denervation. The infusion of nitroglycerin elicits marked hypotension but fails to produce a reflex tachycardia. This absence of reflex tachycardia occurs in spite of direct evidence for sympathetic reinnervation as demonstrated by stimulation of the left and right stellate ganglia. In this animal, tyramine infusion resulted in a slight increase in force of contraction of the atria, right ventricular conus, and left ventricular base. Norepinephrine (0.1 μg) infusion no longer resulted in a profound inotropic supersensitivity in all chambers but did evoke

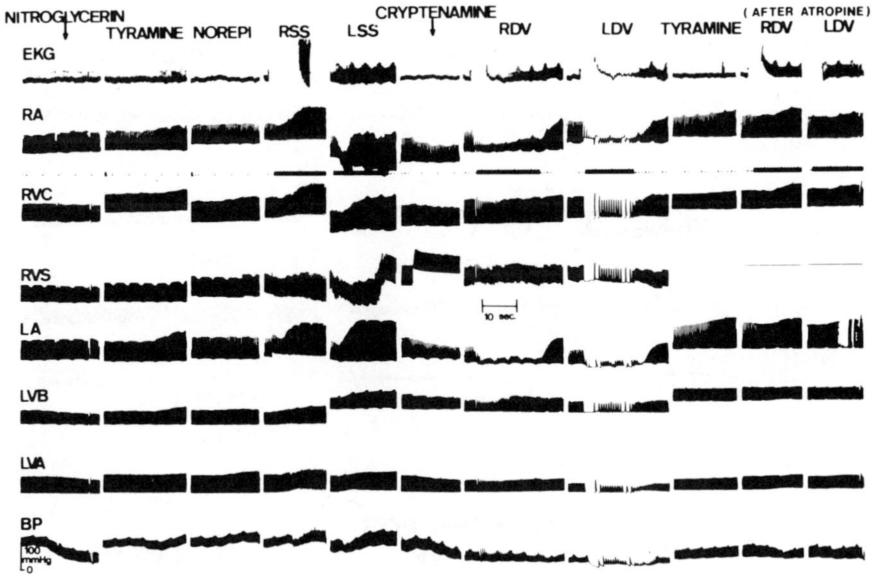

Fig. 12-3. Effects of nerve stimulation and drug administration 6 months after denervation. RVS = right ventricular sinus contractile force. Other abbreviations as in Fig. 12-2.

a response in the left ventricular apex. In this animal, and in other animals studied at a similar period after denervation, right distal vagosympathetic stimulation demonstrated a mixture of sympathetic and parasympathetic reinnervation. As noted in the illustration, there is a force depression in the right and left atria with a simultaneous increase in heart rate and an increase in force of contraction in the left ventricular base. After the administration of atropine, the functional presence of right vagosympathetic fibers was clearly demonstrated. Left distal vagosympathetic stimulation resulted in a profound slowing of the heart and a depression of the force of atrial contraction. Again, the presence of intact vagosympathetic fibers in this nerve was seen during stimulation after the administration of atropine.

Figure 12-4 compares the results of stimulation of the right stellate ganglion and of infusion of norepinephrine and tyramine in an animal during predenervation control studies and 6 months after denervation. Stimulation of the right stellate ganglion in the control period resulted in a marked increase in rate and force of contraction of the left atrium, left ventricular base, and apex. At 6 months, the same stimulation again elicited marked chronotropic effects but a lesser inotropic response in the left atrium and a slight increase in blood pressure. One-fortieth of the control amount of norepinephrine caused a moderate increase in force of contraction in the left ventricular apex with a slight increase in the left ventricular base. Tyramine infusion resulted in release of norepi-

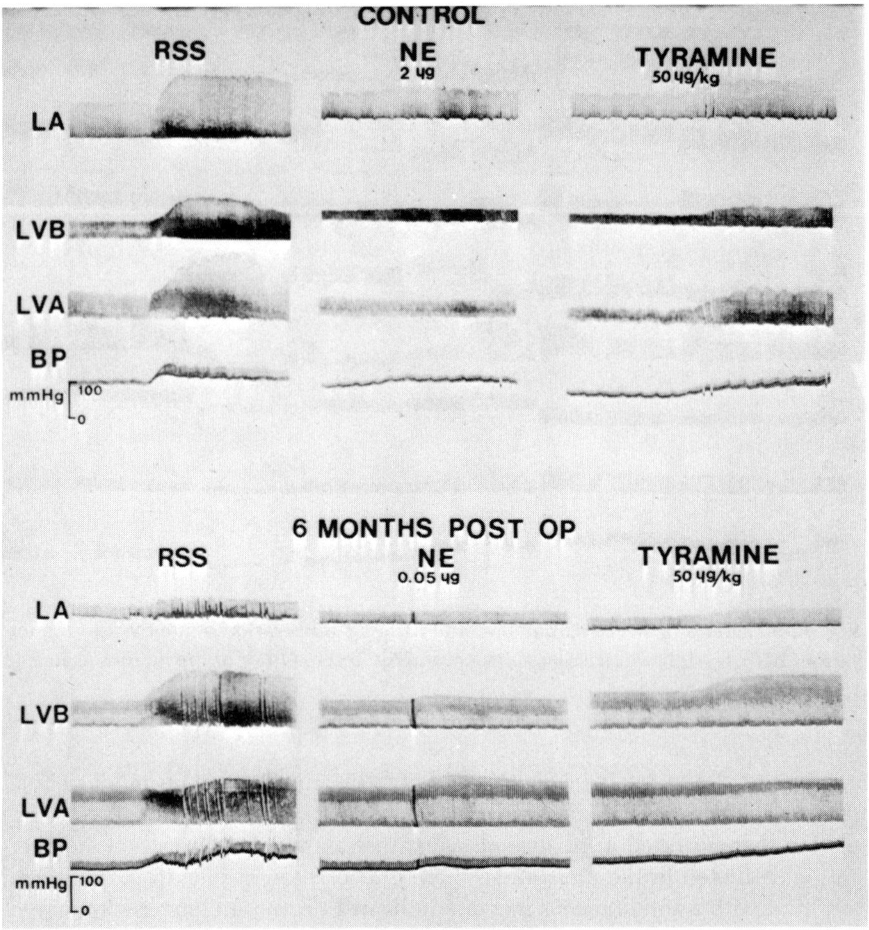

Fig. 12-4. Comparison of right stellate stimulation and norepinephrine (NE) and tyramine infusion postoperatively and 6 months after denervation. Abbreviations as in Fig. 12-2.

nephrine from the ventricular apex during the control period but failed to elicit a response from this area 6 months after denervation.

Studies performed 9 to 12 months after denervation gave evidence that, for the most part, functional reinnervation had taken place. Typical of the results obtained during this period are those from an animal studied 9 months after denervation and illustrated in Figure 12-5. In this animal, stimulation of the right and left stellate ganglia resulted in an increase in heart rate and force of contraction. It should be noted that at this time the most distal portion of the heart, the left ventricular apex, now responds with an increased force of contraction to left stellate ganglion stimulation. Parasympathetic reinnervation is demonstrated by the effects of left and right vagosympathetic trunk stimulation.

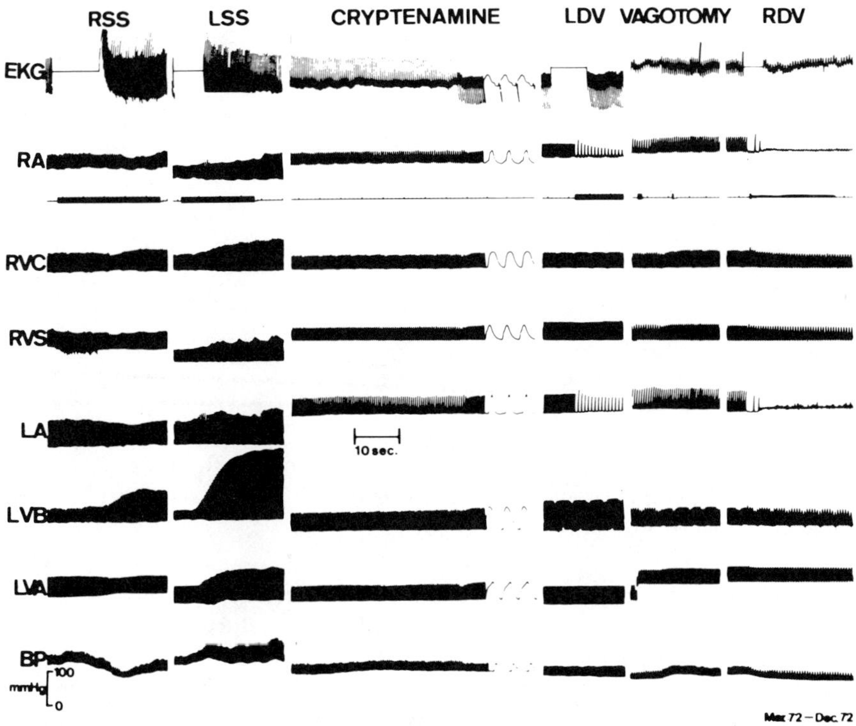

Fig. 12-5. Effects of nerve stimulation and drug administration 9 months after denervation. Abbreviations as in Fig. 12-2 and 12-3.

In addition, at this time, evidence for some afferent reinnervation is seen after the injection of cryptenamine into the pulmonary vein.

Figure 12-6 is a plot of the best line fits, as determined by computer analysis, for the norepinephrine content in eight areas of the 28 hearts analyzed for catecholamine content. Because of the exceptionally low values obtained from samples of the right ventricle, low septal areas, and left ventricular apex, these data have been combined and are represented by the bottom line on the graph. Control values from sham animals and from the literature for the areas studied indicate greater than 2 μg/g for atrial tissue and 1 μg/g for ventricular tissue. This graph demonstrates that the atria, in particular the left atrium, recover their norepinephrine first. This recovery is followed by that in the basal ventricular areas and finally in the apical area. It should be noted, however, that even at 26 months after denervation, norepinephrine levels are still only a small percentage of control values.

From the data presented, it may be concluded that efferent autonomic reinnervation of the surgically denervated heart takes place in a base-to-apex direction and is functionally complete in the dog at about 9 months after denervation. This return of function parallels the return of measurable quantities of myocardial norepinephrine in these areas and is accompanied by a decrease in

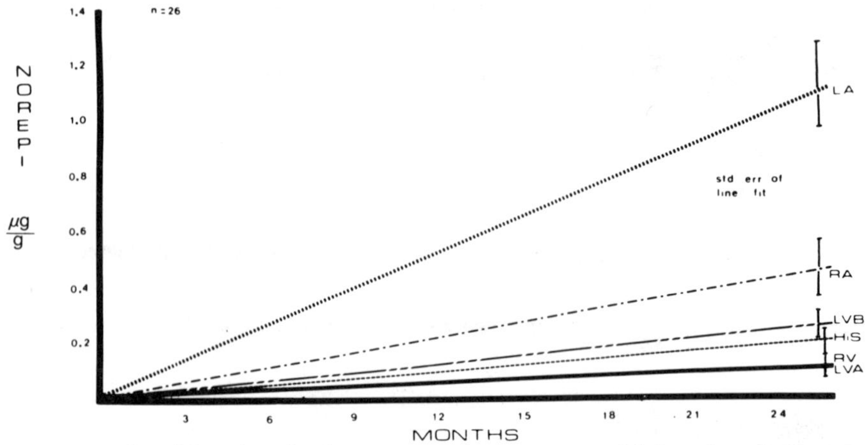

Fig. 12-6. Plot of best line fits for norepinephrine content of left atrium (LA), right atrium (RA), left ventricular apex and base (LVA and LVB), right ventricle (RV), and high interventricular septum (HS).

supersentitivity to exogenous norepinephrine. In accord with these findings, responsiveness to tyramine infusion also parallels the return of the functional response to electrical stimulation.

Data obtained during the electrical stimulation of the distal end of the severed left and right vagosympathetic trunks both before and after the administration of atropine indicate that the right vagosympathetic effects return before the parasympathetic effect and as early as 3 months. These data further indicate that the left vagosympathetic functional reinnervation occurs before that of the right side.

The validity of the use of indirect (reflex) methods of determining reinnervation is questioned because no sympathetic reflex tachycardia to induced hypotension was noted until after 6–9 months, or 3–6 months after the appearance of sympathetic response to direct electrical stimulation.

The Bezold-Jarisch reflex requires perhaps only one of many possible afferent pathways from the heart, and so the return of this reflex on administration of cryptenamine indicates that this particular afferent pathway, at least, has been reestablished 6–9 months after denervation. The return of apparently complete functional reinnervation cannot be quantitatively related to myocardial catecholamine levels. Although functional reinnervation appears to be complete at 9–12 months, catecholamine content of the heart is only a fraction of the normal values at this time and has not reached normal values as late as 1 year after functional reinnervation.

The data obtained after infusion of small doses of norepinephrine suggest that the segmented myocardial supersensitivity to norepinephrine is sequentially reversed during progressive adrenergic reinnervation. Furthermore, these data strongly suggest that the labile tyramine-releasable pool of norepinephrine, although small, is restored and accounts for the acquired evidence for functional reinnervation.

PARTIAL DENERVATION

Sympathectomy

Numerous techniques have been described for total and partial ablation of cardiac sympathetic efferent nerve fibers. As has been mentioned, Franck [43] is credited for the suggestion that sympathetomy would relieve the pain of angina. Various procedures for ablation of sympathetic efferent and afferent nerve pathways were developed consequent to this thesis, and a summary of these procedures and their results was published by Cutler and Fine in 1926 [26]. Although there was some enthusiasm for cardiac denervation in the treatment of angina during the early part of the twentieth century, many cardiologists then and today reflected the conservative attitude of Sir James Mackenzie, who suggested that it would be unfortunate if surgeons should discover an operation to relieve the pain of angina because it would remove the vital danger signal which warns patients that they are overtaxing their hearts. As has subsequently been shown by White and colleagues [120], this is indeed not the case since the sense of painless constriction and dyspnea have been effective detriments for these patients.

Since 1939, with the publication by Arnulf [2] of the theoretical basis and techniques for cardiac denervation, until the advent of the present surgical procedures for myocardial revascularization, there has been intermittent interest in sympathetic denervation of the heart for the treatment of angina. During this interval, techniques for cardiac denervation included paravertebral chemical blockade, posterior rhizotomy, cervical thoracic ganglionectomy, chemical and mechanical epicardiectomy, pericoronary neurectomy, and resection of the preaortic plexus as described by Arnulf. Except for the report by Palumbo [92] in 1963, little has appeared in the literature published in the United States during recent decades regarding the use of sympathectomy in the treatment of angina.

In other countries, notably in France, a resurgence of interest in cardiac denervation has occurred since Prinzmetal's report on variant angina. In addition, there has been increasing interest in the surgical treatment of disturbance of cardiac rhythm by surgical modulation of the autonomic innervation of the heart.

A preliminary report in February 1977, by Grondin and Limet [54], reiterated the rationale for surgical intervention and techniques used successfully in two patients with Prinzmetal's angina. These techniques essentially followed the techniques described for preaortic plexectomy by Arnulf. In March of 1977, Clark et al. [17] reported the surgical treatment of four patients with Prinzmetal's angina in whom medical management had failed. One of these patients was subjected to cardiac autotransplantation while the remaining three underwent stripping of the great vessels. Although pain was completely relieved in the patient undergoing cardiac autotransplantation, coronary spasm persisted following the ergotrate stimulation test. In contrast to this report, Talano et al. [115] reported successful ablation of coronary artery spasm by coronary artery bypass combined with intrapericardial cardiac denervation. Bertrand et al. in

1980 [7] published the results of plexectomy combined with coronary artery bypass for treatment of variant angina, and indicated that the results utilizing this mode of treatment were better than results with bypass alone (86% versus 61%). These authors also noted that the recurrence rate of angina was less when plexectomy was performed in addition to bypass grafting (5% versus 18%). The studies of Bertrand and his associates [6] have now been expanded to include at least 56 patients with variant angina. Fifty-four of these patients survived the operative procedure and during a mean follow up of 27 months (range 3–65 months), 49 patients remained symptom free, two patients had moderate attacks of exertional angina, and two patients (5.6%) had bad results with the continuation of spontaneous angina and characteristic ECG changes.

Of great interest to those considering cardiac denervation as a potential therapeutic modality, is a recent case reported by Bertrand and associates [8] of autotransplantation of the heart for the treatment of severe refractory coronary spasm. In this patient, as in the patient described by Clark et al. [17], spontaneous pain and ECG changes were completely abolished following the operative procedure. In spite of the abolition of pain, Bertrand was able to demonstrate on postoperative coronary arteriography that Methergine still induced coronary vasospasm and appropriate ST segment elevation. Of greater interest, however, is the addendum to this report indicating that some years following cardiac autotransplantation, the patient was readmitted because of the reappearance of spontaneous chest pain at rest. As indicated by the authors, this recurrence of symptoms suggests reinnervation of the autotransplanted heart and raises a question regarding the effective duration of cardiac denervation. These findings of reinnervation of the cardiac autotransplant are in contrast to the lack of evidence for reinnervation in patients undergoing therapeutic homologous cardiac transplantation.

The Arnulf technique includes extended dissection, questionable completeness of sympathetic ventricular denervation, and transection of parasympathetic fibers. Because of this, Medici and Fesani [83] have recently undertaken studies to demonstrate the effectiveness of selective ventricular denervation in patients undergoing coronary artery bypass. Using direct electrical stimulation of the left stellate ganglion and with strain gauge arches sewn to the right atrium and left ventricle, these authors obtained intraoperative, predenervation, and postdenervation recordings (Fig. 12-7). These studies demonstrated that following peripulmonary dissection and transection of the Fold of Marshall along with the adventitia of the left superior pulmonary vein, complete ventricular denervation was accomplished. Medici and Fesani noted the necessity of cutting fibers in the Fold of Marshall and along the left superior pulmonary vein in order to accomplish complete denervation in all cases.

As an understanding of the effects of cardiac innervation on rhythm has evolved, so has the interest in surgical or pharmacological modulation of this input. The role of the autonomic nervous system and the genesis of cardiac dysrhythmias is discussed in detail elsewhere in this book.

Moss and McDonald, in 1971 [84], reported the successful treatment of the

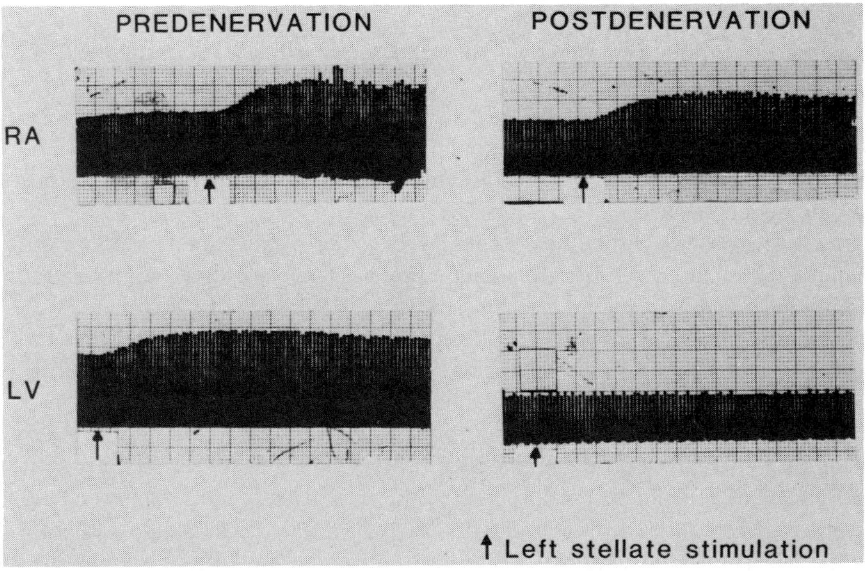

Fig. 12-7. Composite reproduction of intraoperative tracings. RA = strain gauge recordings from right atrium; LV = strain gauge recordings from left ventricle; arrow indicates onset of electrical stimulation of left stellate ganglion prior to (predenervation) and following (postdenervation) selective ventricular denervation.

prolonged QT interval syndrome by unilateral cervical thoracic sympathetic ganglionectomy. The patient described by these authors did well for a period of 4 years, but during the fifth year, gradually and progressively, the QT interval lengthened to approximately 0.60 seconds. This lengthening of the QT interval was once again associated with the onset of palpations. Subsequently, the patient underwent rhizotomy involving T_2 to T_6 on the left with significant shortening of the QT interval. Other investigators [103,105] have similarly reported successful treatment of the long QT syndrome by left stellectomy, and current studies by Schwartz [104] indicate the continuing success of this procedure.

Unilateral and bilateral cardiac sympathectomy has likewise been performed for recurrent ventricular tachycardias. Harken et al. [56] have recently reviewed this subject and cite the success rate of this procedure as being in the range of 50–60%. He notes, however, that although sympathectomy may be inadequate as the sole method of control, it may improve conditions and augment control of ventricular tachyarrhythmias.

Experimentally, if total or near-total depletion of myocardial catecholamines is taken as an index of denervation, then only bilateral stellectomy, caudal cervical ganglionectomy, and resection of the thoracic sympathetic ganglia through T-5 will fulfill this criterion. Of eight dogs with bilateral stellectomy and thoracic ganglionectomy studied by Peiss and associates [93], only four showed complete decentralization of the sympathetic cardiac outflow from the central nervous system. All of the animals exhibited large cardioacceleration responses when the distal cervical vagosympathetic trunk was electrically stimulated after the administration of atropine. Significant residual levels of myocardial catecholamines were measurable in these animals. Changes in cardiac performance after sympathetic denervation have been reported by Essex and associates [42] and are similar to the changes in performance following total cardiac denervation.

In contrast to the difficulties encountered in performing total cardiac sympathetic denervation, ventricular denervation has been readily accomplished in a number of ways. Kaye and associates [63] have described a technique for ventricular sympathetic denervation by dissection of the peripulmonary tissues and transection of the ventrolateral cardiac nerve in dogs, and they have documented depletion of myocardial catecholamines after this procedure to a level comparable to that found after autotransplantation. These authors have also accomplished total ventricular denervation by chemical epicardiectomy [60]. The effects of ventricular epicardiectomy on myocardial contractile force have been compared with the effects noted after stellate ganglionectomy, beta adrenergic blockade, and surgical epicardiectomy and found to be similar [64]. Function studies performed by Pace and associates [90] on epicardiectomized animals indicated that stellate ganglion stimulation in these animals resulted in an elevation of both mean left atrial pressure and left ventricular diastolic pressure; this reverses the normal trend of variations in atrioventricular pressure accompanying this procedure. In addition, epicardiectomy abolishes the char-

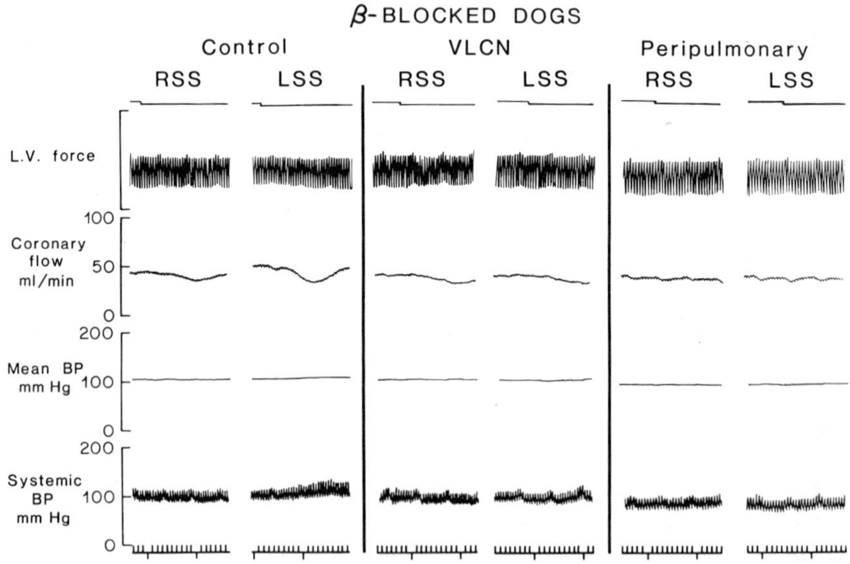

Fig. 12-8. Total coronary blood flow response to stellate stimulation after beta adrenergic blockade. RSS and LSS = right and left stellate ganglia stimulation; VLCN = after transection of ventrolateral cardiac nerve; peripulmonary = after transection of peripulmonary nerves; LV force = left ventricular force.

acteristic augmentation in ventricular function normally associated with stellate ganglion stimulation. Brachfeld and associates [13], who used a procedure similar to the technique of peripulmonary neurectomy for ventricular denervation, have indicated that this procedure results in loss of coronary artery vasoconstrictor tone and a concomitant increase in coronary flow for a given myocardial oxygen consumption. Figure 12-8 demonstrates the effect of ventricular denervation by peripulmonary neurectomy and transection of the ventrolateral cardiac nerve on coronary blood flow during sympathetic stimulation. In dogs placed on right-heart bypass, total coronary venous blood flow was recorded with an electromagnetic flowmeter. After beta blockade, stimulation of the stellate ganglia resulted in coronary vasoconstriction that was abolished by ventricular sympathectomy.

Epicardiectomy or ventricular sympathectomy has additionally been demonstrated to increase the threshold for ventricular fibrillation [97], decrease mortality after coronary occlusion [57,111,118], abolish angina [57], and increase myocardial blood flow and contribute to the development of collateral circulation [68]. Even more specific segmental sympathetic denervation has been described by Geis and Kaye [45], in studies on the distribution of sympathetic fibers in the left ventricular epicardial plexus in dogs, and by Kaye and Randall in studies on the effects of denervation of the anterior descending coronary artery [65]. Hence total cardiac sympathectomy may be performed at regional or segmental levels.

PARASYMPATHECTOMY

The effects of acute bilateral cervical vagosympathectomy on the cardiovascular system of the anesthetized dog have been demonstrated [79]. Attempts to devise a chronic animal model with parasympathetic cardiac denervation have been complicated in most instances by early mortality due to pulmonary and esophagogastric dysfunction [19,107,109,110]. From our experiences in mapping the precise projections of the autonomic nerves onto the heart and defining the paracardiac pathways of these nerves, it has become apparent that the primary sympathetic nerves can be qualitatively isolated from the parasympathetic. However, because of the marked degree of intermingling of fibers from both systems at the level of the caudal cervical ganglion, it is probably impossible to preserve all of the cardiac sympathetic innervation while performing surgical parasympathectomy.

The technique in this procedure is illustrated in Fig. 12-9. Briefly, it consists of ligation and division of the azygos vein and transection of the tissues surrounding the superior vena cava at this level. The pericardial reflection along the superior aspect of the left atrium between the left and right superior pulmonary veins is transected and the intrapericardial portion of the right pulmonary artery is cleaned of connective tissue. Figure 12-10 illustrates pre- and postdenervation intraoperative tracings from an animal subjected to this procedure; it demonstrates lack of cardiac response to parasympathetic stimulation.

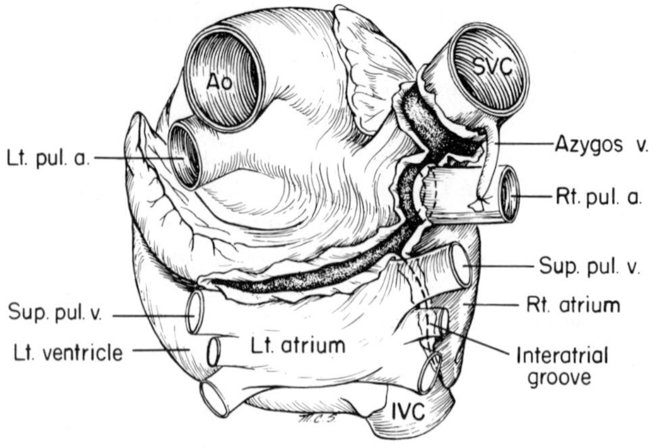

Fig. 12-9. Superior-posterior view of heart, illustrating dissections for parasympathectomy. Ao = aorta; SVC = superior vena cava; IVC = inferior vena cava. (Reproduced through the courtesy of *J. Appl. Physiol.* *38*: 183, 1975)

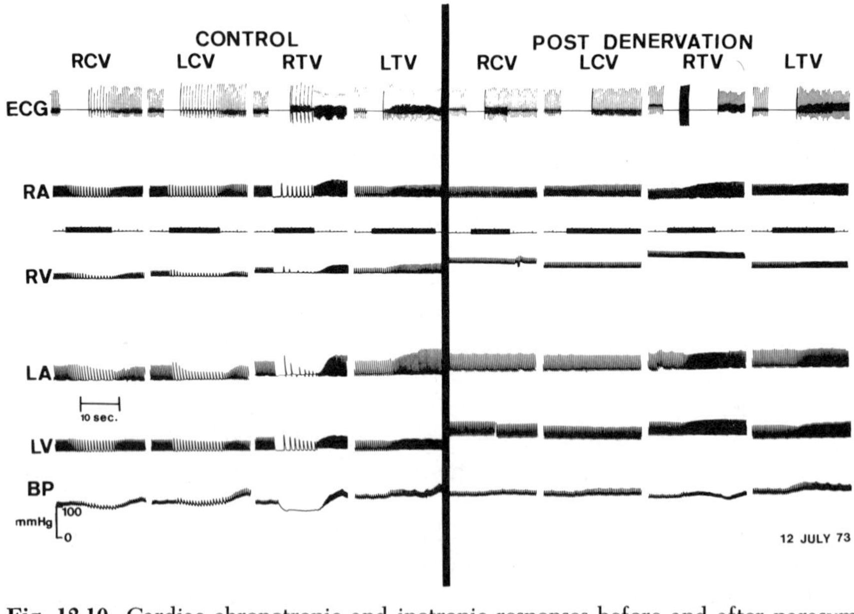

Fig. 12-10. Cardiac chronotropic and inotropic responses before and after parasympathectomy. ECG = limb lead II electrocardiogram; RA = strain-gauge force recording from right atrial appendage; RV = right ventricle; LA = left atrium; LV = left ventricle; BP = femoral blood pressure; RCV = right cervical vagus (cranial to caudal cervical ganglion); LCV = left cervical vagus; RTV = right thoracic vagus (caudal to caudal cervical ganglion); LTV = left thoracic vagus. Stimulation indicated by signal marker. (Reproduced through the courtesy of *J. Appl. Physiol.* *38*: 183, 1975)

In addition, reflex bradycardia induced by norepinephrine infusion and reflex hypotension and bradycardia induced by infusion of a veratrum alkaloid are abolished [61]. The selectivity of the operative procedure for parasympathetic fibers is illustrated in Fig. 12-11. After the procedure, stimulation of the stellate ganglia again demonstrated marked positive inotropic and chronotropic responses and thereby indicated that there is little disruption of the sympathetic innervation of the heart. Postoperative electrocardiograms in animals subjected to this procedure reveal persistent sinus tachycardia at a rate of 140–160 beats per minute.

Significant cardiac dysfunction manifested by overt heart failure has not been seen in animals subjected to this procedure. The heart failure reported after bilateral cervical vagotomy [79,107,109,110] must therefore be attributed to complications arising from extracardiac sources.

The positive inotropic and chronotropic responses of the heart to vagosympathetic stimulation after parasympathectomy can result from either denervation-independent, false reciprocal excitation [73] or to reflex sympathetic activation [99]. False reciprocal excitation is caused by sympathetic fibers incorporated with parasympathectomy fibers in the vagus nerves. Because the described parasympathectomy does not transect sympathetic fibers to the heart, it is possible that the vagosympathetic fibers are also unaffected by the surgery.

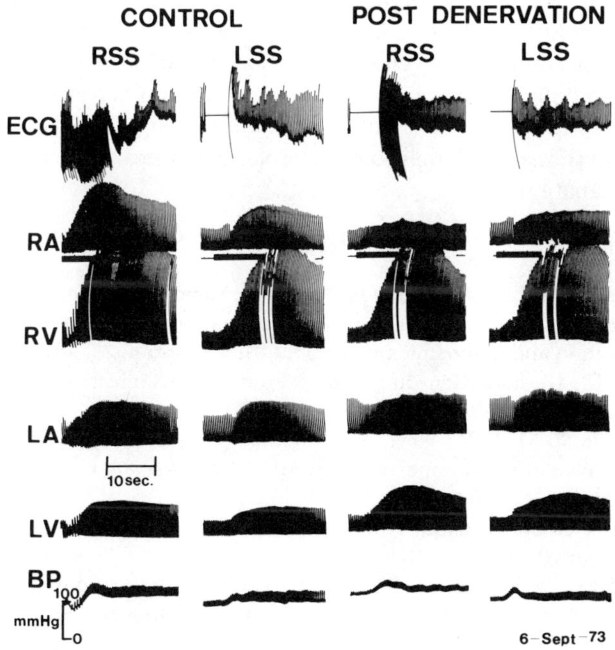

Fig. 12-11. Cardiac responses to right and left stellate ganglia stimulation before and after selective parasympathectomy. RSS = right stellate stimulation; LSS = left stellate stimulation. Other abbreviations as in Fig. 12-10. (Reproduced through the courtesy of *J. Appl. Physiol.* 38: 183, 1975)

An alternate explanation for the postparasympathectomy excitation with vagal stimulation is activation of afferent fibers in the vagus nerves which then induce reflex sympathetic stimulation of the heart [99].

Abolition of the cardiac afferent activity stimulated by left atrial injection of a veratrum alkaloid is also accomplished by this procedure. No other attempts to stimulate receptors located in the heart were made, but it is apparent that this preparation may be of great benefit in attempting to evaluate the role of cardiac afferents in the control of circulatory dynamics and water and electrolyte homeostasis.

The persistent tachycardia after parasympathectomy may result from loss of chronic vagal tone or loss of afferent nerve traffic from volume receptors or cardiac length (or both) and chemoreceptors. Other possible explanations for the tachycardia that follow vagotomy have been reviewed in detail by Cooper and associates [19]. Since in the preparation described above sympathetic cardiac fibers remain intact, postparasympathectomy tachycardia may well reflect an unopposed "normal" sympathetic activity.

Although much knowledge concerning the function of the denervated heart has been gained from studies resulting from the technical development of cardiac transplantation and refinements of techniques of total, regional, and segmental denervation of the heart, much has yet to be learned. Knowledge about the role of cardiac receptors and their efferent nerves is still incomplete. Long-term effects of segmental denervation induced iatrogenically or by disease states have not been elucidated. Interest in the resistance of the denervated heart to disturbances of rhythm after coronary occlusion has been rekindled, and the metabolic consequences of cardiac sympathectomy on coronary occlusive disease require further study. The entire field of autonomic imbalance in the genesis of dysrhythmias and the potential role of surgical intervention require detailed explanation.

REFERENCES

1. Amorim, D. S., J. A. Mello de Oliveira, J. C. Manco, L. Gallo, Jr., J. S. Meira de Oliveira, Chagus' heart disease: first demonstrable correlation between neuronal degeneration and autonomic impairment, *Acta Cardiol.* *28*: 431–440, 1973.
2. Arnulf, G., De la section du plexus préaortique. Justification et technique, *La Presse Med.* *47*: 1635–1638, 1939.
3. Barsamian, E. M., S. W. Jacob, S. C. Collins, O. E. Owen, Preliminary studies on the transplantation of supercooled hearts, *Plast. Reconstr. Surg.* *25*: 405–408, 1960.
4. Beck, W., C. N. Barnard, V. Schrire, Heart rate after cardiac transplantation, *Circulation* *40*: 437–445, 1969.
5. Beck, W., C. N. Barnard, and V. Schrire, Hemodynamic studies in two long-term survivors of heart transplantation, *J. Thorac. Cardiovasc. Surg.* *62*: 315–320, 1971.
6. Bertrand, M. E., Personal communication.
7. Bertrand, M. E., J. M. Lablanche, M. F. Rousseau, H. H. Warembourg, Jr., C. Stankowtak, G. Soots, Surgical treatment of variant angina: use of plexectomy with aortocoronary bypass, *Circulation* *61*: 877–882, 1980.

8. Bertrand, M. E., J. M. Lablanche, P. Y. Tilmant, G. Ducloux, H. Warembourg, Jr., G. Soots, Complete denervation of the heart (autotransplantation) for treatment of severe, refractory coronary spasm, *Am. J. Cardiol.* *47*: 1375–1378, 1981.
9. Bing, R. J., C. Chiba, A. Chrysohou, S. Gudbjarnason, P. L. Wolf, Metabolic, histologic and histochemical aspects of the homografted heart, *Trans. Assoc. Am. Physicians* *74*: 318–330, 1961.
10. Bing, R. J., C. Chiba, A. Chrysohou, P. L. Wolf, S. Gudbjarnason, Transplantation of the heart (editorial), *Circulation* *25*: 273–276, 1962.
11. Bishop, V. S. and L. D. Horwitz, Effects of altered autonomic control on left ventricular function in conscious dogs, *Am. J. Physiol.* *221*: 1278–1282, 1971.
12. Blinks, J. R., Positive chronotropic effect of increasing right atrial pressure in the isolated mammalian heart, *Am. J. Physiol.* *186*: 299–303, 1956.
13. Brachfield, N., R. G. Monroe, R. Gorlin, Effect of pericoronary denervation on coronary hemodynamics, *Am. J. Physiol.* *199*: 174–178, 1960.
14. Cannon, W. B., Studies on the conditions of activity in endocrine glands. V. The isolated heart as an indicator of adrenal secretion induced by pain, asphyxia, and excitement, *Am. J. Physiol.* *50*: 399–432, 1919.
15. Carrel, A. and C. C. Guthrie, The transplantation of veins and organs, *Am. Med.* *10*: 1101–1102, 1905.
16. Chiba, C., P. L. Wolf, S. Gudbjarnason, A. Chrysohou, H. Ramos, B. Pearson, R. J. Bing, Studies on the transplanted heart: its metabolism and histology, *J. Exp. Med.* *115*: 853–866, 1962.
17. Clark, D. A., R. A. Quint, R. L. Mitchell, W. W. Angell, Coronary artery spasm: medical management, surgical denervation, and autotransplantation, *J. Thorac. Cardiovasc. Surg.* *73*: 332–339, 1977.
18. Connaughton, P. J. and F. J. Lewis, Use of glycerol and chloroform in heart preservation by freezing, *Surg. Forum* *12*: 177–179, 1961.
19. Cooper, T., W. M. Daggett, G. G. Nugent, C. R. Hanlon, Selective cardiac vagotomy: surgical preparation and techniques of verification, *J. Thorac. Cardiovasc. Surg.* *52*: 761–768, 1966.
20. Cooper, T., J. W. Gilbert, Jr., R. D. Bloodwell, J. R. Crout, Chronic extrinsic cardiac denervation by regional neural ablation: description of the operation, verification of the denervation and its effects on myocardial catecholamines, *Circ. Res.* *9*: 275–281, 1961.
21. Cooper, T., E. F. Hirsch, V. L. Willman, C. R. Hanlon, Transplantation of the heart: alterations in morphology of heart, *Arch. Surg. (Chicago)* *89*: 915–920, 1964.
22. Cooper, T., M. Jellinek, V. L. Willman, C. R. Hanlon, Metabolism of the transplanted heart, *J. Am. Med. Assoc.* *191*: 304–305, 1965.
23. Cooper, T., V. L. Willman, C. R. Hanlon, Drug responses of the transplanted heart, *Dis. Chest* *45*: 284–287, 1964.
24. Cooper, T., V. L. Willman, M. Jellinek, C. R. Hanlon, Heart autotransplantation: effect on myocardial catecholamines and histamine, *Science* *138*: 40–41, 1962.
25. Corcondilas, A., D. E. Donald, J. R. Shepherd, Assessment by two independent methods of the role of cardiac output in the pressor response to carotid occlusion, *J. Physiol. (Lond.)* *170*: 250–262, 1964.
26. Cutler, E. C. and J. Fine, Sympathectomy in angina pectoris, *J. Am. Med. Assoc.* *86*: 1972–1979, 1926.
27. Demikhov, V. P., *Experimental Transplantation of Vital Organs*, translated by B. Haigh. New York: Consultants Bureau, 1962.

28. Dempsey, P. J. and T. Cooper, Supersensitivity of the chronically denervated feline heart, *Am. J. Physiol. 215*: 1245–1249, 1968.
29. DePasquale, N. P., G. E. Burch, E. Pena, K. Reemtsma, Electrocardiographic studies in homologous canine heart transplantations, *Circ. Res. 16*: 197–202, 1965.
30. Donald, D. E., Myocardial performance after excision of the extrinsic cardiac nerves in the dog, *Circ. Res. 34*: 417–424, 1974.
31. Donald, D. E., D. A. Ferguson, S. E. Milburn, Effect of beta-adrenergic receptor blockade on racing performance of greyhounds with normal and denervated hearts, *Circ. Res. 22*: 127–134, 1968.
32. Donald, D. E., S. E. Milburn, J. T. Shepherd, Effect of cardiac denervation on the maximal capacity for exercise in the racing greyhound, *J. Appl. Physiol. 19*: 849–852, 1964.
33. Donald, D. E. and S. L. Samueloff, Exercise tachycardia not due to blood-borne agents in canine cardiac denervation, *Am. J. Physiol. 211*: 703–711, 1966.
34. Donald, D. E. and J. T. Shepherd, Response to exercise in dogs with cardiac denervation, *Am. J. Physiol. 205*: 393–400, 1963.
35. Donald, D. E. and J. T. Shepherd, Initial cardiovascular adjustment to exercise in dogs with chronic cardiac denervation, *Am. J. Physiol. 207*: 1325–1329, 1964.
36. Donald, D. E. and J. T. Shepherd, Supersensitivity to *l*-norepinephrine of the denervated sinoatrial node, *Am. J. Physiol. 208*: 255–259, 1965.
37. Dong, E., Jr., E. J. Hurley, R. R. Lower, N. E. Shumway, Performance of the heart two years after autotransplantation, *Surgery 56*: 270–273, 1964.
38. Dong, E., Jr., R. R. Lower, E. J. Hurley, N. E. Shumway, Transplantation of the heart, *Dis. Chest 48*: 455–457, 1965.
39. Downie, H. G., Homotransplantation of the dog heart, *Arch. Surg. (Chicago) 66*: 624–636, 1953.
40. Ebert, P. A., The effects of norepinephrine infusion on the denervated heart, *J. Cardiovasc. Surg. 9*: 414–419, 1968.
41. Ebert, P. A. and D. C. Sabiston, Jr., Pharmacologic quantitation of cardiac sympathetic reinnervation, *Surgery 68*: 123–127, 1970.
42. Essex, H. E., J. F. Herrick, E. J. Baldes, F. C. Mann, Effects of exercise on the coronary blood flow, heart rate and blood pressure of traind dogs with denervated and partially denervated hearts, *Am. J. Physiol. 138*: 687–697, 1943.
43. Franck, F., Signification physiologique de la résection du sympathique dans la maladie de Basedow, l'épilepsie, l'idiotie et le glaucome, *Bull. Acad. Med. 41*: 565–594, 1899.
44. Gasser, H. S. and W. J. Meek, A study of the mechanisms by which muscular exercise produces acceleration of the heart, *Am. J. Physiol. 34*: 48–71, 1914.
45. Geis, W. P. and M. P. Kaye, Distribution of sympathetic fibers in the left ventricular epicardial plexus of the dog, *Circ. Res. 23*: 165–170, 1968.
46. Geis, W. P., C. J. Tatooles, M. P. Kaye, W. C. Randall, Complete cardiac denervation without transplantation: a simple and reliable technique, *J. Appl. Physiol. 30*: 289–293, 1971.
47. Gilmore, J. P. and W. M. Daggett, Response of the chronic cardiac denervated dog to acute volume expansion, *Am. J. Physiol. 210*: 509–512, 1966.
48. Glick, G., W. H. Plauth, Jr., E. Braunwald, Circulatory response to hypoxia in unanesthetized dogs with and without cardiac denervation, *Am. J. Physiol. 207*: 753–758, 1964.
49. Glick, G., W. H. Plauth, Jr., E. Braunwald, Role of the autonomic nervous system in the circulatory response to acutely induced anemia in unanesthetized dogs, *J. Clin. Invest. 43*: 2112–2124, 1964.

50. Goodall, M. and N. Kirshner, Effect of cervico-thoracic ganglionectomy on the adrenaline and noradrenalin content of the mammalian heart, *J. Clin. Invest.* *35*: 649–656, 1956.
51. Graham, A. F., D. C. Harrison, J. S. Schroeder, Studies on circulatory response to hypoxia in the denervated transplanted human heart, *Am. J. Med.* *56*: 477–481, 1974.
52. Greenfield, L. J. and P. A. Ebert, Cardiac denervation effect in hypoxia and hypercapnia, *Arch. Surg. (Chicago)* *87*: 717–721, 1963.
53. Gregg, D. E., E. M. Khouri, D. E. Donald, H. S. Lowensohn, S. Pasyk, Coronary circulation in the conscious dog with cardiac neural ablation, *Circ. Res.* *31*: 129–144, 1972.
54. Grondin, C. M. and R. Limet, Sympathetic denervation in association with coronary artery grafting in patients with Prinzmetal's angina, *Ann. Thorac. Surg.* *23*: 111–117, 1977.
55. Guyton, R. A., J. A. Bianco, G. W. Ostheimer, E. A. Shanahan, W. M. Daggett, Adrenergic control of ventricular performance in normal and cardiac-denervated dogs, *Am. J. Physiol.* *223*: 1021–1028, 1972.
56. Harken, A. H., L. N. Horowitz, M. E. Josephson, The surgical treatment of ventricular tachycardia, *Ann. Thorac. Surg.* *30*: 499–508, 1980.
57. Harken, D. E., H. Black, J. F. Dickson, III, H. E. Wilson, III, De-epicardialization: a simple, effective surgical treatment for angina pectoris, *Circulation* *12*: 955–962, 1955.
58. Hunt, R., Direct reflex acceleration of the mammalian heart with some observations on the relations of the inhibitory and accelerator nerves. *Am. J. Physiol.* *2*: 395–470, 1899.
59. Jonsson, G. and C. Sachs, Degenerative and nondegenerative effects of 6-hydroxydopamine on adrenergic nerves, *J. Pharmacol. Exp. Ther.* *180*: 625–635, 1972.
60. Kaye, M. P., G. G. Brynjolfsson, W. P. Geis, Chemical epicardiectomy: a method of myocardial denervation, *Cardiologia* *53*: 139–149, 1968.
61. Kaye, M. P., G. R. Hageman, W. C. Randall, Selective parasympathectomy of the heart, *J. Appl. Physiol.* *38*: 183–186, 1975.
62. Kaye, M. P., G. R. Hageman, W. C. Randall, J. Isobe, One stage cardiac denervation without transplantation, *J. Surg. Res.* *15*: 357–362, 1973.
63. Kaye, M. P., D. V. Priola, J. Coyle, Depletion of ventricular catecholamine levels following peripulmonary neurectomy, *Proc. Soc. Exp. Biol. Med.* *135*: 844–848, 1970.
64. Kaye, M. P. and W. C. Randall, Mechanism of decreased myocardial contractile force after epicardiectomy, *Cardiovasc. Res.* *4*: 154–159, 1970.
65. Kaye, M. P. and W. C. Randall, Coronary artery surgery: could it be better? *Curr. Med. Dialog.* *41*: 531–532, 1974.
66. Kaye, M. P., D. J. Wells, G. M. Tyce, Nerve growth factor enhanced reinnervation of surgically denervated canine heart, *Am. J. Physiol.* *236*: H624–H628, 1979.
67. Kent, K. M. and T. Cooper, The denervated heart: a model for studying autonomic control of the heart, *N. Engl. J. Med.* *291*: 1017–1021, 1974.
68. King, R. D., S. H. Steiner, I. L. Heimburger, Effect of epicardiectomy on myocardial blood flow, *J. Throac. Cardiovasc. Surg.* *51*: 660–666, 1966.
69. Kondo, Y., J. L. Matheny, J. D. Hardy, Autonomic reinnervation of cardiac transplants: further observations in dogs and rhesus monkeys, *Ann. Surg.* *176*: 42–48, 1972.

70. Kontos, H. A., M. D. Thames, R. R. Lower, Responses to electrical and reflex autonomic stimulation in dogs with cardiac transplantation before and after reinnervation, *J. Thorac. Cardiovasc. Surg. 59*: 382–392, 1970.
71. Kontos, H. A., T. Zubair-ul-Hassan, M. D. Thames, R. R. Lower, Circulatory responses to hemorrhage in dogs with cardiac autotransplantation, *Am. J. Physiol. 220*: 621–623, 1971.
72. Leachman, R. D., D. V. P. Cokkinos, R. Cabrera, L. L. Leatherman, D. G. Rochelle, Response of the transplanted, denervated human heart to cardiovascular drugs, *Am. J. Cardiol. 27*: 272–276, 1971.
73. Levy, M. N., Sympathetic—parasympathetic interactions in the heart, *Circ. Res. 29*: 437–445, 1971.
74. Lloyd-Mostyn, R., P. J. Watkins, S. Oram, Autonomic neuropathy and the heart in diabetes (abstr.), *Br. Heart J. 36*: 397, 1974.
75. Lower, R. R., Cardiac transplantation without complete cardiac denervation: the role of afferent receptors, *Am. Heart J. 71*: 841–842, 1966.
76. Lower, R. R., H. A. Kontos, J. C. Kosek, D. H. Sewell, W. H. Graham, Experiences in heart transplantation: technique, physiology and rejection, *Am. J. Cardiol. 22*: 766–771, 1968.
77. Lower, R. R. and N. E. Shumway, Studies on orthotopic homotransplantation of the canine heart, *Surg. Forum 11*: 18–19, 1960.
78. Lower, R. R., R. C. Stofer, N. E. Shumway, Homovital transplantation to the heart, *J. Thorac. Cardiovasc. Surg. 41*: 196–204, 1961.
79. MacCanon, D. M. and S. M. Horvath, Effect of bilateral cervical vagotomy in the dog, *Am. J. Physiol. 189*: 569–572, 1957.
80. Mann, F. C., J. T. Priestley, J. Markowitz, W. M. Yater, Transplantation of the intact mammalian heart, *Arch. Surg. (Chicago) 26*: 219–224, 1933.
81. Marcus, E., S. N. T. Wong, A. A. Luisada, Homologous heart grafts. I. Technique of interim parabiotic perfusion. II. Transplantation of the heart in dogs, *Arch. Surg. (Chicago) 66*: 179–191, 1953.
82. Mayo, C. H., Discussion, *Arch. Surg. (Chicago) 10*: 541, 1925.
83. Medici, D. Personal communication.
84. Moss, A. J. and J. McDonald, Unilateral cervicothoracic sympathetic ganglionectomy for the treatment of long QT interval syndrome, *N. Engl. J. Med. 285*: 903–904, 1971.
85. Mulcahy, J. J., R. L. Malvin, W. P. Geis, The effects of cardiac denervation on body fluids, *Proc. Soc. Exp. Biol. Med. 143*: 265–269, 1973.
86. Napolitano, L., T. Cooper, V. L. Willman, C. R. Hanlon, Fine structures of the heart after transplantation: with special reference to the neural elements *Circulation 29, Suppl. 1*: 81–85, 1964.
87. Norvell, J. E. and R. R. Lower, Degeneration and regeneration of the nerves of the heart after transplantation, *Transplantation 15*: 337–344, 1973.
88. Orlick, A. E., D. R. Ricci, E. L. Alderman, E. B. Stinson, D. C. Harrison, Effects of alpha adrenergic blockade upon coronary hemodynamics, *J. Clin. Invest. 62*: 459–467, 1978.
89. Paasonen, M. K. and O. Krayer, The release of norepinephrine from the mammalian heart by reserpine, *J. Pharmacol. Exp. Ther. 123*: 153–160, 1958.
90. Pace, J. B., W. P. Geis, M. P. Kaye, D. V. Priola, Influence of ventricular epicardiectomy on cardiac responses to stellate ganglion stimulation, *J. Thorac. Cardiovasc. Surg. 58*: 39–47, 1969.

91. Palmer, G. C., H. A. Spurgeon, D. V. Priola, Involvement of adenylate cyclase in mechanisms of denervation supersensitivity following surgical denervation of the dog heart, *J. Cyclic Nucleotide Res. 1*: 89–95, 1975.
92. Palumbo, L. T. and D. J. Lulu, Transthoracic upper dorsal sympathectomy, *Surgery 53*: 563–566, 1963.
93. Peiss, C. N., T. Cooper, V. L. Willman, W. C. Randall, Circulatory responses to electrical and reflex activation of the nervous system after cardiac denervation, *Circ. Res. 19*: 153–166, 1966.
94. Pennock, J. L., P. E. Oyer, B. A. Reitz, S. W. Jamieson, C. P. Bieber, J. Wallwork, E. B. Stinson, N. E. Shumway, Cardiac transplantation in perspective for the future. Survival, complications, rehabilitation, and cost, *J. Thorac. Cardiovasc. Surg. 83*: 168–177, 1982.
95. Potter, L. T., T. Cooper, V. L. Willman, D. E. Wolfe, Synthesis, binding, release and metabolism of norepinephrine in normal and transplanted dog hearts, *Circ. Res. 16*: 468–481, 1965.
96. Priola, D. V., Individual chamber sensitivity to norepinephrine after unilateral cardiac denervation, *Am. J. Physiol. 216*: 604–614, 1969.
97. Ragheb, S and A. Vineberg, The effect of epicardectomy on ventricular fibrillation threshold, *Surgery 55*: 293–298, 1964.
98. Randall, D. C., M. P. Kaye, W. C. Randall, J. V. Brady, K. H. Martin, Response of primate heart to emotional stress before and after cardiac denervation, *Am. J. Physiol. 230*: 988–995, 1976.
99. Randall, W. C. and J. A. Armour, Complex cardiovascular responses to vagosympathetic stimulation, *Proc. Soc. Exp. Biol. Med. 145*: 493–499, 1974.
100. Reemtsma, K., J. P. Delgado, O. Creech, Jr., Transplantation of the homologous canine heart: serial studies of myocardial blood flow, oxygen comsumption, and carbohydrate metabolism, *Surgery 47*: 292–300, 1960.
101. Sayegh, S. F. and O. Creech, Jr., Transplantation of the homologous canine heart, *J. Thorac. Surg. 34*: 692–703, 1957.
102. Schroeder, J. S., Hemodynamic performance of the human transplanted heart, *Transplantation Proc. 11*: 304–308, 1979.
103. Schwartz, P., Experimental reproduction of the long Q-T syndrome (abstr.), *Am. J. Cardiol. 41*: 374, 1978.
104. Schwartz, P., Personal communication.
105. Schwartz, P. and Malliani, A., Electrical alternation of the T-wave: clinical and experimental evidence of its relationship with the sympathetic nervous system and with the long Q-T syndrome, *Am. Heart J. 89*: 45–50, 1975.
106. Seki, S. and G. K. Danielson, Characteristics of cardiac reinnervation in growing calves, *J. Thorac. Cardiovasc. Surg. 62*: 602–607, 1971.
107. Sharpey-Schafer, E., Experiments on the cervical vagus and sympathetic, *Q. J. Exp. Physiol. 12*: 231–301, 1920.
108. Shaver, J. A., D. F. Leon, S. Gray, III, J. J. Leonard, H. T. Bahnson, Hemodynamic observations after cardiac transplantation, *N. Engl. J. Med. 281*: 822–827, 1969.
109. Shepard, R. S. and A. J. Whitty, Bilateral cervical vagotomy: a long-term study on the unanesthetized dog, *Am. J. Physiol. 206*: 265–269, 1964.
110. Sloan, R. D., W. R. Webb, A. L. Meena S. S. Lee, The cause of fatalities in bilateral vagotomies, *Surg. Forum 9*: 427–429, 1959.
111. Stanton, E. J., P. Schildt, C. S. Beck, The effect of abrasion of the surface of the heart upon intercoronary communications, *Am. Heart J. 22*: 529–538, 1941.

112. Steiner, G. and E. Schönbaum, Immunosympathectomy. New York, Elsevier, 1972.

113. Stinson, E. B., R. B. Griepp, D. A. Clark, E. Dong, N. E. Shumway, Cardiac transplantation in man. VIII. Survival and function, *J. Thorac. Cardiovasc. Surg. 60*: 303–319, 1970.

114. Stinson, E. B., R. B. Griepp, J. S. Schroeder, E. Dong, Jr., N. E. Shumway, Hemodynamic observations one and two years after cardiac transplantation in man, *Circulation 45*: 1183–1194, 1972.

115. Talano, J. V., Personal communication.

116. Thames, M. D., Zubair-ul-Hassan, N. C. Brackett, Jr., R. R. Lower, H. A. Kontos, Plasma renin responses to hemorrhage after cardiac autotransplantation, *Am. J. Physiol. 221*: 1115–1119, 1971.

117. Tsakiris, A. G., D. E. Donald, W. J. Rutishauser, N. Banchero, E. H. Wood, Cardiovascular responses to hypertension and hypotension in dogs with denervated hearts, *J. Appl. Physiol. 27*: 817–821, 1969.

118. Vineberg, A. M., A. Becerra, R. S. Chari, The influence of the Vineberg sponge operation upon the hydrostatics of the myocardial circulation in health and disease: evidence of luminal ventricular circulation in the beating heart, *Can. Med. Assoc. J. 85*: 1075–1090, 1961.

119. Wesolowski, S. A. and J. F. Fennessey, Pattern of failure of the homografted canine heart, *Circulation 8*: 750–755, 1953.

120. White, J. C., The neurosurgical treatment of angina pectoris, *J. Chron. Dis. 4*: 388–401, 1956.

121. Willman, V. L., T. Cooper, L. G. Cian, C. R. Hanlon, Autotransplantation of the canine heart, *Surg. Gynecol. Obstet. 115*: 299–302, 1962.

122. Willman, V. L., T. Cooper, L. G. Cian, C. R. Hanlon, Neural responses following autotransplantation of the canine heart, *Circulation 27*: 713–716, 1963.

123. Willman, V. L., T. Cooper, C. R. Hanlon, Return of neural responses after autotransplantation of the heart, *Am. J. Physiol. 207: 187–189, 1964.*

124. Willman, V. L., T. Cooper, G. C. Kaiser, C. R. Hanlon, Cardiovascular response after cardiac autotransplant in primate, *Arch. Surg. (Chicago) 91*: 805–806, 1965.

125. Willman, V. L., J. P. Marjavy, R. Pennell, C. R. Hanlon, Response of the autotransplanted heart to blood volume expansion, *Ann. Surg. 166*: 513–517, 1967.

13

Central Nervous System Regulation of the Heart: An Overview

ROBERT D. WURSTER

This chapter offers general concepts of the organization of central nervous system regions involved in cardiovascular function and should serve as an introduction to the following chapters. Views from the past and present are incorporated, as well as directions which may be opening for future research. The chapter is aimed at non-neuroscientists who may be perplexed by many recent and exciting developments in this field.

CENTERS TO CIRCUITS

Our view of the anatomical basis for central neural control of cardiovascular function has changed markedly over the past twenty years. Formerly, it was thought that integrative control of cardiovascular function was localized in "centers" (Fig. 13-1), such as the medullary vasomotor center [1]. In the 1950's and 1960's, this outlook was broadened to encompass "areas" involved in integration but not necessarily exclusive loci for such integration, for instance, the dual role of the medulla and hypothalamus in cardiovascular control [3].

As the involvement of more central nervous system structures in cardiovascular control was recognized, the concept of "circuits" evolved (Fig. 13-2). Numerous multilevel circuits contained interconnections between spinal, medullary, hypothalamic, limbic and other forebrain structures [4]. It was recognized that lesions restricted to one component of the circuit may alter, but not totally impair function. As in television circuits, removal of a single component may not greatly alter overall performance. Yet, this single component is not "vestigial" or necessarily "redundant." Its removal may produce a deficit only under certain conditions. A specific deficit might occur only when certain frequencies are selected. In the case of the neural control of the cardiovascular

Research supported by NIH Grants HL 27612 and HL 08682. The author wishes to express thanks to C. A. Connelly for reviewing the text and for the use of her figures.

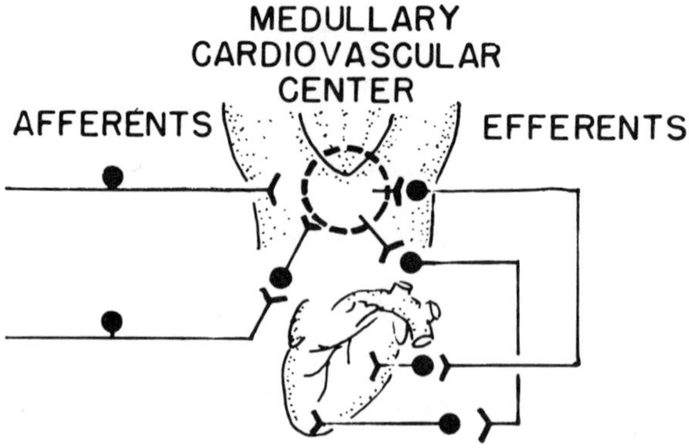

Fig. 13-1. Model of medullary cardiovascular center. Various afferent inputs (left side) are integrated in a special anatomical location or "center" to determine efferent autonomic activity (right side) to the heart.

system, deficits might occur only under certain physiological or pathological conditions, e.g. exercise, emotional stress, etc. It is suggested that no portion of the overall neural circuit can really be considered a "center."

Modern neuroanatomical tracing techniques paved the way for an even more complicated view of these circuits [2]. As each investigator discovers a new, more detailed picture of a small subcomponent, such as the projections to and from the nucleus of the solitary tract, a new layer of complexity evolves. As the

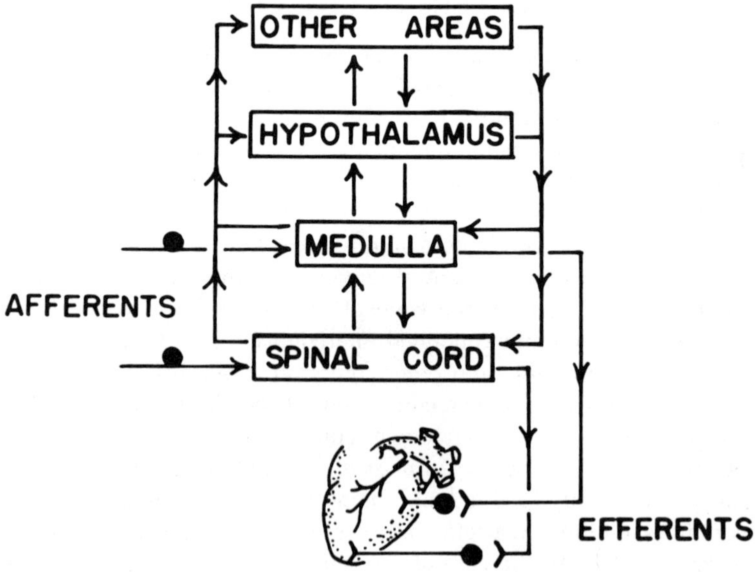

Fig. 13-2. Model of central neural cardiovascular circuits. Efferent autonomic activity to the heart is determined by complex circuits which are interconnected at numerous levels of the central nervous system.

complexity develops, simultaneous, detailed understanding of the functions of the entire control circuit may become more difficult to comprehend. Similarly, the behavior of each component of a complicated electronic circuit may in itself be easy to understand; yet, comprehensive detailed understanding of the entire circuit's function may be difficult. Thus, understanding of an electronic circuit (e.g. the television circuit) is aided by conceptual subdivision of the circuit, e.g. the tuner, high-voltage section, etc. Similarly, understanding of neural control circuits is facilitated by subdividing the circuit into its individual subsections, e.g. blood pressure regulation. Caution must be used in this analytic approach because specific neural circuits may subserve several different functional systems.

Furthermore, the circuits that are revealed may derive from experiments that alter the nature of the circuit, e.g. the anesthetized model. These circuits need to be investigated in the unanesthetized animal model under different behavioral conditions.

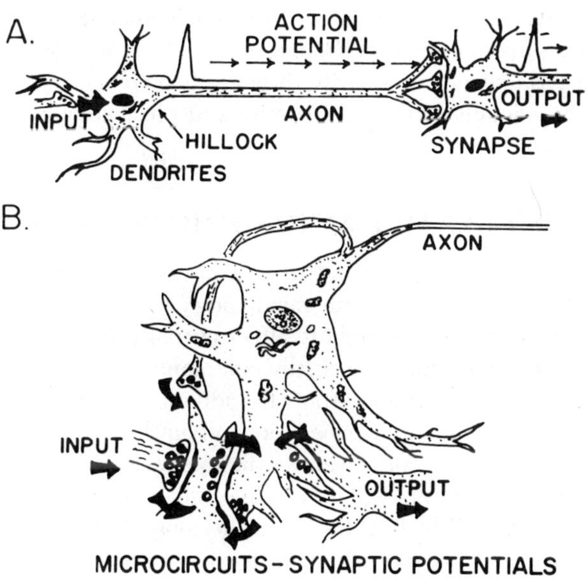

Fig. 13-3. Mechanisms of central nervous system information transmission and integration. (A) Conventional axodendritic or axosomatic synapses (input) alter the excitability of the axon hillock region. When this region reaches threshold a regenerative action potential occurs and spreads along the axon. At the axonal terminal (synapse), a transmitter is released which alters the excitability of the next nerve soma (output). Regenerative action potential transmission provides a faithful information transfer over long distances in an all-or-none or digital form. (B) Microcircuit transmission and integration. Possible complex array of axodendritic and dendrodendritic synapses. By means of feedforward and feedback excitatory and inhibitory synapses, information is integrated and transmitted via several dendrites by microcircuits in a complex, graduated manner. This information is eventually transmitted to a cell body for long-distance transmission (output).

ACTION POTENTIALS AND MICROCIRCUITS

The basic approach has been to record the action potential activity of units involved in cardiovascular control. This has proven useful for some functional neuroanatomical understanding. It assumes that functions of neurons can be understood by the all-or-none properties of the axon hillock region—the physiological site of initiation of action potentials in central nervous system neurons. As with other neuronal systems, the action potential is principally responsible for nondistorted information transmission over long distances (greater than perhaps a millimeter) (Fig. 13-3A) [6]. An important site of integration most likely occurs in the dendrites. Here, transmission of axodendritic and dendrodendritic information occurs. The dendrites are also a likely site for integration via the proposed complex microcircuits (Fig. 13-3B). Unlike the digital coding nature of action potentials, microcircuits may utilize the more powerful analog information processing. This dendritic processing may involve dendrites from a number of neurons with excitatory and inhibitory feedforward and feedback circuit elements. Local membrane potential changes may regulate vesicular and hence, transmitter release, in addition to action potentials. It is possible that certain dendrites may be involved in processing information whose "output" is via other neurons and not necessarily through its own cell body and axon. At the present time, details about the anatomy and physiology of such microcircuitry are not known.

DIFFERENTIAL AUTONOMIC RESPONSES

Early views of autonomic control of the cardiovascular system were, for the most part, quite stereotyped for both vagal and sympathetic outflow. The sympathetic nervous system was thought to affect virtually all cardiovascular effectors in a similar manner under principally emergency circumstances. However, we now recognize that separate outputs to individual cardiovascular effectors, e.g. heart and a particular vascular bed, depend on the particular physiological state (Fig. 13-4). During some states, these effectors may have opposite responses (states A and C in Fig. 13-4) while under other states their outputs would be similar (state B in Fig. 13-4). Furthermore, the role of tonic sympathetic activity in nonemergency situations is widely accepted.

In a similar manner, the iron-clad notion of reciprocal CNS control of sympathetic and parasympathetic outflow to the cardiovascular system has been greatly modified (Fig. 13-5). Although under certain circumstances their activity may be in opposite directions to established "balanced" regulation (states A and B in Fig. 13-5), under other circumstances their separate activities may increase or decrease simultaneously (state C in Fig. 13-5).

PARTY AND PRIVATE LINES

Differential control implies that central nervous system connections may be specific to one specific group of sympathetic preganglionic cell bodies in the spinal

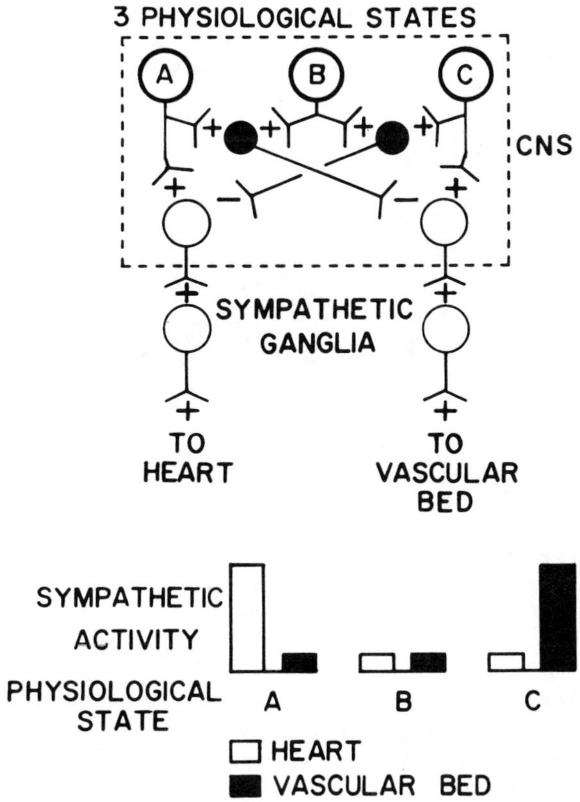

Fig. 13-4. Differential sympathetic control. The central nervous system (schematically represented by structures within the dashed box) may reciprocally or similarly regulate sympathetic outflow to different effector organs, e.g. heart and a particular vascular bed. Portions of the CNS involved in three hypothetical responses or physiological states are represented by A, B, and C. Solid cell bodies indicate inhibitory interneurons; open cell bodies indicate excitatory neurons. Sympathetic activity relative to the effectors during the three physiological states is indicated below by bar graphs. In physiological states A and C reciprocal relationships exist in sympathetic activity, while in B both outputs are similarly inhibited.

cord regulating a particular effector organ, e.g. kidney, heart, etc. Thus, these pathways may be analogous to "private lines" which are used for specific functional responses of the cardiovascular system (Fig. 13-6, states A and D). For example, it is potentially possible that areas of the hypothalamus may be involved in regulation of release of antidiuretic hormone and send axons to the spinal cord which may control sympathetic activity to the kidney and control the activation of the renin—angiotensin system. These descending pathways may constitute "private lines" for these responses. Similar private lines may exist for the heart and other portions of the cardiovascular system. On the other hand, more than one control circuit may utilize the same pathway for regula-

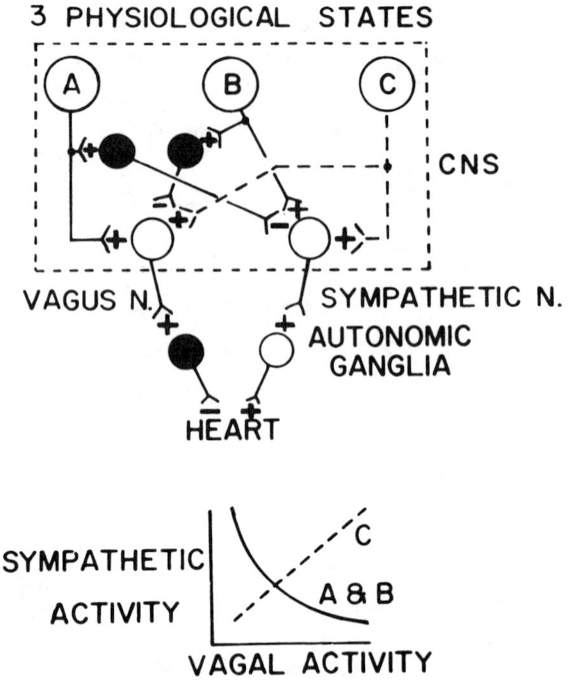

Fig. 13-5. Relationship between sympathetic and vagal activity. Depending on the physiological state (A,B, or C), the central nervous system (schematically represented by the structures within the dashed box) may produce reciprocal and at other times similar changes in sympathetic and vagal activity. Portions of the CNS involved in three different responses or physiological states are indicated by A,B, and C. Inhibitory neurons are indicated by solid cell bodies; open cell bodies indicate excitatory neurons. The relative sympathetic and vagal activity during these three physiological states are indicated below. In physiological states A and B a reciprocal relationship exists, while similar changes in activity occur in C.

tion of a number of autonomic effector organs. These other pathways constitute "party lines" (Fig. 13-6, states B and C).

The use of the radiolabeled 2-deoxyglucose technique and immunohistological techniques on cardiovascular circuits may reveal some of these "private" or "party" lines. 2-deoxyglucose can be administered during a given cardiovascular reflex or during a given behavioral state [5]. The 2-deoxyglucose is taken up by metabolizing neurons relative to their metabolic rate, i.e. the higher the nerve activity, the higher the metabolic uptake. Because this substance is not readily metabolized, it persists intracellularly and can be detected using autoradiographic histological techniques. This allows the tracing of pathways involved in a particular neural response.

The immunohistological techniques allow one to trace neural circuits involving certain transmitters [7]. Specific antibodies are formed either against the transmitter or its synthesizing enzymes. These antibodies are labeled and thus, the pathways of the transmitters can be determined.

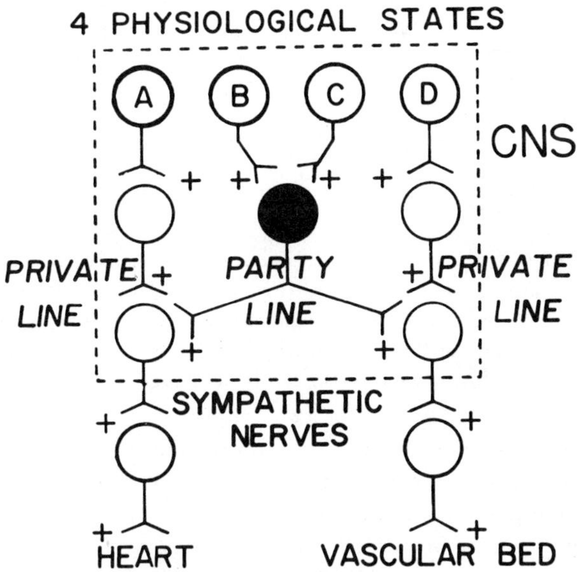

Fig. 13-6. Control of sympathetic output by "private" and "party" lines. The central nervous system (schematically represented as the structures inside the dashed box) has some pathways organized to mediate activity to only one type of sympathetic output (e.g. the heart) and constitutes "private" lines. Other CNS pathways mediate responses to several different types of sympathetic output and constitute "party" lines. Depending on the physiological states (A,B,C, or D), "party" or "private" lines may be activated: states A and D activate "private" lines while states B and C involve "party" lines.

NEURAL RHYTHMS

Peripheral autonomic nerve fibers characteristically have rhythmic activity which may be secondary to rhythmic baroreceptor inputs, relate to the respiratory cycle, or originate elsewhere in the central nervous system (see chapters 15 and 16). What is the importance of such rhythms? If a rhythm is characteristic of certain control systems, this might allow the investigator to locate the cardiovascular control circuits without necessarily knowing the actual anatomical connectivity of the recorded neurons. However, in cardiovascular central nervous system circuits, such rhythms might only be presented in limited regions, e.g. near the bulbospinal outflow areas. It is also possible that noncardiovascular neural control circuits have similar rhythms, which make circuit analysis based on rhythms futile.

The central nervous system may employ circuits which principally process information during the ON phase or OFF phase of the rhythmic changes (Fig. 13-7). Thus, the fundamental frequency of the system would remain unaltered but more or less activity would occur in either the ON or OFF phase, i.e. the system is pulsed at a given frequency and the information is sampled, integrated, and/or delivered during those pulses.

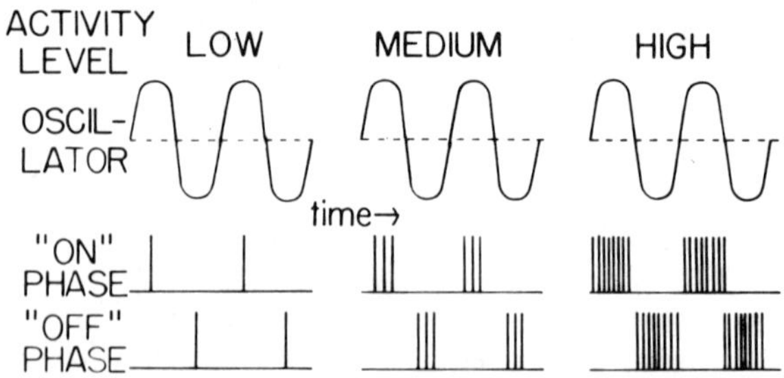

Fig. 13-7. ON phase and OFF phase processing. The fundamental rhythm or oscillator maintains the same frequency while neuronal circuit processes information during the ON -phase or OFF -phase of the oscillator rhythm. Higher levels of activity are indicated by more activity during each phase, not by a change in the oscillator rhythm.

Synchronized, rhythmic systems also improve the safety factor for synaptic transmission. Synchronized activity from different nerves will have a greater probability of temporal summation than would unsynchronized activity. For example, in Fig. 13-8, two axons terminate on one nerve cell and produce excitatory postsynaptic potentials (EPSPs). If the activity in the two axons is synchronized to the same oscillator, the EPSPs may have a high probability of summating and reaching threshold, i.e. producing an action potential. As indicated in the figure, absolute synchronization of the two axons to every oscillation is

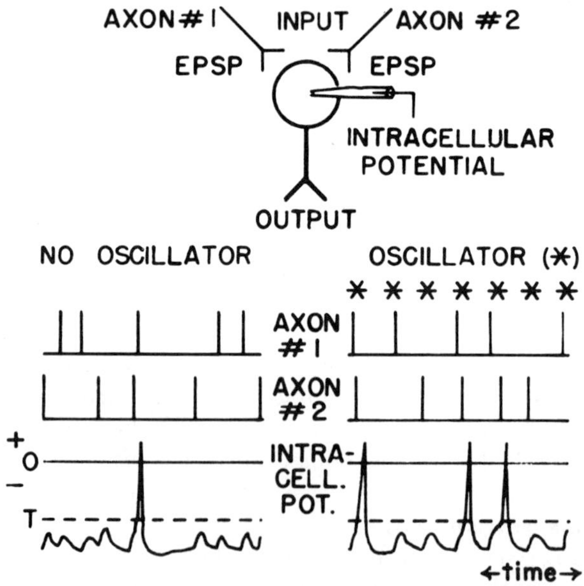

Fig. 13-8. The effects of temporal summation on oscillating (right) and nonoscillating (left) activity of two axon terminals on the output of a third neuron. Below, schematic activity pattern of the two axons and the consequence of their excitatory postsynaptic potentials (EPSPs) on the intracellular potential of the third neuron. Note the higher probability of action potentials with oscillating than with nonoscillating activity.

not necessary. On the other hand, if the two axons fire asynchronously (no oscillator in Fig. 13-8) at the same mean frequency as above, the probability for temporal summation and information transfer by the third nerve would be quite low. It is even possible that one nerve fiber could carry information related to two different systems by having some of its activity synchronized with two different oscillators. Therefore, synchronization may improve transmission of information in central nervous system circuits controlling autonomic outflow to the cardiovascular system, as well as in the autonomic ganglia.

Do cardiovascular effectors, such as the heart and blood vessels demonstrate rhythms similar to autonomic nerves? In the case of parasympathetic vagal effects, the heart can respond very rapidly to changes in vagal activity. Thus, heart rate may change rapidly under vagal regulation, i.e. within a small fraction of a single cardiac cycle. On the other hand, sympathetic responses generally have a much longer delay between alteration in sympathetic activity and the cardiovascular response. Thus, the effects of rapid, rhythmic changes of sympathetic activity are damped out or integrated, while slower rhythmic changes (Traub-Hering and Mayer waves) may still be observed.

The rhythmic oscillations of sympathetic activity with the respiratory cycle are excellent examples of rhythmic activity. (Fig. 13-9). Simultaneous recordings of integrated phrenic nerve activity and the inferior cardiac nerve activity of the cat demonstrate that sympathetic nerve activity often increases before inspiration, reaching its maximum in mid to late inspiration. This activity decreases before phrenic nerve activity begins to diminish at the onset of expiration. It reaches its lowest level early in the expiratory phase and then begins to increase by mid-expiration. If sympathetic activity is increased by baroreceptor hypotension (bilateral carotid artery occlusion in a vagotomized, chloralose-anesthetized cat), the principal increase in sympathetic activity often occurs during expiratory phase with less or no change during the inspiratory phase (Fig. 13-9A). On the other hand, increased respiratory drive, e.g. with increased arterial carbon dioxide levels, results in increased sympathetic activity in the inspiratory phase and little or no changes in activity in the expiratory phase (Fig. 13-9B). Consequently, the rhythmic respiratory oscillations of sympathetic nerves will determine which stimulus will affect sympathetic activity in which phase.

What mechanisms generate the central nervous system rhythms? They basically fall into two categories: delayed negative feedback oscillators and intrinsic oscillators. Fundamentally, a feedback oscillator consists of a group of activated cells that excites another group of cells that subsequently inhibits the initially activated group after a delay (Fig. 13-10A). When the first group of cells is inhibited, their excitation of the inhibitory cells ceases. Hence, after a delay, the inhibition of the initial cell group is withdrawn, allowing these cells to discharge again. Thus, the system begins to oscillate rhythmically. The period of oscillation depends on the delay time for the feedback. For 5 Hz frequency, a delay loop for the feedback would require hundreds of milliseconds. This would either necessitate a chain of hundreds of neurons, a very long delay loop, or extremely slow conduction velocities. There should be groups of interneurons

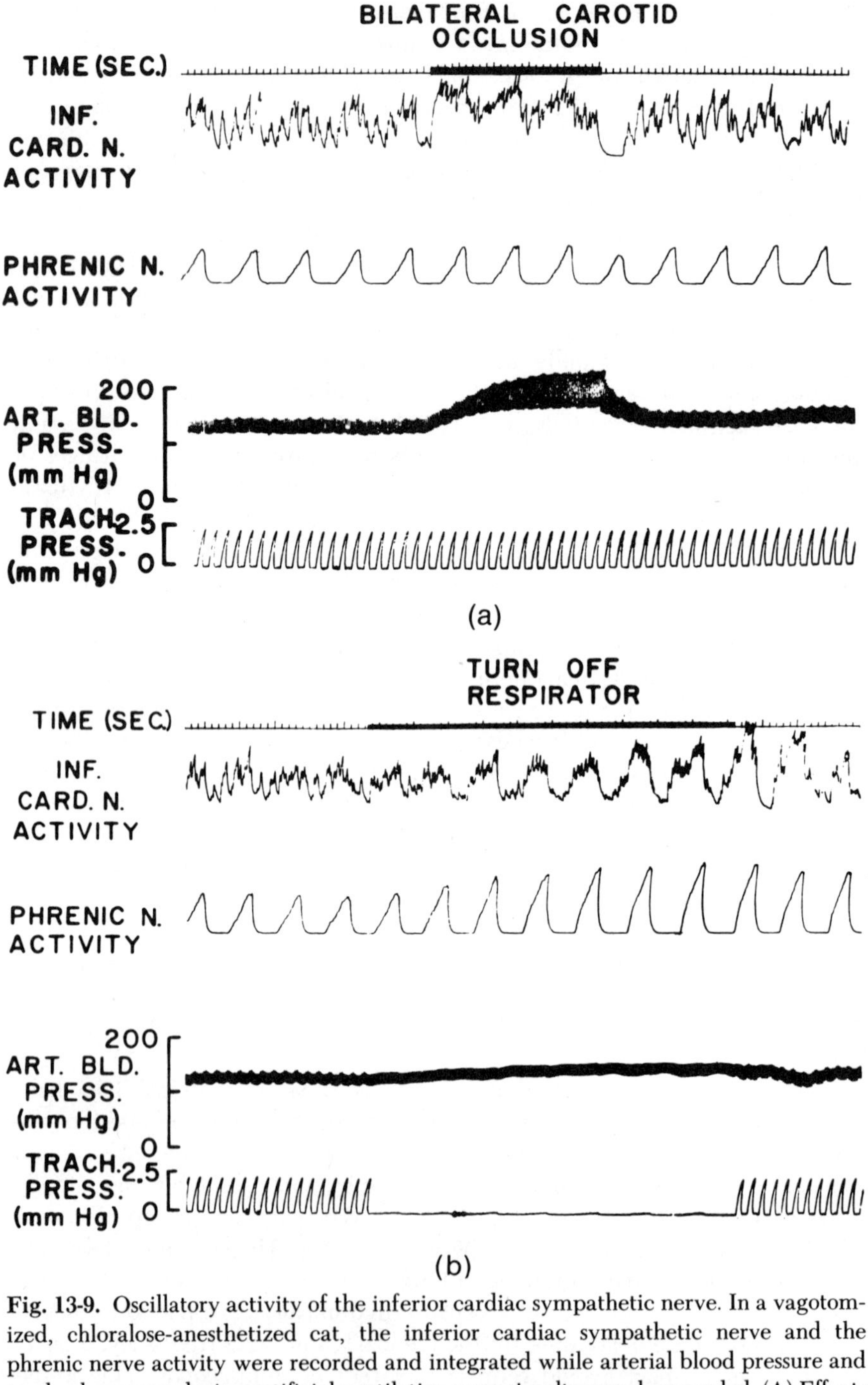

Fig. 13-9. Oscillatory activity of the inferior cardiac sympathetic nerve. In a vagotomized, chloralose-anesthetized cat, the inferior cardiac sympathetic nerve and the phrenic nerve activity were recorded and integrated while arterial blood pressure and tracheal pressure during artificial ventilation were simultaneously recorded. (A) Effects of baroreceptor hypotension (bilateral carotid occlusion). (B) Effects of arterial chemoreceptor activation (turn off respirator). Note: in both A and B increased total sympathetic nerve activity occurred but in different phases of the respiratory cycle.

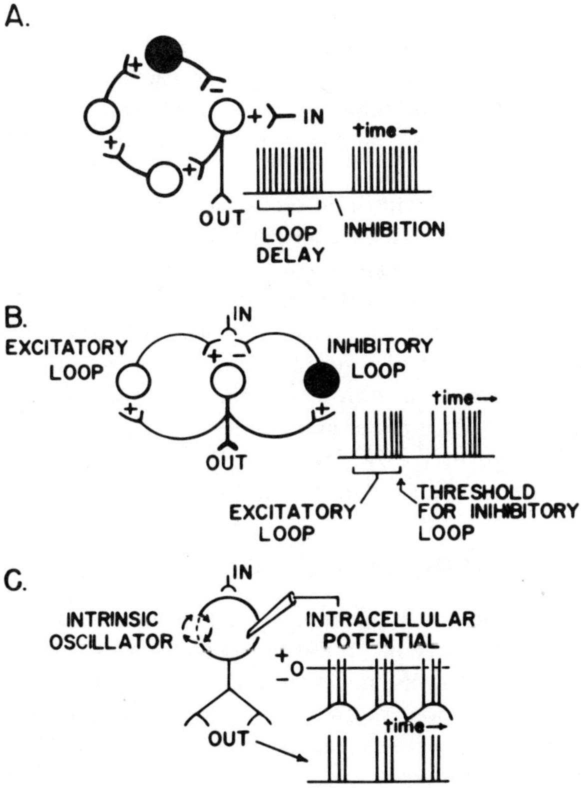

Fig. 13-10. Some models for central neural oscillators which impart rhythmic activity on autonomic nerves. (A) Delayed negative feedback model. With a continuous excitatory input (IN), a chain of excitatory interneurons (open cell bodies) eventually excites an inhibitory interneuron (solid cell body) after a loop delay. After the resulting inhibition of loop, the process repeats itself resulting in an oscillatory output (OUT). (B) Excitatory feedback with a parallel inhibitory loop. The positive or excitatory loop increases the excitation. This excitation summates on an inhibitory loop, which upon reaching threshold, inhibits the excitatory loop. After cessation of the inhibition, the process repeats itself due to a continuous excitatory input (IN) and results in an oscillatory output (OUT). (C) Intrinsic oscillator contained in a cell body, which produces oscillatory changes in the intracellular potential that results in an oscillatory output (OUT).

with the same frequency but with a continuous spectrum of phase shifts representing different portions of the feedback loop. To date, such a spectrum of cell groups has not been recorded to explain these oscillations based on a delayed negative feedback hypothesis.

Another type of negative feedback oscillator is represented in Fig. 13-10B. Due to a positive or excitatory feedback loop (left side) the frequency of discharge increases. This increased activity also summates on an inhibitory neuron (inhibitory loop on right side), which eventually reaches threshold periodically to inhibit the excitatory loop. This is similar to the "OFF switch" oscillator described for respiratory control systems. The period of oscillation depends on the rate of increase of activity (the "gain"), the excitability of the inhibitory neuron (threshold for the the inhibitory loop), and the duration of inhibition. Unlike the negative feedback oscillator in Fig. 13-10A, this system does not require delay loops.

Another possibility is the intrinsic oscillator consisting of pacemaker cells (Fig. 13-10C). These cells may interact via microcircuitry connections such as dendrodendritic synapses, similar to cardiac pacemakers. The oscillation frequency may vary depending on the rate of depolarization of the pacemaker potential and threshold of the pacemaker cell. Such cells probably contain their own feedback system which may relate to the periodic accumulation of extracellular potassium, changes in transmembrane calcium movements, or alterations in ion pumps. Other types of oscillators may be possible or combinations of several mechanisms may exist. However, there is little or no evidence for pacemaker or intrinsic oscillators in the central nervous system.

DYNAMIC SPHERES OF INFLUENCE

Cardiovascular investigators tend to view organization of the central control circuits from the perspective of the cardiovascular system. Other investigators look at the organization of circuits controlling water and electrolytes, respiration, temperature regulation, reproduction, etc. Each group of investigators tends to view these as separate circuits and, in part, they may be correct.

Each functional system may be described as having a neuronal "sphere of influence" including all neurons involved in that control system (Fig. 13-11A). The "sphere of influence" is similar to Sherrington's concept of discharge zones and subliminal fringe; but it should be viewed as having inhibitory, as well as excitatory effects.

The spheres of influence for one functional system may overlap those from another (Fig. 13-11B). One area where this may be demonstrated is in the hypothalamus, although the concept can be represented at other levels. In the hypothalamus, the same neurons may subserve water and electrolyte control, temperature regulation, and cardiovascular functions. What appears to be a thermoregulatory neuron to a temperature regulation physiologist, may be considered part of the water and electrolyte regulation sphere of influence to a renal physiologist. Thus, what a neuron is may depend on the "eyes of the beholder." This should not be surprising since excitatory events, such as exercise, may involve all of these systems.

Other neurons may be part of "private" lines that primarily subserve one functional system. Their private quality may depend on the type and intensity of the stimulus. For example, at high body temperatures, neurons subserving thermoregulatory functions may be part of the blood pressure regulation system. They might inhibit baroreceptor control of heart rate. However, at lower body temperatures, these portions of the thermoregulatory circuit may seem to be a private line for some strictly thermoregulatory function.

One can view these "spheres" as increasing and decreasing continuously

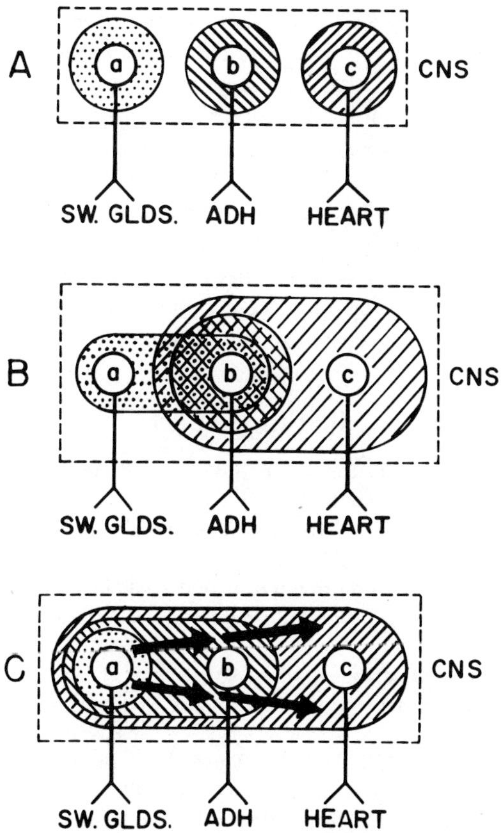

Fig. 13-11. Dynamic spheres of influence. (A) Spheres of influence. Areas of the central nervous system involved in control of particular systems, e.g. sweat glands, antidiuretic hormone release (ADH), and the heart, are schematically represented by areas containing neurons a, b and c, respectively. (B) Overlapping spheres of influence. Control of different functions may involve neuronal circuits which overlap spheres of influence of different effector systems, e.g. thermoregulatory control circuits may overlap sweat gland and antidiuretic hormone control areas of spheres of influence. (C) Dynamic spheres. The effective overlap of control systems may vary from one time to another and from one physiological state to another depending on the intensity of the regulatory drive or stimulus. The CNS is represented by the structures within the dashed boxes.

depending on the total incoming stimuli (Fig. 13-11C). Even the "private lines" may vary their nature by incorporating distribution to other functional circuits. Thus, I view these systems as a highly dynamic expansion and contraction of multiple overlapping spheres.

SIMPLICITY AMONGST COMPLEXITY?

Have our models of the neural control of the cardiovascular system grown too complex for comprehension? The honest answer is yes, if we try to consider the complex, changing role of individual neurons or groups of neurons. Detailed incoming information may be modeled by a computer, but the system would still be beyond our comprehension. The computer model might be useful for predicting behavior of the cardiovascular control system under specific physiological or pathological conditions. For example, what would happen to cardiovascular control if a component structure were inactivated or what would be the predicited consequences of a certain pharmacological manipulation.

How can we simplify our approach to these intricate control systems in man? We must continue to develop general conceptual views of the function within different portions of the cardiovascular neural control circuits. Many, including some proposed in this chapter, may have to be discarded while others will be added as we attempt to conceptualize the system as a whole.

REFERENCES

1. Alexander, R. S., Tonic and reflex functions of medullary sympathetic cardiovascular centers. *J. Neurophysiol.* *9*: 205–217, 1946.
2. Loewy, A. F. and S. McKeller, The neuroanatomical basis of central cardiovascular control. *Fed. Proc.* *39*: 2495–2503, 1980.
3. Manning, J. W., Intracranial representation of cardiac innervation, In *Nervous Control of the Heart*, ed. W. C. Randall. Williams and Wilkins, Baltimore, 1965, pp. 16–33.
4. Peiss, C. N., Concepts of cardiovascular regulation: past, present and future, In *Nervous Control of the Heart*, ed. W. C. Randall. Williams and Wilkins, Baltimore, 1965, pp. 154–197.
5. Sharp, F. R., T. S. Kilduff, H. C. Heller, The 2-deoxyglucose neuroanatomical mapping technique. *Trends in Neurosci.* *4*: 144–147, 1981.
6. Siegler, M. V. S. and M. Burrows, Non-spiking interneurones and local circuits. *Trends in Neurosci.* *3*: 73–77, 1980.
7. Watson, S. J. and H. Akil, Immunocytochemistry—techniques, trials, and tribulations. *Neuroscience Newsletter* *12*: 10–15, 1981.

14

Spinal Cord Control of the Cardiovascular System

SUSAN M. BARMAN

Until recently, the spinal cord was assumed to have only a subordinate role in determining sympathetic outflow, with the medulla considered the main site of integration of activity from supramedullary structures and afferent nerves. However, several observations indicate that information processing in spinal neural circuits can be a major determinant of the level of activity in sympathetic nerves which supply the heart and blood vessels. First, following electrolytic lesions of hypothalamic structures, degenerating fibers are evident in spinal autonomic regions [20,116]. These data suggest that neurons in the spinal cord integrate the activity from medullary and supramedullary nuclei that regulate cardiovascular function. Second, the work of Alexander [3] implies that sympathoinhibition occurs at a spinal locus since sympathetic nerve discharge (SND) increased after cervical cord section in an animal in which blood pressure and SND had been maximally reduced by medullary transection at the level of the obex. Thus, the final output from the central nervous system to the cardiovascular system is determined by the interaction of excitatory and inhibitory inputs to spinal autonomic neurons. Third, activation of somatic and visceral afferent fibers produces reflex responses in sympathetic nerves which do not require the integrity of bulbospinal pathways [71,110]. Fourth, blood pressure gradually returns toward control levels and prominent cardiovascular reflexes can be elicited in chronic spinal animals and man [12,52,56,113,123]. These observations represent remarkable departures from classical views and have led to further studies on the organization of spinal neural circuits in the control of cardiovascular function. This chapter summarizes these investigations.

PREGANGLIONIC SYMPATHETIC NEURONS: THE FINAL COMMON PATHWAY

Information from the central nervous system is transmitted to the cardiovascular system via sympathetic nerves (pre- and postganglionic fibers). The tra-

*The author wishes to thank Dr. R.D. Wurster for reviewing the text.

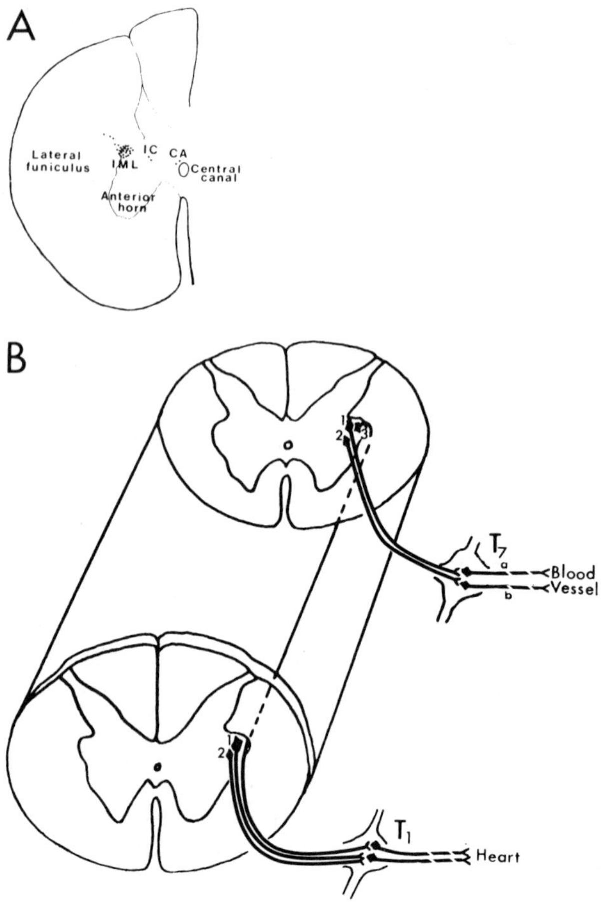

Fig. 14-1. Location and organization of preganglionic sympathetic neurons (PSNs). (A) Location of PSNs in upper thoracic spinal cord as demonstrated by horseradish peroxidase technique. CA, central autonomic nucleus; IC, intercalated nucleus; IML, intermediolateral cell column. (Reproduced through courtesy of *Brain Res. 91*: 126–131, 1975). (B) Schematic of organization of myelinated and unmyelinated PSNs. 1, PSN with myelinated axon; 2, PSN with unmyelinated axon; 3, PSN with long intraspinal axon. At the first thoracic level (T_1) a myelinated and unmyelinated PSN converge on the same postganglionic neuron. At T_7 a myelinated PSN synapses on a postganglionic vasoconstrictor neuron (a) and an unmyelinated PSN synapses on a postganglionic cholinergic vasodilator neuron (b). In addition, a PSN whose cell body is located at T_7 has a long intraspinal axon which projects to T_1. The axon leaves the cord at this level to synapse on a postganglionic neuron.

ditional description of the sympathetic outflow is as follows. Cell bodies of preganglionic sympathetic neurons (PSNs) are located predominantly in the thoracolumbar level of the spinal cord in a region called the intermediolateral cell column (IML). Axons of PSNs are myelinated and leave the spinal cord via the ventral root of the segment in which their cell bodies of origin lie. The PSNs then separate from the ventral root to form the white ramus and synapse on cells located in the sympathetic trunk or peripheral ganglia. The axons of postganglionic neurons are unmyelinated and project to the neuroeffector organs (heart, blood vessels, etc.). The ratio of pre- to postganglionic neurons is between 1:17 and 1:32. With the use of improved research technology in the past few years, much of this classic description has undergone marked changes. Figure 14-1 illustrates many of the new concepts that have developed regarding the organization of PSNs.

Location and Structure of Cell Bodies of PSNs

Retrograde transport of horseradish peroxidase (HRP) into the stellate or superior cervical ganglia of cats [14,16], adrenal medulla of rats [111], and thoracic or lumbar paravertebral ganglia of dogs [35,96] has been used to label cell bodies of PSNs. In addition to locating PSNs in the thoracolumbar cord, neurons were found in the lower cervical spinal cord [14]. Although the majority of cell bodies were indeed located ipsilaterally along the lateral edge of the intermediate gray region (IML), neurons were also labeled in the lateral funiculus, the medial zone of the intermediate gray region or intercalated nucleus, and the central autonomic nucleus which lies dorsolateral to the central canal (Fig. 15-1A). PSNs have also been localized in the ventral horn of cats [14]. A few neurons in the contralateral IML were labeled following injection of HRP into lumbar, but not thoracic, paravertebral ganglia of the dog [96]. Whether PSNs in different loci are involved in different functions (e.g. vasoconstrictor, pilomotor, etc.) has not been critically examined. In this regard, it is interesting to note that, at least in the rat, the cell bodies of PSNs which innervate the hypogastric nerve (i.e. bladder control) are located almost exclusively in the dorsal commissure (a region which approximates the central autonomic nucleus) [54].

Cell bodies of PSNs occur in clusters and vary in shape from round to fusiform with diameters of approximately 8–40 μm. The smaller neurons contain one or two dendrites, while the larger PSNs are multipolar and give rise to two or three large primary dendrites [17]. Close apposition of dendrites of neurons in IML with those in the lateral funiculus or in the more medial regions of the spinal gray was suggested by the work of Chung et al. [16] and Schramm et al. [111]. Thus, one can speculate on the possibility that PSNs located in different autonomic nuclei interact with each other.

Axons of PSNs

The axons of PSNs emanate from one of the large dendrites and then proceed ventrally and travel along the lateral margin of the ventral horn [103]. They do not appear to emit collateral branches. The traditional concept that the axons of all PSNs are myelinated has been challenged by several laboratories. As early as 1918, Ranson and Billingsley [102] noted the presence of unmyelinated preganglionic axons in the cervical sympathetic nerve of the cat. However, they proposed that these fibers were most likely collaterals of preganglionic axons which lost their myelin sheath during the process of branching in peripheral ganglia. In 1932, Duncan [31] found unmyelinated axons in thoracolumbar ventral roots and speculated that they may be axons of PSNs. Perhaps the most convincing anatomical evidence for the existence of PSNs with unmyelinated axons is that provided by Coggeshall and colleagues [21,22,32]. They used electron microscopy to determine the functional categories of unmyelinated axons in white rami from various thoracolumbar cord levels. Approximately one-third of the unmyelinated axons in the white rami degenerated distal to section of the ventral root and thus were considered axons of PSNs. In the mid-thoracic level of the spinal cord approximately 40% of PSNs have axons which are unmyelinated [21].

PSNs with unmyelinated axons have also been identified electrophysiologically. Many investigators [26,44,51,67,76,114] have reported that some PSNs have axonal conduction velocities of less than 2 meters/second, which is indicative of unmyelinated fibers.

Whether PSNs with myelinated and unmyelinated axons subserve different functions is not certain. In this regard, sympathetic cholinergic vasodilatation and piloerection depend upon activation of unmyelinated PSNs, while vasoconstriction results from excitation of myelinated PSNs [39,51]. This separation of function for myelinated and unmyelinated PSNs is illustrated for neurons at T_7 segment in Fig. 14-1B. In contrast, and as depicted for neurons at T_1 segment in Fig. 14-1B, others report that the same postganglionic cell receives input from myelinated and unmyelinated PSNs [26,76,114].

The failure to account for PSNs with unmyelinated axons in earlier studies caused a major error in the calculation of the ratio of pre- to postganglionic neurons. Recently, Brooks-Fournier and Coggeshall [13] calculated a ratio of 1:4 when taking into consideration the large number of unmyelinated PSNs.

Segmental or Intersegmental Organization of PSNs

Controversy surrounds the issue of whether axons of all PSNs leave the spinal cord via the ventral root of the segment in which their cell bodies of origin lie. Chung et al. [14] and Faden and Petras [35] reported that PSNs were labeled over several spinal segments following HRP injection into the stellate or other thoracic paravertebral ganglia which were surgically isolated from the rest of the sympathetic trunk while preserving a single white ramus. These investigators proposed that many axons travelled long distances (up to 12 segments) prior to joining the ventral root and leaving the spinal cord. This projection of a PSN is shown for neuron 3 in Fig. 14-1B. Faden et al [33,34] offered physiological support for this centention; they reported that electrical stimulation of the IML in the lower thoracic and upper lumbar segments of the spinal cord of the cat elicited an increase in heart rate and cardiac contractility which could be abolished by spinal cord transection 2–3 segments rostral to the site of stimulation. The implication from the anatomical and stimulation studies is that control of cardiac function is not limited to a small portion of the upper thoracic cord, but rather, that PSNs throughout the thoracolumbar cord synapse on postganglionic fibers which innervate the heart. PSNs which control cardiac function exit the spinal cord via the T_1–T_5 ventral roots [92].

Recently, several investigators [74,93,106] have independently questioned the existence of this extensive intraspinal preganglionic pathway. When precautions were taken to prevent uptake of HRP into the cut ends of the sympathetic trunk, PSNs were labeled within a restricted level of the spinal cord. Neurons were located within the segment from which the intact white ramus exited the cord and, in some instances, in the caudal portions of the preceding spinal segment. This apparent segmental organization of PSNs makes it difficult to define the basis for the cardiac responses produced by electrical stimulation of the lower thoracic and lumbar spinal cord [33,34]. Either axons of PSNs in this region project long distances before leaving the cord (in contrast to PSNs in more rostral cord segments) or the changes in heart rate and cardiac contractility resulted from activation of an afferent fiber tract which excited PSNs in the upper thoracic cord. Additional experiments are required to resolve the issue of segmental versus intersegmental organization of PSNs.

Spontaneous Discharges of PSNs

A prominent feature of the sympathetic nervous system is the appearance of spontaneously occurring discharges in nerves which innervate the heart and blood vessels. This activity provides the basis for sympathetic nervous system control of resting blood pressure and heart rate. This concept was first recognized by Claude Bernard [11] when he sectioned the cervical spinal cord of an animal and noted a profound fall in blood pressure.

The first recordings of spontaneous activity in the inferior cardiac sympathetic nerve were made by Adrian et al [1] in 1932. As reviewed by Gebber [42,43] the activity of populations of pre- or postganglionic sympathetic nerves is synchronized into bursts or slow waves. Most commonly, these bursts are temporally related to the phases of the cardiac and respiratory cycles. Following baroreceptor denervation (i.e. bilateral section of the carotid sinus, aortic depressor, and vagus nerves) slow waves in SND occur at a frequency of 2-6cps and are no longer locked to the phases of the cardiac cycle. In addition, a 10 cps rhythm [89] and periodic oscillations associated with Mayer waves [100] have been described. The neurogenic bases for these activity patterns are described by Gebber [42,43].

These oscillations in the discharges of whole sympathetic nerve bundles reflect the synchronized firing of a large population of individual units (pre- and postganglionic neurons). The spontaneous activity of individual PSNs has been studied with two methods. Single fibers can be teased from a sympathetic nerve bundle (e.g. cervical and lumbar sympathetic trunk); alternatively, recordings can be made from the soma of PSNs located within the spinal cord. PSNs within the thoracolumbar spinal cord are identified via antidromic activation from stimulation of the peripheral sympathetic nerve bundle. Although the majority of studies have relied on extracellular recording of unit activity, a few investigators have successfully impaled the soma of PSNs and recorded their intracellular action potentials [27,36,91,122]. McLachlan and Hirst [91] successfully impaled the somas of 36 antidromically identified PSNs. In agreement with earlier studies [36,122], the intracellularly recorded action potentials of PSNs were quite long in duration (>5 msec) with a prolonged afterhyperpolarization (25–200 msec). Spontaneous activity took the form of ongoing subthreshold synaptic potentials upon which action potentials were occasionally generated. Excitatory and, in some instances, inhibitory postsynaptic potentials were recorded, thus indicating that the discharges of PSNs depend on the integration of excitatory and inhibitory inputs to these neurons. No evidence for pacemaker-type potentials were found.

There are approximately 40,000 PSNs in the cat spinal cord [57]. Approximately 20–30% of these neurons exhibit background discharges [45,66,67,86] and, thus, are responsible for maintaining the resting level of blood pressure and sympathetic control of cardiac function in the anesthetized, CNS-intact animal. These neurons have characteristically low spontaneous firing rates (0.1–6 Hz), with 90% discharging at frequencies of less than 2 Hz [26,45,66,67,86, 98,112]. Factors which may play a role in determining the number of spontaneously active units at a given time, as well as the firing rate of an individual PSN, include the excitability of the neurons, the degree of synchrony within the driving inputs to these neurons from the brainstem and from somatic and visceral afferents, the level of CO_2 (i.e. chemoreceptor influence), and the level of blood pressure (i.e. baroreceptor influences). The observations that only a small percentage of the total population of PSNs is tonically active at a given time and that the firing frequency of the individual PSN is low attest to the tremendous reserve built into the sympathetic nervous system. That is, marked increases in blood pressure and heart rate can be produced by activating a greater number of PSNs as well as by increasing the firing rate of those neurons that are already spontaneously active.

While cardiac- and respiratory-related discharge patterns are ubiquitous to whole sympathetic nerve bundle recordings, less than two-thirds of the spontaneously active PSNs exhibit such periodicities [26,45,55,86,99,101,112]. Since the spontaneous firing frequency is generally less than the heart rate, the cardiac-related periodicity of PSN activity is most easily detected using computer-aided analysis. As shown by the oscilloscopic records of the spontaneous activity of a PSN (Fig. 14-2-IA), this neuron missed firing in many cardiac cycles. However, post-R wave interval analysis revealed a prominent cardiac-related rhythm in the activity of this unit (Fig. 14-2-IIA). Peak probability of PSN discharge is reached at approximately 175 msec after the R wave. Presumably, the excitatory impulses projecting to this neuron were not sufficiently synchronous during those cardiac cycles in which the unit failed to fire. Other PSNs were therefore responsible for the discharges in postganglionic neurons during those cardiac cycles.

Polosa and colleagues [55,99,101] observed that 50–70% of the spontaneously active units in the upper thoracic spinal cord or in the cervical sympathetic nerve exhibited a respiratory-related discharge pattern in artificially respired, vagotomized cats. The majority of such units reached maximal discharge during

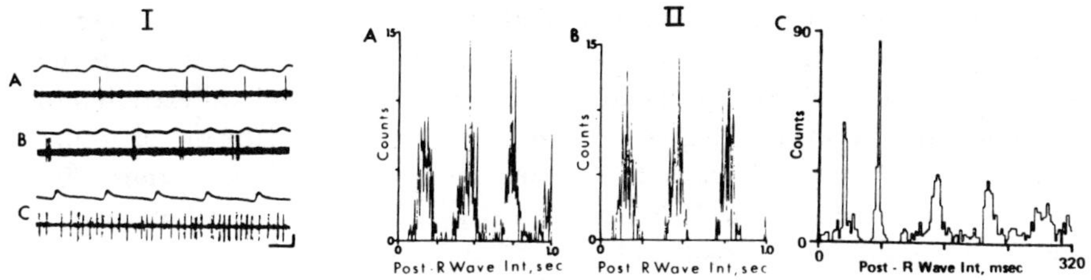

Fig. 14-2. Spontaneous activity patterns of spinal sympathetic neurons located in upper thoracic spinal cord. I. Oscilloscopic records of blood pressure (top traces) and unit activity (bottom traces). (A) Antidromically identified preganglionic sympathetic neuron in the intermediolateral cell column (IML), (B) an excitatory sympathetic interneuron (IN) located in IML, (C) an inhibitory sympathetic IN located in the intermediomedial region. Blood pressure (in mm Hg) was 170/120 (A), 165/115 (B), and 180/125 (C). Horizontal calibration is 150 msec (A) and 200 msec (B, C). Vertical calibration is 100 μV (A, B, and C). II. Post-R wave interval histograms for units shown in I. (A) Sample run was 256 sec. R-R interval was 294 msec. Address bin was 4 msec. (B) sample run was 128 sec. R-R interval was 313 msec. Address bin was 4 msec. (C) number of sweeps was 200. R-R interval was 320 msec. Address bin was 2.5 msec. (Records are modified from *Am. J. Physiol. 231*: 722–733, 1976 and *232*: H657–H665, 1977)

the inspiratory phase of the central respiratory cycle, as monitored by recordings of phrenic nerve activity. These inspiratory-related units were sensitive to changes in end tidal CO_2 (over a range of 1–10%), with increased firing frequency at higher CO_2 levels. A few units reached peak discharge during expiration; these units exhibited higher firing rates at the lower levels of end-tidal CO_2. PSNs whose discharges did not exhibit a respiratory-related pattern were insensitive to changes in CO_2. In addition, Polosa and colleagues found that the CO_2 sensitivity is due to both central and peripheral chemoreceptor activation. They concluded that PSNs receive a major excitatory input from brainstem inspiratory neurons.

The question arises whether those PSNs which exhibit spontaneous activity are functionally distinct from quiescent neurons. In a study of postganglionic neurons, Jänig and colleagues [51,62] proposed that vasoconstrictor neurons are tonically active while pilomotor and cholinergic vasodilator neurons normally are quiescent. Presumably, the same would be true for the PSNs which innervate these distinct groups of postganglionic neurons. However, these data do not imply that all PSNs which supply postganglionic vasoconstrictor neurons are tonically active under basal conditions. Indeed, a large number of quiescent units respond to activation of pressor sites in the medulla [120] and, therefore, may be elements of a vasoconstrictor pathway.

Evoked Responses in PSNs

Does the PSN serve as the final common pathway for cardiovascular responses produced by activation of widely separated vasoactive sites in the medulla and by stimulation of somatic afferents? Taylor and Gebber [120] reported that the same PSN responds to single shocks applied to several distinct nuclei in the medullary reticular formation. Importantly, one-third of the PSNs tested were activated by two distinct excitatory pathways (i.e. pathways which differed in terms of conduction velocity, degree of variability in onset latency of evoked responses, and responsiveness to baroreceptor activation) and, thus, those authors concluded that the PSN can act as the final common pathway at least for these two descending pathways.

Sato [109] studied the convergence of various reflex pathways on 76 spontaneously active lumbar PSNs. He characterized the responses of these PSNs to activation of four major reflex pathways: the spinal, medullary, and suprapontine reflexes mediated via myelinated somatic afferents and the reflex mediated via unmyelinated somatic afferents. Although over 40% of the PSNs responded to activation of at least three of the reflex pathways, nearly 30% responded to activation of only one. Thus, while some units exhibit a high degree of convergence, others show a high degree of specificity. This variation in responsiveness of different PSNs might indicate functionally distinct pools of neurons. In this regard, postganglionic fibers in cutaneous and muscle nerves differ in their responses to afferent nerve stimulation [51,65,72]. That is, cutaneous vasoconstrictor neurons are activated primarily by myelinated afferents, while muscle vasoconstrictor neurons are more readily excited by unmyelinated afferents.

Inhibitory Interaction Among PSNs

Antidromic or orthodromic activation of PSNs is followed by a period of depressed background discharges that can last up to several hundred msec [44,86,87,97]. The origin of this silent period has been debated for a number of years. Polosa and co-workers [86,97] proposed that the depressed excitability is due solely to the recovery process intrinsic to the PSN. This contention is based on the following observations. First, stimuli applied to the whole preganglionic sympathetic nerve trunk which were subthreshold for activation of the PSN under study (but threshold for activation of other PSNs) did not decrease the spontaneous activity recorded from the soma of this neuron. Second, increasing the stimulus intensity above threshold for activation of the axon usually failed to enhance the duration of the silent period of a given neuron. Third, glutamate-induced firing of otherwise quiescent PSNs was also interrupted during antidromic activation; thus, the silent period does not involve a reduction in presynaptic excitatory input.

On the other hand, Lebedev and co-workers [75] suggested that approximately one-third of PSNs with myelinated axons may be under a recurrent inhibitory mechanism. They reported that the soma of some PSNs responded to repetitive stimuli applied to the axons of these neurons only if the interval between shocks was greater than 16 msec, a value which they considered to be greater than the refractory period of the PSN. Furthermore, antidromic activation of one PSN could prevent orthodromic activation (via electrical stimulation of the segmental afferent fiber) of another. These investigators failed to account for the possible involvement of activation of afferents within the sympathetic nerve bundle in the inhibition of PSN discharges. Gebber and Barman [44] considered this problem and reevaluated the inhibitory interaction among PSNs located in T_1–T_3 cord segments. The C_8 through T_3 dorsal root ganglia were extirpated and the sympathetic chain was sectioned between T_3 and T_4 to eliminate the effects produced by stimulation of afferent fibers in the cervical sympathetic nerve which enter the spinal cord via either dorsal or ventral roots. The effects of varying the intensity of a conditioning shock applied to the sympathetic nerve on a response of a PSN whose axon was myelinated (conduction velocity 2.8-8.2 m/sec) to a test antidromic shock were studied. Figure 14-3 shows the results from one such experiment. Trace *a* shows the unconditioned test antidromic response of a PSN whose axonal conduction velocity was 3.2 m/sec. A conditioning shock below threshold for activation of this unit failed to alter the test response (trace b). The interval between the conditioning and test

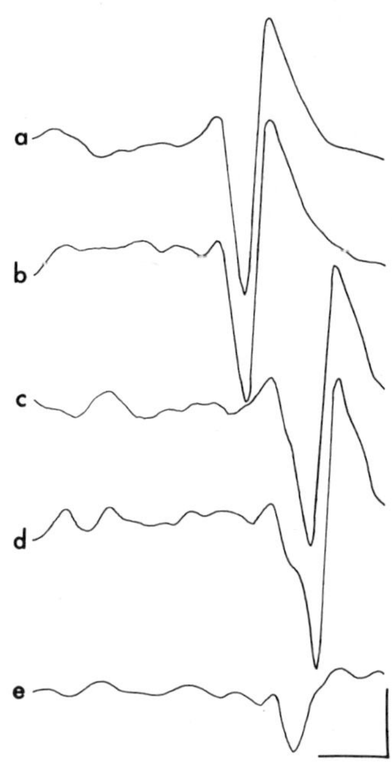

Fig. 14-3. Changes in test antidromic response of a myelinated preganglionic sympathetic neuron (axonal conduction velocity, 3.2 m/sec) produced by conditioning shocks of different intensity. The conditioning and test stimuli were applied to the cervical sympathetic nerve. Traces are normalized averages (16 trials) and show only test response (negativity recorded downward) on an expanded time base. (A) Unconditioned test response, onset latency was 25 ms; (B) test response which was conditioned with a shock (4.8 V) just below threshold for antidromic activation of the unit, C-T interval was 20 msec in this and subsequent traces; (C) test response conditioned with shock (5 V) at threshold for activation of the unit; (D,E) test responses conditioned with suprathreshold shocks; intensity of conditioning shock was 12 V in (D) and 15 V in (E). Vertical calibration is 75 μV; horizontal calibration is 2 msec; address bin was 100 μ sec. (Reproduced through courtesy of *Nervous System and Hypertension*, 1979, pp. 137–145)

shocks was 20 msec. The onset of the test response was delayed by about 2 msec when the conditioning shock was just at threshold for excitation of the PSN (trace c). Moreover, the test spike was fractionated into its initial segment (IS) and soma-dendritic (SD) components (see inflection on the rising phase of the action potential; negativity was recorded downward). Significantly, the SD but not the IS spike was further delayed (trace d) and then blocked (trace e) when the intensity of the conditioning stimulus was increased from threshold to suprathreshold levels. The investigators also noted that blockade of the test response occurred only when the intensity of the conditioning shock was sufficient to recruit PSNs whose axons were unmyelinated (conduction velocity less than 2 m/sec) into the field of antidromic activation. Thus, they speculated that activation of unmyelinated PSNs might inhibit the discharges of neighboring ones whose axons are myelinated. Although the physiological significance of the data remains uncertain, these findings may indicate interaction between functionally distinct groups of PSNs.

SPINAL SYMPATHETIC INTERNEURONS

Several observations imply that interneurons (INs) are contained within spinal circuits which convey information from at least some supraspinal networks and afferent nerves to PSNs. No degeneration is found in IML following lesions of vasoactive sites in the hypothalamus [20,116] and descending sympathetic pathways in the cervical spinal cord [15,104] or dorsal root ganglionectomy [95]. These anatomical studies indicate that information from supraspinal networks and afferent nerves to PSNs is relayed over polysynaptic spinal circuits. Kirchner et al [70] reported that spinal sympathoinhibition evoked by electrical stimulation of the lateral funiculus of the thoracic cord of the cat persisted 4–6 weeks after cervical cord transection. The authors speculated on the existence of a propriospinal pathway for mediating inhibitory influences from supraspinal structures. The implication of these anatomical and physiological studies is that spinal autonomic networks are more complexly organized than originally described. The concept that the spinal cord autonomic network consists solely of PSNs maintains that any spinal information processing would occur at the level of the PSN. The inclusion of one or more interneurons in spinal autonomic circuits allows an additional site for integration of inputs to sympathetic nerves which control the cardiovascular system.

Gebber and colleagues [45,90] provided direct electrophysiological evidence for the existence of spinal sympathetic interneurons in both sympathoexcitatory and sympathoinhibitory networks. In the first study, Gebber and McCall [45] compared the spontaneous discharge pattern of upper thoracic IML neurons which could not be antidromically activated with that of antidromically identified PSNs. Some nonantidromically activated neurons discharged with a prominent cardiac-related component as demonstrated with post-R wave interval analysis (Fig. 14-2 IIB). The pattern of R wave locked activity was similar to that of PSNs (Fig. 14-2 IIA), with maximal activity occurring 160–180 msec after the R wave. In contrast to PSNs which fired with interspike intervals of greater than 75 msec, the nonantidromically activated neurons discharged in bursts or couplets with interspike intervals of 2–20 msec (Fig. 14-2 IB). As was the case for PSNs, the nonantidromically activated neurons missed firing in many cardiac cycles. The responses of these two neuronal types to electrical stimulation of medullary pressor and depressor sites were also compared. Both unit types were activated with similar onset latencies by single shocks applied to medullary pressor sites. This observation led to the conclusion that the nonantidromically activated neurons were INs interposed between the terminals of sympathoexcitatory reticulospinal fibers and PSNs. The discharge of INs and PSNs exhibited two phases of inhibition following short trains of stimuli applied to medullary depressor sites. The early phase most likely indicates inhibition occurring at a spinal locus [121]; and thus, the authors proposed that this component of inhibition is mediated at the level of the IN. However, the existence of pathways which provide for direct inhibition of PSN discharge has not been ruled out. In this regard, Wyszogrodski and Polosa [124] and Kirchner et al. [69] observed that glutamate-induced firing of PSNs was suppressed by stimuli applied to medullary depressor sites, spinal sympathoinhibitory tracts, or somatic afferent nerves. Thus, they postulated that inhibition occurred directly on the PSN. Their data are inconclusive since the glutamate-induced firing of PSNs may have resulted from the action of the drug on closely adjacent INs or the decreased activity of PSNs may have resulted from disfacilitation (via inhibition of INs). Recently, however, using intracellular recording techniques, McLachlan and Hirst [91] occasionally monitored inhibitory postsynaptic potentials in PSNs. Thus, it is possible that descending inhibitory influences onto PSNs may be mediated directly, as well as indirectly via depression of activity of a sympathoexcitatory IN.

In a second study, McCall et al [90] identified spinal INs which most likely were elements of a sympathoinhibitory network. These neurons were located in the medial zone of the intermediate gray regions of the upper thoracic cord. The spontaneous discharges of these neurons were interrupted within one heart beat following bilateral occlusion of the common carotid arteries in cats with sectioned aortic depressor and vagus nerves. This observation suggested that these neurons received driving input from medullospinal projections of the baroreceptor reflex circuit and therefore were spinal sympathoinhibitory interneurons. Two additional observations supported this contention. First, the pattern of R wave-locked activity for these neurons (Fig. 14-2 IIC) was similar to that for some neurons in the nucleus of the tractus solitarius (NTS; primary site of baroreceptor afferent nerve termination). The cardiac-related periodicity exhibited 1 to 4 peaks at intervals of approximately 30, 70, 135, and 210 msec after the R wave. Second, these neurons were activated by electrical stimulation of the NTS. The latency of activation of these neurons (8 ± 1 msec) was 2–3 msec shorter than the onset latency for inhibition of INs and PSNs in IML. Thus, baroreceptor-induced sympathoinhibition may involve activation of spinal INs.

These studies indicate that the spinal autonomic circuits contain at least two categories of INs. Whether the same or different spinal excitatory (or inhibitory)

INs are involved in mediating influences onto PSNs from widely separated vasopressor (or vasodepressor) sites (e.g. hypothalamus, medullary reticular formation, etc.) and from visceral and somatic afferents is a subject for further investigation. In this regard, the spinal sympathoinhibitory INs described above may also be involved in producing the inhibitory effects of cardiac afferent nerve stimulation on SND since these neurons were activated by single shocks applied to the central end of the sectioned inferior cardiac nerve at intensities which decreased blood pressure [90].

ORIGIN OF INPUTS TO SPINAL SYMPATHETIC NEURONS

Both anatomical and electrophysiological studies have indicated that a rather large number of supraspinal structures innervate spinal sympathetic neurons. The fact that various central nervous system nuclei project to spinal autonomic neurons attests to the role of the spinal cord in processing information for cardiovascular control. The neuroanatomical organization of central autonomic pathways involved in control of heart rate and blood pressure was recently reviewed by Loewy and co-workers [77,79,82,83].

Following the injection of HRP into the thoracolumbar cord, neurons were labeled in caudal raphe nuclei [4,80,88,105], nucleus reticularis gigantocellularis [80,88], NTS [4,78], rostral portions of lateral reticular nucleus and of the ventral surface of the medulla [4,80,88,105], the A5 catecholamine region [81], and paraventricular nucleus of the hypothalamus [53,107]. With the exception of the study by Amendt et al [4], no attempt was made to selectively inject the HRP into IML. As a consequence, the results of these studies are not specific for central autonomic pathways. To more carefully assess the neuroanatomical organization of central sympathetic networks, the connections from supraspinal sites to IML have been traced using autoradiography following the injections of tritiated leucine or proline into various nuclei. Labeling of fibers (presumed to be terminals) within the IML occurs subsequent to injection of amino acids into raphe nuclei [8,80,88], nucleus reticularis gigantocellularis and magnocellularis [8,88], ventral surface of the rostral medulla and lateral reticular nucleus [80,88], the A5 catecholamine region [81], pontine reticular formation [61], Kolliker-Fuse [108], and the paraventricular nucleus of the hypothalamus [107].

Dahlstrom and Fuxe [28] noted increased levels of catecholamine in the A1 region following spinal cord section. They interpreted this to be a response to axotomy and concluded that norepinephrine inputs to spinal nuclei (including the IML) arise from cell bodies in the A1 region. In agreement with these findings, Fleetwood-Walker and Coote [38] found that, following lesions of this region, catecholamine concentrations in the IML were markedly attenuated.

Henry and Calaresu [58,59] antidromically activated neurons in the brainstem via electrical stimulation of the IML in the cat. They located neurons in the following nuclei: raphe, paramedian reticular, lateral reticular, and gigantocellularis. Since activation of these same regions led to an increase in heart rate and blood pressure, they speculated that these nuclei are involved in control of cardiovascular function and provide direct input to spinal autonomic neurons.

Although these anatomical and electrophysiological studies are helpful in the identification of those regions which provide input to spinal sympathetic circuits, their description of central autonomic pathways is far from complete. Many other brain regions may be involved in regulating SND, and therefore blood pressure and heart rate, but synapse in those brainstem nuclei which project to the cord. Furthermore, these studies fail to provide information regarding the function (i.e. sympathoexcitatory or sympathoinhibitory) of such pathways or to determine which areas are involved in generating the tonic activity in sympathetic nerves. In Chapter 15, Gebber describes data that provide new insights into these problems.

SPINAL SYMPATHETIC PATHWAYS

Excitatory and inhibitory inputs to spinal sympathetic neurons arise from nearly every level of the neuraxis, as well as from somatic and visceral afferent nerves. The effects on blood pressure, heart rate, or SND produced by electrical stimulation or lesions of the white matter of the cervical or thoracic spinal cord have been used to identify the fiber tracts responsible for mediating these influences. Figure 14-4 I depicts the location of ascending and descending spinal sympathetic pathways.

Descending Sympathoexcitatory Pathways

It is generally agreed that fibers in the dorsolateral funiculus (DLF) of the spinal cord mediate excitatory influences on sympathetic nerves [5–7,40,46,58–60,63,68,115,118,119]. Stimuli applied to this area elicit an increase in SND (Fig. 14-4 IIB) which leads to an elevation in heart rate and blood pressure (Fig. 14-4 IIA). Bilateral lesions of this region produce a marked fall in blood pressure and heart rate, prevent the reflex increase in blood pressure produced by bilateral occlusion of the common carotid arteries or stimuli applied to medullary reticular formation, and abolish the supraspinal component of the somatosympathetic reflex in the anesthetized cat [29,30,40,41,50,115,118]. Both crossed and uncrossed pathways have been localized within the DLF [40,60,119].

Barman and Wurster [6] studied the functional organization of this pathway in the dog. They calculated changes in heart rate and peripheral resistance in the carotid, renal, and femoral vascular beds during electrical stimulation of various loci within the DLF. The site which upon stimulation elicited the maximum change in these parameters was determined. The authors noted that the maximum increases in heart rate and carotid resistance were produced by stimuli applied to the most dorsal aspects of this region; femoral resistance was most affected by activation of the more ventral regions; and renal resistance was maximally increased at an intermediate site. Chung et al. [15] provided anatomical evidence in support of this visceromotor organization of the DLF. They found that following lesions of this area in the cat, fibers exit mainly from the dorsal portion of the tract and the ventral fibers gradually shift dorsally as the pathway proceeds caudally.

Gebber et al [46] characterized two distinct systems within the sympathoex-

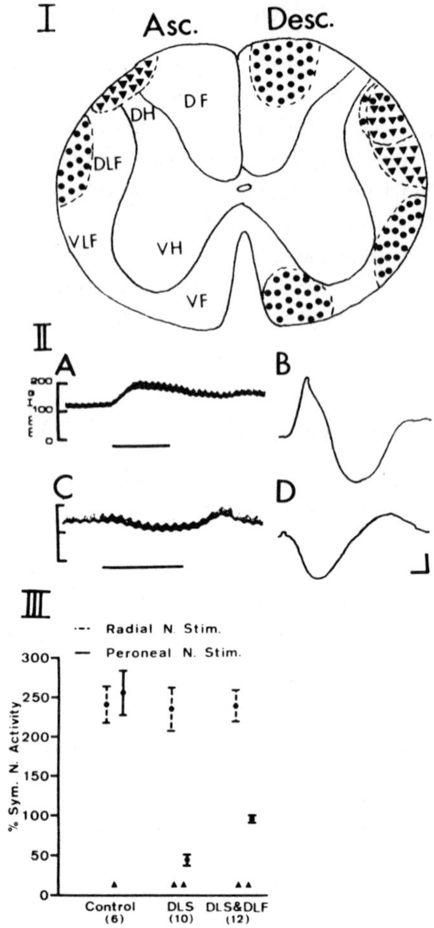

Fig. 14-4. Ascending and descending sympathetic pathways. I. Localization of ascending (left) and descending (right) sympathetic pathways in the cervical spinal cord. Triangles indicate excitatory tracts and circles indicate inhibitory tracts. DF, dorsal funiculus; DH, dorsal horn; DLF, dorsolateral funiculus; VF, ventral funiculus; VH, ventral horn; VLF, ventrolateral funiculus. II. Responses to electrical stimulation of descending pathways. (A) Blood pressure response produced by activation of C_7 DLF. Stimuli (10 V, 0.5 msec in duration) were applied at 50 Hz during the time indicated by the bar. (B) Computer summed (32 trials) evoked potential recorded from the inferior cardiac nerve when shocks (10 V, 0.1 msec) were applied to the C_8 DLF at a rate of one every 2 sec. Address bin was 400 μsec. (C) Blood pressure response produced by activation of C_7 VLF. Stimuli (10 V, 1 msec in duration) were applied at 50 Hz during the time indicated by the bar. (D) Computer-summed (50 trials) inhibition of T_2 preganglionic nerve activity when shocks (8 V, 1 msec in duration) were applied to the C_8 VLF at a rate of 1 every 2 sec. Horizontal calibration is 7.5 sec (A, C), 50 msec (B), and 15 msec (D). Vertical calibration is 5 μV (B), and 10 μV (D). III. Effect of spinal lesions on sympathetic nerve responses to stimulation of afferent nerves. Data are expressed as mean $\pm$ SE of percent sympathetic nerve activity during stimulation compared to spontaneous activity. One triangle indicates no statistically significant difference. Two triangles indicate significant difference of $p < 0.0001$. Number of multifiber preparations recorded in each experiment is shown at bottom. (Panel III was reproduced through courtesy of *Am. J. Physiol. 231*: 786–792, 1976)

citatory pathway in the DLF in control of external carotid SND. The conduction velocity of the first system was $\simeq$2.5 m/sec and the potentials elicited by stimulation of this pathway were blocked by activation of the baroreceptor reflex (i.e. during the pressor response produced by an intravenous injection of norepinephrine). In contrast, the second system had a conduction velocity of $\simeq$5.5 m/sec and the potentials evoked by stimulation of this pathway were not attenuated by increased baroreceptor nerve activity. Since SND is completely abolished during the pressor response to norepinephrine [46,117], they concluded that the baroreceptor nonblockable pathway did not function in the tonic control of SND. In a later study, Taylor and Gebber [120] reported that the same PSN could be activated by stimulation of the two descending pathways.

The role of the sympathoexcitatory pathway in DLF in mediating excitatory drive to spinal sympathetic neurons in conscious dogs has recently been investigated by Geis et al. [47]. They found that there was no difference in blood pressure or heart rate in the resting conscious animal before and after bilateral lesions of this area at low cervical levels. Thus, this pathway does not appear to be responsible for the tonic excitatory influences on the cardiovascular system in the unanesthetized dog. Subsequent complete spinal cord transection at the lower cervical level reduced blood pressure and heart rate during rest; thus, a pathway other than the DLF is responsible for providing tonic excitatory drive to spinal sympathetic neurons in the unanesthetized dog. Geis et al [47] also studied the effects of lesions of the DLF on the cardiovascular responses to exercise and bilateral occlusion of the common carotid arteries. The change in blood pressure and heart rate which normally accompanies decreased pressure in the carotid sinus is prevented by interruption of this pathway. The increase in blood pressure, but not the tachycardia, which results from exercise was also prevented by the lesion.

Descending Sympathoinhibitory Pathways

Pathways which convey inhibitory influences onto spinal sympathetic neurons have been described in four major regions: an area just lateral to the apex of the dorsal horn in the DLF [23–25,29,30,70], the ventrolateral funiculus (VLF) [7,23–25,63,64], the ventral funiculus (VF) [23–25], and in the dorsal funiculus (DF) [23–25]. Figure 14-4 II shows an example of the fall in blood pressure (panel C) and of computer-summed inhibition of SND (panel D) produced by stimuli applied to the sympathoinhibitory fibers within the VLF.

Which of these areas mediates tonic inhibitory influences on background discharges in spinal sympathetic neurons [3] has not been determined. However, the role of inhibitory pathways in tonic modulation of the spinal component of the somatosympathetic reflex has been studied by Dembowsky et al. [29,30]. They showed that the spinal reflex was enhanced following cold block or lesions of the DLF and thus proposed that this region tonically inhibits the discharges of neurons within the spinal reflex arc. However, since these manipulations of the DLF interrupt the excitatory drive to PSNs, the increased magnitude of the spinal reflex may reflect activation of PSNs which were previously in a refractory period due to spontaneous activity rather than to elimination of tonic inhibitory influences.

Coote and MacLeod [25] have attempted to define the origin of the various inhibitory fiber tracts in the spinal cord. They monitored the effect of spinal lesions on the inhibition of a segmental reflex during electrical stimulation of depressor sites in the medulla. Lesions of the DLF prevented sympathoinhibition from activation of the ventrolateral medulla and nucleus raphe pallidus, whereas destruction of the VF prevented the inhibition evoked from stimulation of the ventromedial reticular formation.

Spinal Component of Baroreceptor-Induced Sympathoinhibition

Until recently it was generally assumed that the inhibitory effects on SND produced by baroreceptor activation were mediated solely at supraspinal loci. In 1973, Gebber et al. [46] provided the first direct evidence for a spinal component in the baroreceptor reflex arc. They demonstrated that the evoked responses in sympathetic nerves elicited by single shocks applied to the descending excitatory pathway in the DLF could be markedly attenuated during the pressor response produced by intravenous infusion of norepinephrine. Prior section of the carotid sinus, aortic depressor, and vagus nerves (i.e. baroreceptor denervation) prevented this inhibitory effect. Since this study, others [7,24] have verified a spinal component to baroreceptor-induced sympathoinhibition.

In a later study, Taylor and Gebber [121] characterized two components to the baroreceptor-mediated inhibitory effects on the background discharges in sympathetic nerves. The onset latency and duration of the early phase of inhibition on the splanchnic preganglionic nerve was $\simeq$30 msec and $\simeq$75 msec, respectively. The same parameters for the late phase of inhibition were $\simeq$100 msec and $\simeq$300 msec. Importantly, they showed that an evoked potential on the sympathetic nerve produced by single shocks applied to the DLF could be attenuated during the early, but not the late period of inhibition. Thus, they concluded that the early phase of inhibition was mediated at the level of the spinal cord while the late phase was most likely of medullary origin. The conduction velocity of this spinal pathway was calculated to be approximately 15 m/sec [90].

Coote and MacLeod [24] proposed that the spinal component of the baroreceptor reflex involved activation of slowly conducting ($\simeq$3 m/sec) inhibitory fibers in the region of the DH. This conclusion was based on the observation that lesions of this region prevented the inhibition of a spinal sympathetic reflex produced by increasing pressure in the carotid sinus. Thus, while more rapidly conducting pathways may be involved in mediating the baroreceptor inhibitory influences on the background discharges of spinal sympathetic neurons [121], the somatosympathetic reflex may be modulated by a more slowly conducting inhibitory pathway [24].

Ascending Sympathetic Pathways

Responses in sympathetic nerves which accompany activation of somatic afferent fibers are mediated over spinal and supraspinal reflex arcs [71,110]. In addition, spinal pathways from afferent nerves to medullary cardiac vagal neurons also exist [71]. Pathways within the cord which relay afferent information to supraspinal sites involved in the somatoautonomic reflexes have been described by Wurster and colleagues [18,19,48,73]. Spinal cord lesions were made at mid-lumbar levels to avoid interruption of the efferent limb of the somatosympathetic reflex. The sympathetic nerve and cardiovascular responses to electrical stimulation of the lower lumbar roots were recorded. Lesions of the area surrounding the dorsolateral sulcus (DLS) prevent the evoked excitatory response in sympathetic neurons and the pressor response to stimulation of unmyelinated somatic afferent nerve fibers [18,19]. Lesions of the DLF prevent the inhibition of sympathetic nerve activity and depressor response to activation of myelinated somatic afferent nerve fibers [18,19]. The graph in Fig. 14-4 III depicts the effects of spinal lesions on afferent nerve-induced responses in the cervical sympathetic nerve. The intensity of the shocks applied to the peroneal nerve was sufficient to activate both myelinated and unmyelinated fibers. The control response indicates the summation of excitatory and inhibitory influences of somatic afferent nerve stimulation. Following lesions of the DLS, only the inhibitory effects were recorded. Subsequent ablation of the DLF prevented the depression of SND. The responses which result from radial nerve stimulation were not affected, thus indicating that efferent pathways to the cervical sympathetic nerve remained intact. The region surrounding the DLS is also involved in mediating the somatic afferent nerve-induced inhibition of vagal nerve activity in the cat (48) and the tachycardia produced by exercise in the conscious dog [73].

CARDIOVASCULAR REFLEXES AND SND IN SPINAL PREPARATIONS

Although transection of the spinal cord produces an immediate marked drop in blood pressure and sympathetic nerve activity, near normal levels of resting blood pressure and prominent vasomotor reflexes are observed in chronic spinal animals and man. Sherrington [113] noted that 300 days after low cervical spinal cord section in the dog, mean arterial pressure was 90 mm Hg and could be elevated to over 200 mm Hg by electrical stimulation of afferents in the sciatic nerve. Brooks [12] also noted that in some chronic spinal cats, resting blood pressure levels were 90–100 mm Hg. Furthermore, chronic spinal cats had the ability to compensate for hemorrhage of 10–20% of blood volume. This compensatory response was attenuated, but not abolished, by dorsal root section and adrenalectomy. However, additional section of the ventral roots eliminated the response, thus indicating that the increase in blood pressure was mediated via enhanced activity in sympathetic nerves which supply the cardiovascular system.

Cardiovascular reflexes have also been elicited in patients with spinal cord injury [52,56,123]. Wurster and Randall [123] reported that in patients with spinal lesions above the T_5 level, bladder distension led to an increase in cardiac contractility and blood pressure. In patients with lesions below this level, bladder distension led to vasoconstriction. However, since the lesion was below the outflow to the heart, no cardiac responses were noted.

Prominent cardiocardiac reflexes can be elicited in acute spinal animals [84,85,94]. Electrical, mechanical, or chemical activation of cardiac sympathetic afferent nerves can lead to an increase in sympathetic nerve activity and a tachycardia in acute spinal cats [84,85]. In addition to cardiocardiac reflexes, electrical stimulation of somatic afferents can elicit a reflex discharge in PSNs [9,10,37]. The sympathetic nerve response is most prominent at the segment in which the afferent nerves enter the spinal cord. In some instances, blood pressure was increased during afferent nerve stimulation.

These studies reveal that marked reflex changes in blood pressure and heart rate do not require the integrity of medullospinal pathways. Rather, these reflexes are complete within the spinal cord. In addition to reflexly mediated sympathetic nerve activity, several investigators have reported spontaneous activity in individual PSNs in acute spinal cats [9,10,86]. The firing frequency is low (0.3–1.4 Hz) when compared to that of an intact animal. Some activity also persists in animals with sectioned afferent nerves [86]. These data reveal that spinal neuronal elements are capable of generating activity in PSNs in the absence of supraspinal and afferent influences.

Several observations made by Alexander [2] suggest that activity in the inferior cardiac nerve of the acute spinal cat depends on anoxic stimulation of spinal neurons. First, the nerve was quiescent during hyperventilation. Second, a marked increase in nerve activity was induced by asphyxia in an animal with an isolated cord (i.e. sections at low cervical and mid-thoracic cord levels and dorsal roots cut bilaterally between these segments). Third, this increase in nerve activity was prevented if the spinal cord was destroyed, thus ruling out anoxic activation of ganglia cells. McCall and Gebber [89] and Gootman and Cohen [49,50] also noted that asphyxia enhances SND. Importantly, they noted that the asynchronous activity recorded from whole sympathetic nerve bundles (preganglionic or postganglionic) during normocapnia was transformed into slow waves which occurred at frequencies of 2–3 cps or 10 cps during asphyxia. These data reveal that spinal neuronal networks exist which function to synchronize the discharges of large populations of PSNs at least during stressful situations such as asphyxia.

CONCLUSIONS

The traditional concept that the spinal cord serves solely as a relay station for transmitting information from the medulla to postganglionic neurons innervating the cardiovascular system is no longer tenable. Rather, the data summarized in this chapter indicate that information processing within spinal autonomic networks is an important determinant of the level of SND. The complex organization of spinal autonomic networks is indicated by the existence of INs within sympathoexcitatory and sympathoinhibitory pathways, the multiplicity of projections from supraspinal regions to spinal autonomic networks, and the inhibitory interaction of myelinated and unmyelinated PSNs. Furthermore, spinal autonomic circuits can operate in the absence of driving inputs from the medulla, as indicated by synchronous activity in SND of the acute spinal cat during asphyxia. The data obtained in the past several years should serve as an impetus to promote further research on the organization of spinal autonomic networks.

REFERENCES

1. Adrian, E. D., D. W. Bronk, G. Phillips, Discharges in mammalian sympathetic nerves. *J. Physiol. (London) 74*: 115–133, 1932.
2. Alexander, R. S., The effects of blood flow and anoxia on spinal cardiovascular centers. *Am. J. Physiol. 143*: 698–708, 1945.
3. Alexander, R. S., Tonic and reflex functions of medullary sympathetic cardiovascular centers. *J. Neurophysiol. 9*: 205–217, 1946.
4. Amendt, K., J. Czachurski, D. Dembowsky, H. Seller, Bulbospinal projections to the intermediolateral cell column; a neuroanatomical study. *J. Autonom. Nerv. Sys. 1*: 103–117, 1979.
5. Barman, S. M., T. V. McCaffrey, R. D. Wurster, Cardiovascular and electrophysiological characteristics of sympathetic pathway stimulation. *Am. J. Physiol. 230*: 1095–1100, 1976.
6. Barman, S. M. and R. D. Wurster, Visceromotor organization within descending spinal sympathetic pathways in the dog. *Circ. Res. 37*: 209–214, 1975.
7. Barman, S. M., and R. D. Wurster, Interaction of descending spinal sympathetic pathways and afferent nerves. *Am. J. Physiol. 234*: H223–H229, 1978.
8. Basbaum, A. I., C. H. Clanton, H. L. Fields, Three bulbospinal pathways from the rostral medulla of the cat: an autoradiographic study of pain modulating systems. *J. Comp. Neurol. 178*: 209–224, 1978.
9. Beacham, W. S. and E. R. Perl, Background and reflex discharge of sympathetic preganglionic neurons in the spinal cat. *J. Physiol. (London) 173*: 400–416, 1964.
10. Beacham, W. S. and E. R. Perl, Characteristics of a spinal sympathetic reflex. *J. Physiol. (London) 173*: 431–448, 1964.
11. Bernard, C., Leçons sur la Physiologie et la Pathologie du Systeme Nerveux, Vol. 1, Ballière, Paris, 1863.
12. Brooks, C. McC., The reaction of chronic spinal animals to hemorrhage. *Am. J. Physiol. 114*: 30–39, 1935.
13. Brooks-Fournier, R. and R. E. Coggeshall, The ratio of preganglionic axons to postganglionic cells in the sympathetic nervous system of the rat. *J. Comp. Neurol. 197*: 207–216, 1981.
14. Chung, K., J. M. Chung, F. W. LaVelle, R. D. Wurster, Sympathetic neurons in the cat spinal cord projecting to the stellate ganglion. *J. Comp. Neurol. 185*: 23–30, 1979.
15. Chung, K., J. M. Chung, F. W. LaVelle, R. D. Wurster, The anatomical localization of descending pressor pathways in the cat spinal cord. *Neurosci. Lett. 15*: 71–75, 1979.
16. Chung, J. M., K. Chung, R. D. Wurster, Sympathetic preganglionic neurons of the cat spinal cord: horseradish peroxidase study. *Brain Res. 91*: 126–131, 1975.
17. Chung, K., F. W. LaVelle, R. D. Wurster, Ultrastructure of HRP-identified sympathetic preganglionic neurons in the cat. *J. Comp. Neurol. 190*: 147–155, 1980.

18. Chung, J. M., C. L. Webber, R. D. Wurster, Ascending spinal pathways for the somatosympathetic A and C reflexes. *Am. J. Physiol. 237*: H342–H347, 1979.
19. Chung, J. M. and R. D. Wurster. Ascending pressor and depressor pathways in the cat spinal cord. *Am. J. Physiol. 231*: 786–792, 1976.
20. Ciriello, J. and F. R. Calaresu, Descending hypothalamic pathways with cardiovascular function in the cat: a silver impregnation study. *Exp. Neurol. 57*: 561–580, 1977.
21. Coggeshall, R. E., M. B. Hancock, M. L. Applebaum, Categories of axons in mammalian rami communicantes. *J. Comp. Neurol. 167*: 105–123, 1976.
22. Coggeshall, R. E., C. W. Maynard, L. A. Langford, Unmyelinated sensory and preganglionic fibers in rat L_6 and S_1 ventral spinal roots. *J. Comp. Neurol. 193*: 41–47, 1980.
23. Coote, J. H. and V. H. Macleod, The influence of bulbospinal monoaminergic pathways on sympathetic nerve activity. *J. Physiol. (London) 241*: 453–475, 1974.
24. Coote, J. H. and V. H. Macleod, Evidence for the involvement in the baroreceptor reflex of a descending inhibitory pathway. *J. Physiol. (London) 241*: 477–496, 1974.
25. Coote, J. H. and V. H. Macleod, The spinal route of sympatho-inhibitory pathways descending from the medulla oblongata. *Pfluegers Arch. 359*: 335–347, 1975.
26. Coote, J. H. and D. R. Westbury, Functional grouping of sympathetic preganglionic neurons in the third thoracic segment of the spinal cord. *Brain Res. 179*: 367–372, 1979.
27. Coote, J. H. and D. R. Westbury, Intracellular recordings from sympathetic preganglionic neurones. *Neurosci. Lett. 15*: 171–175, 1979.
28. Dahlstrom, A. and K. Fuxe, Evidence for the existence of monoamine neurons in the central nervous system. II. Experimentally induced changes in the intraneuronal amine levels of bulbospinal neuron systems. *Acta Physiol. Scand. 64(Suppl. 247)*: 7–85, 1965.
29. Dembowsky, K., J. Czachurski, K. Amendt, and H. Seller, Tonic descending inhibition of the spinal somato-sympathetic reflex from the lower brain stem. *J. Autonom. Nerv. Sys. 2*: 157–182, 1980.
30. Dembowsky, K., K. Lackner, J. Czachurski, H. Seller, Tonic catecholaminergic inhibition of the spinal somato-sympathetic reflexes originating in the ventrolateral medulla oblongata. *J. Autonom. Nerv. Sys. 3*: 277–290, 1981.
31. Duncan, D., A determination of the number of unmyelinated fibers in the ventral roots of the rat, cat, and rabbit. *J. Comp. Neurol. 55*: 459–471, 1932.
32. Emery, D. G., H. Ito, R. E. Coggeshall, Unmyelinated axons in thoracic ventral roots of the cat. *J. Comp. Neurol. 172*: 37–48, 1977.
33. Faden, A. I., T. Jacobs, M. Woods, Cardioacceleratory sites in the zona intermedia of the cat spinal cord. *Exp. Neurol. 61*: 301–310, 1978.
34. Faden, A., T. Jacobs, M. Woods, An intraspinal sympathetic preganglionic pathway: physiological evidence in the cat. *Brain Res. 162*: 13–20, 1979.
35. Faden, A. I. and J. M. Petras, An intraspinal sympathetic preganglionic pathway: anatomic evidence in the dog. *Brain Res. 144*: 358–362, 1978.
36. Fernandez de Molina, A., M. Kuno, E. R. Perl, Antidromically evoked responses from sympathetic preganglionic neurones. *J. Physiol. (London) 180*: 321–335, 1965.

37. Fernandez de Molina, A. and E. R. Perl, Sympathetic activity and the systemic circulation in the spinal cat. *J. Physiol. (London) 181*: 82–102, 1965.
38. Fleetwood-Walker, S. M. and J. H. Coote, The contribution of brain stem catecholamine cell groups to the innervation of the sympathetic lateral cell column. *Brain Res. 205*: 141–155, 1981.
39. Folkow, B., B. Johansson, B. Oberg, The stimulation threshold of different sympathetic fibre groups as correlated to their functional differentiation. *Acta Physiol. Scand. 44*: 146–156, 1958.
40. Foreman, R. D. and R. D. Wurster, Localization and functional characteristics of descending sympathetic spinal pathways. *Am. J. Physiol. 255*: 212–217, 1973.
41. Foreman, R. D. and R. D. Wurster, Conduction in descending spinal pathways initiated by somatosympathetic reflexes. *Am. J. Physiol. 228*: 905–908, 1975.
42. Gebber, G. L., Central oscillators responsible for sympathetic nerve discharge. *Am. J. Physiol. 239*: H143–H155, 1980.
43. Gebber, G. L. Bulbospinal control of sympathetic nerve discharge. In *Neural Control of Circulation,* Ed. M. J. Hughes and C. D. Barnes. Academic Press, New York, 1980, pp. 51–80.
44. Gebber, G. L. and S. M. Barman, Inhibitory interaction between preganglionic sympathetic neurons. In *Nervous System and Hypertension,* Eds. by P. Meyer and H. Schmitt. Wiley, New York: 1979, pp. 137–145.
45. Gebber, G. L. and R. B. McCall, Identification and discharge patterns of spinal sympathetic interneurons. *Am. J. Physiol. 231*: 722–733, 1976.
46. Gebber, G. L., D. G. Taylor, L. C. Weaver, Electrophysiological studies on organization of central vasopressor pathways. *Am. J. Physiol. 224*: 470–481, 1973.
47. Geis, G. S., G. Barratt, R. D. Wurster, Role of the descending pressor pathway in the conscious and pentobarbital-anesthetized dog. *Am. J. Physiol. 234*: H152–H156, 1978.
48. Geis, G. S. and R. D. Wurster, Localization of ascending inotropic and chonotropic pathways in the cat. *Circ. Res. 49*: 711–717, 1981.
49. Gootman, P. M. and M. I. Cohen, Origin of rhythms common to sympathetic outflows at different spinal levels. In *Arterial Baroreceptors and Hypertension,* Ed. P. Sleight. Oxford Univ. Press, New York, 1980, pp. 154–160.
50. Gootman, P. M. and M. I. Cohen, Sympathetic rhythms in spinal cats. *J. Autonom. Nerv. Sys. 3*: 379–387, 1981.
51. Grosse, M. and W. Janig, Vasoconstrictor and pilomotor fibres in skin nerves to the cat's tail. *Pfluegers Arch. 361*: 221–229, 1976.
52. Guttman, L. and D. Whitteridge, Effects of bladder distension on autonomic mechanisms after spinal cord injuries. *Brain 70*: 361–404, 1947.
53. Hancock, M. B., Cells of origin of hypothalamo-spinal projections in the rat. *Neurosci. Lett. 3*: 179–184, 1976.
54. Hancock, M. B. and C. A. Peveto, A preganglionic autonomic nucleus in the dorsal gray commissure of the lumbar spinal cord of the rat. *J. Comp. Neurol. 183*: 65–72, 1979.
55. Hanna, B. D., F. Lioy, C. Polosa, Role of carotid and central chemoreceptors in the CO_2 response of sympathetic preganglionic neurons. *J. Autonom. Nerv. Sys. 3*: 421–435, 1981.
56. Head, H. and G. Riddock, The autonomic bladder, excessive sweating, and some other reflex conditions in gross injuries of the spinal cord. *Brain 40*: 188–263, 1917.

57. Henry, J. L. and F. R. Calaresu, Topography and numerical distribution of neurons of the thoraco-lumbar intermediolateral nucleus in the cat. *J. Comp. Neurol. 144*: 205–214, 1972.
58. Henry, J. L. and F. R. Calaresu, Excitatory and inhibitory inputs from medullary nuclei projecting to spinal cardioacceleratory neurons in the cat. *Exp. Brain Res. 20*: 485–504, 1974.
59. Henry, J. L. and F. R. Calaresu, Pathways from medullary nuclei to spinal cardioacceleratory neurons in the cat. *Exp. Brain Res. 20*: 505–514, 1974.
60. Henry, J. L. and F. R. Calaresu, Origin and course of crossed medullary pathways to spinal sympathetic neurons in the cat. *Exp. Brain Res. 20*: 515–526, 1974.
61. Holstege, G., H. G. J. M. Kuypers, R. C. Boer, Anatomical evidence for direct brain stem projections to the somatic motoneuronal cell groups and autonomic preganglionic cell groups in cat spinal cord. *Brain Res. 171*: 329–333, 1969.
62. Horeyseck, G., W. Janig, F. Kirchner, V. Thamer, Activation and inhibition of muscle and cutaneous postganglionic neurones to hindlimb during hypothalamically induced vasoconstriction and atropine-sensitive vasodilation. *Pfluegers Arch. 361*: 231–240, 1976.
63. Illert, M. and M. Gabriel, Descending pathways in the cervical cord of cats affecting blood pressure and sympathetic activity. *Pfluegers Arch. 335*: 109–124, 1972.
64. Illert, M. and H. Seller, A descending sympathoinhibitory tract in the ventrolateral column of the cat. *Pfluegers Arch. 313*: 343–360, 1969.
65. Jänig, W., A. Sato, R. F. Schmidt, Reflexes in postganglionic cutaneous fibres by stimulation of group I to group IV somatic afferents. *Pfluegers Arch. 331*: 244–256, 1972.
66. Jänig, W., and R. F. Schmidt, Single unit responses in the cervical sympathetic trunk upon somatic nerve stimulation. *Pfluegers Arch. 314*: 199–216, 1970.
67. Jänig, W., and P. Szulczyk, Functional properties of lumbar preganglionic neurones. *Brain Res. 186*: 115–131, 1980.
68. Kerr, F. W. and S. Alexander, Descending autonomic pathways in the spinal cord. *Arch. Neurol. 10*: 249–261, 1964.
69. Kirchner, F., D. Kirchner, C. Polosa, Spinal organization of sympathetic inhibition by spinal afferent volleys. *Brain Res. 87*: 161–170, 1975.
70. Kirchner, F., I. Wyszogrodski, C. Polosa, Some properties of sympathetic neuron inhibition by depressor area and intraspinal stimulation. *Pfluegers Arch. 357*: 349–360, 1975.
71. Koizumi, K. and C. McC. Brooks, The integration of autonomic system reactions: A discussion of autonomic reflexes, their control and their association with somatic reactions. *Ergebnisse der Physiologie 67*: 1–68, 1972.
72. Koizumi, K., and A. Sato, Reflex activity of single sympathetic fibres to skeletal muscle produced by electrical stimulation of somatic and vago-depressor afferent nerves in the cat. *Pfluegers Arch. 332*: 283–301, 1972.
73. Kozelka, J. W., J. M. Chung, R. D. Wurster, Ascending spinal pathways mediating somato-cardiovascular reflexes. *J. Autonom. Nerv. Sys. 3*: 171–175, 1981.
74. Kuo, D. C., D. S. Yamasaki, G. M. Krauthamer, Segmental organization of sympathetic neurone of the splanchnic nerve as revealed by retrograde transport of horseradish peroxidase. *Neurosci. Lett. 17*: 11–16, 1980.
75. Lebedev, V. P., V. I. Petrov, V. A. Skobelev, Do sympathetic preganglionic neurones have a recurrent inhibitory mechanism? *Pfluegers Arch. 383*: 91–97, 1980.

76. Lebedev, V. P., A. V. Syromiatnikov, V. I. Skok, The convergence of sympathetic preganglionic fibres on vasomotor neurones of the ganglia in lumbar sympathetic chain. *Neurosci. Lett. 4*: 243–247, 1977.
77. Loewy, A. D., Descending pathways to sympathetic and parasympathetic preganglionic neurons. *J. Autonom. Nerv. Sys. 3*: 265–275, 1981.
78. Loewy, A. D. and H. Burton, Nuclei of the solitary tract: efferent connections to the lower brain stem and spinal cord of the cat. *J. Comp. Neurol. 181*: 421–450, 1978.
79. Loewy, A. D., and S. McKellar, The neuroanatomical basis of central cardiovascular control. *Fed. Proc. 39*: 2495–2503, 1980.
80. Loewy, A. D. and S. McKellar, Serotonergic projections from the ventral medulla to the intermediolateral cell column in the rat. *Brain Res. 211*: 146–152, 1981.
81. Loewy, A. D., S. McKellar, C. B. Saper, Direct projections from the A5 catecholamine cell group to the intermediolateral cell column. *Brain Res. 174*: 309–314, 1979.
82. Loewy, A. D. and J. J. Neil, The role of descending monoaminergic systems in central control of blood pressure. *Fed. Proc. 40*: 2778–2785, 1981.
83. Loewy, A. D., J. H. Wallach, S. McKellar, Efferent connections of the ventral medulla oblongata in the rat. *Brain Res. Rev. 3*: 63–80, 1981.
84. Malliani, A., F. Lombardi, M. Pagani, G. Recordati, P. J. Schwartz, Spinal cardiovascular reflexes. *Brain Res. 87*: 239–246, 1975.
85. Malliani, A., M. Parks, R. P. Tuckett, A. M. Brown, Reflex increases in heart rate elicited by stimulation of afferent cardiac sympathetic nerve fibers in the cat. *Circ. Res. 32*: 9–14, 1973.
86. Mannard, A. and C. Polosa, Analysis of background firing of single sympathetic preganglionic neurons of cat cervical nerve. *J. Neurophysiol. 36*: 398–408, 1973.
87. Mannard, A., P. Rajchgot, C. Polosa, Effect of post-impulse depression on background firing of sympathetic preganglionic neurons. *Brain Res. 126*: 243–261, 1977.
88. Martin, G. F., A. O. Humbertson, C. Laxson, W. M. Panneton, Evidence for direct bulbospinal projections to laminae IX, X, and the intermediolateral cell column. Studies using axonal transport techniques in the North American opossum. *Brain Res. 170*: 165–171, 1979.
89. McCall, R. B. and G. L. Gebber, Brain stem and spinal synchronization of sympathetic nervous discharge. *Brain Res. 89*: 139–143, 1975.
90. McCall, R. B., G. L. Gebber, S. M. Barman, Spinal interneurons in the baroreceptor reflex arc. *Am. J. Physiol. 232*: H657–H665, 1977.
91. McLachlan, E. M. and G. D. S. Hirst, Some properties of preganglionic neurons in upper thoracic spinal cord of the cat. *J. Neurophysiol. 43*: 1251–1265, 1980.
92. Norris, J. E., R. D. Foreman, R. D. Wurster, Responses of the canine heart to stimulation of the first five ventral thoracic roots. *Am. J. Physiol. 227*: 9–12, 1974.
93. Oldfield, B. J. and E. M. McLachlan, The segmental origin of preganglionic axons in the upper thoracic rami of the cat. *Neurosci. Lett. 18*: 11–17, 1980.
94. Pagani, M., P. J. Schwartz, R. Banks, F. Lombardi, A. Malliani, Reflex responses of sympathetic preganglionic neurones initiated by different cardiovascular receptors in spinal animals. *Brain Res. 68*: 215–225, 1974.
95. Petras, J. M. and J. F. Cummings, Autonomic neurons in the spinal cord of the Rhesus monkey: a correlation of the findings of cytoarchitectonics and sympa-

thectomy with fiber degeneration following dorsal rhizotomy. *J. Comp. Neurol.* *146*: 189–218, 1972.
96. Petras, J. M. and A. I. Faden, The origin of sympathetic preganglionic neurons in the dog. *Brain Res.* *144*: 353–357, 1978.
97. Polosa, C., The silent period of sympathetic preganglionic neurons. *Can. J. Physiol. Pharmacol.* *45*: 1033–1045, 1967.
98. Polosa, C., Spontaneous activity of sympathetic preganglionic neurons. *Can. J. Physiol. Pharmacol.* *46*: 887–896, 1968.
99. Preiss, G., F. Kirchner, C. Polosa, Patterning of sympathetic preganglionic neuron firing by the central respiratory drive. *Brain Res.* *87*: 363–374, 1975.
100. Preiss, G. and C. Polosa, Patterns of sympathetic neuron activity associated with Mayer waves. *Am. J. Physiol.* *226*: 724–730, 1974.
101. Preiss, G. and C. Polosa, The relation between end-tidal CO_2 and discharge patterns of sympathetic preganglionic neurons. *Brain Res.* *122*: 255–267, 1977.
102. Ranson, S. W. and P. R. Billingsley, The thoracic truncus sympathicus, rami communicantes and splanchnic nerves in the cat. *J. Comp. Neurol.* *29*: 405–439, 1918.
103. Rethelyi, M., Cell and neuropil architecture of the intermediolateral (sympathetic) nucleus of cat spinal cord. *Brain Res.* *46*: 203–213, 1972.
104. Rethelyi, M., Spinal transmission of autonomic processes. *J. Neural Trans. Suppl.* *11*: 195–212, 1974.
105. Ross, C. A., D. A. Ruggiers, D. J. Reis, Projections to the spinal cord from neurons close to the ventral surface of the hindbrain in the rat. *Neurosci. Lett.* *21*: 143–148, 1981.
106. Rubin, E. and D. Purves, Segmental organization of sympathetic preganglionic neurons in the mammalian spinal cord. *J. Comp. Neurol.* *192*: 163–174, 1980.
107. Saper, C. B., A. D. Loewy, L. W. Swanson, W. M. Cowan, Direct hypothalamo-autonomic connections. *Brain Res.* *117*: 305–312, 1976.
108. Saper, C. B. and A. D. Loewy, Efferent connections of the parabrachial nucleus in the rat. *Brain Res.* *197*: 291–317, 1980.
109. Sato, A., Relative involvement of different reflex pathways in somato-sympathetic reflexes, analyzed in spontaneously active single preganglionic sympathetic units. *Pfluegers Arch.* *333*: 70–81, 1972.
110. Sato, A., and R. F. Schmidt, Somatosympathetic reflexes: Afferent fibers, central pathways, discharge characteristics. *Physiol. Rev.* *53*: 916–947, 1973.
111. Schramm, L. P., J. R. Adair, J. M. Stribling, L. P. Gray, Preganglionic innervation of the adrenal gland of the rat: a study using horseradish peroxidase. *Exp. Neurol.* *49*: 540–553, 1975.
112. Seller, H., The discharge pattern of single units in thoracic and lumbar white rami in relation to cardiovascular events. *Pfluegers Arch.* *343*: 317–330, 1973.
113. Sherrington, C. S., *The Integrative Action of the Nervous System.* Yale University Press, New Haven, 1906.
114. Skok, V. I. and S. S. Heerog, Synaptic delay in superior cervical ganglion of the cat. *Brain Res.* *87*: 343–353, 1975.
115. Smirnov, K. A. and S. L. Potekhina, On localization of the descending vaso-motor pathways in the spinal cord. *Sechenov Physiol. J., U.S.S.R.* *58*: 871–875, 1972.
116. Smith, O. A., Anatomy of central neural pathways mediating cardiovascular functions. In *Nervous Control of the Heart,* Ed. W. C. Randall. Baltimore, Williams and Wilkins, 1965, pp. 34–53.

117. Snyder, D. W. and G. L. Gebber, Relationships between medullary depressor region and central vasopressor pathways. *Am. J. Physiol. 225*: 1129–1137, 1973.
118. Szulczyk, P., Descending spinal sympathetic pathway utilized by somato-sympathetic reflex and carotid chemoreflex. *Brain Res. 112*: 190–193, 1976.
119. Taylor, D. G. and M. J. Brody, Spinal adrenergic mechanisms regulating sympathetic outflow to blood vessels. *Circ. Res. 38(Suppl. II)*: II 10–II 20, 1976.
120. Taylor, D. G. and G. L. Gebber, Sympathetic unit responses to stimulation of the cat medulla. *Am. J. Physiol. 225*: 1138–1146, 1973.
121. Taylor, D. G. and G. L. Gebber, Baroreceptor mechanisms controlling sympathetic nervous rhythms of central origin. *Am. J. Physiol. 228*: 1002–1013, 1975.
122. Wurster, R. D., Spinal sympathetic control of the heart. In *Neural Regulation of the Heart,* ed. by W. C. Randall. Oxford Univ. Press, New York, 1977, pp. 212–246.
123. Wurster, R. D. and W. C. Randall, Cardiovascular responses to bladder distention in patients with spinal transection. *Am. J. Physiol. 228*: 1288–1292, 1979.
124. Wyszogrodski, I. and C. Polosa, The inhibition of sympathetic preganglionic neurons by somatic afferents. *Can. J. Physiol. Pharmacol. 51*: 29–38, 1973.

15

Brainstem Systems Involved in Cardiovascular Regulation

GERARD L. GEBBER

In a remarkable chapter of a predecessor to this book, published in 1965, Peiss [57] outlined many of the problems in understanding the central systems involved in cardiovascular regulation that existed at that time. The anatomic limits of those systems had not been precisely defined, nor in fact was there firm evidence of a neuroanatomic substrate specifically related to cardiovascular control. The origins of bulbospinal sympathetic pathways and preganglionic cardiac vagal neurons were, for the most part, matters of speculation rather than investigation. There was considerable debate as to whether or not the central vasomotor system consisted of a number of independently functioning parallel pathways. No one had yet recorded with confidence from individual brainstem or hypothalamic "sympathetic" neurons. Thus, it was possible only to speculate on the mechanisms involved in generating the basal discharges in sympathetic nerves. The relative roles played by the brainstem and suprabulbar structures such as the hypothalamus in generating these discharges were unclear. Finally, the level(s) of the neuraxis at which the baroreceptor reflexes exerted their influence on sympathetic nerve discharge (SND) was hotly debated.

Peiss' chapter was remarkable in that it accurately predicted the general course of research on central cardiovascular control mechanisms for the next 17 years. Although much remains to be learned, it can be stated with assurance that a number of important breakthroughs have been made during this period. The purpose of this chapter is to describe these breakthroughs and to look toward the future.

HISTORICAL OVERVIEW

The role of the brain in regulating cardiovascular function was first recognized when Bernard [10] demonstrated that transection of the cervical spinal cord led

The research from the author's laboratory contained within this chapter was sponsored by the National Heart and Lung Institute (Grant HL-13187).

to a pronounced fall in blood pressure which was sustained throughout the course of an acute experiment. By implication, it was concluded that supraspinal neural networks were primarily responsible for generating basal autonomic tone to the heart and vasculature.

In the early 1870's, Dittmar [21] and Owsjannikow [56] undertook studies aimed at defining those regions of the brain responsible for basal autonomic tone. Their approach was to study the effects on blood pressure produced by serial transection of the brainstem in the rabbit. Transection of the neuraxis above the caudal third of the pons produced little or no change in blood pressure. From this result, Dittmar and Owsjannikow concluded that the forebrain was not intimately involved in maintaining the resting level of blood pressure. As will be discussed subsequently, our views on this subject have changed. Transections made more caudally revealed that the background discharges in sympathetic nerves arise primarily from networks located in the caudal third of the pons and rostral two-thirds of the medulla (i.e. between sections A and C in Fig. 15-1). This point was demonstrated directly with recordings made from the cervical and inferior cardiac sympathetic nerves of the cat in a later study by Alexander [2].

As an extension of the studies described above, Ranson and Billingsley [60] began an investigation of the location of cardiovascular reactive sites in the brainstem of the cat. They found two discrete areas on the dorsal surface of the medulla (i.e. floor of fourth ventricle) from which blood pressure could be changed with electrical stimulation. A decrease in blood pressure (later shown to result from inhibition of sympathetic nerve traffic) could be elicited from a medial medullary point near the obex. An increase in blood pressure was produced by stimulation of an area somewhat lateral and rostral to the depressor site. Although Ranson and Billingsley were careful not to attribute their results to the activation of functionally discrete and anatomically circumscribed "centers," others were not so cautious in their interpretations. Thus, the misconception of discrete centers for generation and control of basal autonomic tone arose. The pendulum swung to the opposite extreme in 1939 when Wang and Ranson [75] reexplored the brainstem for cardiovascular reactive sites. The depths, as well as the dorsal surface, of the brainstem were electrically stimulated in this study. As shown in Fig. 15-1B, the pressor and depressor points found earlier on the dorsal surface of the medulla by Ranson and Billingsley [60] were not anatomically circumscribed centers but rather the apexes of two "triangles" that extended almost to the ventral surface of the brainstem through the reticular formation. Decreases in blood pressure were produced most often by stimulation of the medial reticular formation. Increases in blood pressure usually were elicited by stimulation of the periventricular gray and lateral reticular formation. These results were thought to indicate that the background discharges in sympathetic nerves were randomly generated within a diffusely interconnected network of brainstem reticular neurons. This concept, as well, is outmoded. As will be discussed subsequently, the brainstem sympathetic generator is complexly organized and inherently capable of synchronizing the discharges of populations of bulbospinal neurons in a periodic fashion. That is, the brainstem

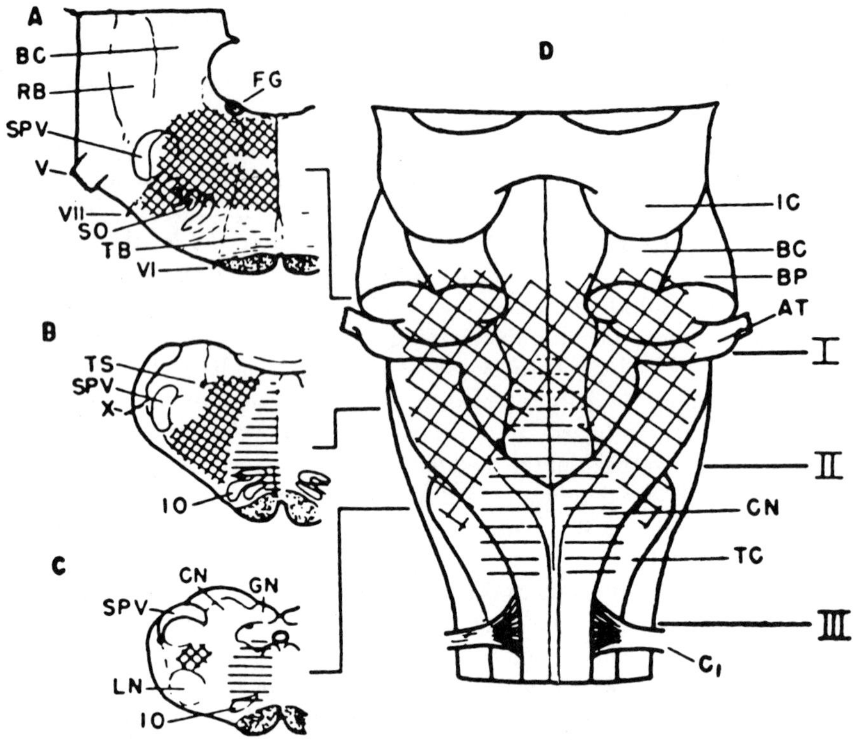

Fig. 15-1. Pressor and depressor regions of brainstem of cat. Pressor region indicated by crosshatching, depressor region by horizontal ruling. (A-C) Frontal sections through medulla at levels indicated by guidelines to D. (D) Pressor and depressor regions projected onto dorsal surface of brainstem. I, II, and III in D are levels of transection discussed by Alexander [2]. AT, auditory tubercle; BC, brachium conjunctiva; BP, brachium pontis; C_1, first cervical nerve; CN, cuneate nucleus; FG, facial genu; GN, gracilis nucleus; IC, inferior colliculus; IO, inferior olivary nucleus; LN, lateral reticular nucleus; RB, restiform body; SO, superior olivary nucleus; SPV, spinal trigeminal tract; TB, trapezoid body; TC, tuberculum cinereum; TS, tractus solitarius; V, VI, and VII, corresponding cranial nerves. (Reproduced through courtesy of *J. Neurophysiol.* 9: 205–217, 1946)

sympathetic network can be viewed as a rhythm generator containing recurrent and reciprocal feedback loops, and perhaps reexcitant pathways.

LOCATION OF BULBOSPINAL SYMPATHETIC NEURONS AND CARDIAC VAGAL PREGANGLIONIC NEURONS

The advent of autoradiographic and retrograde transport techniques, and the use of antidromic stimulation to locate central neurons whose axons project to distant sites have allowed a number of laboratories to define some of the nuclei of origin of bulbospinal sympathetic neurons (see reviews by Calaresu et al. [13] and Loewy [44]) and cardiac vagal preganglionic neurons [14,31,32,47–49,67].

Bulbospinal Sympathetic Pathways. Brainstem regions which contain the somata of bulbospinal sympathetic neurons are shown in Fig. 15-2. The spinal intermediolateral nucleus (IML) which contains preganglionic sympathetic neurons receives serotonergic inputs directly from the caudal raphe nuclei of the pons and medulla (i.e. magnus, obscurus, and pallidus), a norepinephrine

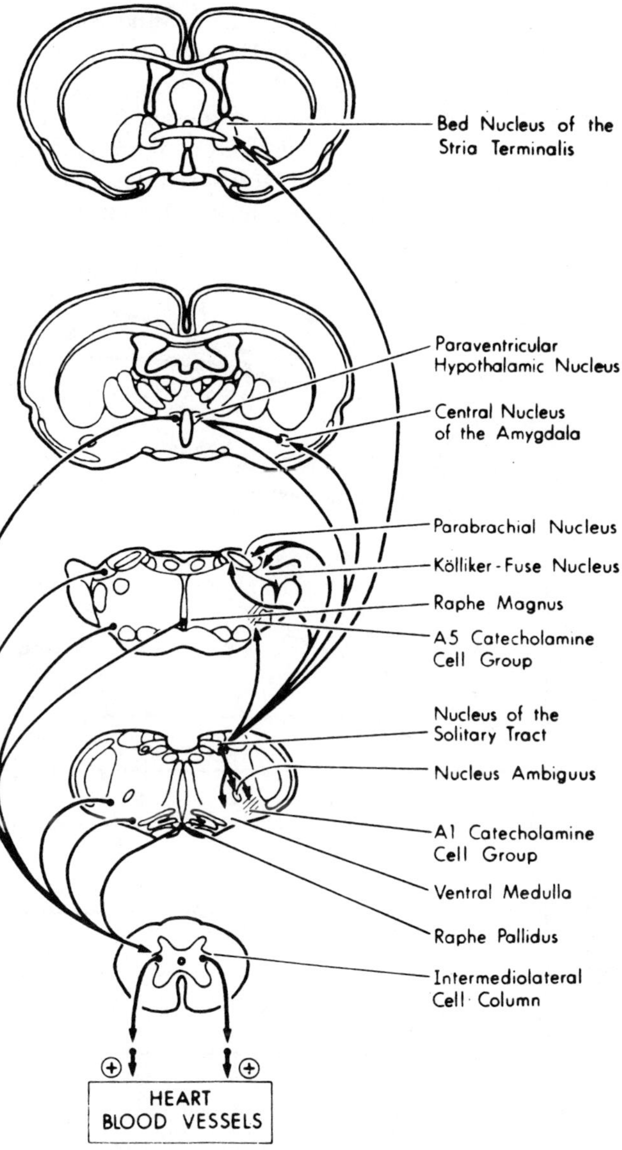

Fig. 15-2. Schematic showing some of the efferent connections of NTS as well as brainstem and hypothalamic regions which directly innervate the spinal IML. See text for description. (Reproduced through courtesy of *J. Autonom. Nerv. Sys.* 3: 265–275, 1981)

input from the A5 cell group in the pons, and an epinephrine input from the C1 cell group in the medulla. Additional brainstem regions containing neurons whose axons project to IML include the nucleus of the tractus solitarius (NTS), chemosensitive ventral medullary surface, and the Kölliker-Fuse nucleus of the pons. Neurons of the paraventricular hypothalamic nucleus also project to IML in the spinal cord. That at least some of these parallel bulbospinal pathways converge onto the same preganglionic sympathetic neurons in IML has been demonstrated by Taylor and Gebber [70]. They showed that individual preganglionic neurons in the upper thoracic IML of the cat exhibited two distinct response patterns to electrical stimulation of pressor sites in the lateral hypothalamus, medulla, and dorsolateral funiculus of the cervical spinal cord—a short latency response which could not be blocked during baroreceptor reflex activation, and a longer latency response which was sensitive to blockade by the baroreceptor reflexes.

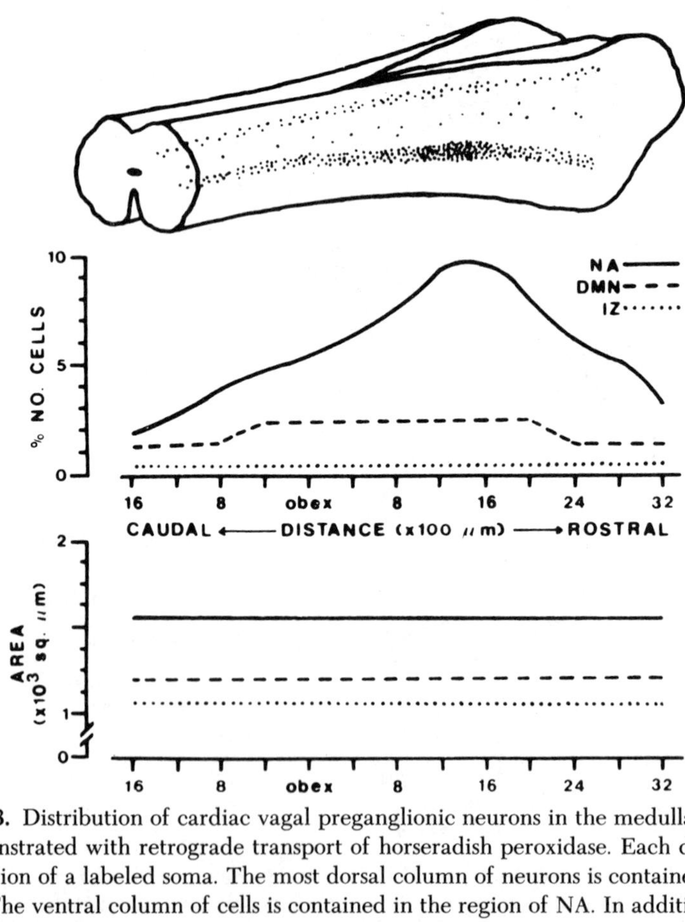

Fig. 15-3. Distribution of cardiac vagal preganglionic neurons in the medulla of a cat as demonstrated with retrograde transport of horseradish peroxidase. Each dot shows the location of a labeled soma. The most dorsal column of neurons is contained within DMN. The ventral column of cells is contained in the region of NA. In addition, some cells are labeled in an intermediate zone (IZ) located between DMN and NA. Graphs show the longitudinal and size distribution of labeled somata. (Reproduced through courtesy of *J. Autonom. Nerv. Sys.* 3: 437–450, 1981)

Cardiac Vagal Preganglionic Neurons. Brainstem regions of origin of cardiac vagal preganglionic neurons are shown in Fig. 15-3. The map is based on the results obtained by Geis et al. [31,32] with retrograde transport of horseradish peroxidase injected into the cat heart. Only the right vagus was intact in their experiments. Somata of cardiac vagal preganglionic neurons were located ipsilateral to the right vagus in the dorsal motor nucleus of nerve X (DMN), nucleus ambiguus (NA), and an intermediate zone between DMN and NA. The NA contained 72% of the total number of cell bodies while 19% were found in the DMN. The results obtained with retrograde transport of horseradish peroxidase are somewhat at odds with those obtained by McAllen and Spyer [47] using the technique of antidromic stimulation. These workers were able to antidromically activate cardiac vagal preganglionic neurons in NA, but not in DMN with shocks applied to the thoracic cardiac vagal nerves. More recently, however, Ciriello and Calaresu [14] have been successful in antidromically activating neurons in NA, DMN, and the intermediate zone with shocks applied to the cardiac vagal branches of the cat thoracic vagus. In addition, they reported antidromic activation of some neurons in the NTS. Thus, there is both anatomic and electrophysiologic data which support the concept of parallel cardiac vagal pathways. That such pathways are organized according to physiological function is strongly indicated by the work of Geis et al. [31]. These workers found that electrical stimulation of NA decreased heart rate but had no direct effect on ventricular contractile force. In contrast, stimulation of DMN led to a decrease in the force of ventricular contraction, but did not change heart rate. Their experiments were performed on cats subjected to beta-adrenergic blockade.

Whereas investigations employing transport techniques and antidromic activation have increased our knowledge of autonomic representation in the brainstem, the reader surely will recognize that such studies fail to provide information on a number of important questions. First, which of the parallel pathways (both sympathetic and cardiac vagal) participate in generating the basal discharges in autonomic nerves? Second, which bulbospinal sympathetic pathways subserve excitatory function and which subserve inhibitory functon? Third, how are the interneuronal circuits which control the activity of bulbospinal sympathetic neurons and cardiac vagal preganglionic neurons organized? As discussed in the following section, some inroads have been made in answering these questions.

BASAL AUTONOMIC TONE

Sympathetic Tone

One of the least understood aspects of autonomic neurophysiology concerns the manner in which the basal discharges in sympathetic nerves are generated. Our laboratory has approached this problem by studying the neural circuitry involved in generating the 2–6 cps rhythm (normally entrained to the cardiac cycle by the baroreceptor reflexes) in SND of the cat. The 2–6 cps rhythm is ubiquitous to SND under a wide variety of experimental conditions including hypocapnia, asphyxia, and extremes of body temperature. As shown in Fig. 15-

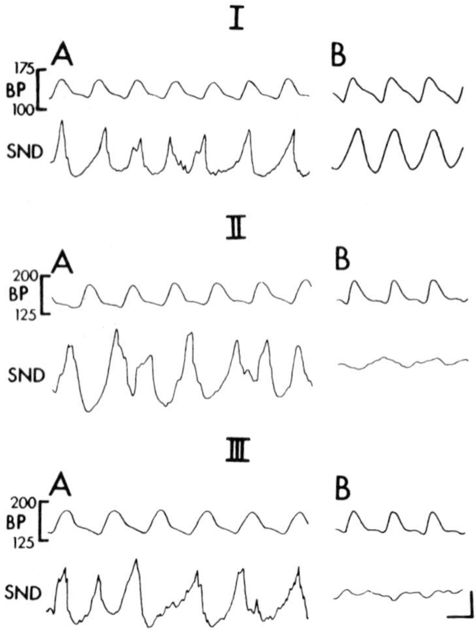

Fig. 15-4. Characteristics of splanchnic SND before and after baroreceptor denervation and after midcollicular decerebration. I. Baroreceptor reflexes intact. (A) oscilloscopic records of blood pressure in mm Hg (top) and splanchnic SND (bottom). Negativity is recorded an an upward deflection in this and subsequent figures. (B) R wave-triggered computer averaged records (64 trials). Sequence of traces same as in A. Address bin is 1 msec. II. Same but after baroreceptor denervation. R wave-triggered average of SND is essentially flat due to disruption of phase relations between 2–6 cps slow wave and the cardiac cycle. III. Same, but after midcollicular decerebration. Note the persistence of 2–6 cps slow waves in SND. Horizontal calibration is 200 msec. Vertical calibration is 100 μV for SND. (Reproduced through courtesy of *Am. J. Physiol. 239* (*Regulatory Integrative Comp. Physiol. 8*): R42-R47, 1980)

4, the rhythm persists in SND after baroreceptor denervation [5,25,26,71] and is not eliminated by decerebration at the midcollicular level [5]. The 2–6 cps rhythm in SND, however, is eliminated by acute transection of the neuraxis at the medullospinal junction [50]. From these results, we have suggested that the ubiquitous 2–6 cps rhythm is representative of the fundamental organization of the brainstem sympathetic generator [5,25]. If this assumption is accepted, it becomes important to determine how the rhythm (and, thus, a significant proportion of the basal discharges in sympathetic nerves) is generated.

Several possibilities arise concerning the mechanisms responsible for the 2–6 cps rhythm in SND. It might be generated by a group of brainstem neurons with inherent pacemaker activity. Alternatively, the rhythm might arise as the consequence of network interactions. For instance, the rising phase of the 2–6 cps burst of SND (recorded as as a slow wave using a wide preamplifier bandpass) might result from the synchronous discharges of one group of brainstem neurons while the falling phase might be due to active inhibition produced by the synchronous discharges of a second group of brainstem neurons. Such neuronal networks might interact directly to form a rhythm generator. Additional neuronal networks might be involved in switching from the excitatory to the inhibitory (and vice versa) phase of SND. Consideration of these possibilities requires the identification of those neuronal types which comprise the brainstem sympathetic generator. We have approached this problem by using the method of spike-triggered averaging [6,7,26,55]. That is, the spikes of single brainstem neurons (recorded extracellularly with metal microelectrodes) are used to trigger the computation of an average of accompanying changes in the activity of a sympathetic nerve bundle (usually the inferior cardiac postganglionic sympathetic nerve). This method has allowed us to locate single neurons in the dorsolateral medullary reticular formation [6] and caudal raphe nuclei [55] with naturally occurring discharges which are synchronized to the cardiac-related rhythm in SND.

A problem arises in distinguishing which brainstem neurons with cardiac-related activity are actually contained in networks responsible for basal SND. Progress is impeded by the fact that a number of functionally distinct brainstem systems share baroreceptor input. For instance, the baroreceptor reflexes influence cortical activity [9], respiratory function [63,], and somatomotor reflexes [20] in addition to autonomic nerve activity. Thus, the cardiac-related rhythm in SND might be temporally related to that in the discharges of a number of functionally distinct brainstem neurons. We have approached this problem by searching the brainstem for neurons with sympathetic nerve-related activity in baroreceptor-denervated cats [7,26,55]. This approach has enabled us to locate brainstem neurons with 2–6 cps activity locked to that in inferior cardiac SND, but not to the cardiac cycle. Such neurons (located in dorsolateral medullary reticular formation and caudal raphe nuclei) fall into two categories—those with activity locked to the rising phase of the 2–6 cps slow wave in SND and those whose discharges are locked to the falling phase of inferior cardiac sympathetic nerve activity. An example of a spike-triggered average of SND for a unit whose discharges were locked to a point early on the rising phase of the slow wave is shown in Fig. 15-5. In this case, midsignal spike-triggered averaging was employed. The average of SND is constructed from data acquired prior to as well as after the discharge of the brainstem unit (A). The occurrence of the unit spike is at time 0 in the average of SND. The portion of the average to the left of time 0 is for inferior cardiac nerve activity which preceded unit spike occurrence, while that to the right of time 0 is for SND which followed unit discharge. The average of SND in panel A contains a rhythmic component in the 2–6 cps range both in activity which preceded and followed the midsignal spike trigger. The period of this rhythm was the same as that in the autocorrelograms of the discharges of the brainstem unit (B) and inferior cardiac nerve (C). Identical periodicities in the autocorrelograms and spike-triggered

354

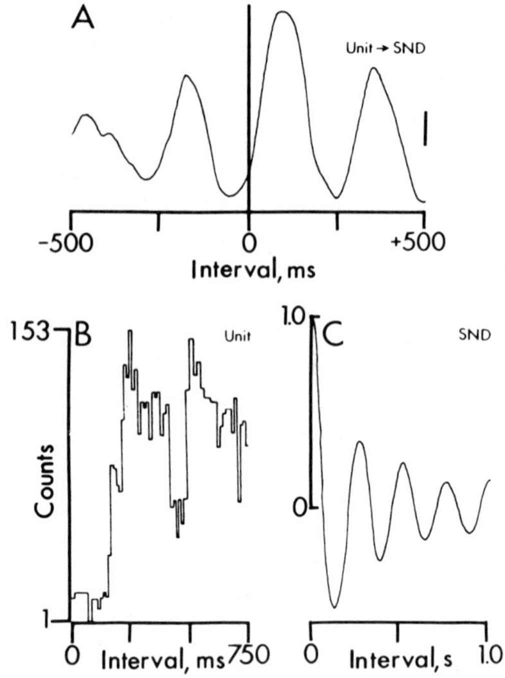

Fig. 15-5. Relationship between the discharges of a brainstem neuron and inferior cardiac nerve activity in a baroreceptor-denervated cat. (A) Midsignal spike-triggered average of inferior cardiac SND (1200 trials). Unit spike occurrence is at zero lag. Address bin is 1 msec. Vertical calibration is 5 μV. (B) Autocorrelogram of unit discharges. Address bin is 12 msec. Analysis based on 2432 spikes. (C) Autocorrelogram of inferior cardiac SND. Analysis time was 40 sec. Address bin is 10 msec. (Reproduced through courtesy of *Am. J. Physiol. 240 (Regulatory Integrative Comp. Physiol. 9)*: R348-R355, 1981)

average clearly indicate that the 2–6 cps rhythms in unit and inferior cardiac nerve activity were locked to each other. Thus, it seems reasonable to assume that such neurons either were contained in or received inputs from the brainstem oscillator responsible for the 2–6 cps rhythm in SND of the baroreceptor-denervated cat.

Although our results in baroreceptor-denervated cats were encouraging, we were still left with the problem of how to identify elements of the brainstem sympathetic network under more natural circumstances, i.e. when the baroreceptor homeostatic reflex mechanism is not interrupted. With this purpose in mind, we developed a test which allowed us to distinguish brainstem sympathetic neurons in the baroreceptor-innervated cat from other neuronal types which also exhibit a cardiac-related discharge pattern. The test is based on the fact that it is possible to shift the phase relations between the pulse synchronous components of baroreceptor nerve activity and the SND by changing heart rate with ventricular pacing [24]. Thus, it was reasoned that the temporal relations between brainstem sympathetic unit activity and the discharges of peripheral sympathetic nerves should not be affected during changes in heart rate which shift the phase relations between baroreceptor and sympathetic nerve activity. As a corollary, we predicted that the temporal relations between SND and the discharges of other types of brainstem neurons exhibiting cardiac-related activity (such as interneurons in the afferent limb of the baroreceptor reflex arc) should be altered during changes in heart rate. As detailed in our recent study [55], we were successful in distinguishing such neuronal types.

Identification of those cell types which comprise the brainstem sympathetic network is only the first step in understanding how the 2–6 cps rhythm is generated. The second step is to define the network interactions which underlie the genesis of oscillatory activity, and thus a major component of the basal discharges in sympathetic nerves. The phenomena which require explanation include: (1) synchronization of the discharges of those neurons responsible for the rising (i.e. excitatory) phase of the 2–6 cps sympathetic nerve slow wave, (2) synchronization of activity of those neurons responsible for the falling (i.e. inhibitory) phase of the slow wave, and (3) switching from the excitatory to the inhibitory phase and vice versa. We have recently begun to study the underlying mechanisms responsible for these phenomena using crosscorrelation analysis to examine the short-term interactions (millisecond time scale) between brainstem sympathetic neurons. Neuronal interactions which occur on a short time scale (indicative of mono- and/or oligosynaptic connections) ultimately result in periodic firing of sympathetic nerves on a longer time scale (hundreds of milliseconds in the case of 2–6 cps rhythm).

A working model of those brainstem circuits involved in the genesis of the 2–6 cps rhythm in SND and its entrainment to the cardiac cycle by the baroreceptor reflexes is shown in Fig. 15-6. Unit types are as defined in experiments in which spike-triggered averaging and post-R wave interval analysis were used to identify brainstem sympathetic neurons. The unit types are:

S_eR neurons. Units with cardiac-realted activity whose discharges are synchronized to a point on the rising phase of the 2–6 cps slow wave in SND.
S_iR neurons. Same as above, except that unit discharge is synchronized to a point on the falling phase of the 2–6 cps slow wave SND.
SE neurons. Units with activity related to SND and which receive input from forebrain (FB) regions as evidenced by synchronization of their discharges to EEG rhythms. As discussed by Gebber and Barman [26], such neurons are believed to provide inputs to S_eR and S_iR neurons.
B neurons. Interneurons in afferent limb of the baroreceptor reflex arc. Unlike S_eR and S_iR units whose discharges remain locked to SND during shifts in phase relations between the pulse synchronous components of baroreceptor nerve activity and SND, the discharges of B neurons remain locked to the cycle of baroreceptor nerve activity.

Off-Switch neurons (O.S.). These neurons are unique in that they appear to receive activating inputs both from the baroreceptors and from elements of

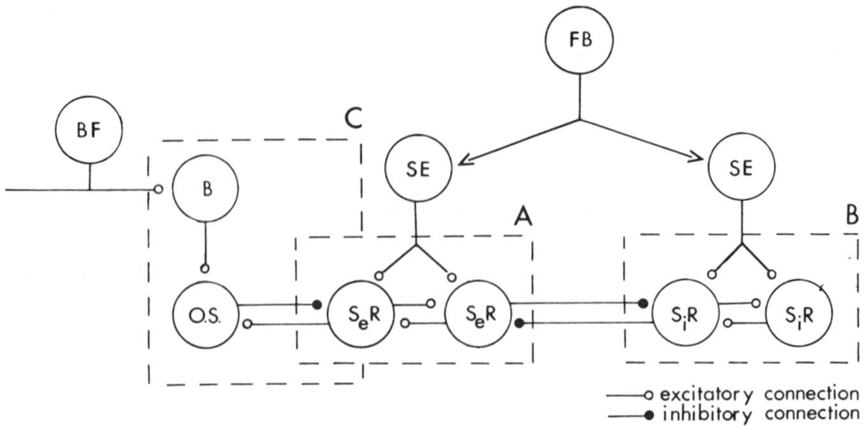

Fig. 15-6. Working model of brainstem sympathetic generator. B, interneuron in afferent limb of baroreceptor reflex; BF, baroreceptor fiber; FB, forebrain; O.S., Off-Switch neuron which may help to terminate the rising (i.e. excitatory) phase of 2–6 cps slow wave in SND; S_eR and S_iR, neurons with spontaneous activity related to SND and R wave of ECG. Discharges of S_eR neurons are synchronized to points on the rising phase of sympathetic nerve slow wave. Discharges of S_iR neurons are synchronized to points on the falling (i.e. inhibitory) phase of slow wave in SND. SE, units with activity related to SND and cortical rhythms; Circuit A, responsible for synchronization of discharges of S_eR units; Circuit B, responsible for synchronization of discharges of S_iR units; Circuit C contains a recurrent inhibitory loop which may be responsible for termination of excitatory phase of SND. Interactions between circuits A and B may also participate in switching from the rising to falling phase (and vice versa) of sympathetic nerve slow wave. Proposed neuronal interconnections are described in the text.

the efferent network responsible for the 2–6 cps rhythm in SND (Morrison and Gebber, unpublished observations). Such neurons may be contained in a recurrent inhibitory loop which acts to switch the phase of SND from excitation to inhibition.

The model contains a number of hypothetical circuits that are currently being scrutinized using unit → unit crosscorrelation analysis. Circuit A is for the synchronization of the discharges of S_eR neurons in order to form the rising phase of the 2–6 cps slow wave in SND. Synchronization might occur via direct excitatory synaptic connections between S_eR neurons (one-way or reciprocal) and/or via the sharing of common input (perhaps from SE neurons). Circuit B is for the synchronization of the discharges of S_iR neurons responsible for the falling phase of SND. Potential mechanisms for synchronization in circuit B are the same as in circuit A. One-way or reciprocal inhibition between S_eR and S_iR neurons in circuits A and B are considered as possible mechanisms for phase switching as is the recurrent inhibitory loop in circuit C. The candidate for the Off-Switch neuron in circuit C is the type of unit that is excited both by baroreceptor input and by elements (presumably S_eR) of the sympathetic generator.

The discharge level of these neurons gradually increases during the development of the rising phase of the sympathetic nerve slow wave, presumably due to excitatory input from S_eR neurons. S_eR unit discharge is terminated when O.S. unit activity reaches a critically high level. Baroreceptor inputs also excite the O.S. neuron, and thus may influence the timing of S_eR unit cutoff (i.e. phase switching). Regarding this point, the duration of the rising phase of the sympathetic nerve slow wave is prolonged when the interval between successive baroreceptor nerve cycles is lengthened by slowing ventricular rate [55]. The reader surely will recognize that the recurrent inhibitory loop in circuit C is analogous to that which has been postulated [16] to play a role in inspiratory cutoff (i.e. loop containing inspiratory neurons of the I_α and I_β type).

Periodicities in addition to or in place of the 2–6 cps rhythm (normally related in a 1:1 fashion to the cardiac cycle) may appear in the basal discharges of sympathetic nerves. A 10 cps rhythm which occasionally is locked in a 3:1 relation to the cardiac cycle in the baroreceptor-innervated cat has been reported by Cohen and Gootman [17] and Green and Heffron [34]. Subsequent work by McCall and Gebber [50] demonstrated a 10 cps periodic component in autocorrelograms of renal SND during asphyxia in cats with a transected spinal cord. Thus, it appears that spinal as well as brainstem sympathetic networks are inherently capable or rhythm generation.

The basal discharges of sympathetic nerves often exhibit a slow rhythmic component with the period of the respiratory cycle which is superimposed on the more rapid 2–6 cps rhythm. Part of the slow rhythm in SND arises from the inhibitory influence of pulmonary inflation afferents of the vagus nerve [18]. However, a strong respiratory-related periodicity persists in SND after bilateral vagotomy in paralyzed, pneumothoracotomized and artificially ventilated cats. This rhythm is generally assumed to be extrinsically imposed on the brainstem sympathetic generator by elements of the respiratory oscillator [17,40,58]. This view has been challenged by Barman and Gebber [3]. Their results support the hypothesis that the slow periodic components in SND and phrenic nerve activity of vagotomized cats are generated by independent brainstem oscillators normally coupled to each other. They noted that changes in respiratory rate (as monitored from the phrenic nerve in paralyzed, vagotomized, and artificially ventilated cats) were accompanied by dramatic shifts in the phase relations between phrenic and sympathetic nerve activity. Specifically, the level of SND was highest during inspriation at respiratory rates around 30 cycles/min. In contrast, SND was most prominent during expiration at respiratory rates around 20 cycles/min. These results make it difficult to accept the notion that the respiratory-related periodicity in SND is directly imposed on central sympathetic networks by elements of the brainstem respiratory oscillator. If such was the case, then the phase relations between phrenic and sympathetic nerve activity should have been independent of respiratory rate. The independent oscillators hypothesis is further supported by the observation that the slow periodic component in SND often persisted when the rhythmic discharge pattern of the phrenic nerve disappeared during hyperventilation [3]. This observation suggests that the neuronal types that comprise the slow sympathetic oscillator are less apt to lose their rhythmic discharge pattern during hyperventilation than are those neurons that comprise the respiratory oscillator. In summary, it appears that the central sympathetic generating system is organized into a number of hierarchically arranged oscillators located both in the brainstem and spinal cord.

Cardiac Vagal Tone

Although current concepts on the mechanisms responsible for basal SND remain, in large part, hypothetical in nature, even less is known about the origins of basal activity in cardiac vagal preganglionic neurons. The discharges of single cardiac vagal preganglionic neurons located in the region of NA [48,49,67] and of the thoracic cardiac vagal nerves [41–43] exhibit both cardiac- and respiratory-related rhythms. The traditional view for the origin of such activity is as follows. The dominant factor thought to be responsible for basal cardiac vagal activity is driving input of baroreceptor origin [41,42]. Baroreceptor drive is generally assumed to be mediated over a pathway containing synaptic stations in NTS and NA (see review by Spyer [67]). Peripheral chemoreceptor drive is also thought to participate in generating cardiac vagal tone under certain conditions. The respiratory-related rhythm in cardiac vagal discharge is believed to arise as the result of inhibitory influences mediated by the respiratory oscillator during inspiration [41,42]. Reciprocity of cardiac vagal and sympathetic nerve activity is believed to arise from opposing influences mediated by the baroreceptors and respiratory oscillator on the two systems. There is increasing evidence which suggests that the above described scheme is much too simple. First, Kollai and Koizumi [41] have demonstrated that, although decreased, cardiac vagal tone persists after all baro- and chemoreceptor inputs to the central nervous system are eliminated. Residual activity is synchronous with the respiration. Thus, cardiac vagal tone, to a degree, appears to be maintained via central mechanisms. Second, Kollai and Koizumi [41,42] have also shown that, under certain conditions, the cardiac vagal and sympathetic nerves may respond to reflex stimuli in a nonreciprocal fashion. Finally, the recent work of McAllen and Spyer [49] and Spyer [67] indicates that a simple disynaptic medullary circuit (baroreceptor afferent → NTS → NA) cannot account, under natural circumstances, for the pulse-related activity of cardiac vagal preganglionic neurons. These investigators found that the interval between the onsets of the pulse synchronous components of carotid sinus baroreceptor nerve activity (in the cat with sectioned aortic nerves) and of the discharges of antidromically identified cardiac vagal preganglionic neurons in NA could be as long as 100 msec. They argued that such an interval is much too long to be explained by transmission over a disynaptic medullary pathway as had been generally assumed to be the case. Thus, it is clear that the traditional view on the baroreceptor pathway responsible for cardiac vagal activation is outmoded.

BARORECEPTOR REFLEXES

There has been a significant expansion of our knowledge of the central neural mechanisms responsible for mediation and modulation of the baroreceptor reflexes over the past two decades. The immensity of the problem coupled with the various experimental approaches used to study the baroreceptor reflexes has prompted the author to divide this section into three subject areas. These are: (1) anatomical connections and input–output relationships of the NTS, (2) neuraxis levels of sympathoinhibition of baroreceptor reflex origin, and (3) modulation of the baroreceptor reflexes. A brief discussion of baroreceptor reflex control of the cardiac vagus has already been presented. The reader is referred to a recent review by Spyer [67] who has dealt with this aspect in great detail.

The primary site of termination of carotid sinus and aortic nerve baroreceptor afferents is the NTS which lies in the dorsal medulla (see Fig. 15-2). Specifically, such afferents appear to terminate in three regions of NTS: dorsal NTS, medial NTS, and commissural nucleus (see review by Loewy [44]). The efferent projections of the NTS have been studied with electrophysiological [11,12,37,53] and anatomic techniques [15,45,62]. As recently summarized by Loewy [44], the NTS projects to a number of regions involved in cardiovascular regulation. As shown in Fig. 15-2, four of these regions (paraventricular hypothalamic nucleus, Kölliker-Fuse nucleus, A5 catecholamine cell group, and chemosensitive ventral medullary surface) project directly to the spinal IML. Three regions (paraventricular hypothalamic nucleus, central amygdaloid nucleus, and A5 cell group) which receive input from NTS, in turn project to DMN of nerve X. In addition, NTS directly projects to the spinal IML and to NA.

Surprisingly few NTS neurons in the region of baroreceptor afferent termination exhibit the pulse synchronous discharge pattern characteristic of bararceptor afferents [37,51,52,54,68]. Rather, the majority of NTS neurons with cardiac-related activity exhibit a polymodal distribution of discharges in relation to the R wave of the ECG [51,52,68]. For instance, McCall et al. [51] showed that the post-R wave interval histograms of the discharges of individual NTS neurons exhibited as many as five distinct peaks within the cardiac cycle (Fig. 15-7). The timing of only the second peak in the unit histogram was clearly consistent with that of the pulse synchronous component of the discharges of myelinated baroreceptor fibers in the carotid sinus nerve, which in the cat begins approximately 70 msec after the R wave [24]. The earlier and later peaks were not of aortic baroreceptor or vagal origin since these nerves had been sectioned by McCall et al. [51]. The polymodal distribution of the discharges of such neurons during the cardiac cycle points to the complexity of synaptic arrangement within the medullary nucleus of baroreceptor fiber termination. Thus, it appears that NTS functions as an information processing "center" rather than as a simple relay station in the baroreceptor reflex arc. The intrinsic organization of baroreceptor circuits in NTS, however, remains a topic for future investigation.

The NTS is richly innervated by fibers containing a variety of putative transmitters. Currently, the two serious candidates for the synaptic transmitter

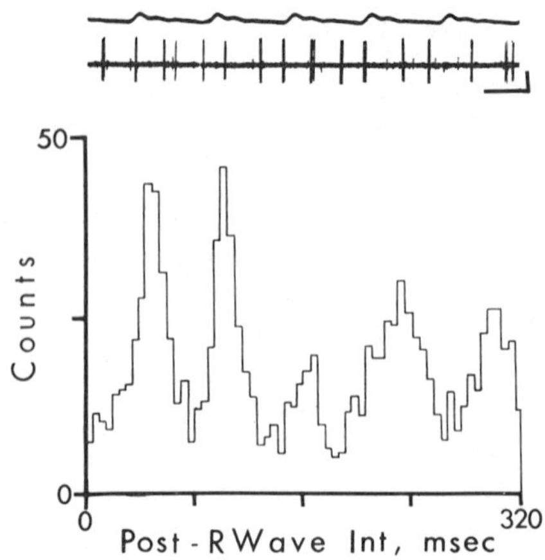

Fig. 15-7. Polymodal post-R wave interval histogram of discharges of a single NTS neuron on time scale of one cardiac cycle. Number of trials was 500. Address bin is 5 msec. Oscilloscopic traces of blood pressure (175/110 mm Hg) and unit discharges are shown above histogram. Horizontal calibration is 200 msec. Vertical calibration is 100 μV. (Reproduced through courtesy of *Am. J. Physiol. 232 (Heart Circ. Physiol. 1)*: H657-H665, 1977)

released from the terminals of baroreceptor afferents are glutamic acid [61] and substance P [33]. Other potential transmitter substances present in NTS are norepinephrine, dopamine, epinephrine, serotonin, and several neuropeptides (see review by Reis et al. [61]). All of these substances except glutamic acid and substance P appear to arise from neurons whose cell bodies are located within the central nervous system [61]. Evidence for a role of norepinephrine in modulating baroreceptor reflex responsiveness has been provided by Reis' laboratory [65,69]. The norepinephrine input to NTS arises from the A2 and possibly the A1 cell groups in the medulla. As demonstrated by Snyder et al. [65], destruction of the A2 cell group by local injection of the neurotoxin 6-hydroxydopamine leads to persistent lability of arterial pressure. This observation suggests that noradrenergic neurons of the A2 group modulate transmission in NTS baroreceptor circuits.

The levels of the neuraxis at which baroreceptor-induced sympathoinhibition is mediated was first subjected to direct investigation in 1973. At that time, Gebber et al. [30] reported that sympathetic nerve responses elicited by electrical stimulation of descending excitatory tracts in the dorsolateral funiculus of the cat cervical spinal cord were partly inhibited upon baroreceptor reflex activation. This observation indicated that sympathoinhibition of baroreceptor reflex origin is mediated, at least in part, at the spinal level. Subsequent experiments performed by Gebber and McCall [28] demonstrated that the inhibition is mediated on spinal interneurons which are interposed between the terminals of bulbospinal sympathoexcitatory tracts and the preganglionic neuron in IML. A review of descending spinal pathways involved in transmitting sympathoinhibitory influences of baroreceptor reflex origin is contained in chapter 14 by Barman.

Taylor and Gebber [71] have provided direct evidence for a brainstem as well as a spinal component of baroreceptor-induced inhibition of basal SND. They observed two periods of inhibition of SND produced by short trains of stimuli applied to the carotid sinus nerve or intramedullary components of the baroreceptor reflex arc in the cat. The onset latency of the early period of inhibition of splanchnic nerve activity was approximately 30 msec, while that of the late period of inhibition was approximately 100 msec. The early inhibition lasted approximately 70 msec, while the late period of inhibition had a duration of approximately 300 msec. Splanchnic nerve responses produced by stimuli applied to descending sympathoexcitatory tracts in the dorsolateral funiculus of the cervical spinal cord were blocked during the early phase of inhibition of basal SND, but not during the late phase. This observation led to the conclusion that the early period of inhibition of basal SND occurred in the spinal cord, while the late phase of inhibition occurred at a supraspinal level (i.e. a site rostral to the point of activation of descending bulbospinal tracts in the cervical spinal cord). Both phases of inhibition were unaltered by midcollicular decerebration [71]. Thus, the late phase of inhibition appeared to be mediated in the brainstem. As reviewed by Gebber [25], subsequent studies demonstrated that the late phase of inhibition acts to entrain the 2–6 cps rhythm of brainstem origin in a 1:1 relation to the cardiac cycle for the purpose of frequency limitation. The spinal component of inhibition, on the other hand, functions as an amplitude modulator (i.e. determines the number of active preganglionic neurons in each cardiac-related cycle of SND).

The failure of midcollicular decerebration to reduce the early and late periods of baroreceptor-induced sympathoinhibition does not preclude a role of forebrain loops in the control of cardiovascular function by this important homeostatic reflex mechanism. Indeed, Hilton and Spyer [36] have demonstrated that lesions of the anterior hypothalamus attenuate the reduction in blood pressure produced by baroreceptor reflex activation. That the change in baroreceptor reflex responsiveness was due to interruption of a bulbo-forebrain loop in the reflex arc is suggested by the fact that it is possible to alter anterior hypothalamic unit discharge rate with natural or electrical stimulation of the baroreceptor nerves [12,66,72]. Furthermore, the recent work of Barman and Gebber [8] provides evidence that at least some of the hypothalamic neurons responsive to baroreceptor nerve activation are contained in networks that govern the discharges of sympathetic nerves. They used spike-triggered averaging to locate hypothalamic neurons with naturally occurring discharges related to inferior cardiac nerve activity. Post-R wave interval analysis revealed that some of these neurons also exhibited cardiac-related activity (Fig. 15-8). That the cardiac-related discharges of hypothalamic units arose as the consequence of baroreceptor inputs was indicated by the observation that hypothalamic neurons exhibiting such activity could not be located in cats with sectioned carotid sinus, aortic depressor, and vagus nerves. Units with activity locked to the 2–6 cps rhythm in SND of the baroreceptor-denervated cat were located in the same hypothalamic regions in which neurons with sympathetic nerve- and cardiac-related activity were found in the baroreceptor-innervated cat. Thus, it is likely that at least some of the hypothalamic units with sympathetic nerve- and cardiac-related activity in the baroreceptor-innervated cat were contained in sym-

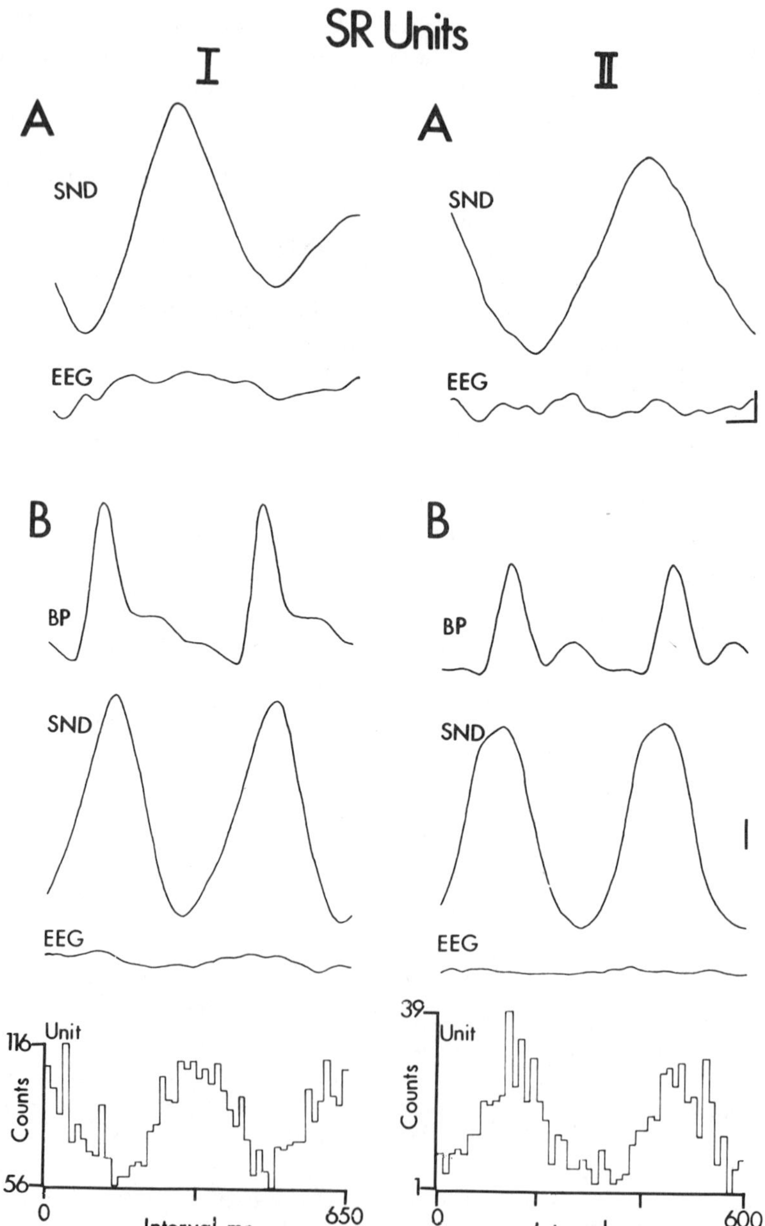

pathetic networks. Based on these data, Barman and Gebber [8] concluded that the hypothalamus plays a role in generating the basal discharges in sympathetic nerves, and that some hypothalamic sympathetic neurons are under baroreceptor reflex control.

It is now firmly established that at least the cardiac vagal component of the baroreceptor reflexes can be strongly influenced by inputs from the forebrain and other regions. Inhibition of baroreceptor-induced vagal bradycardia can be produced by electrical stimulation of the posterolateral hypothalamus [22,29,35], inferior olive [64], and somatic afferent nerves [59]. Recently, Barman and Gebber [4] presented evidence that the hypothalamic system is tonically active in anesthetized cats and that inhibition of vagal bradycardia induced by hypothalamic stimulation is mediated by GABA or a GABAergic-like substance. Facilitation of baroreceptor-induced vagal bradycardia can be produced by electrical activation of the anterior hypothalamus, septal nuclei, and corticomedial nucleus of the amygdala [27,39].

Important issues concerning forebrain modulation of the baroreceptor reflexes remain unresolved. First, whether or not forebrain regions that influence the cardiac vagal reflex also modulate baroreceptor-induced sympathetic responses is controversial. A number of investigators [22,23,29] ascribe to the view that baroreceptor-induced sympathoinhibition is unaffected upon stimulation of forebrain regions that inhibit or facilitate the cardiac vagal reflex. Coote et al. [19] disagree. They claim that electrical stimulation of some sites within the hypothalamus suppressed both the sympathetic and cardiac vagal responses produced by raising carotid sinus pressure, while activation of other hypothalamic sites suppressed only the cardiac vagal component of the reflex. It is important to note that blood pressure was elevated to a higher level during stimulation of those hypothalamic sites purported to block the sympathetic component of the baroreceptor reflex (see Figs. 3 and 4 in [19]). This observation leaves open the possibility that "blockade" of the sympathetic component resulted from powerful hypothalamic-induced excitation which broke through an unimpeded baroreceptor mechanism rather than to true neural inhibition of an interneuronal element in the sympathoinhibitory limb of the baroreceptor reflex arc. Thus, it is the opinion of this author that the question of whether the

---

Fig. 15-8. Relationships among hypothalamic unit discharges, inferior cardiac SND, EEG activity, and R wave of ECG in baroreceptor-innervated cats. Traces in I and II are from different animals. IA, IIA. Spike-triggered averages (1954 trials in IA; 550 trials in IIA) of SND (top) and EEG activity (bottom). Address bin is 0.8 msec. Vertical calibration for SND is 10 μV (IA), 20 μV (IIA); for EEG is 5 μV. Horizontal calibration is 40 ms. IB, IIB: R-wave-triggered analysis (1400 trials in IB; 1227 trials in IIB). Traces are from top to bottom: averages of arterial pulse wave, inferior cardiac SND and EEG activity, and histogram of unit spikes. Address bin for averages is 1.3 msec in IB and 1.2 msec in IIB. Address bin for histograms is 13 msec in IB and 12 msec in IIB. Blood pressure (mm Hg) is 200/100 in IB and 185/120 in IIB. Vertical calibration for SND is 40 μV and for EEG is 10 μV. (Reproduced through courtesy of *Am. J. Physiol. (Regulatory Integrative Comp. Physiol.) 242*: R34-R43, 1982)

hypothalamus is involved in modulating the sympathoinhibitory component of the baroreceptor reflexes remains open.

Although it is generally believed that hypothalamic-induced inhibition of the cardiac vagal component of the baroreceptor reflexes occurs, at least in part, in NTS [1,46,73], the synaptic mechanism involved is controversial. Weiss and Crill [75] reported that stimulation of the posterolateral hypothalamus leads to depolarization of the terminals of carotid sinus afferents in NTS. Thus, they have suggested presynaptic inhibition at the level of the baroreceptor afferent terminal as the mechanism for hypothalamic-induced inhibition of the cardiac vagal reflex. However, Jordan and Spyer [38] have not been able to repeat the results of Weiss and Crill. Thus, they attribute the suppression of carotid sinus nerve-induced NTS unit activation produced by hypothalamic stimulation [1,46] to a postsynaptic inhibitory process.

A final issue to be resolved is whether or not the forebrain regions that act to facilitate or inhibit the cardiac vagal component of the baroreceptor reflexes are contained in positive and negative feedback loops, respectively. Two possibilities arise. First, the neuronal elements in the forebrain regions responsible for modulation of the reflex may themselves be directly influenced by baroreceptor input. In this case, a positive and/or negative feedback loop would exist. Alternatively, the forebrain circuits responsible for inhibition or facilitation of the cardiac vagal reflex may be activated by nonbaroreceptor input. In this case, modulation by the forebrain would be strictly feedforward in nature. It is known that inhibition or facilitation of the cardiac vagal reflex can be produced upon electrical activation of hypothalamic regions containing neurons which receive baroreceptor input [8,12,29,39,66]. However, whether such neurons are contained in the networks responsible for modulation of the baroreceptor reflexes remains to be determined.

REFERENCES

1. Adair, J. R. and J. W. Manning, Hypothalamic modulation of baroreceptor afferent unit activity. *Am. J. Physiol. 229*: 1357–1364, 1975.
2. Alexander, R. S., Tonic and reflex functions of medullary sympathetic cardiovascular centers. *J. Neurophysiol. 9*: 205–217, 1946.
3. Barman, S. M. and G. L. Gebber, Basis for synchronization of sympathetic and phrenic nerve discharges. *Am. J. Physiol. 231*: 1601–1607, 1976.
4. Barman, S. M. and G. L. Gebber, Picrotoxin- and bicuculline-sensitive inhibition of cardiac vagal reflexes. *J. Pharmacol. Exp. Ther. 209*: 67–72, 1979.
5. Barman, S. M. and G. L. Gebber, Sympathetic nerve rhythm of brain stem origin. *Am. J. Physiol. 239 (Regulatory Integrative Comp. Physiol. 8)*: R42-R47, 1980.
6. Barman, S. M. and G. L. Gebber, Brain stem neuronal types with activity patterns related to sympathetic nerve discharge. *Am. J. Physiol. 240 (Regulatory Integrative Comp. Physiol. 9)*: R335-R347, 1981.
7. Barman, S. M. and G. L. Gebber, Problems associated with the identification of brain stem neurons responsible for sympathetic nerve discharge. *J. Autonom. Nerv. Sys. 3*: 369–377, 1981.

8. Barman, S. M. and G. L. Gebber, Hypothalamic neurons with activity patterns related to sympathetic nerve discharge. *Am. J. Physiol. (Regulatory Integrative Comp. Physiol.), 242*: R34-R43, 1982.
9. Baust, W. and H. Heinemann, The role of the baroreceptors and of blood pressure in the regulation of sleep and wakefulness. *Exp. Brain Res. 3*: 12–24, 1967.
10. Bernard, C., *Leçons sur la Physiologie et la Pathologie du Système Nerveux*, Vol. 1. Baillière, Paris, 1863.
11. Biscoe, T. J. and S. R. Sampson, Field potentials evoked in the brain stem of the cat by stimulation of the carotid sinus, glossopharyngeal, aortic and superior laryngeal nerves. *J. Physiol. (London) 209*: 341–358, 1970.
12. Calaresu, F. R. and J. Ciriello, Projections to the hypothalamus from buffer nerves and nucleus tractus solitarius in the cat. *Am. J. Physiol. 239 (Regulatory Integrative Comp. Physiol. 8)*: R130-R136, 1980.
13. Calaresu, F. R., A. A. Faiers, and G. J. Mogenson, Central neural regulation of heart and blood vessels in mammals. *Prog. Neurobiol. 5*: 1–35, 1975.
14. Ciriello, J. and F. R. Calaresu, Distribution of vagal cardioinhibitory neurons in the medulla of the cat. *Am. J. Physiol. 238 (Regulatory Integrative Comp. Physiol. 7)*: R57-R64, 1980.
15. Ciriello, J. and F. R. Calaresu, Autoradiographic study of ascending projections from cardiovascular sites in the nuclei tractus solitarii in the cat. *Brain Res. 186*: 448–453, 1980.
16. Cohen, M. I., Neurogenesis of respiratory rhythm in the mammal. *Physiol. Rev. 59*: 1105–1173, 1979.
17. Cohen, M. I. and P. M. Gootman, Periodicities in efferent discharges of splanchnic nerve of the cat. *Am. J. Physiol. 218*: 1092–1101, 1970.
18. Cohen, M. I., P. M. Gootman, J. L. Feldman, Inhibition of sympathetic discharge by lung inflation. In *Arterial Baroreceptors and Hypertension*, Ed. P. Sleight. Oxford Univ. Press, Oxford, 1980, p. 161–167.
19. Coote, J. H., S. M. Hilton, J. F. Perez-Gonzalez, Inhibition of the baroreceptor reflex on stimulation in the brain stem defence centre. *J. Physiol. (Lond.) 288*: 549–560, 1979.
20. Coote, J. H. and V. H. Macleod, Evidence for the involvement in the baroreceptor reflex of a descending pathway. *J. Physiol. (Lond.) 241*: 477–496, 1974.
21. Dittmar, C., Über die Lage des sogenannten Gefasscentrums der medulla oblongata. *Ber. Verh. Saechs. Wiss. Leipzig Math. Phys. Kl. 25*: 449–479, 1873.
22. Djojosugito, A. M., B. Folkow, P. H. Kylstra, L. Lisander, R. S. Tuttle, Differentiated interaction between hypothalamic defense reaction and baroreceptor reflexes. *Acta Physiol. Scand. 78*: 376–385, 1970.
23. Folkow, B., B. Lisander, R. S. Tuttle, S. C. Wang, Changes in cardiac output upon stimulation of the hypothalamic defense area and the medullary depressor area in the cat. *Acta Physiol. Scand. 72*: 220–233, 1968.
24. Gebber, C. L., Basis for phase relations between baroreceptor and sympathetic nervous discharge. *Am. J. Physiol. 230*: 263–270, 1976.
25. Gebber, G. L., Central oscillators responsible for sympathetic nerve discharge. *Am. J. Physiol. 239 (Heart Circ. Physiol. 8)*: H143-H155, 1980.
26. Gebber, G. L. and S. M. Barman, Sympathetic-related activity of brain stem neurons in baroreceptor-denervated cats. *Am. J. Physiol. 240 (Regulatory Integrative Comp. Physiol. 9)*: R348-R355, 1981.
27. Gebber, G. L. and L. R. Klevans, Central nervous system modulation of cardiovascular reflexes. *Fed. Proc. 31*: 1245–1252, 1972.

28. Gebber, G. L. and R. B. McCall, Identification and discharge patterns of spinal sympathetic interneurons. *Am. J. Physiol. 231*: 722–733, 1976.
29. Gebber, G. L. and D. W. Snyder, Hypothalamic control of baroreceptor reflexes. *Am. J. Physiol. 18*: 124–131, 1970.
30. Gebber, G. L., D. G. Taylor, L. C. Weaver, Electrophysiological studies on organization of central vasopressor pathways. *Am. J. Physiol. 224*: 470–481, 1973.
31. Geis, G. S., J. W. Kozelka, R. D. Wurster, Organization and reflex control of vagal cardio-motor neurons. *J. Autonom. Nerv. Sys. 3*: 437–450, 1981.
32. Geis, G. S. and R. D. Wurster, Horseradish peroxidase localization of cardiac vagal preganglionic somata. *Brain Res. 182*: 19–30, 1980.
33. Gillis, R. A., C. J. Helke, B. L. Hamilton, W. P. Norman, D. M. Jacobowitz, Evidence that substance P is a neurotransmitter of baro- and chemoreceptor afferents in nucleus tractus solitarius. *Brain Res. 181*: 476–481, 1980.
34. Green, J. H. and P. F. Heffron, Observations on the origin and genesis of a rapid sympathetic rhythm. *Arch. Int. Pharmacodyn, Ther. 169*: 403–411, 1967.
35. Hilton, S. M., Inhibition of baroreceptor reflexes on hypothalamic stimulation. *J. Physiol. (Lond.) 165*: 56–67, 1963.
36. Hilton, S. M. and K. M. Spyer, Participation of the anterior hypothalamus in the baroreceptor reflex. *J. Physiol. (Lond.) 218*: 271–293, 1971.
37. Humphrey, D. R., Neuronal activity in the medulla oblongata of cat evoked by stimulation of the carotid sinus nerve. In *Baroreceptors and Hypertension*, Ed. P. Kezdi. Pergamon, New York, 1967, p. 131–167.
38. Jordan, D. and K. M. Spyer, Studies on the excitability of sinus nerve afferent terminals. *J. Physiol. (Lond.) 297*: 123–134, 1979.
39. Klevans, L. R. and G. L. Gebber, Facilitatory forebrain influence on cardiac component of baroreceptor reflexes. *Am. J. Physiol. 219*: 1235–1241, 1970.
40. Koizumi, K., H. Seller, A. Kaufman, C. McC. Brooks, Pattern of sympathetic discharges and their relation to baroreceptor and respiratory activities. *Brain Res. 27*: 281–294, 1971.
41. Kollai, M. and K. Koizumi, Reciprocal and non-reciprocal action of the vagal and sympathetic nerves innervating the heart. *J. Autonom. Nerv. Sys. 1*: 33–52, 1979.
42. Kollai, M. and K. Koizumi, Cardiovascular reflexes and interrelationships between sympathetic and parasympathetic activity. *J. Autonom. Nerv. Sys. 4*: 135–148, 1981.
43. Kunze, D. L., Reflex discharge patterns of cardiac vagal efferent fibres. *J. Physiol. (Lond.) 222*: 1–15, 1972.
44. Loewy, A. D., Descending pathways to sympathetic and parasympathetic preganglionic neurons. *J. Autonom. Nerv. Sys. 3*: 265–275, 1981.
45. Loewy, A. D. and H. Burton, Nuclei of the solitary tract: efferent connections to the lower brain stem and spinal cord of the cat. *J. Comp. Neurol. 181*: 421–450, 1978.
46. McAllen, R. M., The inhibition of the baroreceptor input to the medulla by stimulation of the hypothalamic defence area. *J. Physiol. (Lond.) 257*: 45–46, 1976.
47. McAllen, R. M. and K. M. Spyer, The location of cardiac vagal preganglionic motoneurones in the medulla of the cat. *J. Physiol. (Lond.) 258*: 187–204, 1976.
48. McAllen, R. M. and K. M. Spyer, Two types of vagal preganglionic motoneurones projecting to the heart and lungs. *J. Physiol. (Lond) 282*: 353–364, 1978.
49. McAllen, R. M. and K. M. Spyer, The baroreceptor input to cardiac vagal motoneurones. *J. Physiol. (Lond.) 282*: 365–374, 1978.

50. McCall, R. B. and G. L. Gebber, Brain stem and spinal synchronization of sympathetic nervous discharge. *Brain Res. 89*: 139–143, 1975.
51. McCall, R. B., G. L. Gebber, and S. M. Barman, Spinal interneurons in the baroreceptor reflex arc. *Am. J. Physiol. 232 (Heart Circ. Physiol. 1)*: H657-H665, 1977.
52. Middleton, S., C. N. Woolsey, H. Burton, J. E. Rose, Neural activity with cardiac periodicity in medulla oblongata of cat. *Brain Res. 50*: 297–314, 1973.
53. Miura, M. and D. J. Reis, Termination and secondary projections of carotid sinus nerve in the cat brain stem. *Am. J. Physiol. 217*: 142–153, 1969.
54. Miura, M. and D. J. Reis, The role of the solitary and paramedian reticular nuclei in mediating cardiovascular reflex responses from carotid baro- and chemoreceptors. *J. Physiol. (London) 223*: 525–548, 1972.
55. Morrison, S. F. and G. L. Gebber, Classification of raphe neurons with cardiac-related activity. *Am. J. Physiol. (Regulatory Integrative Comp. Physiol.). 243*: R49-R59, 1982.
56. Owsjannikow, P. Die tonischen und reflectorischen Centren der Gefassnerven. Ber. Verh. *Saechs. Wiss. Leipzig Math. Phys. Kl. 23*: 135–147, 1871.
57. Peiss, C. N., Concepts of cardiovascular regulation: past, present and future. In *Nervous Control of the Heart*, Ed. W. C. Randall, Williams and Wilkins, Baltimore, 1965, p. 154–197.
58. Preiss, G., F. Kirchner, C. Polosa, Patterning of sympathetic preganglionic neuron firing by the central respiratory drive. *Brain Res. 87*: 363–374, 1975.
59. Quest, J. A. and G. L. Gebber, Modulation of baroreceptor reflexes by somatic afferent stimulation. *Am. J. Physiol. 222*: 1251–1259, 1972.
60. Ranson, S. W. and P. R. Billingsley, Vasomotor reactions from stimulation of the floor of the fourth ventricle. *Am. J. Physiol. 41*: 85–90, 1916.
61. Reis, D. J., A. R. Granata, M. H. Perrone, W. T. Talman, Evidence that glutamic acid is the neurotransmitter of baroreceptor afferents terminating in the nucleus tractus solitarius (NTS). *J. Autonom. Nerv. Sys. 3*: 321–334, 1981.
62. Ricardo, J. A. and E. T. Koh, Anatomical evidence of direct projections from the nucleus of the solitary tract to the hypothalamus, amygdala and other forebrain structures in the rat. *Brain Res. 153*: 1–26, 1978.
63. Richter, D. W. and H. Seller, Baroreceptor effects on medullary respiratory neurones of the cat. *Brain Res. 86*: 168–171, 1975.
64. Smith, O. A. and M. A. Nathan, Inhibition of carotid sinus reflex by inferior olive. *Science 154*: 674–675, 1966.
65. Snyder, D. W., M. A. Nathan, D. J. Reis, Chronic lability of arterial pressure produced by selective destruction of the catecholamine innervation of the nucleus tractus solitarii in the rat. *Circ. Res. 43*: 662–671, 1978.
66. Spyer, K. M., Baroreceptor sensitive neurones in the anterior hypothalamus of the cat. *J. Physiol. (Lond.) 224*: 245–257, 1972.
67. Spyer, K. M. Neural organization and control of the baroreceptor reflex. *Rev. Physiol. Biochem. Pharmacol. 88*: 24–124, 1981.
68. Stroh-Werz, M., P. Langhorst, H. Camerer, Neuronal activity with cardiac rhythm in the nucleus of the solitary tract in cats and dogs. I. Different discharge patterns related to the cardiac cycle. *Brain Res. 133*: 65–80, 1977.
69. Talman, W. T., D. Snyder, D. J. Reis, Chronic lability of arterial pressure produced by destruction of A2 catecholaminergic neurons in rat brainstem. *Circ. Res. 46*: 842–853, 1980.
70. Taylor, D. G. and G. L. Gebber, Sympathetic unit responses to stimulation of cat medulla. *Am. J. Physiol. 225*: 1138–1146, 1973.

71. Taylor, D. G. and G. L. Gebber, Baroreceptor mechanisms controlling sympathetic nervous rhythms of central origin. *Am. J. Physiol. 228*: 1002–1013, 1975.
72. Thomas, M. R. and F. R. Calaresu, Responses of single units in the medial hypothalamus to electrical stimulation of the carotid sinus nerve in the cat. *Brain Res. 44*: 49–62, 1972.
73. Thomas, M. R. and F. R. Calaresu, Medullary sites involved in hypothalamic inhibition of reflex vagal bradycardia in the cat. *Brain Res. 80*: 1–16, 1974.
74. Wang, S. C. and S. W. Ranson, Autonomic responses to electrical stimulation of the lower brain stem. *J. Comp. Neurol. 71*: 437–455, 1939.
75. Weiss, G. K. and W. E. Crill, Carotid sinus nerve; primary afferent depolarization evoked by hypothalamic stimulation. *Brain Res. 16*: 269–272, 1969.

16

Mechanisms of Cardiac Pain: Processing of Cardiac Afferent Information in Ascending Spinal Pathways

ROBERT D. FOREMAN

Cardiac receptors continually "sense" the function of the heart, and send information along vagal and sympathetic pathways to the central nervous system [4,18,26,27,30,33,57,78,98]. This information can activate sympathetic preganglionic efferent fibers to elicit cardiovascular reflexes in local segments [19,53,64,66–68,81], as well as distant segments such as the kidney [83,84,106–108]. In addition, vagal preganglionic activity can be reflexly inhibited [88].

The frequency of impulses in these afferent fibers changes in response to mechanical deformation and to application of noxious stimuli such as bradykinin and coronary artery occlusion. Central neural mechanisms mediating cardiac afferent responses are beginning to emerge. In this chapter, after a brief review of stimuli from the heart and related structures, spinal cord structures transmitting this information to the brain and interactions with somatic and vagal afferent inputs will be described. Responses to cardiac nociceptive stimuli or "cardiac pain" will be emphasized.

SYMPATHETIC AFFERENT FIBERS

Although he defined the sympathetic nervous system as motor in function, Langley [54] appreciated and described afferent fibers coursing through sympathetic nerves and their white communicating rami as "afferent sympathetic fibers." Because they did not produce obvious reflex responses like the depressor nerve, Langley concluded that sympathetic afferent fibers were of little significance. Over the past 20 years, however, accumulated data have demonstrated that sympathetic afferent fibers elicit important reflex responses and do mediate

The scientific experiments were supported by Grants #HL22732, HL27260, and Research Career Development Award #HL00557 from the National Heart, Lung, and Blood Institute of the National Institutes of Health.

The author wishes to thank W. S. Ammons, R. W. Blair, H. L. Stone, R. Thies, and R. D. Wurster for reviewing the text and M. Martindale for the photography.

sensation. Such fibers, sensitive to mechanical deformation and noxious stimulation, are found throughout the cardiopulmonary region. Myelinated afferent fibers have receptors located in the ventricles and atria [69,105], aorta [65,101], superior and inferior vena cavae [105], pulmonary vessels [52,58,76], and in or near the coronary vessels [16,17,106].

Myelinated afferent fibers are usually spontaneously active and their discharge pattern is synchronous with cardiac rhythmicity [18]. Pressure changes within the chambers of the heart and blood vessels increase the activity in the sympathetic afferent fibers [69,102,104,105]. Impulses do not necessarily occur with each cardiac cycle, but when they appear, the discharge rate varies from one to three spikes entrained with the cardiac cycle.

In comparison to the myelinated afferent fibers, unmyelinated fibers exhibit an irregular discharge pattern that does not entrain with the cardiac rhythm [21]. No more than one spike occurs with a cardiac cycle and not every cycle generates a spike. Receptors of these afferent fibers are sensitive to mechanical changes in the heart and may provide tonic input to the central nervous system for neural control of circulation [21,64]. These afferents are also excited during coronary artery occlusion [21].

Sympathetic afferent fibers not only transmit information relating to pressure changes in the cardiopulmonary region, but also noxious stimulation changes such as coronary artery occlusion and application of algesic chemicals. What are the possible peripheral mechanisms that could provide the central nervous system with information about cardiac nociception? Two hypotheses have been described. One hypothesis states that increased sympathetic afferent activity associated with cardiac pain may be comprised of two components [8]. One is the mechanoreceptors that increase their discharge rate at a threshold that could be sensing innocuous information; therefore, they may not have a pure nociceptive function. The other component is the unmyelinated and slowly conducting A-delta fibers which have chemosensitive endings. They are sensitive to the algesic chemicals such as bradykinin, but are insensitive to mechanical deformation. Fibers with chemosensitive endings are primarily unmyelinated, and seem to be suitable for cardiac nociception.

The second hypothesis is that a high discharge rate of spontaneously active ventricular unmyelinated fibers provides the information necessary for cardiac nociception [59]. These authors believe that the intensity of the stimulus provides the central nervous system with information concerning cardiac pain. These fibers are sensitive to mechanical probing of the receptive field site. One group of slowly conducting fibers may be sensitive to mechanical manipulation while the other may be sensitive primarily to algesic chemicals. Both groups of afferent fibers may play a role in activating the central nervous system. However, their role cannot be understood without examining the neurons and pathways known to be involved in the transmission of pain and in associated cardiovascular adjustments. An analysis of cell activity during mechanical deformation and the application of noxious chemicals may indicate whether mechanoreceptors, chemosensitive endings, or both provide important inputs for cells of the central nervous system.

SPINAL NEURONS WITH SYMPATHETIC AFFERENT INPUT

Methodology and Visceral Input

Processing of afferent cardiopulmonary information in spinal neurons was first assessed by recording from spinal neurons excited by electrical stimulation of sympathetic afferent fibers [39], and determining whether these units were activated by coronary artery occlusion or manipulation of the heart and surrounding structures [42,43]. To study pathways to the brainstem which mediate cardiac pain and reflexes, spinothalamic and spinoreticular cell bodies in the spinal cord were identified in anesthetized cats and monkeys (Fig. 16-1).

Activity of spinal cells of the spinothalamic and spinoreticular tracts in the lower thoracic region has been studied with regard to somatic [1,3,23,38,40,41,44,71,73,113,114] and visceral afferents [41,47,74]. Spinoreti-

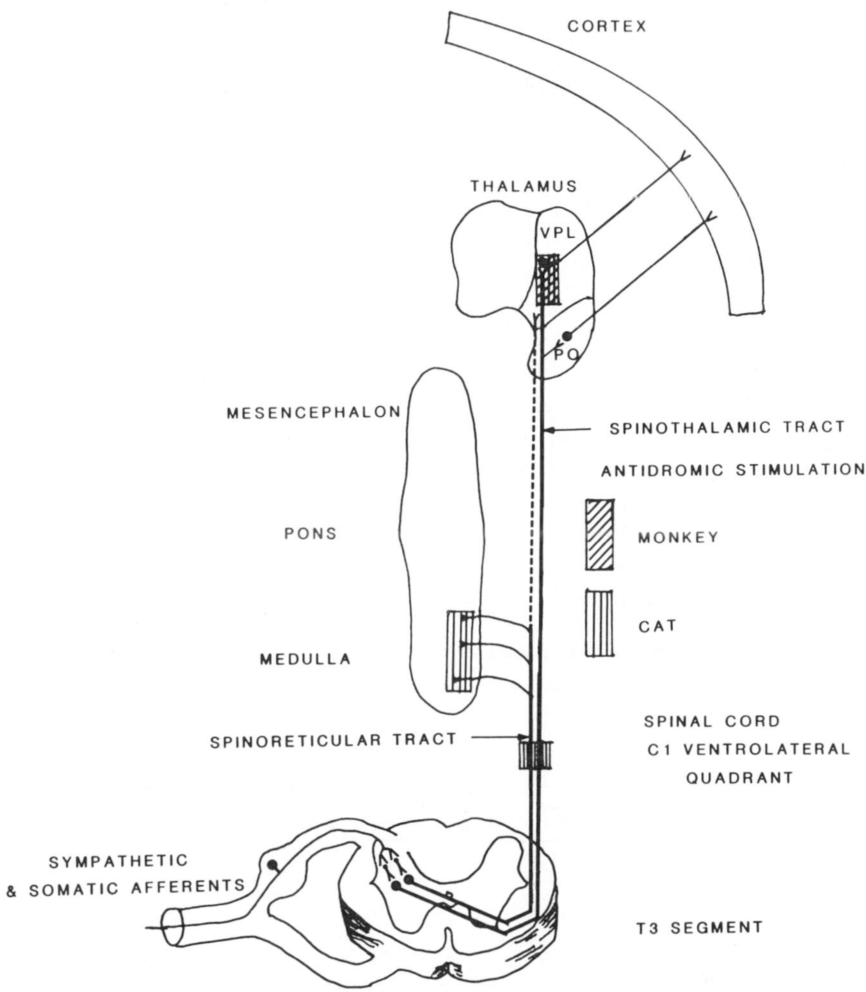

Fig. 16-1. Schematic diagram of spinothalamic and spinoreticular pathways.

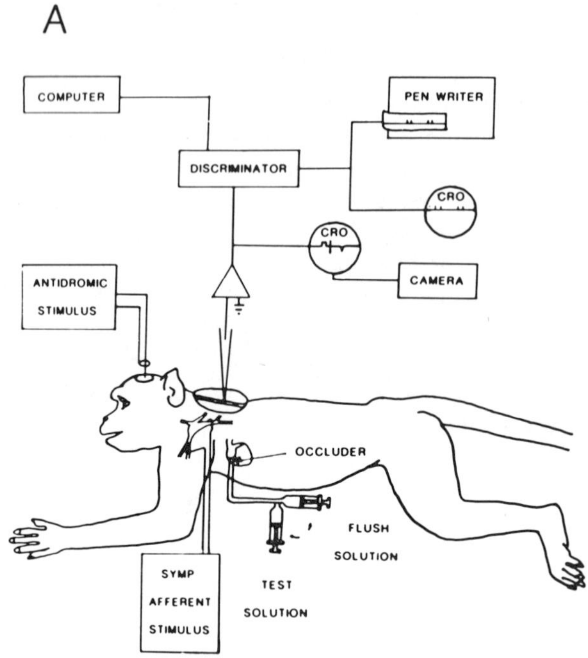
A
COMPUTER
PEN WRITER
DISCRIMINATOR
CRO
CRO
CAMERA
ANTIDROMIC STIMULUS
OCCLUDER
FLUSH SOLUTION
TEST SOLUTION
SYMP AFFERENT STIMULUS

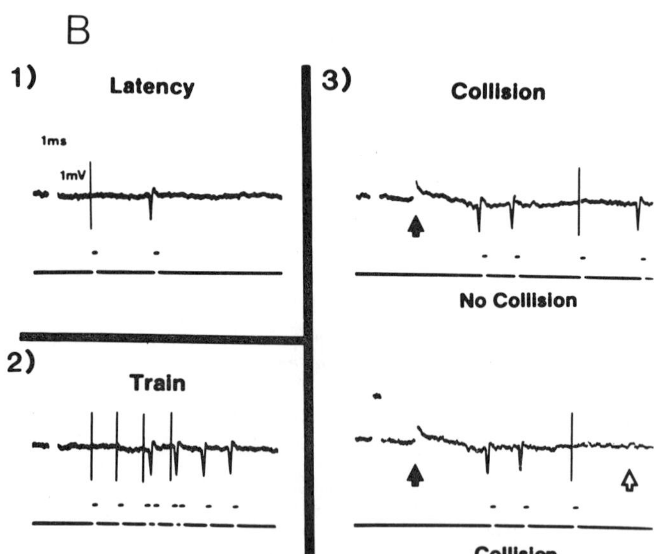
B
1) Latency
1ms
1mV
2) Train
3) Collision
No Collision
Collision

cular activity originates from larger and more complex somatic receptive fields than spinothalamic activity, although many fields are similar [38,71,73]. Spinal cell bodies of these pathways were identified by antidromic activation from electrical stimulation in the contralateral, ventrolateral quadrant of the first cervical spinal segment, from electrical stimulation of the medullary reticular formation, and from the thalamus [12,100]. This antidromic activity must have a constant latency, Fig. 16-2B(1), be able to follow a train of impulses at 333 Hz, Fig. 16-2B(2), and demonstrate occlusion of an antidromically produced action potential with one that is orthodromically produced by afferent stimulation, Fig. 16-2B(3).

Electrical stimulation of sympathetic afferent fibers is first used to determine whether the cell receives visceral input from the cardiopulmonary region. A bipolar electrode is placed on the sympathetic chain, with one hook on the ansa subclavia or between the stellate ganglion and the T_2 white ramus communicans. The other pole of the electrode is placed on the chain behind the T_3 white ramus communicans. In our studies on the spinothalamic tract, both A-delta and C fibers excited the cells. This is consistent with studies showing that impulses generated by receptors of the heart are transmitted to the spinal cord via A-delta [5,6,19,34,69,105] and C fibers [8,21,59,89,103]. However, not every cell received both types of input. Forty percent of the spinothalamic tract cells received both A-delta and C-fiber input, 50% received only A-delta input, and 10% received only C-fiber input [12]. Spinoreticular tract cells also received A-delta and C-fiber input, but for these cells A-delta fibers excited 17%, A-delta and C fibers excited 70%, and C fibers excited 14%. Results of these studies show that spinothalamic and spinoreticular tract cells receive sympathetic afferent inputs but the exact innervation cannot be predicted by studying individual afferent fibers.

Effects of Coronary Artery Occlusion

Sympathetic afferent fibers are excited approximately 10 to 20 seconds following the onset of experimental coronary occlusion [14,16,19,21,104] and partici-

---

Fig. 16-2. Experimental setup (A) and tests for antidromic activation (B) of cells of origin of ascending pathways. A concentric bipolar electrode was placed in the thalamus to excite the cells of origin of the spinothalamic tract antidromically. Sympathetic afferent fibers were excited with a bipolar electrode placed distal and proximal to the stellate ganglion. Extracellular potentials recorded with a microelectrode were sent to a discriminator and from there to recording devices. Tests for antidromic stimulation are shown in B. The upper tracing is the microelectrode recording and the lower tracing the signal from a window discriminator. The first pulse in each trace is the calibration signal. The vertical line in each trace is the shock artifact from the antidromic stimulus. Tests include constant latency (1), a high-frequency train (2), and collision (3). The filled arrow points out the shock artifact for stimulation of the afferents. The open arrow indicates the expected location for the spike which was blocked because of collision.

pate in cardiac reflexes [17,19,36,62,70]. Thus, during coronary artery occlusion, sympathetic afferent fibers project to the spinal cord, but it is not known whether such activity is transmitted to the medullary reticular formation and thalamus. To determine if this information is conducted to the brain by spinoreticular and spinothalamic tracts, the effects of occlusion of either the left main coronary artery or the left circumflex and left anterior descending artery were examined. Cells that responded to coronary occlusion were separated into three groups [42]. Cell activity changed following onset of occlusion according to

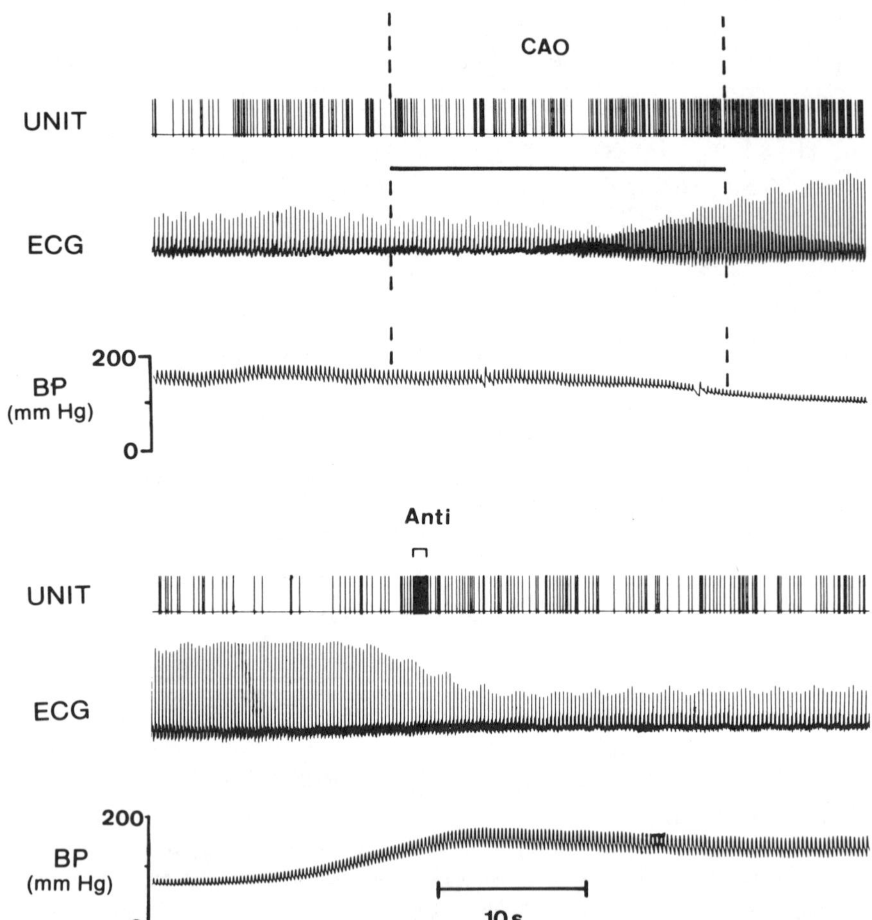

Fig. 16-3. Response of a cell to coronary artery occlusion of the left anterior descending branch of the coronary artery. The top trace is cell activity, the second trace is ECG, and the third trace is aortic blood pressure. The length of the occlusion is marked with a horizontal bar and the dotted lines. The bottom traces are a continuation of the top traces. The word "anti" and the bar underneath it shows the response of the cell to antidromic stimulation of the cell's axon in the contralateral ventrolateral quadrant of the C_1 spinal cord.

latency; the groups were (1) immediate, (2) late, and (3) both immediate and late. Five of 17 cells increased their discharge rate at the onset of the occlusion (immediate group) (Fig. 16-3). This response suggests that change in activity might be due to deformation of receptors within or near the coronary artery. Ten of 17 cells that responded to coronary artery occlusion increased their discharge rate following the onset of the occlusion (late group). The configuration of the ECG changed just before or at the same time the activity of this group of cells increased. On the average, the ECG changed 12 seconds after onset of occlusion. These cells were most likely excited by ischemia produced during the arterial occlusion. Two cells responded both immediately upon occlusion and then increased their firing rate with the change in ECG configuration (both immediate and late group). Twelve cells did not respond to coronary artery occlusion. In studies of spinothalamic tract neurons, seven of 14 cells responded 9 seconds after onset of coronary artery occlusion [2].

Effects of Bradykinin

The effects of injecting bradykinin, an algesic agent, on spinothalamic and spinoreticular tract cells were studied because bradykinin is found in increased amounts in the effluent of the coronary sinus following coronary artery occlusion [49,51]. Bradykinin also produces pseudaffective responses, with indication of pain, when injected into the canine heart [45]. Furthermore, sympathetic afferent fibers are excited when bradykinin is injected into the heart or dripped on the epicardium [8,59,77].

For bradykinin injection (2 μg/Kg), one cannula was placed in the left atrial appendage and another near the aortic arch or in the brachiocephalic artery. When bradykinin was injected into the left atrium, it could either stimulate receptors directly or excite them after entering the coronary circulation. The cannula placed near the aortic arch was used for control injections to insure that other areas of the peripheral circulation were not causing cells of the ascending pathways to increase their discharge rate. Bradykinin excited 30 of 41 spinothalamic tract cells tested. Cell activity increased 15 seconds after injection into the left atrium. The average peak increase in cell activity was 14 Hz [13]. Intrapericardial lidocaine blocked the increased discharge rate following bradykinin injections. Therefore, our results show that bradykinin activates receptors of the heart, transmitting their information to the spinal cord via sympathetic afferent fibers. One cannot predict whether the response was produced by chemosensitive receptors, mechanosensitive receptors, or both. After the discharge rate of 13 cells increased following bradykinin injections, the discharge pattern changed to a cardiac rhythm and then eventually returned to a random pattern.

Role in Cardiac Pain

The most common cause of cardiac pain (angina pectoris) is chronic ischemic heart disease, although other diseases of the heart and thorax produce similar symptoms [22,25]. A major complicating factor in angina pectoris is the referral of pain to somatic structures in the restrosternal, precordial anterior thoracic, or anterior cervical regions of the chest; in the left or right shoulder, arm, wrist, or hand; or in one or both jaws and sometimes including the teeth or posterior region of the lungs [48].

Several theories have been advanced to explain the phenomenon of referred pain. According to the "convergence-facilitation" theory of Mackenzie [60], sensory impulses originating from the visceral organ, in this case the heart, are transmitted to gray matter of the spinal cord. These impulses facilitate, but do not discharge neurons that conduct information to the brain. Mackenzie [60] thought that visceral afferent fibers have no connection with the spinothalamic tract. The enhanced excitability of cells makes it easier for them to reach threshold with fewer impulses arriving from somatic structures. Thus, sensory impulses normally arriving from the skin do not cause the cells to discharge, but after being facilitated by the visceral input, the cells increase their discharge rate, thus causing somatic pain. Therefore, visceral pain should not occur after the inputs from somatic structure are interrupted or anesthetized. Infiltration of procaine in the area of the sternum failed to abolish the referred pain in a patient exhibiting angina pectoris with pain referral to the sternum [55]. Other investigators studying various viscera in humans have obtained similar results with the same technique [15,110,111,116,117]. In animals, denervation of the area of reference failed to abolish the referred pain when the gall bladder was distended [32] or the coronary arteries were occluded [112]. Although Weiss and Davis [109] relieved referred cutaneous pain under certain conditions, the pain usually spreads to the fringes of the anesthetized area if the stimulus is increased. However, Wolf et al. [115] failed to confirm these experiments on the viscera of the abdomen.

Branching of a spinal neuron to innervate a somatic structure and a visceral organ could provide another mechanism for explaining referred pain [6,91]. Branching might provide part of the explanation but it is unlikely that all the visceral afferent fibers are branches of a spinal neuron that also project to somatic structures. The most logical explanation is the convergence-projection theory [85,90]. Afferent fibers from visceral and somatic structures converge, either monosynaptically or polysynaptically, onto spinothalamic tract cells [12,13].

In cats we tested the hypothesis that referred pain occurring during angina pectoris results from impingement of both somatic and sympathetic afferent fiber inputs onto the same cell. Every cell was excited both by sympathetic and somatic inputs. Figure 16-4 illustrates two major categories of somatic fields. Cells were classified according to their responsiveness to somatic manipulation including blowing hair, touching or pinching skin or skin and muscle, and noxious cold. The highest percentage of cells (94%) were classified as high threshold because they responded to high threshold stimuli, that is, pinching the skin or skin and muscle (Fig. 16.4, C and D). Cells with wide dynamic range responded with a low discharge rate to hair movement or touch, but discharged vigorously to pinching the skin or skin and muscle (Fig. 16.4, A and B); they represented 6% of the population of cells antidromically activated from the C_1 ventrolateral

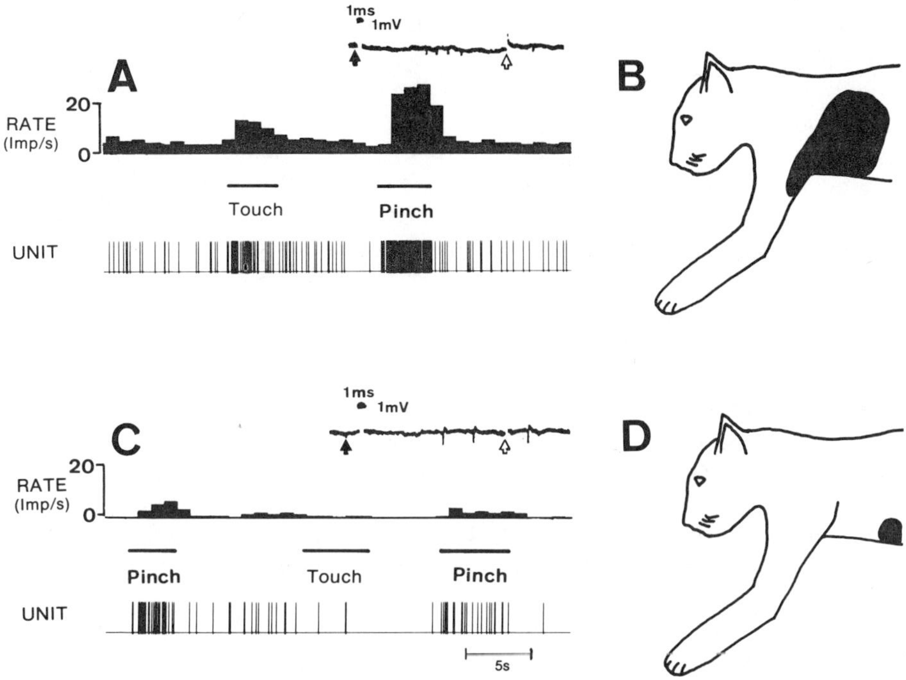

Fig. 16-4. Electrical stimulation of sympathetic afferent fibers and mechanical manipulation of somatic fields. The upper tracing represents the rate of discharge and the lower tracing is the cell activity recorded after the extracellular potential triggered the window discriminator. The response of cell classified as wide dynamic range is shown in A and its location is represented in B. A cell classified as high threshold is shown in C and its receptive field is illustrated in D. The horizontal bar is the period of stimulation. Insets above A and C are oscilloscope tracings illustrating the responses of the cell to electrical stimulation of sympathetic afferent fibers (stimulus artifact marked with filled arrow) and antidromic activation of the cell (stimulus artifact marked with an open arrow) from the C_1 contralateral anterolateral quadrant of the spinal cord.

quadrant of the spinal cord and the spinoreticular pathway. Figure 16-4 illustrates the approximate locations of the somatic fields for exciting two cells obtained by stimulating the ventrolateral quadrant of the spinal cord. Receptive fields are similar to the somatic regions that patients often describe in angina pectoris and other thoracic visceral disease.

Classification of somatic fields for spinothalamic tract cells was somewhat different in the monkey [12]. Of the spinothalamic tract cells studied, 64% were only high threshold, 26% were wide dynamic range, and 10% were high-threshold inhibitory. In the latter category, activity of the cells was inhibited when the hair was blown, but accelerated during a noxious skin pinch. In studies of the spinothalamic tract cells located on the left side of the spinal cord in the monkey, the somatic field was often large and included the left side of the chest and the left arm, even at times the hand and wrist. None of the fields extended to the neck and jaws. The receptive fields correlated well with locations for referred pain described in human patients. We have not studied the somatic input onto spinothalamic tract cells located on the right side of the spinal cord. Thus, sympathetic afferent fibers may continually send signals to the spinal cord, but during angina pectoris the discharge rate increases gradually [63]. In addition, specific chemosensitive endings may become excited [8]. Afferent impulses excite spinothalamic tract cells which then send signals to the thalamus and from there to areas of the brain involved with the conscious perception of pain. In addition to the activity arriving from the heart, somatic afferent impulses, from nociceptors and innocuous receptors, are transmitted to the spinothalamic tract cells [24].

Under normal circumstances for the first 30 to 50 years of life, the spinothalamic tract transmits nociceptive information from somatic structures, since these structures regularly interact with a hostile external environment. At the onset of angina pectoris the afferent impulses which arise from the heart excite the spinothalamic tract cells that also received somatic input. When the information reaches the higher brain structures, it is interpreted as coming from the somatic structures because the brain has "learned" the somatic location from previous experience. Thus, the pain is *referred* to somatic structures but the true origin of the pain is the heart. Although the theory of a "learned" experience sounds like a plausible explanation, there are no experimental data to either support or refute it.

Referred pain associated with angina pectoris is deep and poorly localized. Muscles, periosteum, and joints produce the same deep, poorly localized pain sensations [55]. Why would such poorly localized pain be a common complaint in patients suffering from angina pectoris? It may be that the sympathetic afferent fibers synapse on spinothalamic tract cells that receive their primary somatic afferent input from muscle and deep structures. In our studies on the spinothalamic tract we found many cells that received muscle input as well as cutaneous input. Thus, there may be a relationship between the types of cells excited (visceral and somatic) and particular receptive fields.

Effects of Arrhythmias

Nonpainful sensation also may arise from the heart, e.g. a sensation associated with an arrhythmia or a skipped beat (a premature ventricular contraction) [48,86]. Sympathetic afferent activity, particularly of C fibers, may be altered during ventricular ectopic beats or fibrillation [67,87]. These abnormal ventricular beats may reflexly excite sympathetic efferent fibers [5] and provide sensory input to the central nervous system.

To test if this arrhythmia-induced afferent activity affects ascending pathways in the cat, left ventricular ectopic beats were produced late in diastole by electrical stimulation of the left ventricle while the left atrium was paced [11]. A left ventricular electrogram was also recorded.

The response of a spinoreticular tract cell to such an ectopic stimulus is shown in Fig. 16-5A. The ectopic stimulus delivered at the arrow produced an ectopic

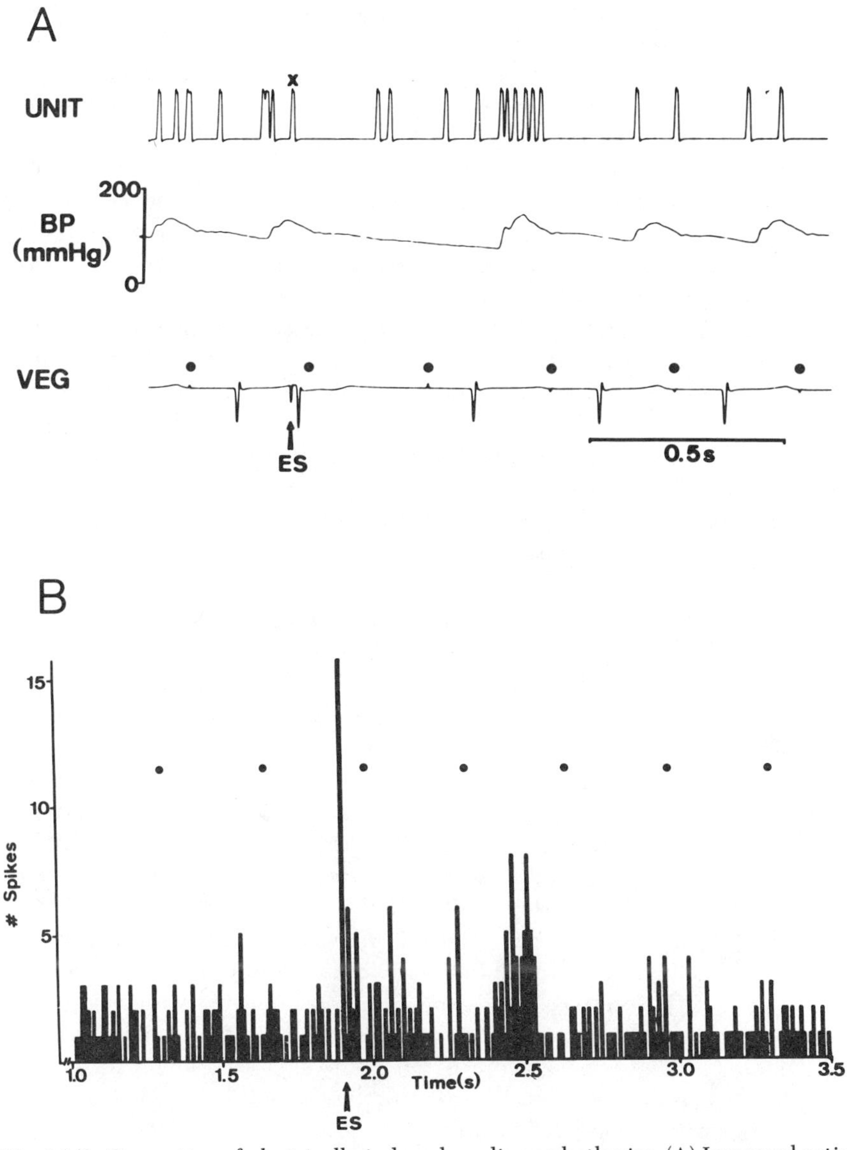

Fig. 16-5. Generation of electrically induced cardiac arrhythmias. (A) Increased activity following an ectopic beat. The upper trace is cell activity. Each upward deflection represents a single action potential. The middle trace is aortic blood pressure (BP), and the bottom trace is the ventricular electrogram (VEG). Dots above VEG indicate the pacing stimulus. The ectopic stimulus (ES) is applied at the arrow. Spike marked with an X (upper trace) is the ES artifact. The pacing rate was 185 beats/min; the ES was delivered 280 msec after the pacing stimulus. (B) The poststimulus histogram showing increased cell activity results from an arrhythmia. The ES was applied 285 msec after the sixth pacing stimulus in a 15-beat period; the histogram was generated from 25 consecutive repetitions of the 15-beat cycle. ES artifact triggered the discriminator. Note the increased cell activity approximately 0.4 sec after the ES.

beat that did not generate an arterial pressure pulse; coincidently, with the subsequent augmented pressure pulse, the cell responded with a burst discharge. Generally, cells responded to the abnormal beat with a burst of one to three spikes; however, such bursts were sometimes difficult to separate from spontaneous activity. To aid in the analysis of these data, poststimulus histograms were compiled with a computer by accumulating 25 consecutive epochs, each consisting of 14 heartbeats. The ectopic stimulus was delivered after the sixth beat in each period. Summed responses of a neuron to this pattern of stimuli is presented in Fig. 16-5B. Note that the discharge was associated with the potentiated beat as described in Fig. 16-5A.

These results provided the first demonstration that some neurons in the central nervous system are sensitive to cardiac events associated with arrhythmias. Since increased cell activity was coincident with the potentiated beat, the stimulus was probably stretch of mechanoreceptors associated with the prolonged R–R interval. This afferent information may provide the cardiovascular regions in the medullary reticular formation with data about the status of the heart. The input may provide mechanism for initiating cardiovascular adjustments to compensate for impaired cardiac function.

SYMPATHETIC AND VAGAL INTERACTION

Vagal Afferents and Their Reflexes

Vagal afferent fibers are found in cardiopulmonary regions similar to the locations of sympathetic afferent fibers. The myelinated fibers arise primarily from the atria and the venoatrial junctions [31,82,99], but a few myelinated afferent fibers arise from the ventricles and coronary arteries [29,33]. Vagal afferent C fibers have their sensory endings in all chambers of the heart [7,29,75,92,97,99].

Unmyelinated afferent vagal fibers can be roughly classified into two groups. One group is mechanoreceptor sensitive and is present in the atria [93,99] and ventricles [79,92,97]. The second group of unmyelinated afferent fibers has chemosensitive endings and is found in the ventricles [29,92], as well as veins, atria, and arteries [28]. Receptors in this category are stimulated with a number of exogenous chemicals and also with naturally occurring substances including bradykinin [56] and prostaglandin E_2 [9]. Unmyelinated afferent fibers in the vagi are excited during coronary artery occlusion and during changes in segment length of the ventricle [95,96].

Vagal afferent fibers from the cardiopulmonary region exert a tonic inhibition on the vasomotor regions of the central nervous system [99]. Interruption of their traffic increases heart rate and blood pressure, while stimulation of the unmyelinated fibers decreases these cardiovascular parameters [79,80,99]. Furthermore, excitation of vagal afferent fibers inhibits activity in the cardiac sympathetic efferent fibers [88].

Effects of Vagal Afferent Activity on Ascending Spinal Afferent Activity

In addition to vagal and sympathetic efferent influences on the heart, vagal afferent activity can alter the ascending spinal afferent activity in the T_1 to T_5

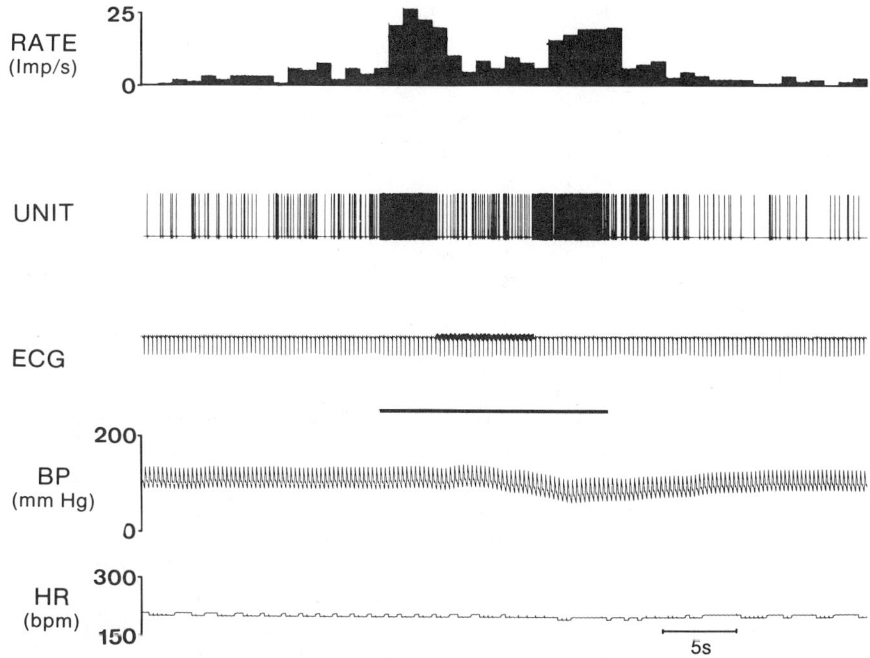

Fig. 16-6. Inhibition of a spinal neuron's response to noxious pinch during electrical stimulation of vagal afferent fibers. Unit is the individual spikes recorded from the cell. The black horizontal bar is the period of the noxious pinch. The increased noise in the ECG trace represents the period of vagal afferent fiber stimulation.

portion of the spinal cord. The effects of stimulation of the proximal end of the left cervical vagus on activity in spinal cells were studied with both somatic and visceral afferent inputs [94]. Of 51 cells recorded, 26 were inhibited, 6 were excited, 2 exhibited both effects, and 17 were unaffected. As illustrated in Fig. 16-6, this inhibition could block even the effects of noxious cutaneous stimulation on somatic and visceral-activated spinal neurons. The horizontal bar represents the length of time the skin and muscle of the left upper arm were pinched. Approximately 4 sec following onset of the noxious pinch, the cardiac branch of the vagus nerve was stimulated, as shown by the stimulus artifact appearing on the ECG tracing. Immediately at the onset of vagal stimulation, cell activity decreased and continued to be inhibited throughout the stimulus period. Following cessation of the vagal stimulation, activity of the cell increased until the noxious pinch was removed. Thus, inhibition of the cell activity produced by a noxious stimulus affected spinal neurons, spinoreticular tract cells, and spinothalamic tract cells.

In Fig. 16-7, the effects of vagal stimulation on sympathetic afferent input are illustrated using conditioning-testing techniques. Experiments were done on cells of origin of the monkey spinothalamic tract as follows. A conditioning stimulus applied to vagal afferent fibers was held at a constant interval after the onset of the histogram. The test stimulus applied to sympathetic afferent fibers was moved to different intervals following the conditioning stimulus. A histo-

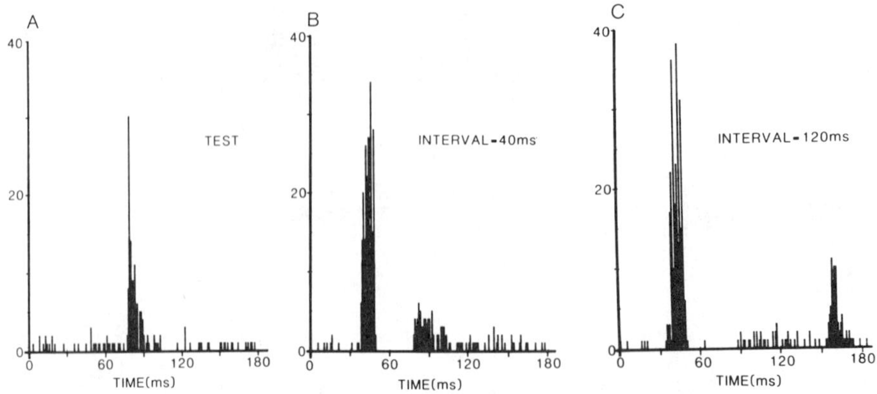

Fig. 16-7. Inhibition of activity from a spinothalamic tract cell produced by stimulating the vagi at different intervals preceding the stimulation of sympathetic afferents. The histograms represent 50 repetitions of the stimuli. (A) Test stimulus, electrical stimulation of the sympathetic afferent fibers. (B) Increased cell activity elicited following the test stimulus (73 msec) is conditioned with electrical stimulation of the vagus nerves 40 msec previously. (C) The test stimulus is moved from 7 msec to 153 msec delay, producing a conditioning–test interval of 120 msec. The lack of spikes following the conditioning stimulus demonstrates that spontaneous activity is also inhibited. The large peak occurring at 33 sec in B and C was produced by the shock artifacts of the vagal stimulus.

gram was generated by summing the conditioning and the testing responses for 50 repetitions. The first histogram shows cell activity produced with the test stimulus alone. The next histogram illustrates the effects of conditioning the response obtained from the test stimulus after an interval of 40 sec. A comparison of the test responses clearly shows that cell activity is markedly decreased following the conditioning stimulus. If the interval between the conditioning and testing stimulus was 120 msec, cell activity following the test stimulus was greater than that observed at the 40 msec interval, but it was still less than control. An interval of approximately 200 msec was needed before the test response returned to the same amplitude as the test stimulus alone. These results indicated that vagal afferent fibers were capable of modulating activity of the cell when sympathetic afferent fibers were stimulated. Again, spinal neurons, spinoreticular tract cells, and spinothalamic tract cells showed similar responses. In some preliminary studies, we have also noted that increased cell activity produced by either injecting bradykinin into the heart or occluding the left coronary artery could be decreased when afferent fibers were stimulated.

Mechanisms for Vagal Inhibition

What are the probable mechanisms whereby the vagal afferents modulate activity of cells of origin of ascending pathways, including spinoreticular and spinothalamic pathways? A schematic diagram of the interaction between vagal afferent fibers and ascending pathways is illustrated in Fig. 16-8. Vagal afferent

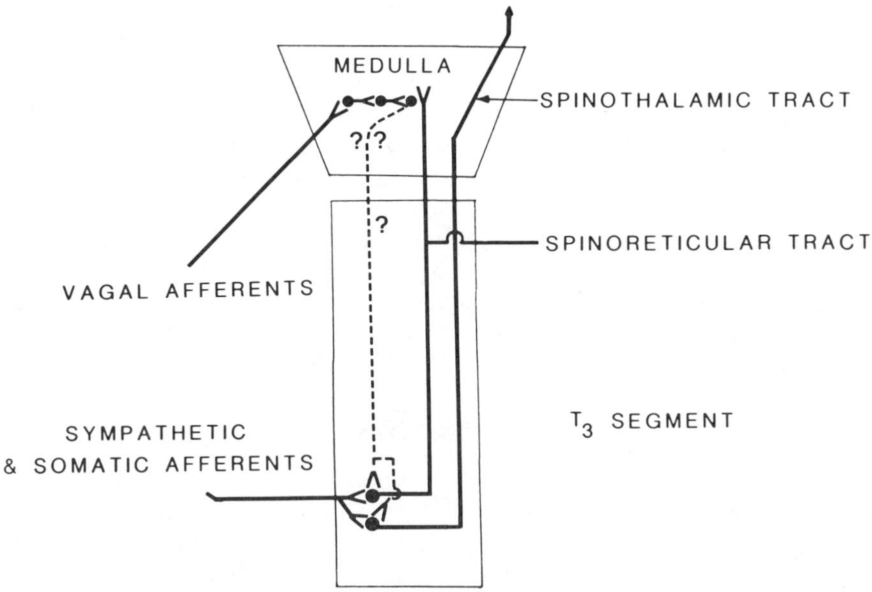

Fig. 16-8. Schematic diagram of a proposed interaction between the vagal afferent fibers and their projections to the cells of origin of ascending pathways. The question marks indicate that the connections between the vagal afferents and the cells of origin are unknown. The sites of termination of the descending pathways on the cells of origin (postsynaptic inhibition) or the afferent terminals (presynaptic inhibition) are also unknown.

fibers enter the brainstem at the level of the medulla. However, connections between the cells of origin of descending pathways and vagal afferents within the medulla have not been determined. Inhibition and occasional excitation may occur via pathways originating from the nucleus raphe magnus, nucleus gigantocellularis, and the periaqueductal gray. Previous investigators have shown that spinal neurons are inhibited during electrical stimulation of the nucleus raphe magnus [10,37,72], and the periaqueductal gray of the midbrain [20,56], and inhibited or excited from nucleus gigantocellularis [46]. Another area for interaction might include the nucleus tractus solitarius. Additional study is needed before any light can be shed on the involvement of these areas in vagal–sympathetic interaction.

Several other questions concerning the vagal interaction with ascending pathways remain to be answered. Does vagal stimulation affect the activity of ascending pathways and thereby modulate the sympathetic efferent activity? Is the inhibition of activity from vagi similar to the inhibition produced by electrical stimulation of the raphe magnus and medial brainstem? What is the role of vagal afferent fibers in controlling or intensifying cardiac pain? Does the inhibition produced by vagal afferents interact with reflexes associated with normal cardiovascular adjustments?

Based on our studies of vagal–sympathetic interaction, the role of the cardiocardiac and cardiosympathetic reflexes should be reexamined [19,35,36,70]. It is conceivable that these reflexes may become functional as the electrical activity transmitted via the descending pathways is decreased or increased. Activity transmitted in the vagi, as well as the carotid sinus nerve and aortic nerve, could possibly modify the behavior of this reflex. Although there may be segmental cardiosympathetic reflexes, other reflexes may be dominated by the spinoreticular pathways which ascend into the medulla, and then activate descending pathways which synapse either monosynaptically or via interneurons onto sympathetic preganglionic neurons. At this time all these connections are speculative, but they should demonstrate the importance of studying the activity of pathways in the central nervous system.

CONCLUSIONS

The heart is a source of afferent activity transmitted to the central nervous system via sympathetic and vagal afferent fibers. The cardiac sympathetic activity converges with somatic afferents to act upon common ascending pathways to the thalamus and brainstem reticular formation. These pathways most likely mediate sensations of cardiac pain, as well as innocuous cardiac sensations. Vagal afferent activity produces predominantly inhibition of ascending spinal afferent activity in addition to other cardiovascular reflex activity.

REFERENCES

1. Albe-Fessard, D. A. Levante, Y. Lamour, Origin of spino-thalamic tract in monkeys. *Brain Res. 65*: 503–509, 1973.
2. Ammons, W. S., R. W. Blair, R. D. Foreman, Responses of primate cells to coronary artery occlusion. (Abst.) *Fed. Proc. 41*: pp. 1517, #7288, 1982.
3. Applebaum, A. E., J. E. Beall, R. D. Foreman, W. D. Willis, Organization and receptive fields of primate spinothalamic tract neurons. *J. Neurophysiol. 38*: 572–586, 1975.
4. Armour, J. A., Physiological behavior of thoracic cardiovascular receptors. *Am. J. Physiol. 225*: 177–185, 1973.
5. Armour, J. A., R. D. Wurster, W. C. Randall, Cardiac reflexes. In *Neural Regulation of the Heart,* ed. W. C. Randall. New York, Oxford Univ. Press, pp. 157–186, 1977.
6. Bahr, R., H. Blumberg, W. Janig, Do dichotomizing afferent fibers exist which supply visceral organs as well as somatic structures? A contribution to the problem of referred pain. *Neurosci. Lett. 24*: 25–28, 1981.
7. Baker, D. G., H. M. Coleridge, J. C. G. Coleridge, Vagal afferent C fibres from the ventricle. In *Cardiac Receptors,* ed. R. Hainsworth, C. Kidd, R. J. Linden. Cambridge University Press, Cambridge, England, pp. 117–137, 1979.
8. Baker, D. G., H. M. Coleridge, J. C. G. Coleridge, T. Nerdrum, Search for a cardiac nociceptor: stimulation by bradykinin of sympathetic afferent nerve endings in the heart of the cat. *J. Physiol. (Lond.) 306*: 519–536, 1980.

9. Baker, D. G., M. P. Kaufman, H. M. Coleridge, J. C. G. Coleridge, Prostaglandin E_2 stimulates vagal chemically-sensitive C-fiber endings in the heart and great vessels (abst.) *Fed. Proc.* *38*: 1322, 1979.
10. Beall, J. E., R. F. Martin, A. E. Applebaum, and W. D. Willis, Inhibition of primate spinothalamic tract neurons by stimulation in the region of nucleus raphe magnus. *Brain Res.* *114*: 328–333, 1976.
11. Blair, R. W., T. Shimizu, V. S. Bishop, The role of vagal afferents in the reflex control of the left ventricular refractory period in the cat. *Circ. Res.* *46*: 378–386, 1980.
12. Blair, R.W., R. N. Weber, R. D. Foreman, Characteristics of primate spinothalamic tract neurons receiving viscerosomatic convergent inputs in T_3–T_5 segments. *J. Neurophysiol.* *46*: 797–811, 1981.
13. Blair, R. W., R. N. Weber, R. D. Foreman, Responses of thoracic spinothalamic neurons to intracardiac injection of bradykinin in the monkey. *Circ. Res.*, *51*: 83–94, 1982.
14. Bosnjak, A. J., E. J. Zuperku, R. L. Coon, J. P. Kampine, Acute coronary occlusion and cardiac sympathetic afferent nerve activity. *Proc. Soc. Exp. Biol. Med.* *161*: 142–148, 1979.
15. Boyden, E. A. and L. G. Rigler, Localization of pain accompanying faradic excitation of stomach and duodenum in healthy individuals. *J. Clin. Invest.* *13*: 833–851, 1934.
16. Brown, A. M., Excitation of afferent cardiac sympathetic nerve fibers during myocardial ischemia. *J. Physiol. (Lond.)* *190*: 35–53, 1967.
17. Brown, A. M., Coronary pressor reflexes. *Am. J. Cardiol.* *44*: 849–851, 1979.
18. Brown, A. M., Cardiac reflexes. In *Handbook of Physiology*, Sec. 2, The Cardiovascular System, Vol. 1. The Heart, Eds. R. M. Berne and N. Sperelakis. Bethesda, Md., Am. Physiol. Soc., pp. 653–676, 1979.
19. Brown, A. M. and A. Malliani, Spinal sympathetic reflexes initiated by coronary receptors. *J. Physiol. (Lond.)* *212*: 685–705, 1971.
20. Carstens, E., M. Fraunhoffer, M. Zimmermann, Serotonergic mediation of descending inhibition from midbrain periaqueductal gray, but not reticular formation of spinal nociceptive transmission in the cat. *Pain* *10*: 149–167, 1981.
21. Casati, R., F. Lombardi, A. Malliani, Afferent sympathetic unmyelinated fibres with left ventricular endings in cats. *J. Physiol. (Lond.)* *292*: 135–148, 1979.
22. Christie, L. G. and R. C. Conti, Systematic approach to evaluation of angina-like chest pain: pathophysiology and clinical testing with emphasis on objective documentation of myocardial ischemia. *Am. Heart J.* *102*: 897–912, 1981.
23. Chung, J. M., D. R. Kenshalo Jr., K. D. Gerhart, W. D. Willis, Excitation of primate spinothalamic neurons by cutaneous C-fiber volleys. *J. Neurophysiol.* *42*: 1354–1369, 1979.
24. Cohen, H. The mechanism of visceral pain. *Trans. Med. Soc. London*, *64*: 65–99, 1944.
25. Cohn, Peter F. and E. Braunwald, Chronic coronary artery disease. In *Heart Disease: A Textbook of Cardiovascular Medicine*, Vol. 2, Ed. E. Braunwald. W. B. Saunders, Philadelphia, 1980, pp. 1387–1436.
26. Coleridge, J. C. G. and H. M. Coleridge, Chemoreflex regulation of the heart. In *Handbook of Physiology*, Sec. 2; The Cardiovascular System, Vol. 1, The Heart, Eds. R. M. Berne and N. Sperelakis. Washington, D. C., American Physiol. Society, pp. 653–676, 1979.

27. Coleridge, H. M. and J. C. G. Coleridge, Cardiovascular afferents involved in regulation of peripheral vessels. *Ann. Rev. Physiol. 42*: 413–427, 1980.
28. Coleridge, H. M., J. C. G. Coleridge, A. Dangel, C. Kidd, J. C. Luck, P. Sleight, Impulses in slowly conducting vagal fibers from afferent endings in the veins, atria, and arteries of dogs and cats. *Circ. Res. 33*: 87–97, 1973.
29. Coleridge, H. M., J. C. G. Coleridge, C. Kidd, Cardiac receptors in the dog, with particular reference to two types of afferent endings in the ventricular wall. *J. Physiol. (Lond.) 174*: 323–339, 1964.
30. Coleridge, H. M., J. C. G. Coleridge, C. Kidd, Afferent innervation of the heart and great vessels: a comparison of the vagal and sympathetic components. *Acta Physiol. Pol 29 (suppl. 17)*: 55–79, 1978.
31. Coleridge, J.C. G., A. Hemingway, R. L. Holmes, R. J. Linden, The location of atrial receptors in the dog: a physiological and histological study. *J. Physiol. (Lond.) 136*: 174–197, 1957.
32. Davis, L., L. J. Pollock, T. T. Stone, Visceral pain. *Surgery, Gynecology and Obstetrics 55*: 418–427, 1932.
33. Donald, D. E., and J. T. Shepherd, Reflexes from the heart and lungs: physiological curiosities or important regulatory mechanisms. *Cardiovascular Res. 12*: 449–469, 1978.
34. Emery, D. G., R. D. Foreman, R. E. Coggeshall, Categories of axons in the inferior cardiac nerve of the cat. *J. Comp. Neurol. 177*: 301–310, 1978.
35. Felder, R. B. and M. D. Thames, Disagreement on the reflex sympathetic activity elicited by experimental coronary occlusion (Letter to the Editor). *Circ. Res. 47*: 628–630, 1980.
36. Felder, R. B. and M. D. Thames, The cardiocardiac sympathetic reflex during coronary occlusion in anesthetized dogs. *Circ. Res. 48*: 685–692, 1981.
37. Fields, H. L., A. I. Basbaum, D. H. Clanton, S. D. Anderson, Nucleus raphe magnus inhibition of spinal cord dorsal horn neurons. *Brain Res. 126*: 441–453, 1977.
38. Fields, H. L., C. H. Clanton, S. D. Anderson, Somatosensory properties of spinoreticular neurons in the cat. *Brain Res. 120*: 49–66, 1977.
39. Foreman, R. D., Viscerosomatic convergence onto spinal neurons responding to afferent fibers located in the inferior cardiac nerve. *Brain Res. 137*: 164–168, 1977.
40. Foreman, R. D., A. E. Applebaum, J. E. Beall, D. L. Trevino, W. D. Willis, Responses of spinothalamic tract neurons to electrical stimulation of hindlimb peripheral nerves. *J. Neurophysiol. 38*: 132–145, 1975.
41. Foreman, R. D., M. B. Hancock, W. D. Willis, Responses of spinothalamic tract cells in the thoracic spinal cord of the monkey to cutaneous and visceral inputs. *Pain 11*: 149–162, 1981.
42. Foreman, R. D. and C. A. Ohata, Effects of coronary artery occlusion on thoracic spinal neurons receiving viscerosomatic inputs. *Am. J. Physiol. 238*: H667–H674, 1980.
43. Foreman, R. D., C. A. Ohata, K. D. Gerhart, Neural mechanisms underlying cardiac pain. In *Neural Mechanisms in Cardiac Arrhythmias*. Eds. P. J. Schwartz, A. M. Brown, A. Malliani, A. Zanchetti. Raven Press, New York, pp. 191–207.
44. Foreman, R. D., R. F. Schmidt, W. D. Willis, Effects of mechanical and chemical stimulation of fine muscle afferents upon primate spinothalamic tract cells. *J. Physiol. (Lond.) 286*: 215–231, 1979.

45. Guzman, F., C. Braun, R. K. S. Lim, Visceral pain and the pseudaffective response to intra-arterial injection of bradykinin and other algesic agents. *Arch. Int. Pharmacodyn. Ther. 136*: 353–83, 1962.
46. Haber, L. H., R. F. Martin, J. M. Chung, W. D. Willis, Inhibition and excitation of primate spinothalamic tract neurons by stimulation in region of nucleus reticularis gigantocellularis. *J. Neurophysiol. 43*: 1578–1593, 1980.
47. Hancock, M. B., R. D. Foreman, W. D. Willis, Convergence of visceral and cutaneous input onto spinothalamic tract cells in the thoracic spinal cord of the cat. *Exp. Neurol. 47*: 240–248, 1975.
48. Harrison, T. R. and T. J. Reeves, Patterns and causes of chest pain. In *Principles and Problems of Ischemic Heart Disease*. Chicago, Year Book Medical Publishers. Inc., 1968, pp. 197–204.
49. Hashimoto, K., M. Hirose, S. Furukawa, H. Haya kawa, E. Kimura, Changes in hemodynamics and bradykinin concentration in coronary sinus blood in experimental coronary artery occlusion. *Jap. Heart J. 18*: 679–689, 1977.
50. Kaufman, M. P., D. G. Baker, H. M. Coleridge, J. C. G. Coleridge, Stimulation by bradykinin of afferent vagal C-fibers with chemosensitive endings in the heart and aorta of the dog. *Circ. Res. 46*: 476–484, 1980.
51. Kimura, E., K. Hashimoto, S. Furukawa, H. Haya kawa, Changes in bradykinin level in coronary sinus blood after the experimental occlusion of a coronary artery. *Am. Heart J. 85*: 635–647, 1973.
52. Kostreva, D. R., E. J. Zuperku, G. L. Hess, R. L. Coon, J. P. Kampine, Pulmonary afferent activity recorded from sympathetic nerves. *J. Appl. Physiol. 39*: 37–40, 1975.
53. Kostreva, D. R., G. L. Hess, E. J. Zuperku, J. Neumark, R. L. Coon, J. P. Kampine, Cardiac responses to stimulation of thoracic afferents in the primate and canine. *Am. J. Physiol. 231*: 1279–1284, 1976.
54. Langley, J. N. The autonomic nervous system. *Brain 26*: 1–26, 1903.
55. Lewis, T. *Pain*. Macmillan Press Ltd, London, 192 pages, 1942.
56. Liebeskind, J. C., G. Guilbaud, J. M. Besson, J. L. Oliveras, Analgesia from electrical stimulation of the periaqueductal gray matter in the cat: behavioral observations and inhibitory effects on spinal cord interneurons. *Brain Res. 50*: 441–446, 1973.
57. Linden, R. J., Reflexes from the heart. *Prog. Cardiovas. Dis. 18*: 201–221, 1975.
58. Lombardi, F., A. Malliani, M. Pagani, Nervous activity of afferent sympathetic fibres innervating the pulmonary veins. *Brain Res. 113*: 197–200, 1976.
59. Lombardi, F., P. Della Bella, R. Casati, A. Malliani, Effects of intracoronary administration of bradykinin on the impulse activity of afferent sympathetic unmyelinated fibers with left ventricular endings in the cat. *Circ. Res. 48*: 69–75, 1981.
60. Mackenzie, J., Some points bearing on the association of sensory disorders and visceral disease. *Brain:16*: 321–354, 1893.
61. Malliani, A., Disagreement on the reflex sympathetic activity elicited by experimental coronary occlusion. (Reply to Letter to the Editor). *Circ. Res. 47*: 627, 1980.
62. Malliani, A. and F. Lombardi, Neural reflexes associated with myocardial ischemia. In *Neural Mechanisms in Cardiac Arrhythmias*, Eds. P. J. Schwartz, A. M. Brown, A. Malliani, A. Zanchetti. New York, Raven Press, pp. 209–219, 1978.

63. Malliani, A. and F. Lombardi, Consideration of the fundamental mechanisms eliciting cardiac pain. *Am. Heart J. 103*: 575–578, 1982.
64. Malliani, A., F. Lombardi, M. Pagani, G. Recordati, P. J. Schwartz, Spinal cardiovascular reflexes. *Brain Res. 87*: 239–246, 1975.
65. Malliani, A. and M. Pagani, Afferent sympathetic nerve fibres with aortic endings. *J. Physiol. (Lond.) 263*: 157–169, 1976.
66. Malliani, A., M. Pagani, G. Recordati, P. J. Schwartz. Spinal sympathetic reflexes elicited by increases in arterial blood pressure. *Am. J. Physiol. 220*: 128–134, 1971.
67. Malliani, A., M. Parks, R. P. Tuckett, A. M. Brown, Reflex increases in heart rate elicited by stimulation of afferent cardiac sympathetic nerve fibers in the cat. *Circ. Res. 32*: 9–14, 1973.
68. Malliani, A., D. F. Peterson, V. S. Bishop, A. M. Brown, Spinal sympathetic cardiocardiac reflexes. *Circ. Res. 30*: 158–166, 1972.
69. Malliani, A., G. Recordati, P. J. Schwartz, Nervous activity of afferent cardiac sympathetic fibres with atrial and ventricular endings. *J. Physiol. (Lond.) 229*: 457–469, 1973.
70. Malliani, A., P. J. Schwartz, A. Zanchetti, A sympathetic reflex elicited by experimental coronary occlusion. *Am. J. Physiol. 217*: 703–709, 1969.
71. Maunz, R. A., N. G. Pitts, B. W. Peterson, Cat spinoreticular neurons: locations, responses and changes in responses during repetitive stimulation. *Brain Res. 148*: 365–379, 1978.
72. McCreery, D. G., J. R. Bloedel, E. G. Hames, Effects of stimulating in raphe nuclei and in reticular formation on response of spinothalamic neurons to mechanical stimuli. *J. Neurophysiol. 42*: 166–182, 1979.
73. Menétrey, D., A. Chaouch, J. M. Besson, Location and properties of dorsal horn neurons at origin of spinoreticular tract in lumbar enlargement of the rat. *J. Neurophysiol. 44(5)*: 862–877, 1980.
74. Milne, R. J., R. D. Foreman, G. J. Giesler Jr., and W. D. Willis, Convergence of cutaneous and pelvic visceral nociceptive inputs onto spinothalamic neurons. *Pain 11*: 163–183, 1981.
75. Muers, M. F. and O. Sleight, Action potentials from ventricular mechanoreceptors stimulated by occlusion of the coronary sinus in the dog. *J. Physiol. (Lond.) 221*: 283–309, 1972.
76. Nishi, K., M. Sakanashi, F. Takenaka, Afferent fibres from pulmonary arterial baroreceptors in the left cardiac sympathetic nerve of the cat. *J. Physiol. (Lond.) 240*: 53–66, 1974.
77. Nishi, K., M. Sakanashi, F. Takenaka, Activation of afferent cardiac sympathetic nerve fibers of the cat by pain producing substances and by noxious heat. *Pflugers Arch. 372*: 53–61, 1977.
78. Oberg, B., Overall cardiovascular regulation. *Ann. Rev. Physiol. 38*: 537–570, 1976.
79. Oberg, B. and P. Thorén, Circulatory responses to stimulation of medullated and non-medullated afferents in the cardiac nerve in the cat. *Acta Physiol. Scand. 87*: 121–132, 1973.
80. Oberg, B. and S. White, Circulatory effects of interruption and stimulation of cardiac vagal afferents. *Acta Physiol. Scand. 80*: 383–394, 1970.
81. Pagani, M., P. J. Schwartz, R. Banks, F. Lombardi, and A. Malliani, Reflex response of sympathetic preganglionic neurones initiated by different cardiovascular receptors in spinal animals. *Brain Res. 68*: 215–225, 1974.

82. Paintal, A. S., Vagal sensory receptors and their reflex effects. *Physiol. Rev. 53*: 159–227, 1973.
83. Purtock, R. V., J. H. von Colditz, J. L. Seagard, F. O. Igler, E. J. Zuperku, J. P. Kampine, Reflex effects of thoracic sympathetic afferent nerve stimulation on the kidney. *Am. J. Physiol. 233 (Heart Circ. Physiol. 2)*: H580–H586, 1977.
84. Reimann, K. A. and L. C. Weaver, Contrasting reflexes evoked by chemical activation of cardiac afferent nerves. *Am. J. Physiol. 239*: H316–H325, 1980.
85. Ruch, T. C., Pathophysiology of Pain. In *Neurophysiology*, Ed. T. C. Ruch, H. D. Patton, J. W. Woodbury, A. L. Towe. Saunders, Philadelphia, pp. 350–368, 1961.
86. Scherf, D. and L. J. Boyd, *Cardiovascular Diseases*. Grune and Stratton, New York, pp. 637–638, 1958.
87. Schwartz, P. J., R. D. Foreman, H. L. Stone, A. M. Brown, Effect of dorsal root section on the arrhythmias associated with coronary occlusion. *Am. J. Physiol. 231*: 923–928, 1976.
88. Schwartz, P. J., M. Pagani, F. Lombardi, A. Malliani, A. M. Brown, A cardiocardiac sympathovagal reflex in the cat. *Circ. Res. 32*: 215–220, 1973.
89. Seagard, J. L., H. J. Pederson, D.R. Kostreva, K. L. Van Horn, J. F. Cusick, J. P. Kampine, Ultrastructural identification of afferent fibers of cardiac origin in thoracic sympathetic nerves in the dog. *Am. J. Anat. 153*: 217–232, 1978.
90. Selzer, M. and W. A. Spencer, Convergence of visceral and cutaneous afferent pathways in the lumbar spinal cord. *Brain Res. 14*: 331–348, 1969.
91. Sinclair, D. C., G. Weddell, W. H. Feindel, Referred pain and associated phenomena. *Brain 71*: 184–212, 1948.
92. Sleight, P. and J. G. Widdicombe, Action potentials in fibres from receptors in the epicardium and myocardium of the dog's left ventricle. *J. Physiol. (Lond.) 181*: 235–258, 1965.
93. Thames, M. D., D. E. Donald, J. T. Shepherd, Behavior of cardiac receptors with nonmyelinated vagal afferents during spontaneous respiration in cats. *Circ. Res. 41*: 694–701, 1977.
94. Thies, R. and R. D. Foreman, Descending inhibition of spinal neurons in the cardiopulmonary region by electrical stimulation of vagal afferent nerves. *Brain Res. 207*: 178–183, 1981.
95. Thorén, P., Left ventricular receptors activated by severe asphyxia and by coronary artery occlusion. *Acta Physiol. Scand. 85*: 455–463, 1972.
96. Thorén, P. N., Activation of left ventricular receptors with nonmedullated vagal afferent fibers during occlusion of a coronary artery in the cat. *Am. J. Cardiol. 37*: 1046–1051, 1976.
97. Thorén, P. N., Characteristics of left ventricular receptors with nonmedullated vagal afferents in cats. *Circ. Res. 40*: 415–421, 1977.
98. Thorén, P., Role of cardiac vagal C-fibers in cardiovascular control. *Rev. Physiol. Biochem. Pharmacol. 86*: 1–94, 1979.
99. Thorén, P. N., D. E. Donald, J. T. Shepherd, Role of heart and lung receptors with nonmedullated vagal afferents in circulatory control. *Circ. Res. Suppl. II 38*: II2–II9, 1976.
100. Trevino, D. L., J. D. Coulter, W. D. Willis, Location of cells of origin of spinothalamic tract in lumbar enlargement of the monkey. *J. Neurophysiol. 36*: 750–761, 1973.
101. Uchida, Y., Afferent aortic nerve fibres with their pathways in cardiac sympathetic nerves. *Am. J. Physiol. 228*: 990–995, 1975.

102. Uchida, Y., Afferent sympathetic nerve fibres with mechanoreceptors in the right heart. *Am. J. Physiol. 228*: 223–230, 1975.
103. Uchida, Y., K. Kamisaka, S. Murao, H. Ueda, Mechanosensitivity of afferent cardiac sympathetic nerve fibers. *Am. J. Physiol. 226*: 1088–1093, 1974.
104. Uchida, Y. and S. Murao, Excitation of afferent cardiac sympathetic nerve fibers during coronary occlusion. *Am. J. Physiol. 226*: 1094–1099, 1974.
105. Ueda, H., Y. Uchida, K. Kamisaka, Distribution and responses of the cardiac sympathetic receptors to mechanically induced circulatory changes. *Jap. Heart J. 10*: 70–81, 1969.
106. Weaver, L. C., Cardiopulmonary sympathetic afferent influences on renal nerve activity. *Am. J. Physiol. 233 (Heart Circ. Physiol. 2)*: H592–H599, 1977.
107. Weaver, L. C., L. M. Danos, R. S. Oehl, R. L. Mechler, Contrasting reflex influences of cardiac afferent nerves during coronary occlusion. *Am. J. Physiol. 240*: H620–H629, 1981.
108. Weaver, L. C., L. J. Macklem, K. A. Reimann, R. L. Meckler, R. S. Oehl, Organization of thoracic sympathetic afferent influences on renal nerve activity. *Am. J. Physiol. 237 (Heart Circ. Physiol. 2)*: H44–H50, 1979.
109. Weiss, S. and D. Davis, Significance of afferent impulses from skin in mechanism of visceral pain, skin infiltration as useful therapeutic measure. *Am. J. Med. Sci. 176*: 517–536, 1928.
110. White, J. C., Conduction of visceral pain. *New Eng. J. Med. 246*: 686–691, 1952.
111. White, J. C., Conduction of pain in man: observations on its afferent pathways within the spinal cord and visceral nerves. *Arch. Neurol. Psychiat. 71*: 1–23, 1954.
112. White, J. C., W. E. Garrey, J. A. Atkins, Cardiac innervation: experimental and clinical studies. *Arch. Surg. 26*: 765–786, 1933.
113. Willis, W. D., R. A. Maunz, R. D. Foreman, J. D. Coulter, Static and dynamic responses of spinothalamic tract neurons to natural stimulation of hindlimb. *J. Neurophysiol. 37*: 358–372, 1974.
114. Willis, W. D., D. L. Trevino, J. D. Coulter, R. A. Maunz, Responses of primate spinothalamic tract neurons to natural stimulation of hindlimb. *J. Neurophysiol. 37*: 358–372, 1974.
115. Wolf, S, H. G. Wolff, and H. Goodell, Unpublished observations, quoted in Wolff and Hardy (116).
116. Wolff, H. G. and J. D. Hardy, On the nature of pain. *Physiol. Rev. 27*: 167–199, 1947.
117. Woolard, H. H., J. E. H. Roberts, E. A. Carmichael, An inquiry into referred pain. *Lancet 1*: 337–338, 1932.

17

Neural Control of the Heart in the Intact Conscious Animal with Implications Concerning the Etiology of Cardiovascular Disease

DAVID C. RANDALL and ORVILLE A. SMITH

Changes in an individual's environment or psychological state can profoundly affect his cardiovascular system, and the neural mechanisms responsible for this interaction are coming under increasingly closer examination in the laboratory. Experiments on anesthetized animals have provided the indispensable base from which to launch corollary studies in awake, intact subjects—experiments that are not compromised by the presence of anesthetics but that pose challenges of their own. This chapter summarizes much of what is known about the neural control of the heart in unanesthetized animals. Possible biobehavioral bases of selected cardiovascular diseases are briefly reviewed. Since this is a discussion of neural mechanisms, regulatory properties intrinsic to the circulation, such as the Frank-Starling mechanism, are not directly examined. Attention will be focused primarily on the heart rather than the peripheral circulation.

Before beginning, it may be well to ask, what are we looking for? Can we expect to locate regions within the brain that generate coordinated patterns of neural activity which control the visceral and somatic responses of an organism to changing environmental demands? This would be a tempting quest for several reasons. First, electrical stimulation of select loci within the central nervous system produces apparently coordinated patterns of overall somatic activity resembling those observed during natural behavior. Secondly, there are also areas within the brain where stimulation evokes blood pressure (BP) and heart rate (HR) changes similar to those actually recorded from behaving animals. As an added enticement, regions from which behavioral responses may be evoked often overlap those giving rise to cardiovascular responses [1,34,63]. Some investigators feel that these data support the concept of "centers" within the brain and have coined the corollary term "central command" to describe the patterned neural activity that presumably emanates from these areas. Though

Portions of this work have been supported by NIH grants HL19343 to the University of Kentucky and RR-00166 and HL16910 to the University of Washington.

there is no scientific concensus in this regard, even the most conservative researchers would probably agree that the nervous system is *somehow* anatomically and functionally organized to produce an integrated cardiovascular response pattern which, in turn, provides the necessary metabolic support for the associated on-going activity of the organism. Let us adopt this general viewpoint as our initial orientation to the available experimental data, and attempt to discern more clearly the nature of this organization.

METHODOLOGICAL CONSIDERATIONS

Use of the intact, unanesthetized animal poses formidable problems in experimental design and data interpretation due to the seemingly unlimited behavioral repertoires of even the simplest organisms, and the enormous complexity of the nervous system. The natural response, of course, has been to simplify the problem as much as possible. With respect to behavior, while it is true that an infinite variety is possible in a subject *freely* interacting with its environment, there are much simpler, more basic behavior *patterns* upon which attention has been closely focused. To be of use in any experiment, each pattern must meet a number of requirements [65]: (1) the characteristics (such as onset, duration, and magnitude) of the behavior must be well defined; (2) one must be able to evoke the response repeatedly and reliably; (3) the animal preparation must be capable of providing sufficient numbers of different patterns to meet the objectives of the experiment; and (4) cardiovascular and neural variables which discriminate one behavior pattern from another must be measured.

It seems useful at this point to consider in detail several of these behavioral paradigms. Classical or Pavlovian conditioning has been commonly used in a number of experiments. Typically, some neutral signal, a tone or light, for example, is presented to the subject. At first this evokes an orienting response (OR) such as a HR change, head movement, etc.; the OR disappears as the animal habituates to the stimulus. In classical aversive conditioning, this signal, or conditional stimulus (CS^+), is then following by an unavoidable electric shock, the unconditional stimulus (UCS). With repeated pairings, presentation of the CS^+ evokes a conditional response (CR) which, in many species, consists of tachycardia and an increase in BP [20,44]. Another tone (or color of light) that is never paired with shock, the CS^-, serves as an experimental control for sensitization or generalization [41]. In a related paradigm, called the conditional emotional response (CER), the CS^+ may be presented while the subject is pressing a lever to receive food; the animal typically slows or stops lever pressing during the CS^+, but not the CS^-.

Of the two major difficulties identified earlier, perhaps the behavioral problem seems the most tractable. But what of the enormous complexity of the brain? Once again, the preparation may, at least to a degree, be tailored to the needs of the experiment. For example, studies of the peripheral autonomic control of the heart often demand elaborate instrumentation to measure a number of variables of cardiac function. This tends to require large animals, and the mammal is the obvious subject of choice; the sophistication of the analysis of nervous mechanisms, however, may be somewhat limited. At the other end of the scale, analyses of cellular events underlying cardiovascular adjustments to environmental perturbations often require experimental animals with a less complex central nervous system. Here, the invertebrates, some of which have nervous systems whose neurons and neuronal interconnections have been partially described by circuit diagrams, come into prominence, and, as we shall see, beautiful analyses of neural mechanisms have been forthcoming. Of course, the subject's behavioral and cardiovascular responses are simpler and less dynamic than in mammals. In other experiments the bird has proven to be useful, possessing some of the advantages of each of the previously mentioned preparations. As the field continues to develop we hope to see a convergence of these several approaches wherein detailed analyses of cardiovascular, behavioral, and neuronal mechanisms are possible within a given preparation.

DIENCEPHALIC AND TELENCEPHALIC SYSTEMS

The Hypothalamus

Electrical stimulation within specific regions of the hypothalamus evokes profound cardiovascular changes [60] and behaviors reminiscent of those seen during naturally occurring emotions [39]. Furthermore, changes in BP, HR, and the distribution of cardiac output in unanesthetized rhesus monkeys during stimulation of hypothalamic pressor areas [18] are similar to those observed in the same species during classical conditioning [48]. The numerous experiments dealing with the "defense response" have also clearly shown this dual involvement of portions of the diencephalon [25].

Recent experiments in the baboon [65] are helping to clarify the role of the hypothalamus in cardiac control during emotional conditioning. Figure 17-1 illustrates changes in several cardiovascular variables recorded from chronically instrumented baboons performing a lever-pressing task. Before the lesion (left panel), the learned response evoked by the conditional stimulus included increases in HR, BP, and terminal aortic flow; renal blood flow decreased, and the animal stopped pressing the lever. The baboon was then anesthetized and an electrode passed into the hypothalamus to a position where electrical stimulation evoked qualitatively similar cardiovascular changes; an electrolytic lesion was made at this precise location and at the corresponding area on the opposite side of the brain. The critical region has a dorsoventral extent of 2 mm; the perifornical area just rostral to the intrahypothalamic route of the columns of the fornix is probably the key site [65]. The right panel of the figure illustrates a trial after the animal had recovered from surgery. The cardiovascular components of the response were virtually eliminated, but the animal still failed to press the lever, just as before. Figure 17-2 from a computer analysis of several such experiments confirms the observation that lesioning in this area of the hypothalamus profoundly decreased the cardiovascular response to the CS^+ (left panel). It is remarkable, however, that the cardiovascular response during lever pressing (right panel) and during exercise (not shown) was not significantly

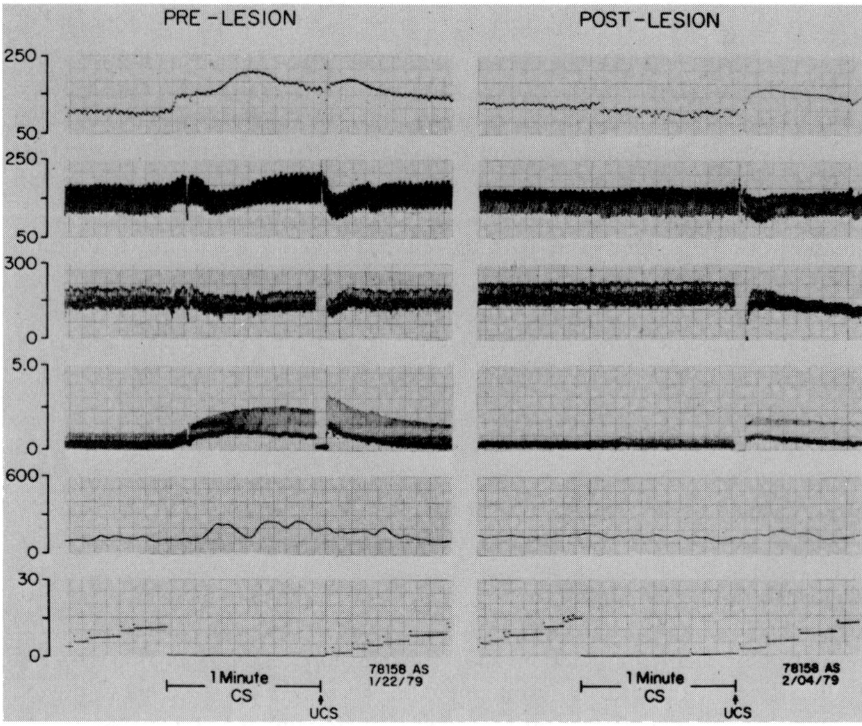

Fig. 17-1. Effect of bilateral hypothalamic lesions on conditioned cardiovascular response to shock during lever pressing in baboon. Postlesion trial was conducted 1 week following placement of lesions; the cardiovascular conditional response was virtually eliminated, although the animal continued to stop lever-pressing during the conditional stimulus. (From Smith et al. [65] by permission from *Fed. Proc.*)

different from control. This indicates that this region of the hypothalamus controls the cardiovascular response associated with emotional behavior but not the corresponding responses to exercise or lever pressing. Nor is the area uniquely responsible for generating the emotional response to the CS^+, at least insofar as is indicated by the animals' continuing failure to press the lever—they were simply unable to produce the autonomic manifestation of that response. Other preliminary data [26] indicate that it *may* be possible to similarly attenuate the cardiovascular response to exercise by placing a lesion in another region of the diencephalon near the subthalamic nuclei.

Similar studies [12] have been undertaken in the pigeon. As in the mammal, the avian hypothalamus is notably cardioactive [34]. When compared with appropriate control groups, birds with extensive or moderate bilateral damage restricted to the posterior hypothalamus exhibited markedly smaller HR increases during classical aversive conditioning. Another group with anterior hypothalamic lesions also showed performance deficits with respect to controls, though less severe than in birds with posterior lesions. There were no significant baseline heart rate differences between the several groups. The investigators

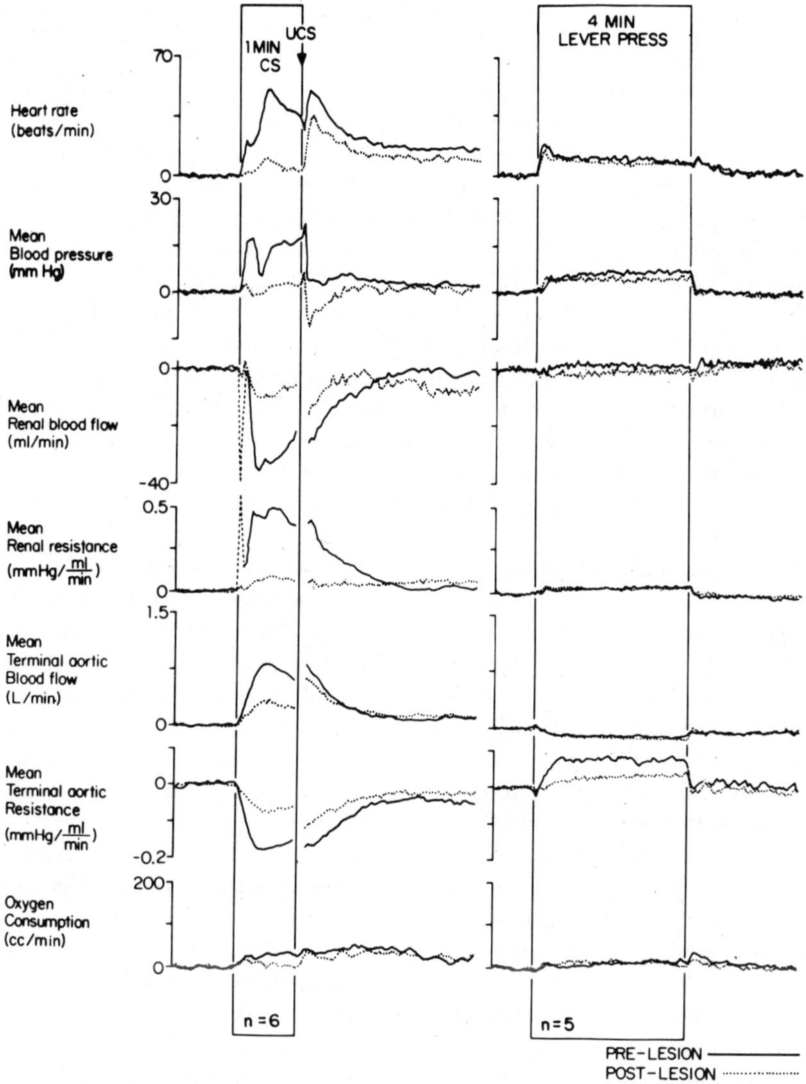

Fig. 17-2. Effect of hypothalamic lesions on composite conditional response (left) and lever press (right). Data are from five prelesion and five postlesion trials for six baboons, and show average percent of control. The conditional changes in heart rate, blood pressure, renal flow, renal resistance, and terminal aortic flow were significantly smaller postlesion. The response pattern during lever pressing remained essentially unchanged before and after lesioning. (From Smith et al. [65] by permission from *Fed. Proc.*)

suggested that the most critical region includes the terminal fields of the projection from the posterior-medial archistriatum, which is the avian homologue of the amygdala in the limbic archistriatum. In any case, it is clear in the bird, as in the primate, that hypothalamic damage severely limits the animal's ability to express classically conditioned HR responses.

The Telencephalon

The identification of hypothalamic loci critically involved in the integration of cardiovascular adjustments to changing behavioral conditions does not necessarily imply that these are autonomous regions. The hypothalamus is particularly noted for its multiple ascending and descending connections, and it has, in fact, been argued [2] that the critical role of this structure is to refine or modulate expression of primitive behavior patterns arising from elsewhere within the brain. Limbic structures such as the lateral septum, the amygdala, the subcallosal gyrus, and the subiculum of the hippocampal formation, as well as fibers from the substantia innominata and pre and supraoptic nuclei, project to the region of the baboon brain previously implicated (Figs. 17-1 and 17-2) in the control of cardiac function. It has not been possible to mimic the cardiovascular response to hypothalamic stimulation by electrical activation of these afferent fibers in the anesthetized baboon [66]; however, activation of certain of these structures, including the diagonal band of Broca, the septum and the amygdala, facilitates the cardiovascular response to submaximal hypothalamic stimulation.

The corresponding situation in pigeon has been examined by lesioning the posterior-medial region of the archistriatum (homologous to the mammalian amygdala) or its projection to the hypothalamus, the tractus occipitomesencephalicus, pars hypothalami [11]. These loci are the most cardioactive regions of the avian telencephalon [34], and their destruction markedly attenuates a previously learned conditional cardioacceleration. In contrast, extensive destruction of certain other regions of the pigeon brain which produce marked HR and/or BP changes upon electrical stimulation, including the septum, had little or no influence on the development of the conditional HR response.

Other telencephalic areas, particularly the frontal cortex, have been implicated in the regulation of cardiac function in unanesthetized animals. The monkey's cardiovascular CR can be reestablished after hypothalamic lesion with continued training, but it is permanently eliminated by subsequent prefrontal lobectomy [62]. Prefrontal lobectomy alone temporarily eliminates the lever-press suppression and attenuates the characteristic BP response [35]. Using another approach to the question, Skinner and Yingling [56] have reported the progressive development of conditional changes in slow-wave electrical potentials recorded from bipolar, chronically implanted electrodes in the frontal cortex of cats during classical aversive conditioning. They report that the changes in these conditioned frontal cortex potentials during acquisition are closely correlated with the development of the conditional HR response. Cryogenic blockade of the inferior thalamic peduncle which connects the frontal cortex to the thalamic reticular formation abolished the conditional slow-wave potential and HR responses while leaving behavioral components intact. The authors did note, however, that cooling this region of the brain elevated the baselines of both physiological variables, which would tend to obscure the conditional responses in each.

Until recently it has not been possible to study the *neuronal* basis per se of cardiovascular control during behavioral conditioning due to the lack of appropriate experimental models. Cohen and his collaborators have now undertaken this task in pigeon. The preparation consists of an immobilized bird maintained on artificial respiration and mounted in a stereotaxic instrument. The behavioral paradigm is composed of successive 6-second periods of control, CS^+ (light), and recovery; the UCS is a 500-msec footshock [22]. The conditional response is a monotonic increase in HR with a latency of approximately one second and maximal values in the fifth or sixth second of the CS^+ [13]. Their neuronal recordings have centered on the principal optic nucleus, one of several brain regions which receives visual signals from the retina. This area corresponds approximately to the dorsal lateral geniculate nucleus of the mammal, and projects to the visual Wulst region of the avian brain (homologue of the mammalian occipitostriate cortex). Not only is the principal optic nucleus retino-recipient, but the majority of its cells also respond to ascending somatic signals activated by the UCS footshock [21]. This means that sensory information from both the conditional and unconditional stimuli has already converged at this level in the bird's central nervous system.

The retinal ganglion cells that transmit CS^+ information monosynaptically to the principal optic nucleus behave as a largely homogeneous population which responds to light onset with a transient burst of impulses [16,17] having a maximum latency of 20 msec and a duration of 80 msec [71]. The visual input to principal optic nucleus is consequently quite uniform and stable over repeated light presentations. Principal optic nucleus neurons respond to CS^+ at latencies ranging from 24 to 70 msec (average = 38 msec), some increasing (type I), and some decreasing (type II) their discharge [21]. Any given unit's response to footshock can also be classified as type I or II; response latency ranges from 60 to 300 msec [21]. As training proceeds a subgroup of the principal optic nucleus neurons (i.e. those which are type I to light but type II to shock) show progressive enhancement of their firing frequency during the first 500 msec of CS^+ [21]. As a group, the birds developed a significant conditional tachycardia within 20 trials. The corresponding training-induced increase in firing from this subpopulation of principal optic nucleus neurons tends to parallel the acquisition of the HR conditional response in a manner reminiscent of the slow-wave potentials described earlier. A number of synapses certainly intervene between these retino-recipient neurons and the final motor outflow controlling HR, but it may, in fact, eventually prove possible to subject the main elements of the entire system to this type of analysis, thus considerably enhancing our understanding of the phenomenon at the cellular level.

BRAINSTEM SYSTEMS

The brainstem is a major crossroads for ascending and descending sensory and motor pathways. Caudal projections from the hypothalamic locus previously implicated in cardiac control during emotion include pathways through: (1) the periventricular gray of the midline; (2) zona incerta; (3) a region dorsal to the substantia nigra; and (4) a band of fibers just dorsal to the optic tract which joins the fibers from the zona incerta and seems to terminate in the dorsal tegmentum medial to the medial lemniscus [61,65]. Some of these projections descend to the medulla and perhaps even as far as the spinal cord [61]. Pathways traversing the brainstem in carnivores thought to mediate the defense response have been described as well [14]. Several specific brainstem loci previously shown to be cardioactive from experiments in anesthetized animals have now also been studied in awake subjects. For example, it has been long known that electrical stimulation of the ventromedial medulla suppresses cardiovascular sympathetic tone. It now appears [5] that lesions involving the raphe region of the rostral medulla result in a significant increase in the HR orienting response to light and the HR change during classical and sensitization conditioning in pigeon; this is consistent with the hypothesis that such lesions interrupt sympathoinhibitory pathways which modulate the HR response during such behavioral situations.

Eventually, descending pathways must terminate on parasympathetic and sympathetic cardiac preganglionic neurons. The former are thought to reside in nucleus ambiguus and/or the dorsal motor nucleus of the vagus (DMNV) in mammal (see chapter 14 for details) and in a specific region of DMNV in pigeon [9,10,52]. Sympathetic outflow arises from the intermediolateral cell column in mammal (see chapter 15) or the column of Terni immediately dorsal to the central canal in pigeon [33] where the ganglion cells are associated with the last three cervical segments, ganglia 12–14. In this regard, it has recently been possible to record from single vagal [22] and sympathetic [6] cardiac neurons in pigeon throughout the course of classical aversive conditioning. Conditioning consisted of 40 lightshock pairings, while the sensitization control group received 40 unpaired light- and footshock presentations. The average conditional HR changes for both groups of birds are shown in Fig. 17-3A. There was a significant divergence of response between the two groups with the conditioning birds showing cardioacceleration. The vagal preganglionic cardiac neurons in DMNV showed a decrease in discharge within the first 500 msec in response to the *first* light presentation; this represents the vagal component of the *orienting* HR response. This decrease was maintained throughout the 6-second light presentation. Note (Fig. 17-3B) that the magnitude of this *decrease* in vagal firing *in*creased during the course of conditioning but *de*creased in the pigeons subjected to sensitization testing. Early in training the response latencies for both groups were approximately 120–159 msec; later, the latency in the conditioning group decreased to about 80–119 msec while it increased in the sensitization group to 160–199 msec. In another study [6] the cardiac sympathetic postganglionic cells were found to respond to the CS^+ with a latency of about 100 msec; the response consisted of a short spike train followed by a brief depression of discharge and subsequent return to maintained activity levels. The phasic burst lasted only about 300–400 msec. Simulating this discharge pattern with electrical stimulation of the right cardiac nerves, which are the primary sympathetic nerves controlling cardiac chronotropism in pigeon [33], evokes a tachycardia of 4–6 seconds duration that closely resembles the behaviorally conditioned HR response [6].

A number of observations and generalizations have been made by Cohen and

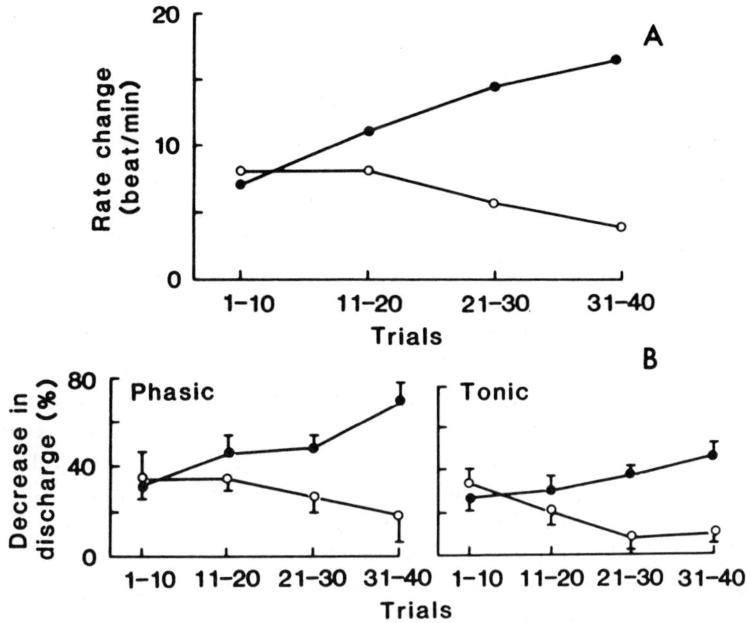

Fig. 17-3. (A) Mean differences between heart rates during CS^+ vs. preceding control for pigeons receiving conditioning (●, n = 13) or sensitization (○, n = 10) training. Each data point is group mean for block of 10 trials. (B) Mean ± SE decrease in discharge of vagal cardiac neurons during first 500 msec (phasic) and last 5500 msec (tonic) response periods during conditioning (n = 10) and sensitization (n = 8) in same pigeons as in A. (From Gold and Cohen [22] by permission of *AAAS*)

his collaborators on the basis of these findings: (1) the data demonstrate a synergistic interaction between the sympathetic and parasympathetic components of the autonomic nervous system during conditioning; (2) the short duration of the unit responses when compared to the duration of the CS^+, and the replication of the CR by a corresponding nerve stimulation, indicate that the maintenance of the conditional HR response over the 6 second CS^+ is primarily a function of a nonlinear input–output relationship between the neuron's discharge and the SA node's ultimate response; (3) since both vagal and sympathetic neurons respond to the light on the first presentation, which is undoubtedly the basis of the HR orienting response, the effect of associative conditioning training is to increase the probability of occurrence and the magnitude of these responses; (4) changes in the discharge characteristics of these neurons with training generally parallel the development of the CR, confirming the close coupling between the two events; (5) based on the difference in latency between the retinal ganglion response time and that of the cardiac sympathetic and parasympathetic neurons, the central processing time is very short, being $\leq$ 60 msec for the vagal cardiac motor neurons; and, (6) this short latency seems to eliminate the possibility of a significant role for feedback from peripheral receptors in mediating the conditional response.

We must at least briefly consider the baroreflex in this section since the mediation of this homeostatic mechanism is often associated with the medulla, although other regions of the brain are also important. Since one often observes simultaneous increases in both HR and BP during various behaviors, it is obvious that the "gain" and/or "setpoint" of this reflex must have been changed under these circumstances. Several aspects of this issue have been studied, including the ability of the hypothalamic defense response to modulate the carotid sinus baroreflex [30] and behaviorally associated changes in the nature of the HR component of the reflex [64,68]. Most of these experiments ultimately devolve to a central issue: does the baroreflex still possess the ability to regulate BP at a level appropriate to the organism's needs under any given circumstance? Data (Fig. 17-4), from Nathan et al. [42] address this issue using classical aversive conditioning in cats. That is, lesioning the nucleus of the solitary tract (NTS), which is the primary projection point for baroreceptor afferents, eliminates the bradycardia to a pressor dose of norepinephrine. The lesions also increase the size of the conditional BP response. This is confirmed in the comparative records (Fig. 17-4) which compare average BP conditional responses in cats with NTS vs. sham lesions. As previously indicated, this suggests that the baroreflex normally buffers the conditional BP increase. It should be possible to examine this issue more critically using recently published techniques for controlling intrasinus pressure in awake animals [67,68,70].

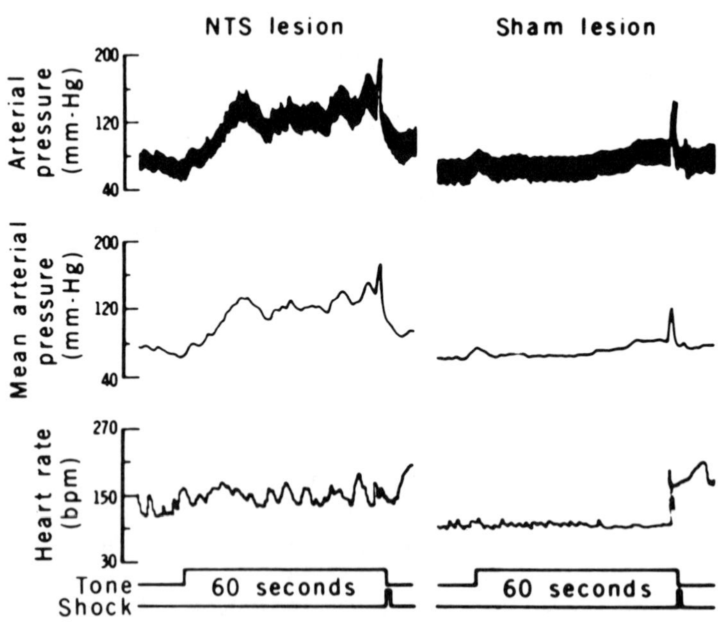

Fig. 17-4. Conditional cardiovascular response of a cat with NTS lesion (Lt) and cat with sham lesion (Rt); bottom traces indicate onset and duration of CS^+ and UCS. Responses for mean changes from baseline for NTS lesion group (n = 4) and sham lesion (n = 4). Average conditional pressor response for NTS lesion group was five times that of the sham lesioned cats. (From Nathan et al. [42]) by permission of *AAAS*)

THE AUTONOMIC NERVOUS SYSTEM

Behavioral conditioning procedures have also proven useful in the study of sympathetic and parasympathetic control of cardiac chronotropism, inotropism, and dromotropism. Neurally mediated increases in each of these variables permits the heart to function more quickly and forcefully when the organism faces environmental challenges. Several aspects of this subject were previously examined by the authors [46,63] as well as in a recent literature review [20] so that the following, for the most part, need be only a brief update.

Cardiac Chronotropism

Heart rate changes observed during transitions from one behavioral state to another are controlled exclusively by the autonomic nervous system, including the catecholamine secretions of the adrenal gland, as is indicated by the following: (1) Surgical cardiac denervation [45] or administration of propranolol and atropine [51] in rhesus monkey markedly attenuates or eliminates the tachycardia observed during classical aversive conditioning; and (2) reinnervation of the previously denervated heart is associated with reemergence of these conditional changes [45]. The relative involvement of the sympathetic and parasympathetic systems in the conditioned HR response is species specific, but in pigeon [8], monkey [43,51], and dog [3,4], there is an initial decrease in parasympathetic tone and an elevation in sympathetic tone. The increased sympathetic drive is principally responsible for the conditional tachycardia in pigeon [8]. In the dog, cardio-selective β-blockade markedly blunts or eliminates the short-latency conditional peak in HR and reduces the overall magnitude of the response by more than 50% [4]. During the latter half of a 1-minute CS^+ in monkey, HR tends to decrease toward control while other indices of sympathetic tone, such as the maximal rate of change of left ventricular pressure [$d(LVP)/dt_{max}$], remain elevated; this suggests that the relationship between the two divisions of the autonomic nervous system may reverse from the initial situation—sympathetic tone remaining elevated while parasympathetic progressively increases [46]. Animals which typically show freezing behavior in prey/predator interactions probably differ from the above schema [20]. Finally, the observation that right, but not left, stellectomy in dog decreases the resting and maximal exercise HR [54] corroborates reports from anesthetized animals that the right cardiac nerves exert more influence on cardiac chronotropism than do the left (cf. chapters 3 and 4).

Cardiac Inotropism

The role of the autonomic nervous system in mediating changes in myocardial inotropism in unanesthetized animals has been more difficult to assess than HR control, but a reasonably clear picture has emerged. This has been accomplished in intact animals by measuring $d(LVP)/dt$ or myocardial isometric contractile force. Administration of propranolol [43] or surgical cardiac denervation [45] markedly reduces or eliminates the usual large increases in these variables seen during classical conditioning. β-blockade is also known to eliminate the increase in d(LVP)/dt during shock avoidance [23]. Section of the left dorsal and ventral ansa subclavia eliminates the increase in d(LVP)/dt otherwise observed during a similar avoidance routine [19], thus confirming the ascendant role of the left cardiac nerves in the regulation of cardiac inotropism, at least as is reflected in these common indices.

A-V Nodal Conduction

Another important aspect of overall cardiac function concerns the ability of the A-V node to faithfully conduct atrial depolarization through to the His-Purkinje conduction system. It is well known that stimulating the appropriate cardiac sympathetic nerves increases A-V conduction velocity, whereas parasympathetic stimulation slows, or may even block, conduction (cf. chapters 3 and 4). However, the relative involvement of these regulatory mechanisms in modulating the cardiac dromotropic state in intact animals has received little attention. Thomas et al. [69] have confirmed that the cardiac nerves do play a significant role in modulating A-V conduction in the intact dog. Using 24-hour Holter ECG monitoring, they determined the average daily HR in a group of control dogs and dogs previously subjected to complete surgical cardiac denervation. The hearts of these dogs were then paced via implanted right atrial electrodes at a rate 30–40/min greater than the previously determined average HR. They again monitored the dogs' heart rates for 24 hours. Normally innervated dogs had frequent episodes of varying degrees of A-V block, particularly during periods of minimal activity. The denervated group showed no deviation from the paced atrial rhythm. The difference between the two groups probably resulted principally from the absence of parasympathetic inhibition of the A-V node in the denervated group.

Skinner et al. [58,59] have used classical appetitive conditioning in awake, chronically instrumented dogs to further examine this phenomenon. Their paradigm consisted of a 30-second tone for CS^+ followed by 30 seconds of food delivery; another tone without food served as CS^-. Figure 17-5 illustrates the HR responses of these dogs to the CS^+ and CS^- tones with and without β-blockade (propranolol, 1.0 mg/kg). There was a modest, but significant, increase in HR during CS^+ but not CS^-, followed by larger increases during food delivery. Left ventricular pressure and d(LVP)/dt (not shown) were also significantly increased over control for both periods. β-blockade completely eliminated the increase in HR and d(LVP)/dt during the CS^+, indicating that these responses were mediated almost exclusively by the sympathetic cardiac nerves; propranolol also eliminated the increase in d(LVP)/dt otherwise observed during food delivery. Electrical bipolar pacing was then used to produce a linear increase in atrial rate from 110/min to 180/min over an average of 11½ seconds; this "ramp function" was imposed during control and during the middle of the 30-second CS^+/CS^- and food/no-food periods. The mean difference between the paced atrial rate and the actual corresponding ventricular rate (from ventricular

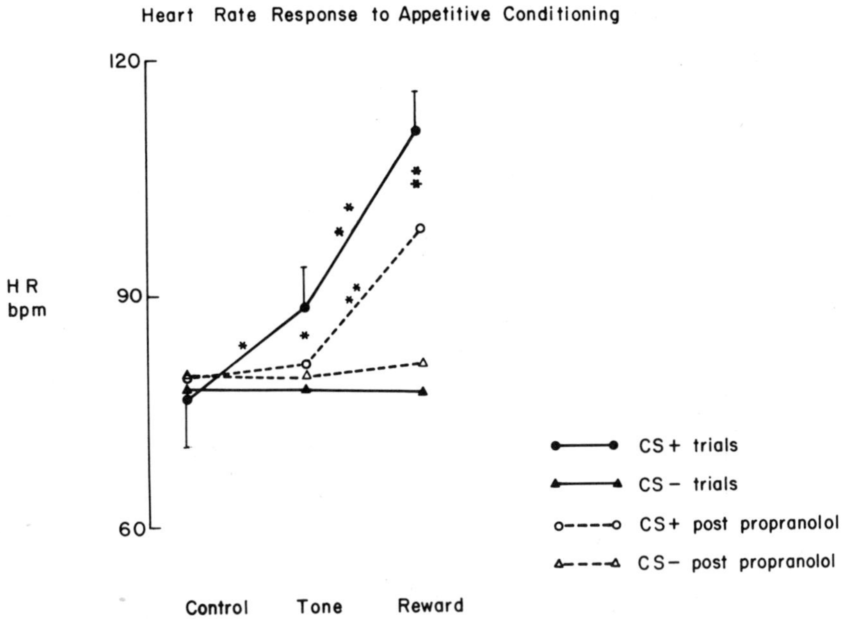

Fig. 17-5. Average (n = 7) heart rate increase for dogs during classical appetitive conditioning with and without β-adrenergic blockade. Increase in heart rate during CS^+ was mediated by increased sympathetic activity; response during food resulted from both increased sympathetic and decreased parasympathetic drive. There were no significant changes during CS^-. ° = $p < .05$; °° = $p < .01$ (From Skinner et al. [59] by permission)

pressure) was then computed over the duration of the progressively increasing atrial pacing function as an index of A-V conduction. Figure 17-6 plots this mean difference for each situation. This index was large during control for all four conditions, indicating that the A-V node did not faithfully conduct the paced atrial depolarization because of frequent A-V block probably associated with a relatively long nodal functional refractory period. The difference decreased during CS^+ (non-β-block), and, for food delivery, was almost zero, indicating a near 1:1 conduction. β-blockade eliminated the increase in conduction during CS^+, suggesting that this aspect of the response had been sympathetically mediated. The mean difference did, however, decrease during food, suggesting the presence of yet another mediating factor, quite probably a parasympathetic withdrawal. It is important to remember that these changes in the mean difference were not directly influenced by the conditional and unconditional HR changes since the ramp-like pacing signal was forcing the A-V node to see the same stimulus pattern across all three periods. Although this index of A-V conduction does not provide an actual measurement of the conduction time, which is certainly one important aspect of nodal function, it does clearly indicate that the entire transmission process is under active neural control in the intact, unanesthetized dog.

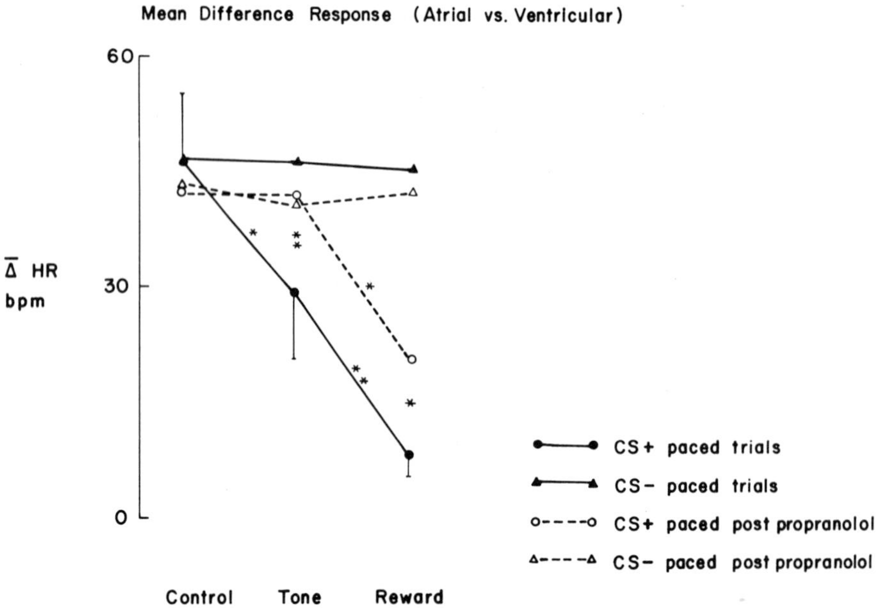

Fig. 17-6. Mean difference between paced atrial heart rate and corresponding ventricular rate during appetitive conditioning before and after β-blockade for same dog as Fig. 18-5. Mean difference of zero indicates 1:1 A-V nodal conduction. Mean difference decreased during CS^+ and food delivery suggesting a neurally mediated increase in dromotropic state. There were no significant changes during CS^-. ° = $p < .05$, °° = $p < .01$. (From Skinner et al. [59] by permission)

CENTRAL COMMAND AND POSSIBLE DIRECTIONS FOR FUTURE RESEARCH

The issue of central command was mentioned briefly in the introduction to this chapter, but we have not overtly come to grips with the concept. A number of ingenious experiments, particularly with isometric exercise, have indicated that some sort of centrally organized patterning of visceral and somatic motor output probably exists. But these experiments do not tell us much about the neurophysiological substrate of this phenomenon. Every preparation has its intrinsic limitations; with regard to the *neuronal* basis of cardiac regulation, possibilities which were only glimpsed in mammalian experiments are beginning to be realized in avian studies. Brief consideration of some related invertebrate experiments may offer another glimpse into future possibilities, particularly regarding the issue of central command.

The advantage of most currently used invertebrate preparations is that their central nervous systems contain many neurons which can be specifically identified in every animal; the connections between these neurons and/or their peripheral target organs also seem to be reliably the same from animal to animal [27]. The neural control of the heart has been studied in the marine mollusk *Aplysia californica*, an animal whose heart, like man's, has a myogenic pacemaker and cardioaccelerator and decelerator nerves. Mayeri et al. [37] have identified seven motoneurons in this animal which appear to account for the major portion of the neural control of the cardiovascular system. Two of these increase HR, two decrease HR, and three increase vasomotor tone. For example, repetitive firing of one of the cardioaccelerator neurons (designated RB_{HE}) by intracellular stimulation increases HR as much as 100%; gradual hyperpolarization of the same cell can virtually stop the heart. Others have different, but demonstrable and unique effects on cardiovascular function. None of the seven motoneurons seems capable of endogenous spike activity, and none is directly interconnected to any other of the seven. However, extensive coordination of their firing patterns results from the action of several identified interneurons [29]. For example, one of these, known as interneuron I or cell L10, excites some followers (not all of which are cardiac motoneurons), inhibits others, and makes a conjoint excitatory–inhibitory synaptic connection to a third type. More specifically, excitation of L10 excites RB_{HE} and inhibits one of the heart and vasculature motor neurons. These investigators suggest that L10 is a *command cell* whose activation produces a *fixed-action pattern* resulting in *coordinated* changes in cardiac and vascular function. What is of particular interest for the present discussion is that interactions between L10 and other interneurons appear to integrate cardiovascular, respiratory, and motor behavior. One stereotyped pattern elaborated by these interneurons consists of contraction of the gill, siphon mantle shelf, and parapodia with inhibition of HR and vasomotor tone; this produces increased circulation of seawater through the mantle cavity and the concomitant pumping of blood into the quiescent heart by the gill [29].

The concept of central command, presumably emanating from somewhere within a specific region of the central nervous system, has been difficult to test experimentally in mammals. Might not these invertebrate experiments suggest the shape of discoveries yet unmade? It is, after all, certain that cardiovascular adjustments are finely tuned under normal circumstances to match an animal's behavior, be it man or sea slug. Although a hypothalamic cognate of L10 may not be identified for many years—if ever—in the mammalian brain, should we be surprised if an identifiable nuclear group appears to possess the attributes of a "command cell"? Intracellular recordings which are reminiscent of those in *Aplysia* are already underway to determine the nature of interneuronal interactions during HR conditioning in pigeon [28] and we may anticipate that the vertebrate, even the mammalian, preparation will continue to develop in this direction. Conversely, the recent demonstration that *Aplysia* is capable of associative learning [7,32] may permit this species to be accorded as much respect as the bird in future studies of the control of cardiovascular function in behaving animals.

POSSIBLE ROLE OF BIOBEHAVIORAL FACTORS IN THE ETIOLOGY OF CARDIOVASCULAR DISEASE

It is apparent that the data presented above have implications vis-à-vis the possible biobehavioral basis of certain cardiovascular diseases. We will focus attention briefly on two such issues—behaviorally induced premature ventricular contraction (PVC) and increases in coronary vascular resistance.

Ventricular Premature Contraction

Sudden cardiac death is presumably due to ventricular arrhythmias culminating in ventricular fibrillation (VF). Under appropriate physiological conditions, especially preexisting myocardial ischemia, subjecting an animal to various environmental challenges has been associated with the onset of PVC which may progress into VF [31,40,47,50]. Since electrical stimulation of sympathetic nerves can also trigger arrhythmias, the hypothesis that behavioral situations known to produce sympathetic arousal might be potentially arrhythmogenic arises rather naturally. This suggestion is buttressed by the observation [57] that cryogenic blockade of the pig's diencephalon at selected points within the frontocortical brainstem pathway prevents stress-related VF following coronary occlusion. The current challenge is to determine more precisely how neural mechanisms enter into the etiology of cardiac arrhythmias.

Recent evidence from behaviorally trained monkeys indicates that high sympathetic tone per se does not necessarily produce the most potentially arrhythmogenic condition in the presence of existing myocardial infarction (47). Figure 17-7, for example, illustrates a conditioning trial in a monkey previously subjected to occlusion of the left anterior descending coronary artery. The animal

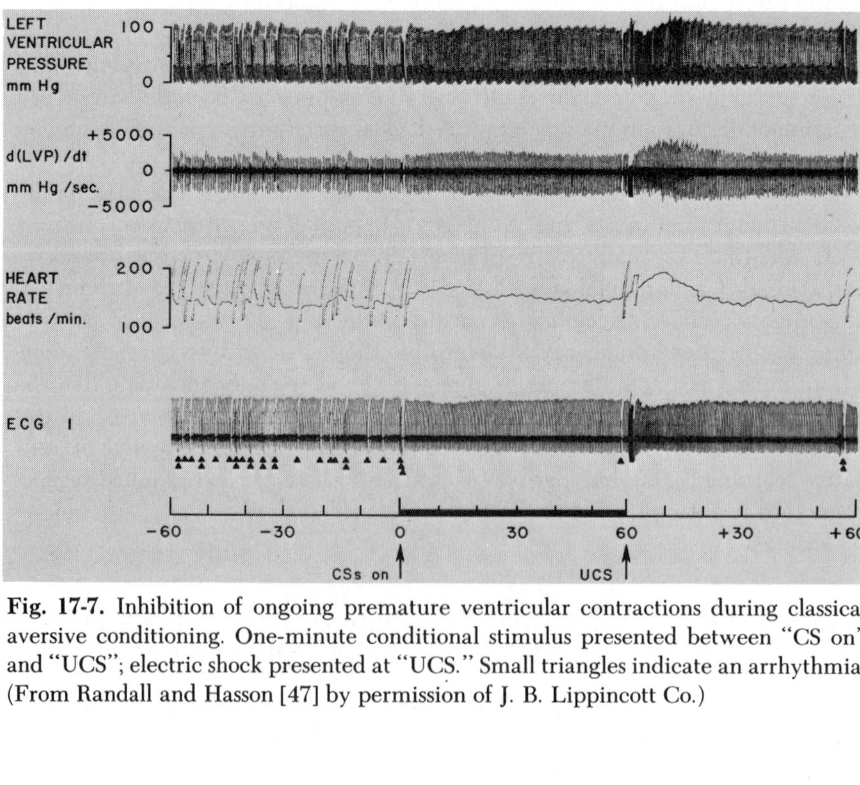

Fig. 17-7. Inhibition of ongoing premature ventricular contractions during classical aversive conditioning. One-minute conditional stimulus presented between "CS on" and "UCS"; electric shock presented at "UCS." Small triangles indicate an arrhythmia. (From Randall and Hasson [47] by permission of J. B. Lippincott Co.)

was experiencing PVC's during the minute prior to presentation of the conditional stimulus; instances of two or even three successive premature contractions occurred while the monkey was sitting quietly during this control period. Rather than exacerbating these on-going PVC's, presentation of the CS^+ with its attendant increase in sympathetic and decrease in parasympathetic tone resulted in virtual cessation of the arrhythmias. These and other data led to the hypothesis [47] that only certain *patterns* of nervous activity—such as concomitant increases in *both* sympathetic and parasympathetic tone—markedly increase PVC occurrence; these, in turn, may be associated with specific behavioral states in any given subject. The following data suggest that unilateral sympathetic discharge from the *left* stellate ganglion may specifically facilitate arrhythmias in intact dogs: (1) following unilateral right stellectomy (RSG_x), cats experience arrhythmias during emotional stress [53]; whereas (2) left stellectomy protects dogs subject to two-stage left anterior descending coronary occlusion from VF [55]. Presumably, the arrhythmias in the RSG_x animals were associated with behaviorally induced increases in sympathetic nerve traffic via the surviving left sympathetic pathways. One particularly important pathway may involve the ventrolateral cardiac nerve which originates from the left stellate ganglion since dogs whose hearts are completely denervated except for this nerve experience arrhythmias during exercise [49]. It is possible that these behavioral data also support the concept of autonomic imbalance discussed elsewhere in this volume.

In summary, although the relationship between emotion and cardiac arrhythmias defies simplistic analysis, there are a number of trends which suggest that certain behavioral situations may be more dangerous in this regard than others [47]. The same complexity appears to hold for the neural basis of these arrhythmias: although the sympathetic nervous system is clearly causally involved, its exact role remains unclear.

Myocardial Ischemia

Another serious health problem is inadequacy of myocardial blood supply in many individuals. Myocardial metabolic demand has long been thought to be a primary determinant of coronary vascular tone, but, as described in chapter 8, neural factors are now known to be of considerable importance as well. This raises the obvious question of whether there are behaviorally mediated changes in coronary blood flow and/or coronary vascular resistance (CVR).

Figure 17-8 illustrates conditional changes in several cardiovascular variables, including late diastolic CVR, for a 30-second control, CS^+, and post-UCS recovery period; data are mean values from eight dogs [4]. Note that there is an initial conditional *in*crease in late diastolic CVR despite large concomitant increases in HR and smaller increases in BP and d(LVP)/dt, all of which tend to increase myocardial metabolism. Although this increase in resistance was transient for the group of animals as a whole, one animal was identified which experienced a *progressive* elevation in late diastolic CVR throughout the entire 30 seconds

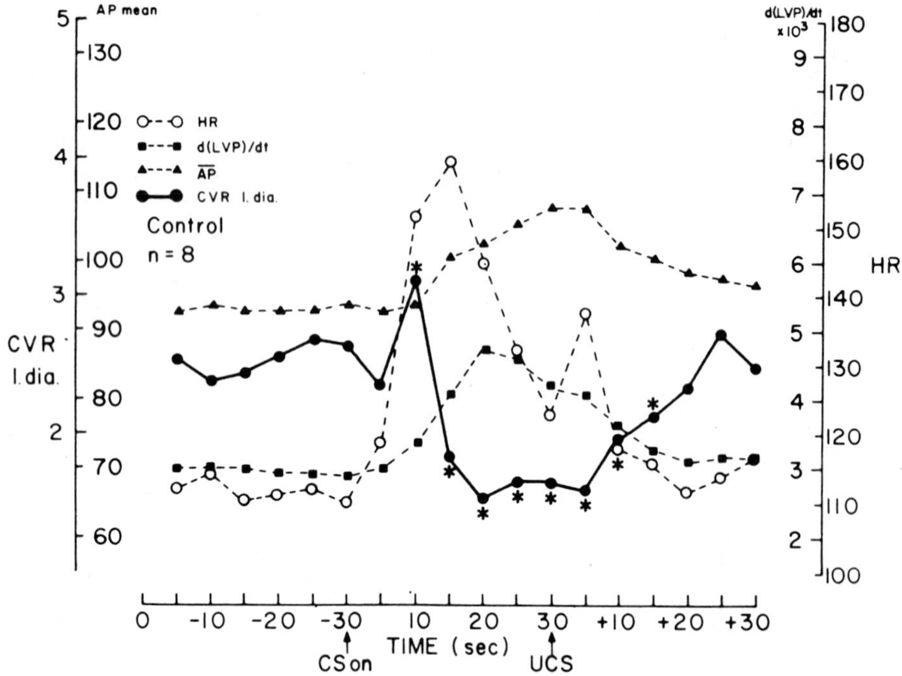

Fig. 17-8. Average conditional response to shock in dog. Thirty second CS⁺ presented between "CS on" and "UCS." Note significant learned increase in late diastolic coronary vascular resistance (CVR) shown [4] to be mediated by increases in a α-adrenergic drive. ° = $p < .01$, shown for l. dia. CVR only. (From Billman and Randall [4] by permission of American Heart Assoc.)

of the CS^+ [3], suggesting that there may be a subpopulation of subjects who are especially vulnerable in this regard. Administration of the α-antagonist phentolamine not only eliminated this aspect of the CR in all animals, but actually reversed it since late diastolic CVR was significantly decreased relative to control for the corresponding time during the CS^+ following drug administration [4]. No significant increases in CVR were observed during a CS^-. The adrenergically mediated conditional increase in CVR is reminiscent of other experiments showing that coronary neural vasoconstrictor activity limits exercise-induced increases in coronary blood flow [24,38].

Although the experiments above do not demonstrate ischemia-induced myocardial lesions subsequent to exercise and aversive conditioning, it has, in fact, been shown that exceedingly demanding behavioral tasks can produce these effects in monkeys [15]. The data in this chapter do, however, demonstrate the existence of a neural/behavioral mechanism which might mediate such changes under appropriate conditions, particularly if there is a subpopulation of susceptible individuals, such as people with "Type A" personalities, comparable to the aberrant dog described previously.

Implications for the Practice of Clinical Medicine

Emotional stress has long been implicated in the etiology of many diseases. We can expect rapid advances in understanding the biobehavioral factors underlying cardiac disease as additional controlled studies of the relevant emotional, environmental, and physiological factors are undertaken. For instance, it seems important to determine what behavioral paradigms and physiological manipulations can be performed to increase and prolong the conditional elevations in CVR just described. With this information it would then become possible to design effective countermeasures to behaviorally induced cardiovascular diseases.

REFERENCES

1. Ángyán, L., Cardiovascular effects of septal, thalamic, hypothalamic and midbrain self-stimulation. *Physiol. Behav. 20*: 217–226, 1978.
2. Bernston, G. G., Organization of brainstem behavioral systems. *Brain Res. Bull. 1*: 471–483, 1976.
3. Billman, G. E. and D. C. Randall, Classic aversive conditioning of coronary blood flow in mongrel dogs. *Pavlovian J. Biol. Sci. 15*: 93–101, 1980.
4. Billman, G. E. and D. C. Randall, Mechanisms mediating the coronary vascular response to behavioral stress in the dog. *Circ. Res. 48*: 214–223, 1981.
5. Cabot, J. B., D. M. Goff, D. H. Cohen, Enhancement of heart rate responses during conditioning and sensitization following interruption of raphe-spinal projections. *J. Neurosci. 1*: 760–770, 1981.
6. Cabot, J. B., D. H. Cohen, D. M. Goff, Discharge patterns of sympathetic postganglionic neurons innervating the heart during the development of a conditioned heart rate response. (In preparation).
7. Carew, T. J., E. T. Walters, E. R. Kandel, Associative learning in a simple reflex of *Aplysia*. *Soc. Neurosci. Abstr.* 7: 383, 1981.
8. Cohen, D. H. and L. H. Pitts, Vagal and sympathetic components of conditioned cardioacceleration in the pigeon. *Brain Res. 9*: 15–31, 1968.
9. Cohen, D. H., A. M. Schnall, R. L. Macdonald, L. H. Pitts, Medullary cells of origin of vagal cardioinhibitory fibers in the pigeon. I. Anatomical studies of peripheral vagus nerve and the dorsal motor nucleus. *J. Comp. Neurol. 140*: 299–320, 1970.
10. Cohen, D. H. and A. M. Schnall, Medullary cells of origin of vagal cardioinhibitory fibers in the pigeon. II. Electrical stimulation of the dorsal motor nucleus. *J. Comp. Neurol. 140*: 321–342, 1970.
11. Cohen, D. H., Involvement of the avian amygdalar homologue (archistriatum posterior and mediale) in defensively conditioned heart rate change. *J. Comp. Neurol. 160*: 13–36, 1975.
12. Cohen, D. H. and R. L. Macdonald, Involvement of the avian hypothalamus in defensively conditioned heart rate change. *J. Comp. Neurol., 167*: 465–480, 1976.
13. Cohen, D. H. and D. M. Goff, Conditioned heart-rate change in the pigeon: analysis and prediction of acquisition patterns. *Physiol. Psychol. 6*: 127–141, 1978.
14. Coote, J. H., S. M. Hilton, A. W. Zbrozyna, The ponto-medullary area integrating the defense reaction in the cat and its influence on muscle blood flow. *J. Physiol. 229*: 257–274, 1973.

15. Corley, K. C., F. O'M. Shiel, H. P. Mauck, L. S. Clark, J. H. Barber, Myocardial degeneration and cardiac arrest in squirrel monkey: physiological and psychological correlates. *Psychophysiol. 14*: 322–328, 1977.
16. Duff, T. A. and D. H. Cohen, Retinal afferents to the pigeon optic tectum: discharge characteristics in response to whole field illumination. *Brain Res. 92*: 1–19, 1975.
17. Duff, T. A. and D. H. Cohen, Optic chiasm fibers of the pigeon: discharge characteristics in response to whole field illumination. *Brain Res. 92*: 145–148, 1975.
18. Forsyth, R. P., Hypothalamic control of the distribution of cardiac output in the unanesthetized rhesus monkey. *Circ. Res. 26*: 783–794, 1970.
19. Galosy, R. A. and L. K. Clarke, The effect of left dorsal and ventral ansa subclavian transection on cardiac changes during behavioral stress in dogs. *Physiol. Behav. 25*: 195–203, 1980.
20. Galosy, R. A., L. K. Clarke, M. R. Vasko, I. L. Crawford, Neurophysiology and neuropharmacology of cardiovascular regulation and stress. *Neurosci. Biobehav. Rev. 5*: 137–175, 1981.
21. Gibbs, C. M., D. H. Cohen, J. Broyles, A. Solina, Conditioned modification of avian dorsal geniculate neurons is a function of their response to the unconditioned stimulus. *Soc. Neurosci. Abstr. 7*: 752, 1981.
22. Gold, M. R. and D. H. Cohen, Modification of the discharge of vagal cardiac neurons during learned heart rate change. *Science 214*: 345–347, 1981.
23. Grignolo, A., K. C. Light, P. A. Obrist, Beta-adrenergic influence on cardiac dynamics during shock-avoidance in dogs. *Pharm. Biochem. Behav. 14*: 313–319, 1981.
24. Gwirtz, P. A. and H. L. Stone, Coronary blood flow and myocardial oxygen consumption after alpha adrenergic blockade during submaximal exercise. *J. Pharm. Exp. Ther. 217*: 92–98, 1981.
25. Hilton, S. M., Hypothalamic control of the cardiovascular responses in fear and rage. In *The Scientific Basis of Medicine,* 1965, Annual Reviews. Athlone Press, London, pp. 217–238.
26. Hobbs, S. F. Central command in exercise; Parallel activation of the cardiovascular and motor systems by descending command signals, In *Circulation, Neurobiology and Behavior,* Ed. O. A. Smith, R. A. Galosy, and S. M. Weiss. Elsevier Biomedical, New York, pp. 217–231, 1982.
27. Kandel, E., *Cellular Basis of Behavior*. W. H. Freeman, San Francisco, 1976,
28. Klein, M. N. Personal communication.
29. Koester, J., E. Mayeri, G. Liebeswar, E. R. Kandel, Neural control of circulation in *Aplysia*. II. Interneurons. *J. Neurophysiol. 37*: 476–496, 1974.
30. Kumada, M., L. P. Schramm, R. A. Altmansberger, K. Sagawa, Modulation of carotid sinus baroreceptor reflex by hypothalamic defense response. *Am. J. Physiol. 228*: 34–45, 1975.
31. Lown, B., R. A. DeSilva, R. Lenson, Roles of psychologic stress and autonomic nervous system changes in provocation of ventricular premature complexes. *Am. J. Cardiol. 41*: 979–985, 1978.
32. Lukowiak, K. and C. Sahley, The *in vitro* classical conditioning of the gill withdrawal reflex of *Aplysia californica*. *Science 212*: 1516–1518, 1981.
33. Macdonald, R. L. and D. H. Cohen, Cells of origin of sympathetic pre and postganglionic cardioacceleratory fibers in the pigeon. *J. Comp. Neurol. 140*: 343–358, 1970.

34. Macdonald, R. L. and D. H. Cohen, Heart rate and blood pressure responses to electrical stimulation of the central nervous system in the pigeon *(Columbia livia)*. *J. Comp. Neurol., 150*: 109–136, 1973.
35. Marshall, L. B. and O. A. Smith, Prefrontal control of conditioned suppression and associated cardiovascular variables in the monkey *(Macaca mulatta)*. *J. Comp. Physiol. Psychol. 88*: 21–35, 1975.
36. Marshall, L. B., A.R. Zeiner, O. A. Smith, Development of conditioned supression and associated cardiovascular responses in the monkey. *Physiol. Behav., 20*: 441–446, 1978.
37. Mayeri, E., J. Koester, I. Kupfermann, G. Liebeswar, E. R. Kandel, Neural control of circulation in *Aplysia*. I. Motoneurons. *J. Neurophysiol. 37*: 458–475, 1974.
38. Murray, P. A. and S. F. Vatner, Alpha-adrenoceptor attenuation of the coronary vascular response to severe exercise in the conscious dog. *Circ. Res. 45*: 654–660, 1979.
39. Nakao, H., Emotional behavior produced by hypothalamic stimulation. *Am. J. Physiol. 194*: 411–418, 1958.
40. Natelson, B. H. and N. A. Cagin, The role of shock predictability during aversive conditioning in producing psychosomatic digitalis toxicity. *Psychosom. Med. 43*: 191–197, 1981.
41. Nathan, M. A. and O. A. Smith, Jr. Differential conditional emotional and cardiovascular responses—a training technique for monkeys. *J. Exp. Anal. Behavior 11*: 77–82, 1968.
42. Nathan, M. A., L. W. Tucker, W. H. Severini, D. J. Reis, Enhancement of conditioned arterial pressure responses in cats after brainstem lesions. *Science 201*: 71–73, 1978.
43. Randall, D. C. and O. A. Smith, Ventricular contractility during controlled exercise and emotion in the primate. *Am. J. Physiol. 226*: 1051–1059, 1974.
44. Randall, D. C., J. V. Brady, K. H. Martin, Cardiovascular dynamics during classical appetitive and aversive conditioning in laboratory primates. *Pavlovian J. Biol. Sci. 10*: 66–75, 1975.
45. Randall, D. C., M. P. Kaye, W. C. Randall, J. V. Brady, K. H. Martin, Reponse of primate heart to emotional stress before and after cardiac denervation. *Am. J. Physiol. 230*: 988–995, 1976.
46. Randall, D. C., Neural control of the heart in the intact nonhuman primate. In *Neural Regulation of the Heart*, Ed. W. C. Randall. Oxford University Press, New York, pp. 380–408, 1977.
47. Randall, D. C. and D. M. Hasson, Cardiac arrhythmias in the monkey during classically conditioned fear and excitement. *Pavlovian J. Biol. Sci. 16*: 97–107, 1981.
48. Randall, D. C., C. M. Cottrill, E. P. Todd, M. A. Price, C. C. Wachtel, Cardiac output and blood flow distribution during rest and classical aversive conditioning in monkey. *Psychophysiol. 19*: 490–497, 1982.
49. Randall, W. C., J. X. Thomas, D. E. Euler, G. J. Rozanski, Cardiac dysrhythmias associated with autonomic nervous system imbalance in the conscious dog. In Eds. Schwartz, P. J., A. M. Brown, A. Malliani, A. Zanchetti. *Neural Mechanisms in Cardiac Arrhythmias*, Raven Press, New York, pp. 123–138, 1978.
50. Rosenfeld, J., M. R. Rosen, B. F. Hoffman, Pharmacologic and behavioral effects on arrhythmias that immediately follow abrupt coronary occlusion: a canine model of sudden coronary death. *Am. J. Cardiol. 41*: 1075–1082, 1978.

51. Schoenfeld, W. N., R. M. Kadden, P. J. Tremont, M. R. McCullough, W. A. Steele, Effects of pharmacological autonomic blockade upon cardiac rate and blood pressure conditioned and unconditioned response in *Macaca mulatta*. *J. Autonom. Nerv. Sys.* *2*: 365–375, 1980.
52. Schwaber, J. S. and D. H. Cohen, Electrophysiological and electron microscopic analysis of the vagus nerve of the pigeon, with particular reference to the cardiac innervation. *Brain Res.* *147*: 65–78, 1978.
53. Schwartz, P. J. and H. L. Stone, Unilateral stellectomy and sudden death. In *Neural Mechanisms in Cardiac Arrhythmias*, Eds. Schwartz, P. J., A. M. Brown, A. Malliani, A. Zanchetti, Raven Press, New York, pp. 107–122, 1978.
54. Schwartz, P. J. and H. L. Stone, Effects of unilateral stellectomy upon cardiac performance during exercise in dogs. *Circ. Res.* *44*: 637–645, 1979.
55. Schwartz, P. J. and H. L. Stone, Left stellectomy in the prevention of ventricular fibrillation caused by acute myocardial ischemia in conscious dogs with anterior myocardial infarction. *Circulation 62*: 1256–1265, 1980.
56. Skinner, J. E. and C. D. Yingling, Central gating mechanisms that regulate event-related potentials & behavior. A neural model for attention. In *Prog. Clin. Neurophysiol.* (Ed. J. E. Desmedt) *1*: 70–96. S. Karger, Basel, 1977.
57. Skinner, J. E. and J. C. Reed, Blockade of frontocortical-brainstem pathway prevents ventricular fibrillation of ischemic heart. *Am. J. Physiol., 240*: H156–H163, 1981.
58. Skinner, T. L., S. R. Vallance, D. C. Randall, K. L. Park, C. L. Fischer. Effects of behaviorally conditioned changes in autonomic tone on A-V transmission in the dog. *The Physiologist 24*: 22, 1981.
59. Skinner, T. L., The effect of behaviorally mediated changes in neural activity on the atrio-ventricular transmission process. Univ. Kentucky MS thesis, 1982.
60. Smith, O. A., Jr., S. J. Jabbur, R. F. Rushmer, E. P. Lasher, Role of hypothalamic structures in cardiac control. *Physiol. Rev. 40*: 136–141, 1960.
61. Smith, O. A., Jr. Anatomy of central neural pathways mediating cardiovascular functions. In *Nervous Control of the Heart*, Ed. W. C. Randall. Williams & Wilkins, Baltimore, pp. 34–53, 1965.
62. Smith, O. A., Jr., M. A. Nathan, N. P. Clarke, Central nervous system pathways mediating blood pressure changes. In *Hypertension*, Vol. 16: *Neural Control of Arterial Pressure*, Ed. J. E. Wood. American Heart Association, New York: pp. 9–22, 1967.
63. Smith, O. A., Reflex and central mechanisms involved in the control of the heart and circulation. *Ann. Rev. Physiol. 36*: 93–124, 1974.
64. Smith, O. A., C. A. Astley, A. R. Hohimer, R. B. Stephenson, Behavioral and cerebral control of cardiovascular function. In *Neural Control of Circulation*, Eds. J. J. Hughes and C. D. Barnes. Academic Press, New York, pp. 1–21, 1980.
65. Smith, O. A., C. A. Astley, J. L. DeVito, J. M. Stein, K. E. Walsh, Functional analysis of hypothalamic control of the cardiovascular responses accompanying emotional behavior. *Fed. Proc. 39*: 2478–2494, 1980.
66. Smith, O. A., C. A. Astley, J. L. DeVito, Stimulation of rostral afferents to the hypothalamic area controlling the cardiovascular response to emotion. *Fed. Proc. 40*: 522, 1981.
67. Stephenson, R. B. and D. E. Donald, Reversible vascular isolation of carotid sinuses in conscious dogs. *Am. J. Physiol. 238*: H809–H814, 1980.

68. Stephenson, R. B., O. A. Smith, A. M. Scher, Baroreceptor regulation of heart rate in baboons during different behavioral states. *Am. J. Physiol. 241*: R277–R285, 1981.
69. Thomas, J. X., Jr., W. C. Randall, M. J. Barber, J. F. Moran, A-V conduction in the conscious dog. *The Physiologist 22*: 123, 1979.
70. Walgenbach, S. C. and D. E. Donald, Baroreflex regulation of blood pressure during rest and exercise in conscious dogs. *The Physiologist, 24*: 23, 1981.
71. Wild, J. M. and D. H. Cohen, Invariance of retinal output during visual learning. Submitted for publication.

18

Neural Control of the Heart and Coronary Circulation During Exercise

STEPHEN F. VATNER

Exercise is associated with rapid cardiovascular adjustments that are mediated by the autonomic nervous system. In fact, substantial increases in heart rate and myocardial contractility occur even with the anticipation of exercise. During severe exercise heart rate rises rapidly to reach a level over 300 beats/min in the dog, 200 beats/min in man, and to an intermediate peak value in subhuman primates. Similar three- to fivefold increases in myocardial contractility occur with maximal exercise. These factors are responsible in part for the four- to fivefold increases in cardiac output that occur and which provide the necessary blood flow and oxygen delivery to the exercising musculature, including the heart. Autonomic adjustments during exercise occur in the heart, coronary circulation, and peripheral circulations. This chapter emphasizes two of these aspects; autonomic control of ventricular function and autonomic control of the coronary circulation during exercise.

AUTONOMIC CONTROL OF LEFT VENTRICULAR FUNCTION

During near maximal exercise in dogs running spontaneously in the field, heart rate rises fourfold to 300 beats/min. Myocardial contractility also rises approximately fourfold to levels between 12,000 and 15,000 mm Hg/sec (Fig. 18-1) [20,22]. To a major extent these are the mechanisms, which permit the four- to fivefold increases in cardiac output that occur during exercise and which are required to perfuse the exercising musculature (Fig. 18-2). In man the percent increases in cardiac output are somewhat less, as the heart rate can rise only to 200 beats/min during maximal exercise, although the contribution of stroke volume is slightly more important than observed in lower species [3,7].

The question arises as to whether the changes in heart rate and myocardial contractility are autonomically mediated or are due to metabolic changes.

Supported in part by U.S. Public Health Service Grant HL15416, HL17459, and HL23724.

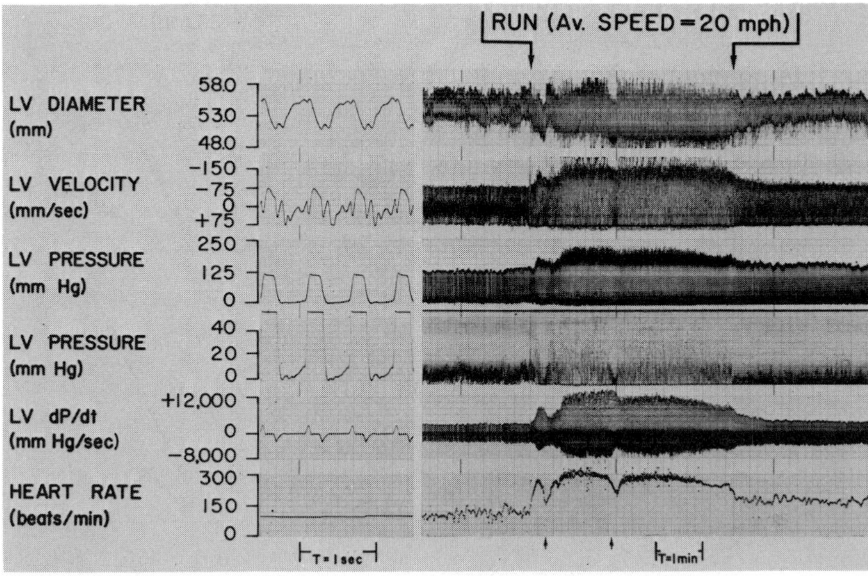

Fig. 18-1. A typical response to intense exercise for phasic left ventricular diameter (epicardial), velocity, pressure, diastolic pressure, dP/dt, and heart rate. Intense exercise was associated with a modest rise in left ventricular end-diastolic diameter and a fall in end-systolic diameter. (Reprinted with permission of *J. Clin. Invest.* *51*: 3052–3060, 1972)

There are several lines of evidence, which point to neural factors responsible for these changes. The fact that maximal values of heart rate and myocardial contractility are achieved rapidly during exercise and even begin before exercise starts, points to factors other than metabolic ones, e.g. activation of autonomic nerves. More important, after beta-adrenergic receptor blockade, exercise results in a limited rise in heart rate (approximately 50% of the normal value) and almost no increase in myocardial contractility (Fig. 18-3) [20,22].

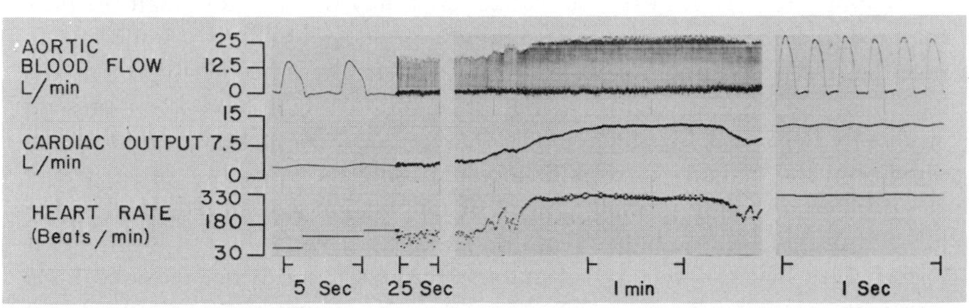

Fig. 18-2. A typical response of aortic blood flow measured and telemetered during intense exercise. The phasic waveforms representing instantaneous stroke volume during exercise at the right played back at fast paper speed can be contrasted to the ones at the left before exercise. The slow rise in mean aortic blood flow (cardiac output) is due to the RC filter having an 8 second time constant. (Reprinted with permission of *J. Clin. Invest.* *51*: 3052–3060, 1972)

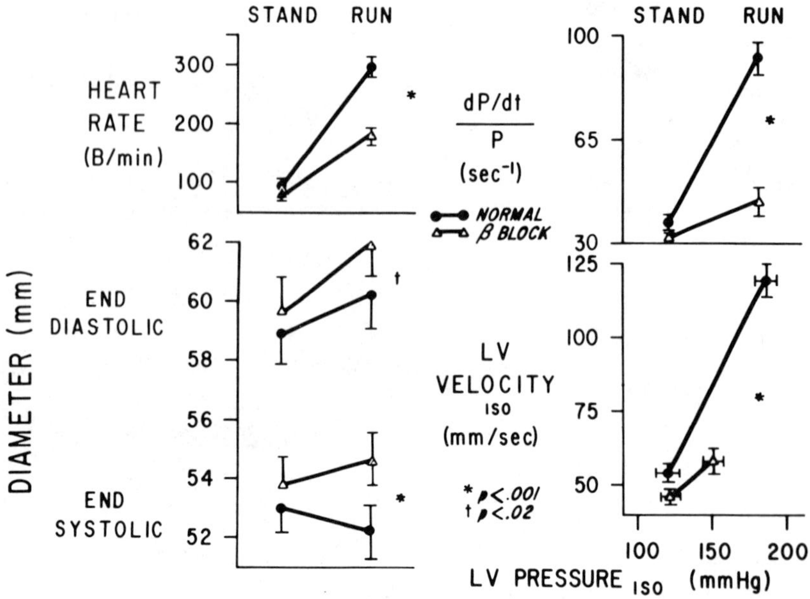

Fig. 18-3. Average ± SE values standing, at rest, and during steady-state intense exercise for seven dogs studied in both spontaneous rhythm and after 1.0 mg/kg propranolol. The values attained during intense exercise that were significantly different are noted. (Reprinted with permission of *J. Clin. Invest. 51*: 3052–3060, 1972)

Blocking neural response, then, impairs the response of cardiac output to exercise and ultimately the ability to perform exercise. Those experiments in man and animals have both pointed out an important role for the beta-adrenergic nervous system in the response to exercise [7,20,22].

Experiments by Donald, Shepherd, and co-workers, have demonstrated that an intact cardiac autonomic nervous innervation is not essential to the exercise response [5,6]. In fact, in the studies in dogs with denervated hearts, the maximum ability to perform exercise was affected only trivially, although the time required to achieve maximal heart rate was prolonged [5,6]. It is important to note that the experiments of Donald and Shephard have been criticized on the basis that incomplete cardiac neural denervation might have been present. Studies by Peiss et al. [4], suggested that a significant component of innervation remains in the majority of dogs denervated using the technique of Cooper et al. [19]. Perhaps, only a small amount of innervation is required to allow the heart to respond normally to stress such as exercise. Regardless, it is important to recognize that the majority of autonomic innervation is not required for a seemingly normal response to intense exercise. These observations suggest that other compensatory mechanisms exist, which can be called into play in the absence of an intact autonomic nervous system.

One of these compensatory mechanisms is the Frank-Starling mechanism [2,9,18,23]. It plays an exceedingly important role in regulating cardiac performance in isolated cardiac muscle strips, isolated hearts, and in open-chest, anesthetized preparations. In the intact, conscious animal or man, the Frank-Starling mechanism appears of lesser importance and is overshadowed or masked by the concomitant tachycardia [2,23]. As long as heart rate can rise normally during exercise, the increases in LV end-diastolic size and concomitant increases in LV stroke shortening and stroke volume (Frank-Starling mechanism) tend to be offset (Fig. 18-4) [20,22]. The role of the Frank-Starling mechanism is somewhat more prominent when examined in man during upright exercise than during supine exercise [7]. This is because the baseline values for cardiac end-diastolic dimensions decrease upon assuming the upright posture, and therefore can increase further during exercise. In summary, the Frank-Starling mechanism plays only a minor role in regulating ventricular stroke shortening and stroke volume during normal exercise. However, that role might be enhanced considerably in the presence of disease states or cardiac neural ablation, and particularly in cases where baseline heart rate is already elevated. In the absence of normal cardiac innervation, it is also conceivable that metabolic adjustments occur, which allow more intense exercise under conditions of limited blood flow and oxygen delivery.

While the beta-adrenergic component of the sympathetic nervous system plays an important role during normal exercise, there is little evidence that parasympathetic regulation of cardiac performance is of major significance. In

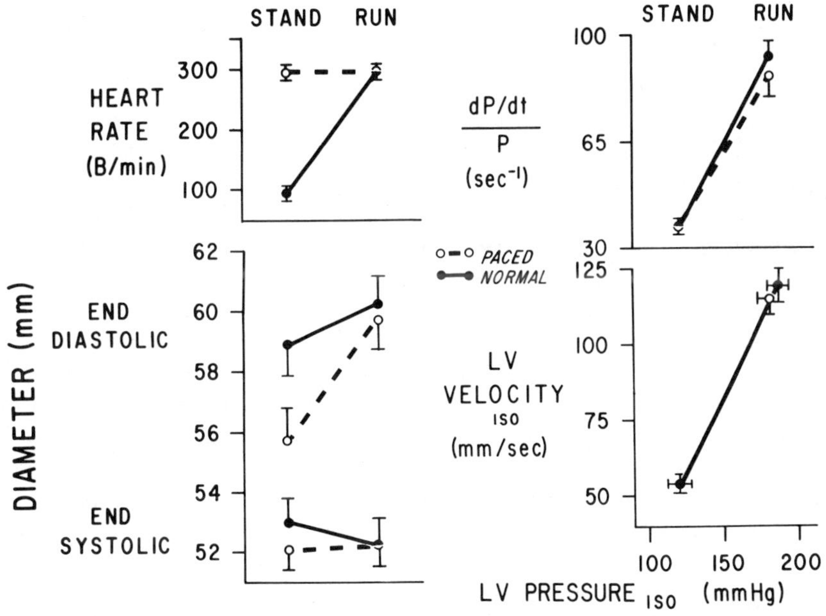

Fig. 18-4. The average ± SE values standing, at rest, and during intense exercise for seven dogs studied both in spontaneous rhythm and after heart rate had been elevated at rest to exercise levels with electrical stimulation of the atria. None of the values attained during steady-state intense exercise were significantly different in these two states. (Reprinted with permission of *J. Clin. Invest. 51*: 3052–3060, 1972)

fact, if the parasympathetic nervous system were activated, then a decrease in heart rate should occur, but, in fact, resting parasympathetic activity is withdrawn and heart rate rises during exercise. Thus, it appears that the vagus is turned off during exercise. Moreover, responses to exercise are essentially identical in the presence and absence of parasympathetic blockade with atropine, indicating the relative lack of importance of this system in mediating responses to exercise.

NEURAL CONTROL OF THE CORONARY VASCULAR BED DURING SEVERE EXERCISE

The coronary circulation is primarily regulated by the changes in myocardial metabolic demands. At any given perfusion pressure, myocardial oxygen consumption and consequently coronary blood flow and vascular resistance are regulated by changes in heart rate, LV wall tension, and myocardial contractility. It is only when these metabolic factors have been accounted for that neural and humoral mechanisms can be considered. The role of sympathetic is much more important during exercise that the parasympathetic. The latter plays an important role in regulating the coronary circulation at rest, but during exercise, as noted above, is turned off.

The ways in which the sympathetic nervous system regulates the coronary circulation during exercise are interconnected. First, it is important to keep in mind the two major subdivisions of the adrenergic nervous system, the alpha and beta. Both the alpha and beta adrenergic systems have at least two functions with separate receptors and are referred to as $alpha_1$, $alpha_2$, and $beta_1$, $beta_2$. The adrenergic system can be activated by sympathetic nerves, which release norepinephrine at the nerve ending, or by circulating catecholamines from the adrenal medulla, which release both norepinephrine and epinephrine. Norepinephrine and epinephrine are similar in that they both contain alpha-stimulating properties, but differ in that norepinephrine contains $beta_1$ stimulating properties, while epinephrine stimulates both $beta_1$ and $beta_2$ adrenergic receptors. The $alpha_1$ receptors are postjunctional, and when stimulated constrict blood vessels in the coronary as well as systemic circulation [8,21,24]. The $alpha_2$ receptors are prejunctional, and when stimulated act as a negative feedback mechanism by reducing the release of norepinephrine from the neuron terminal [15]. The $beta_1$ receptors, when stimulated are responsible for adrenergically mediated increases in heart rate and myocardial contractility, while their role in vascular regulation remains controversial. In contrast, the $beta_2$ receptors are located primarily in blood vessels, and as far as the cardiovascular system is concerned, when stimulated result in arteriolar dilation [10,12,16,25].

Clearly the major response of the coronary vascular bed to exercise is the marked dilation that occurs in the coronary bed (Fig. 18-5), which is the primary mechanism by which oxygen is provided to the exercising heart. This is necessary because the oxygen extraction is almost maximally complete at rest and can be enhanced only slightly during exercise. Thus, an increase in coronary blood flow is the most prominent mechanism by which oxygen supply can

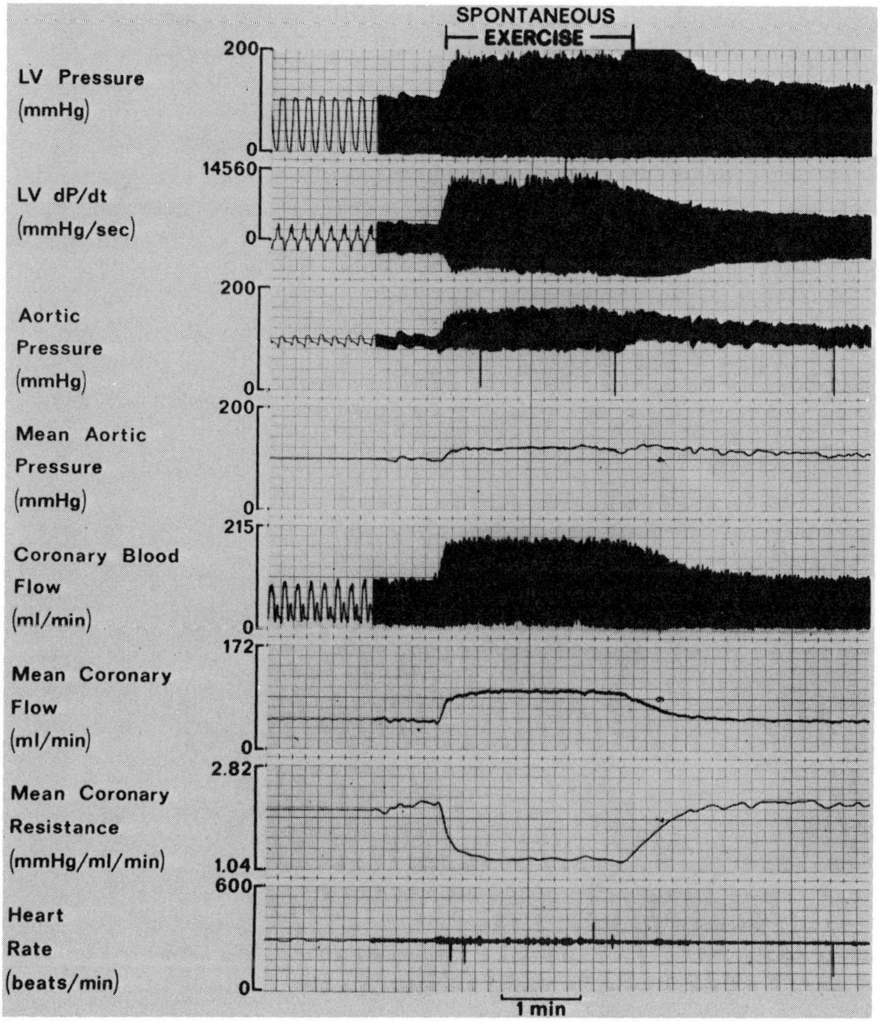

Fig. 18-5. Characteristic responses of the measured variables to a period of intense, free-ranging exercise over a 0.5-mile hilly course in the absence of any pharmacological blocking agent. Maximum speed of 20 miles/hour was attained by this dog during the course of the exercise period. Heart rate was held constant at approximately 300 beats/min by electrical pacing. (Reprinted with permission of *Circulation Research 45*: 654–660, 1979)

increase. Normally the coronary vascular bed responds with a fourfold increase in coronary blood flow during the stress of intense exercise. This is required to provide oxygen for the increased myocardial metabolic demands induced by increases in heart rate, ventricular wall tension, and myocardial contractility. As pointed out above, the increases in heart rate and myocardial contractility are due to neural factors and thus in many ways the coronary vascular response to exercise can be considered neurally mediated, albeit, secondarily to metabolic demands. However, it is important to emphasize the secondary rather than primary nature of the coronary vascular response. By far the major response of the coronary circulation to exercise is an increase in coronary blood flow and decrease in coronary vascular resistance secondary to the augmented myocardial metabolic demands.

The increases in myocardial metabolic demands are generated primarily from $beta_1$ adrenergic increases in cardiac contractility, cardiac rate, and wall tension. While the coronary circulation is endowed with $beta_2$ adrenergic receptors, which when stimulated result in coronary vasodilation [16,17,25], the extent to which these are activated during exercise is not known. It is unlikely that $beta_2$ adrenergic coronary vasodilation occurs during exercise secondary to increased cardiac neural activity, since experiments with electrical stimulation of cardiac nerves failed to demonstrate appreciable $beta_2$ adrenergic vasodilation [12]. However, increases in circulating epinephrine could mediate $beta_2$ adrenergic coronary vasodilation during exercise.

The extent to which alpha adrenergic modulation of the coronary vascular response to exercise occurs was recently examined in our laboratory [17]. Since the coronary bed is innervated by alpha adrenergic receptors, it could respond to the prevailing increased levels of sympathetic drive to the heart with alpha adrenergic coronary constriction. If this occurred, then alpha adrenergically mediated vasoconstriction induced by neural mechanisms could attenuate the metabolic vasodilation that occurs during exercise. To address this possibility, we examined responses to exercise in dogs in the presence and absence of alpha

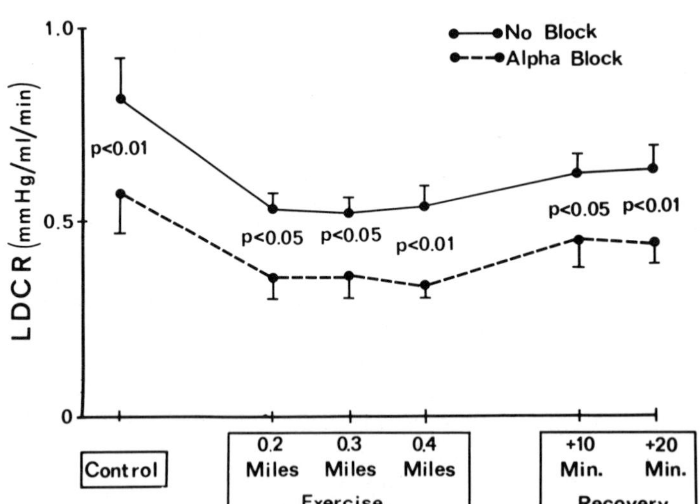

Fig. 18-6. Average (± SEM) values of late diastolic coronary resistance (LDCR) in nine dogs with α-receptor activity intact (no block), and after blockage of α-receptor activity (α block) while standing quietly prior to exercise, at 0.2, 0.3, and 0.4 mile during the exercise period and 10 and 20 minutes after cessation of exercise. Heart rate was held constant at approximately 300 beats/min by electrical pacing. (Reprinted with permission of *J. Clin. Invest.* *51*: 3052–3060, 1972)

adrenergic receptor blockade with phentolamine. After pretreatment with phentolamine coronary vascular resistance fell to significantly lower levels during exercise than in the absence of alpha adrenergic receptor blockade (Fig. 18-6). However, these experiments are inconclusive, due to concomitant changes in heart rate and myocardial contractility, that might have complicated the interpretation of the data. To avoid these complicating factors, the animals were pretreated with beta adrenergic receptor blockade, and heart rate was held constant. Under these conditions it was observed that significantly greater increases in coronary blood blow and decreases in coronary vascular resistance occurred in the presence of combined alpha and beta adrenergic receptor blockade than with beta adrenergic blockade alone (Fig. 18-7). These studies support the hypothesis that there is alpha adrenergic activation during exercise, which can attenuate the metabolic vasodilation that occurs during this stress. Studies by Gwirtz and Stone [11], and by Heyndrickx et al. [13] further support this hypothesis in that they measured arterial and coronary sinus oxygen contents at rest and during exercise. They both observed that there was a widening of cor-

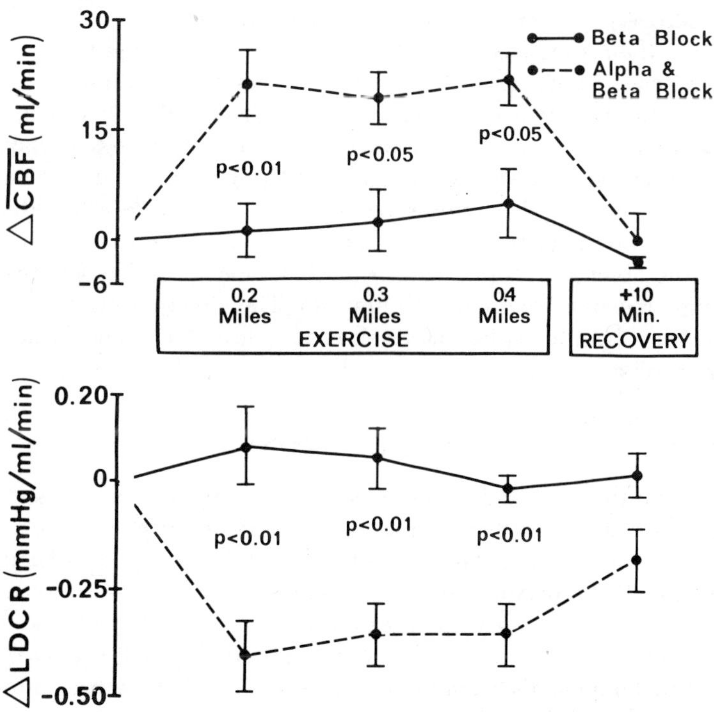

Fig. 18-7. Average (± SEM) changes in mean left circumflex coronary blood flow (Δ CBF) (top) and late diastolic coronary resistance (Δ LDCR) (bottom) of nine dogs during spontaneous exercise at 0.2, 0.3, and 0.4 mile and 10 minutes after cessation of exercise following pretreatment with propranolol with α-receptor activity intact (β block) and following blockade of α-receptor activity (α and β block). Heart rate was held constant at approximately 190 beats/min by electrical pacing. (Reprinted with permission of *J. Clin. Invest. 51*: 3052–3060, 1972)

onary A-V O_2 difference during exercise, particularly noticeable in the presence of beta adrenergic blockade, and which was abolished by pretreatment with alpha adrenergic receptor blockade. Thus, the alpha adrenergically mediated vasoconstriction results in additional oxygen extraction across the heart during exercise. In addition Aung-Din et al. demonstrated alpha-adrenergic coronary constriction during static hindlimb exercise as well [1].

The results of these experiments have potential clinical relevance. It is known that angina pectoris is frequently elicited by exercise. It is generally thought that this pathological situation is mediated by increases in myocardial metabolic demands that occur in excess of myocardial blood supply. It is not generally thought that neural mechanisms play any major role in mediating angina pectoris during exercise. However, it is conceivable that under certain conditions alpha-adrenergic vasoconstriction may act in concert with enhanced metabolic demand to reduce the blood supply of an area that is rendered ischemic during exercise.

The above evidence for the role of $alpha_1$ adrenergic receptors during exercise has recently been complemented by studies demonstrating a function for $alpha_2$ adrenergic receptors during exercise. Prejunctional $alpha_2$ adrenergic receptors, when stimulated, inhibit norepinephrine release at the sympathetic nerve endings [15]. It appears that during moderate exercise $alpha_2$ stimulation attenuates the rise in norepinephrine, and consequently LV dP/dt, for any given increase in coronary blood flow [14]. Experiments in dogs during exercise by Heyndrickx and co-workers demonstrated a significantly greater rise in LV dP/dt and heart rate during exercise after $alpha_2$ blockade with either phentolamine or yohimbine (which blocks $alpha_2$ receptors) as opposed to that occurring in the absence of alpha adrenergic blockade or during selective $alpha_1$ adrenergic receptor blockade with prazosin. The $alpha_2$ mechanism may protect the heart by attenuating the levels of myocardial norepinephrine attained during exercise.

CONCLUSIONS

The stress on the heart and coronary bed imposed by severe exercise is met by a variety of compensatory mechanisms. The major efferent autonomic mechanisms involve activation of both the beta adrenergic and alpha adrenergic arms of the sympathetic nervous system. The other major branch of the autonomic nervous system, the parasympathetic arm, plays little efferent role, since its major effect is one of withdrawal of vagal restraint. While it is clear that these neural and humoral mechanisms are considerable, their precise importance under normal conditions is not established, since there are other secondary compensatory mechanisms which can be called upon in the absence of autonomic influences.

Thus, despite extensive research that has involved control of the heart and coronary circulation during exercise, more questions remain than have been answered. Questions of major importance are: (1) What are the afferent signals responsible for mediating the autonomic adjustments to exercise? (2) What is the role of receptors and/or nerves in the central nervous system, which might be capable of initiating exercise responses in the presence or absence of afferent input? (3) How are the autonomic mechanisms altered in the presence of cardiovascular disease, e.g. myocardial hypertrophy, cardiac failure, and coronary arterial spasm?

REFERENCES

1. Aung-Din, R., J. H. Mitchell, J. C. Longhurst, Reflex alpha-adrenergic coronary vasoconstriction during hindlimb static exercise in dogs, *Circ. Res. 48*: 502–509, 1981.
2. Boettcher, D. H., S. F. Vatner, G. R. Heyndrickx, E. Braunwald, Extent of utilization of Frank-Starling mechanism in conscious dogs, *Am. J. Physiol. 3*: H338-H345, 1978.
3. Chapman, C. B., J. N. Fisher, J. J. Sproule, Behavior of stroke volume at rest and during exercise in human beings, *J. Clin. Invest. 39*: 1208–1213, 1960.
4. Cooper, T., J. W. Gilbert, Jr., R. D. Bloodwell, J. R. Crout, Chronic extrinsic cardiac denervation by regional neural ablation: description of the operation, verification of denervation and its effects on myocardial catecholamines, *Circ. Res. 9*: 275–281, 1961.
5. Donald, D. E. and J. T. Shepherd, Response to exercise in dogs with cardiac denervation, *Am. J. Physiol. 205*: 393–400, 1963.
6. Donald, D. E., S. E. Milburn, J. T. Shepherd, Effect of cardiac denervation on the maximal capacity for exercise in the racing greyhound, *J. Appl. Physiol. 19*: 849–852, 1964.
7. Epstein, S. E., B. F. Robinson, R. L. Hakler, E. Braunwald, Effects of beta-adrenergic blockade on the cardiac response to maximal and submaximal exercise in man, *J. Clin. Invest. 44*: 1745–1753, 1965.
8. Feigl, E. O., Control of myocardial oxygen tension by sympathetic coronary vasoconstriction in the dog, *Circ. Res. 37*: 88–95, 1975.
9. Frank, O., Zur dynamik des herzmuskels, Z. *Biol. 32*: 370–437, 1895.
10. Gross, G. J. and E. O. Feigl, Analysis of coronary vascular beta receptors in situ, *Am. J. Physiol. 228*: 1909–1913, 1975.
11. Gwirtz, P. A. and H. L. Stone, Coronary blood flow and myocardial oxygen consumption after alpha adrenergic blockade during submaximal exercise, *J. Pharmacol. Exp. Ther. 217*: 92–98, 1981.
12. Hamilton, F. N. and E. O. Feigl, Coronary vascular sympathetic beta-receptor innervation, *Am. J. Physiol. 230*: 1569–1576, 1976.
13. Heyndrickx, G. R., P. Muylaert, J. L. Pannier, Alpha-adrenergic control of oxygen delivery to myocardium during exercise in conscious dogs, *Am. J. Physiol. 242*: H805-H809, 1982.
14. Heyndrickx, G. R., J. P. Vilaine, E. Moerman, I. Leusen, Presynaptic $alpha_2$ adrenoreceptor regulation of myocardial performance during exercise in conscious dogs, *Circulation 66*: 1014, 1982 (abstr.).
15. Langer, S. Z., Presynaptic receptors and their role in the regulation of transmitter release, *Br. J. Pharmacol. 60*: 481–497, 1977.
16. McRaven, D. R., A. L. Mark, F. M. Abboud, H. E. Mayer, Responses of coronary vessels to adrenergic stimuli, *J. Clin. Invest. 50*: 773–778, 1971.

17. Murray, P. A., S. F. Vatner, Alpha-adrenergic attenuation of the coronary vascular response to severe exercise in the conscious dog, *Circ. Res. 45*: 654–660, 1979.
18. Patterson, S. W. and E. H. Starling, On the mechanical factors which determine the output of the ventricles, *J. Physiol. (Lon.) 48*: 375–379, 1914.
19. Peiss, C. N., T. Cooper, V. L. Willman, W. C. Randall, Circulatory responses to electrical and reflex activation of the nervous system after cardiac denervation, *Circ. Res. 19*: 153–166, 1966.
20. Vatner, S. F., D. Franklin, C. B. Higgins, T. Patrick, E. Braunwald, Left ventricular response to severe exertion in untethered dogs, *J. Clin. Invest. 51*: 3052–3060, 1972.
21. Vatner, S. F., C. B. Higgins, E. Braunwald, Effects of norepinephrine on coronary circulation and left ventricular dynamics in the conscious dog, *Circ. Res. 34*: 812–823, 1974.
22. Vatner, S. F. and M. Pagani, Cardiovascular adjustments to exercise: hemodynamics and mechanisms, In *Progress in Cardiovascular Diseases*. 19: 91–108, 1976.
23. Vatner, S. F. and D. H. Boettcher, Regulation of cardiac output by stroke volume and heart rate in conscious dogs, *Circ. Res. 42*: 557–561, 1978.
24. Vatner, S. B., M. Pagani, W. T. Manders, A. D. Pasipoularides, Alpha adrenergic vasoconstriction and nitroglycerine vasodilation of large coronary arteries in the conscious dog, *J. Clin. Invest. 65*: 5–14, 1980.
25. Vatner, S. F., T. H. Hintze, P. Macho, Regulation of large coronary arteries by beta adrenergic mechanisms in the conscious dog, *Circ. Res. 51*: 56–66, 1982.

19

The Rationale for Therapeutic Cardiac Denervation

WALTER C. RANDALL, JOHN X. THOMAS, JR., and ROLF M. GUNNAR

Technology requisite for therapeutic denervation of the human heart is now available, even to the extent of cardiac transplantation. Reference is made repeatedly in this book (chapters 3,4,10–12) to applications of denervation, partial or complete, for the treatment of human cardiac disease states. Kaye (chapter 12) discusses denervation in the treatment of vasospasm and ventricular tachyarrhythmias, while Schwartz (chapter 10) illustrates the role of sympathectomy in cases of sympathetic imbalance. In view of dramatic improvements in diagnostic evaluations of specific cardiac disease states, as well as the emergence of surgical and/or pharmacological therapies, it seems appropriate at this juncture to briefly review selected clinical situations in which cardiac denervation merits consideration. It is our opinion that *selective* denervation of highly restricted portions of the heart will evolve in the immediate future (chapter 3), and that specific treatment of both abnormal A-V junctional conduction problems, and conditions currently blanketed under sick sinus syndrome, debilitating bradydysrhythmias, etc., may be accomplished. Besides the potential therapeutic benefit of denervation in rhythm disturbances, we shall also explore the rationale for applying this technique to functional disturbances such as coronary vasospasm, focal ischemia, etc.

Attempts to denervate the heart in the treatment of variant angina or as an adjunct to coronary bypass surgery have been successful in several different hospitals [2,18,22]. The combination of coronary arterial bypass grafting with partial denervation of the heart in order to prevent arterial spasm was first described by Arnulf [1], and later employed by Grondin and Limet [22] and Bertrand et al. [4,5], in patients with Prinzmetal's angina. Therapeutic results have not proved universally successful, perhaps because of different surgical

Experimental data were supported by grants from the National Institutes of Health, HL08682, HL27595, The Bane Charitable Trust of Chicago, and the James DePauw Fund of Chicago.

approaches, varying degrees of completeness of denervation [38], and wide variability in symptom complexes in patients tested.

In theory, denervation of the heart may be expected to contribute significantly to relief of ischemic pain, protect against electrical instability, remove vasoconstrictor tone, and perhaps conserve oxygen utilization. A systematic review of indications for therapeutic cardiac denervation and its application to selected patients has not been made. In fact, chapter 11 presents some arguments against using cardiac denervation in human patients. Therefore, in this chapter we will present a rationale supporting cardiac denervation (complete or partial) in treatment of carefully selected cases of cardiac disease.

Previously, dependable denervation has been difficult to achieve and, short of cardiac transplantation, many procedures may actually endanger innervation of extracardiac tissues. The recent development of an intrapericardial approach to cardiac denervation [52] provides a relatively simple technical accomplishment of either total or selectively partial denervation, with the ability to confirm completeness of denervation at the time of surgery. It insures against concurrent denervation of other thoracic or abdominal organ systems. It would be of great interest, in fact, to know how much denervation is inadvertently accomplished during conventional aortocoronary bypass surgery. Dissection around the base of the aorta and pulmonary arteries, exposure of the superior surfaces of the atria, and dissection in the region of the coronary arteries may result in considerable denervation of the heart, an important concern which, to our knowledge, has not been adequately evaluated. Indeed, relief of anginal pain has been reported frequently to outlast patency of the grafts, suggesting that at least some afferent denervation occurs. The early reports of 90% relief of symptoms with only 85% graft patency would support the hypothesis that relief of symptoms occurs by some mechanism other than vascular bypass of the obstruction.

At present, considerable controversy exists over the effectiveness of surgical revascularization versus medical therapy in the treatment of coronary artery disease. In either group of patients, routine postoperative and postmedical therapy follow-up tests have indicated four categories of patients classified according to perception of anginal pain by the patient and demonstrable electrocardiographic ST segmental changes: (1) ischemic ST segment with no angina, (2) ischemic ST with angina, (3) no ischemic ST with no angina, and (4) inconclusive treadmill tests. Mnayer et al. [47] found that in the medically treated group, only 9% of the patients fell into the first category, while in the surgically treated group, there was an alarming 59% of the patients. This finding is also consistent with the hypothesis that coronary bypass surgery may result in considerable afferent denervation.

Given the technical feasibility of thoroughly safe, consistent surgical denervation at the time of bypass or associated cardiac surgery, what are some of the reasons for considering such therapy? There is a growing body of scientific evidence that demands further examination of this procedure as a possible alternative therapy in each of the following clinical entities: (1) severe alpha-adrenergic-mediated coronary vasospasm, (2) intractable ventricular tachydysrhythmia and fibrillation, (3) severe anginal pain, (4) myocardial ischemia with absence of collaterals, and (5) protection from impending infarction. Let us consider the role and possible influence of cardiac denervation in each of these important clinical conditions.

CORONARY VASOSPASM OF NEURAL ORIGIN

Since Prinzmetal's report on variant angina in 1959 [51], much interest in its underlying causes and its treatment has arisen [16,20,43,55,61]. The occurrence of symptoms during periods of quiet rest, or even sleep, indicates a functional mechanism quite different from that responsible for exertional angina, and indicates active vasomotor tone as its fundamental cause [9,10,25,32,45,49]. Many investigators have been able to demonstrate spasm involving long segments of the proximal conduit arteries at angiography, and some have reported prompt and complete relief by means of alpha-adrenergic blocking agents [35,44,46, 62]. While spasmodic features of coronary occlusion and infarction have been well described, they have been largely ignored by those who firmly believe in mechanical obstruction (plaque or thrombi) as the causative mechanism. Even those authorities who believe in vasospasm as a likely cause of acute myocardial infarction frequently ignore the possible implication of alpha-adrenergic constriction [26]. In acute episodes, vasospasm may actually be confused with coronary thrombosis, platelet plugging, or downstream vasoconstriction that progressively spreads proximally to develop into an angiographically demonstrable spasm. A previously existing plaque would serve to exacerbate the condition.

As in Raynaud's and other vasospastic diseases [11], denervation should be expected to prevent or abolish arterial spasm of sympathetic origin. Indeed, sympathetic cardiac denervation has been advocated at various times [1,37] to interrupt pain fibers in patients with angina pectoris. Schwartz describes in detail the possible advantages of complete or partial sympathectomy in treatment of sympathetic imbalance in the heart (see chapter 10). Grondin and Limet [22] and Bertrand et al. [4,5] have recently reported good to excellent results in combining sympathetic denervation with coronary artery grafting. Since the variant forms of angina involve a wide spectrum of coronary vascular disease, ranging from apparently normal appearing vessels to severely restricted ones, cardiac denervation should be considered among possible therapeutic regimens. Even in the absence of vasospasm as the precipitating factor in ischemia, it has been suggested that localized release of norepinephrine during ischemia can produce localized spasm [60]. This could potentially further limit flow and has been shown to be eliminated by local infiltration with procaine, which presumably produces localized denervation [21].

INTRACTABLE VENTRICULAR TACHYDYSRHYTHMIA

In patients with intractable ventricular arrhythmia, cardiac denervation should be considered as a potentially life-saving procedure. Employing a chloralose anesthetized dog model after vagotomy and sinus node clamping, Martins recently demonstrated that the sympathetic nerves directly increase rates of spontaneous ventricular tachycardia resulting from 24-hour myocardial ischemia [42]. Stellate ganglionectomy or local chemical sympathectomy (epicardial phenol application) markedly reduced the incidence of tachycardic complexes. Decreased incidence of fibrillation after sympathectomy was first reported by Harris et al. [24]. Ebert and colleagues [15] demonstrated the remarkable protection against fatal arrhythmia following coronary artery ligation in the denervated dog heart afforded by sympathectomy.

Employing animal models, Lown and Verrier [39] manipulated the sympathetic neural inut to influence cardiac vulnerability to electrical instability and fibrillation. During ischemia, they found that such input may be a sufficient stimulus to trigger fibrillation. Psychological stress, even of brief duration, can profoundly reduce the threshold for fibrillation and result in major disorders in rhythm. These authors cite references claiming significant reduction in incidence of sudden death by use of beta-adrenergic blocking drugs. It may be true that cause-and-effect relationships may exist between myocardial tissue catecholamine levels and electrical instability of ventricular tissue. Ebert observed that adequate time must elapse between cardiac denervation (which results in depletion in myocardial catecholamines) and reduction in electrical vulnerability. Many investigations have demonstrated a direct relationship between ventricular fibrillation thresholds and electrical excitation within the sympathetic nervous system [32,57,58]. The simultaneous creation of myocardial ischemia further exaggerates the instability [6,40,7]. Harken et al. [23] recently reviewed surgical attempts to treat ventricular tachycardia in humans by sympathectomy [17,38,48,63] and reported typically successful "arrhythmia control" in 50–60% of patients.

Thus, there is ample evidence for an intrinsic relationship between myocardial excitability, ischemia, and levels of sympathetic tone. In a heart in which such electrical instability cannot be adequately controlled by pharmacological therapy, denervation would appear to be a viable alternative or adjunct to ventricular aneurysmectomy-bypass procedures.

RELIEF OF ANGINAL PAIN

In patients with severe anginal pain, particularly if it is not associated with intense exertional stresses, interruption of the afferent pathways within sympathetic cardiac nerves for such pain would be a direct therapeutic intervention. Such surgical treatment was recognized and proposed at the turn of the century by Francois Franck [19]. Kaye has carefully reviewed the arguments for and against this approach to the treatment of anginal pain in chapter 12, with particular reference to the summary of Cutler and Fine in 1926 describing the merits of sympathectomy as applied early in the twentieth century [12]. Kaye also refers to the fundamental argument that transection of pain pathways results in removal of pain as a "danger signal" which potentially warns patients that their heart is being "overtaxed." White and Bland [50] reported that in some patients subjected to various forms of denervation, referred pain persisted at the jaw with the onset of ischemic events. Actually, the precise mechanisms of cardiac pain are still not understood (chapter 16), and only if nerve traffic can be clearly demonstrated in the afferent cardiac nerves during appropriate ischemic stimulation can we be certain that elimination of pain can be accomplished by denervation. However, the relief of pain following cardiac denervation might result from a combination of afferent denervation and the previously described [3,28,30] salutary effects during ischemic episodes.

CARDIAC INNERVATION AND COLLATERAL RESISTANCE

Chronic ventricular sympathectomy results in increased perfusion of ischemic myocardium following acute coronary occlusion (see chapter 11). Thus, after coronary ligation in hearts that have been surgically denervated 2 weeks previously, contractile force in myocardium supplied by the occluded vessel was maintained at a higher level than in control, acutely denervated, or sham-denervated hearts [56]. Moreover, tracer microsphere studies directly demonstrate that after coronary ligation in ventricles that had been surgically sympathectomized 2 weeks earlier, perfusion of the ischemic myocardium (distal to the ligation) was 200–400% of that in controls [27]. The increased perfusion was thought to be due to increased collateral blood flow secondary to reduced resistance in anastomotic collateral channels. Jones et al. employed Scheel's isolated dog heart preparation to measure directional collateral resistances in both acutely and chronically denervated hearts. The major coronary arteries were perfused separately during maximum vasodilation (adenosine), and collateral resistances were measured. In chronically sympathectomized hearts, all collateral resistances were 47–65% less than in controls [29]. This suggests that the increased perfusion is a time dependent mechanism and not simply due to the interruption of existing vasoconstrictor tone to the coronary vessels. It has been suggested that removal of sympathetic innervation to the ventricle may stimulate the development of collateral vessels, although the mechanism(s) involved remain obscure.

PROTECTION AGAINST IMPENDING INFARCTION

Recent laboratory data document an important autonomic influence on the ischemic myocardium. Following coronary occlusion, administered catecholamines increase infarct size [13,34], impair contractile function [8], increase ST segment elevation [41], and profoundly alter myocardial metabolism [53,59]. Conversely, after coronary occlusion propranolol or practolol reduce infarct size [36,41,53], ST segment elevation [36,41], serum enzyme levels of CPK [50] and coronary microvascular injury [33]. Thus it appears that after coronary occlusion, enhanced adrenergic activity has deleterious effects, while blockage of adrenergic activity has beneficial results.

All of the above data were based on acute or immediate effects, and other experiments suggest that even more dramatic protection is afforded by long-term cardiac denervation. Thus, coronary occlusion in hearts denervated 2 weeks earlier resulted in much smaller infarct size [28] than was documented in normally innervated hearts. The reduction in infarct size was associated with diminished ST segment elevation following occlusion in the chronically denervated heart [3], increased perfusion to the ischemic region in the chronically sympathectomized heart, and decreased production of lactate by the ischemic denervated heart [30].

Finally, comparisons have been made in contractile force in the ischemic zone (during localized coronary arterial occlusion) of three groups of animals: (1) controls, (2) acutely denervated hearts, and (3) chronically denervated hearts. Following occlusion, contractile force in the ischemic area decreased by 67% in the control group, 74% in the acutely denervated group, but only 22% ($p < 0.001$) in the chronically denervated group. Infarct size was only 4% of left ventricular weight in chronically denervated dog hearts as compared to 20.1% in the control group and 16.2% in the acutely denervated group. Thus, chronic cardiac denervation in the experimental model limits infarct size, results in maintenance of contractile function, and enhanced levels of collateral blood flow.

In addition, as detailed in chapter 11, myocardial oxygen consumption is reduced by approximately 25% in the chronically denervated heart. It has been theorized that this reduction in oxygen demand (increased efficiency) contributes significantly to the salutary effects of denervation witnessed during myocardial ischemia. In the clinical setting of angina pectoris in a patient with both large and small vessel disease, revascularization could circumvent the danger created by large vessel lesions. However, the patient's prognosis might be jeopardized by the presence of lesions in the small vessels. Small vessel disease in angina has not been documented as an anatomical entity, but there may be changes in vascular resistance, a *functional* abnormality. We suggest that cardiac denervation would improve the prognosis because of the beneficial effects outlined above. Furthermore, we propose that denervation at the time of revascularization may also reduce the incidence and severity of perioperative myocardial infarction. These dramatic effects certainly warrant careful consideration for application of surgical denervation in the human patient.

CONCLUSIONS

Compelling reasons for either partial or complete cardiac denervation can be developed in each of five clinical circumstances, in addition to cases of serious sympathetic imbalance and in patients at risk of sudden death as discussed in Chapters 10 and 20. While the concept of therapeutic denervation has occasionally surfaced during the past several years, adequate surgical technology and better functional understanding of vasospasm have evolved only recently. Many questions have not been resolved simply because appropriate clinical experience has not accumulated. These remaining concerns include hypersensitivity to circulating autonomic transmitters, incidence and time course of reinnervation, functional responsiveness of the cardiovascular and sensory systems following denervation, and the potential possibility of unequal regrowth of neurons to different parts of the heart. However, the successful performance of cardiac transplantation in human subjects, at least for several years, proves that the results of denervation will not be catastrophic but could provide many years of improved quality of life.

REFERENCES

1. Arnulf, G., De la section du plexus preaortique: justification et technique, *Presse Med. 47*: 1635–1638, 1939.
2. Arnulf, G., Les operations de denervation de coronaries, In *Chirurgie des Coronaires*, ed. G. Arnulf. Paris: Masson, p. 197, 1965.
3. Barber, M. J., D. E. Euler, J. X. Thomas, W. C. Randall, Changes in blood flow and S-T segment during coronary arterial occlusion in denervated and nondenervated canine hearts, *Am.J.Cardiol. 45*: 973–978, 1980.
4. Bertrand, M. E., J. M. LaBlanche, M. F. Rousseau, H. H. Warembourg, Jr., C. Stankowtak, C. Soots, Surgical treatment of variant angina: use of plexectomy with aortocoronary bypass, *Circulation 61*: 877–881, 1980.
5. Bertrand, M. E., J. M. LaBlanche, P. Y. Tilmant, Treatment of Prinzmetal's variant angina. Role of medical treatment with nifedipine and surgical coronary revascularization combined with plexectomy, *Am.J.Cardiol. 47*: 174–178, 1981.
6. Brown, A. M., Excitation of afferent cardiac sympathetic nerve fibers during myocardial ischemia, *J.Physiol. (Lond.) 190*: 35–53, 1967.
7. Corbalan, R., R. L. Verrier, B. Lown, Differing mechanisms for ventricular vulnerability during coronary artery occlusion and release, *Am. Heart J. 92*: 223–230, 1976.
8. Ceremuzynski, L., K. Herbaczynska-Cedro, B. Broniszwska-Ardelt, J. Nauman, B. Wozniewicz, J. Lawecki, Evidence for detrimental effect of adrenaline infused to healthy dogs in doses imitating spontaneous secretion after coronary occlusion, *Cardiovasc. Res. 12*: 179–189, 1978.
9. Cheng, T. O., T. Bashour, G. A. Kelser, Jr., L. Weiss, J. Bacos, Variant angina of Prinzmetal with normal arterial arteriograms: a variant of the variant, *Circulation 47*: 476–485, 1973.
10. Clark, D. A., R. A. Quint, J. Bolen, J. S. Schroeder, The angiographic demonstration of coronary artery spasm in patients with suspected variant angina: method and therapeutic implications, *Am. J. Cardiol. 35*: 127, 1975.
11. Coffman, J. D. and W. T. Davies, Vasospastic diseases: a review, *Prog. Cardiovasc. Dis. 18*: 123–145, 1975.
12. Cutler, E. C. and J. Fine, Sympathectomy in angina pectoris, *J. Am. Med. Assoc. 86*: 1972–1979, 1926.
13. Davidson, S., P. R. Maroko, E. Braunwald, Effects of isoproterenol on contractile function of the ischemic and anoxic heart, *Am. J. Physiol. 227*: 439–443, 1974.
14. DuPont, E., C. E. Jones, B. S. Leudecke, E. E. Smith, Chronic ventricular sympathectomy: effect on myocardial perfusion after ligation of the circumflex artery in dogs, *Circ. Shock 6*: 323–331, 1979.
15. Ebert, P. A., R. B. Vanderbeck, R. J. Allgood, D. C. Sabiston Jr., Effect of chronic cardiac denervation on arrhythmia after coronary artery ligation, *Cardiovasc. Res. 4*: 141–147, 1970.
16. Endo, M., I. Kanda, S. Hosoda, H. Hayashi, K. Hirosawa, S. Konno, Prinzmetal's variant form of angina pectoris. Reevaluation of mechanisms, *Circulation 52*: 33–37, 1975.

17. Estes, E. H. and H. L. Iziar, Recurrent ventricular tachycardia: a case successfully treated by bilateral cardiac sympathectomy, *Am. J. Med. 31*: 493–497, 1961.
18. Fesani, F., G. Barboso, S. Saccani, F. Chiodo, R. Campodonica, D. Medici, F. Effendy, F. Cucchini, La denervazione simpatica ventricolo-coronarica in associazione alla rivascolarizzazione diretta nel trattamento della ischemia coronarica, *Est. da Min. Caridoangiol. 27*: 677–681, 1979.
19. Francois-Franck, C. A., Signification physiologique de la resection du sympathique dans la malodie de basedow, l'epilepsie, l'idiote et le glaucome, *Bull. Acad. Med. 41*: 556–594, 1899.
20. Gaasch, W. H., A. V. Adyanthaya, V. H. Wang, E. Pickering, M. A. Quinones, J. K. Alexander, Prinzmetal's variant angina: hemodynamic and angiographic observations during pain, *Am. J. Cardiol. 35*: 683–690, 1975.
21. Grayson, J. and B. A. Lapin, Observations on the mechanisms of infarction in the dog after experimental occlusion of the coronary artery. *Lancet 1*: 1284–1288, 1966.
22. Grondin, C. M. and R. Limet, Sympathetic denervation in association with coronary artery grafting in patients with Prinzmetal's angina, *Ann. Thor. Surg. 23*: 111–117, 1977.
23. Harken, A. H., L. N. Horowitz, M. E. Josephson, The surgical treatment of ventricular tachycardia, *Ann. Thor. Surg. 30*: 499–508, 1980.
24. Harris, A. S., A. Estandia, R. F. Tillotson, Ventricular ectopic rhythms and ventricular fibrillation following cardiac sympathectomy and coronary occlusion, *Am. J. Physiol. 165*: 505–512, 1951.
25. Hart, N. J., M. E. Silverman, S. B. King, Variant angina pectoris caused by coronary artery spasm, *Am. J. Med. 56*: 269–274, 1974.
26. Hellstrom, H. R., Coronary artery vasospasm: the likely immediate cause of acute myocardial infarction, *Br. Heart J. 41*: 426–432, 1979.
27. Jones, C. E., L. Y. Beck, E. DuPont, G. E. Barnes, Effects of coronary ligation on the chronically sympathectomized dog ventricle, *Am. J. Physiol. 235*: H429-H434, 1978.
28. Jones, C. E., M. D. Devouse, Sr., J. X. Toomas, Jr., E. DuPont, The effect of chronic cardiac denervation on infarct size following acute coronary occlusion, *Am. Heart J. 95*: 738–746, 1978.
29. Jones, C. E. and K. W. Scheel, Reduced coronary collateral resistance after chronic ventricular sympathectomy, *Am. J. Physiol. 238*: H196-H201, 1980.
30. Jones, S. B. and J. X. Thomas, Lactate production in the ischemic denervated heart, *Fed. Proc. 37*: 417, 1978.
31. Kaye, M. P. and W. C. Randall, Cardiac denervation with aortocoronary bypass (letter to editor), *Circulation 62*: 1389, 1980.
32. Kevin, N. and C. A. Macleod, Coronary artery spasm associated with variant angina pectoris, *Br. Heart J. 36*: 224–227, 1974.
33. Kloner, R. A., M. C. Fishbein, R. S. Cotran, E. Braunwald, P. R. Maroko, The effect of propranolol on microvascular injury in acute myocardial ischemia, *Circulation 55*: 872–880, 1977.
34. Lesch, M., Inotropic agents and infarct size: theoretical and practical considerations, *Am. J. Cardiol. 37*: 508–513, 1976.
35. Levene, D. L. and M. B. Freeman, Alpha adrenoceptor-mediated coronary artery spasm, *J. Am. Med. Assoc. 236*: 1018–1022, 1976.
36. Libby, P., P. R. Maroko, J. W. Covell, C. I. Mallock, E. Braunwald, Effect of practolol on the extent of myocardial ischemic injury after experimental coronary

occlusion and its effects on ventricular function in the normal and ischemic heart, *Cardiovasc. Res.* 7: 167–173, 1973.

37. Lindgren, I. and H. Olivecrona, Surgical treatment of angina pectoris, *J.Neurosurg.* 4: 19–39, 1947.
38. Lloyd, R., R. Okada, J. Stagg, R. Anderson, B. Hattler, F. Marcus, The treatment of recurrent ventricular tachycardia with bilateral cervico-thoracic sympathetic ganglionectomy, *Circulation 50*: 382–388, 1974.
39. Lown, B. and R. L. Verrier, Neural activity and ventricular fibrillation, *N. Eng. J. Med. 294*: 1165–1170, 1976.
40. Malliani, A., P. J. Schwartz, A. Zanchetti, A sympathetic reflex elicited by experimental coronary occlusion, *Am. J. Physiol. 217*: 703–709, 1969.
41. Moroko, P. R., J. K. Kjekshus, B. E. Sobel, T. Watanabe, J. W. Covell, J. Ross, Jr., E. Braunwald, Factors influencing infarct size following experimental coronary artery occlusion, *Circulation 43*: 67–82, 1971.
42. Martins, J. B., Sympathetic nerves directly modulate rate of ventricular tachycardia in dogs with 24-hour old myocardial infarction, *Circulation 66*: Suppl. II, Oct., II-130, 1982.
43. McAlpine, R. N., A. A. Kattus, A. B. Alvaro, Angina pectoris at rest with preservation of exercise capacity. Prinzmetal's angina, *Circulation 47*: 946–958, 1973.
44. Maseri, A., A. L'Abbate, A. Pesola, C. Michelassi, M. Marzilli, M. DeNes, Regional myocardial perfusion in patients with atherosclerotic coronary artery disease at rest and during angina pectoris induced by tachycardia, *Circulation 55*: 423–433, 1977.
45. Maseri, A., A. Pesola, A. Marzilli, S. Serveri, O. Parodi, A. L'Abbate, A. M. Ballestra, G. Maltintri, D. M. DeNes, A. Biagini, Coronary vasospasm in angina pectoris, *Lancet 1*: 713–717, 1977.
46. Maseri, A., R. Mimmo, S. Chierchia, C. Marchesi, A. Pesola, A. L'Abbatte, Coronary artery spasm as a cause of acute myocardial ischemia in man, *Chest 68*: 625–633, 1975.
47. Mnayer, M., R. A. Chahine, A. E. Raizner, Mechanisms of angina relief in patients after coronary artery bypass surgery, *Br. Heart J.* 39: 605–609, 1978.
48. Nitter-Hauge, S. and O. Storstein, Surgical treatment of recurrent ventricular tachycardia, *Br. Heart J. 35*: 1132–1135, 1973.
49. Oliva, P. B., D. E. Potts, R. G. Pluss, Coronary arterial spasm in Prinzmetal angina, *N. Eng. J. Med. 288*: 745–751, 1973.
50. Peter, T., R. M. Norris, E. D. Clark, M. K. Heng, B. N. Singh, B. Williams, D. R. Howell, P. K. Ambler, Reduction of enzyme levels by propranolol after acute myocardial infarction, *Circulation 57*: 1091–1095, 1978.
51. Prinzmetal, M., R. Kennamer, T. Wada, N. Bor, Angina pectoris. 1. A variant form of angina pectoris. Preliminary report., *Am. J. Med. 27*: 375–388, 1959.
52. Randall, W. C., M. P. Kaye, J. X. Thomas, M. J. Barber, Intrapericardial denervation of the heart, *J. Surg. Res. 29*: 101–109, 1980.
53. Reimer, K. A., M. M. Rasmussen, R. B. Jennings, On the nature of protection by propranolol against myocardial necrosis after temporary coronary occlusion in dogs, *Am. J. Cardiol. 37*: 520–527, 1976.
54. Shatney, C. H., D. J. Maccarter, R. C. Lillehei, Effects of allopurinal, propranolol and methylprednisolone on infarct size in experimental myocardial infarction, *Am. J. Cardiol. 37*: 572–580, 1976.
55. Shubrooks, S. J., Jr., J. M. Bete, A. M. Hutter, Jr., P. C. Block, M. Buckley, W. M. Daggett, E. D. Mundth, Variant angina pectoris: clinical and anatomic spectrum and results of coronary bypass surgery, *Am. J. Cardiol. 36*: 142–147, 1975.

56. Thomas, J. X., C. E. Jones, D. E. Euler, W. C. Randall, Comparison of effects of acute coronary occlusion in acutely and chronically denervated canine hearts, *Am. J. Cardiol. 41*: 364, 1978.
57. Verrier, R. L., P. L. Thompson, B. Lown, Ventricular vulnerability during sympathetic stimulation: role of heart rate and blood pressure, *Cardiovasc. Res. 8*: 602–610, 1974.
58. Verrier, R. L., A. Calvert, B. Lown, Effect of posterior hypothalamic stimulation on ventricular fibrillation threshold, *Am. J. Physiol. 228*: 923–927, 1975.
59. Waldenstrom, A. P., A. C. Hjalmarson, L. Thornell, A possible role of noradrenaline in the development of myocardial infarction, *Am. Heart J. 95*: 43–57, 1978.
60. White, J. C. and E. F. Bland, The surgical relief of severe angina pectoris. Methods employed and end results in 83 patients, *Medicine 27*: 1–42, 1948.
61. Yasue, H., M. Touyama, M. Shimamoto, H. Kato, S. Tanaka, F. Akiyama, Role of autonomic nervous system in pathogenesis of Prinzmetal's variant form of angina, *Circulation 50*: 534–539, 1974.
62. Yasue, H., M. Touyama, H. Kato, F. Akiyama, Prinzmetal's variant form of angina as a manifestation of alpha-adrenergic receptor-mediated coronary artery spasm: documentation by coronary arteriography, *Am. Heart J. 91*: 148–155, 1976.
63. Zipes, D. P., B. Festoff, S. F. Schall, C. Cox, W. C. Sealy, A. G. Wallace, Treatment of ventricular arrhythmia by permanent atrial pacemaker and cardiac sympathectomy, *Ann. Int. Med. 68*: 591–597, 1968.

20

Clinical Significance of Neural Control of the Heart

THOMAS N. JAMES

To balance supply and demand is as important to human health as it is to the success of any national economy. Optimal maintenance of the circulation is essential to this balance, for without an adequate blood supply no organ system of the body can long survive. Neural control of the circulation normally assures that a proper blood supply is maintained, permitting the heart to make prompt adjustments in its performance during most usual physiological challenges. In this book the discussion is limited to neural influences on the heart, with the recognition that the neural control of the peripheral circulation is of closely related clinical importance.

Some investigators have been misled by the observation that a transplanted heart, necessarily devoid of its normal neural connections (at least in the early postoperative period), behaves in a generally satisfactory way. Without belaboring whether this unusual example can in any way be considered optimal cardiac performance, the more important consideration is that virtually all other human hearts are powerfully influenced by their nerves whether we ordinarily choose to think much about that or not. Furthermore, the cardiac actions of most medications, the effects of ions and hormones on the heart, and the functional interplay between the brain and the heart are all to a great extent mediated by the cardiac nerves. Finally, reflexes that powerfully influence blood pressure or cardiac performance may originate inside or outside the heart, but in either case both the afferent and efferent components require neural mediation.

There is now dawning a new appreciation of the possibility that the nerves of the heart can themselves be the site of structural abnormalities which may collectively be designated either as primary or secondary cardioneuropathies. Primary cardioneuropathies are those in which the disease is predominantly or exclusively within the cardiac nerves or ganglia and the rest of the heart is

Research has been supported by the National Heart, Lung and Blood Institute (Program Project Grant HL 11,310 and SCOR on Ischemic Heart Disease HL 17,667) and by the Daniel Webster Cline Memorial Fund.

spared; examples include forms of ganglionitis and neural degeneration observed in rare cases of sudden, unexpected death [26,27,29,30,47]. The true incidence of this type of abnormality may be more unrecognized than rare, since it is seldom considered. Secondary cardioneuropathies include those diseases which damage nerves of the heart as part of a broader problem; examples include not only ischemic damage as part of the focal injury occurring during the obstruction of coronary blood flow, but also the significant involvement of cardiac nerves or their target structures in any systemic disease, such as lupus erythematosus, rheumatoid arthritis or amyloidosis.

Neural target structures in the heart are not spared during most systemic diseases, and when such structures are damaged, their expected normal response to neural influence is significantly deranged. For example, one form of experimental reflex heart block can be produced simply by selective interruption of vagal influence on the sinus node with about ten micrograms of atropine, permitting varying periods (including prolonged ones) of complete heart block to occur during any reflex vagal event [31]. While this circumstance is not a direct example of cardioneuropathy, it illustrates how randomly distributed focal lesions in the heart can disorganize its neural control. Reflex heart block thus produced is a neurally mediated paradox in which the AV (atrioventricular) junction is structurally and functionally normal but responds in a potentially harmful way because another structure (sinus node) does not participate as it should during a vagal reflex.

To introduce a discussion of cardioneuropathies, it is useful to review in a clinical context those normal components of cardiac function which are influenced by the nerves of the heart. These include the rate at which the heart beats, the rhythm by which the rate is determined, the conduction of any supraventricular rhythm to the ventricles, the speed and pattern of repolarization both in the atria and ventricles, the vigor and sequence of myocardial contraction both in the atria and ventricles, and the magnitude and distribution of coronary blood flow. Full discussions of each of these subjects are available in other chapters of this book. Few, if any, of these processes are influenced individually by the cardiac nerves; therefore, it is important to remember that many or most perturbations will occur concomitantly. Little is known of what actually determines each segment of an overall cardioneural response, except as would be anticipated as a consequence of focal disease. An example of this disparity is the fact that a powerful cardiogenic hypertensive chemoreflex studied experimentally in the dog is characterized by an immediate brief but powerful sympathetic stimulation of the ventricles; however, coronary blood flow during this period is unaffected, i.e. exhibits no change except as is reflected by a surge in flow due to the sudden aortic hypertension [54].

FUNCTIONS OF THE HEART NORMALLY INFLUENCED BY ITS NERVES

Neural Influence on Cardiac Rate

Every medical student is appropriately impressed that the vagus nerve slows the heart while its sympathetic nerves accelerate it. Of course the clinical situation is more complex than that. Many cardiovascular reflexes engage both the vagal and sympathetic efferent paths simultaneously. Furthermore, accurate prediction of any response assumes that the structures normally governing the origination and propagation of the cardiac impulse are operating appropriately and retain their responsiveness to the abundant innervation [16]. While few of those complexities apply very often under normal conditions, the physician usually must deal with a patient who is sick. In the patient with heart disease the manner of sympathetic neural acceleration of the heart, even if it is simple sinus tachycardia, will have a different net effect depending on whether the ventricles are concomitantly stimulated in a normal way and, even if stimulated, whether they are capable of responding appropriately. Other distortions can occur if there is complicating valvular stenosis or incompetence, and if the peripheral vascular resistance is higher or lower than normal.

Except as may be produced by local disease affecting the sinus node [24] or by circulating substances having a positive chronotropic action, virtually all other examples of sinus tachycardia are mediated by the sympathetic nervous system. This may be a direct mediation due to increased sympathetic neural traffic, or an indirect one when vagal influence is diminished, permitting the sympathetic effect to predominate even if its neural traffic in absolute terms does not change. The appropriateness of cardiac acceleration must be judged in the context of all concomitant neural and non-neural effects and associated diseases.

Much the same can be said of vagal slowing, which may be either beneficial or harmful depending in part on the degree of slowing, whether atrial repolarization is concomitantly distorted sufficiently to induce atrial fibrillation, and whether associated cardiac defects or diseases coexist. Acetylcholine normally released by the vagal terminals will suppress both sinus rhythm and AV junctional rhythm [15,49,51], but in addition to its negative chronotropic effect, acetylcholine also has a negative dromotropic action, which will be discussed later.

Neural Influence on Cardiac Rhythm

Under normal circumstances the sinus node is the dominant pacemaker in the mammalian heart, so that cardiac slowing or acceleration is usually mediated by changes in the rate of sinus rhythm. Another major pacemaking system exists in the AV junction, which is also powerfully influenced by the autonomic nerves [19,28,49,51]. In the dog these two centers account for most normal forms of stable cardiac rhythm. However, there are some foci which can act as subsidiary centers of supraventricular automaticity [42], also influenced by autonomic nerves, and these too must be considered in assessing neural influence on cardiac rhythm. Whether these other atrial centers can be the source of prolonged periods of stable rhythm, or whether they have clinical counterparts in humans is presently uncertain.

Although both the sinus node and AV junction are under sympathetic neural influence, there is experimental evidence that AV junctional rhythm is more dependent on this influence than is sinus rhythm [50]. In the absence of adre-

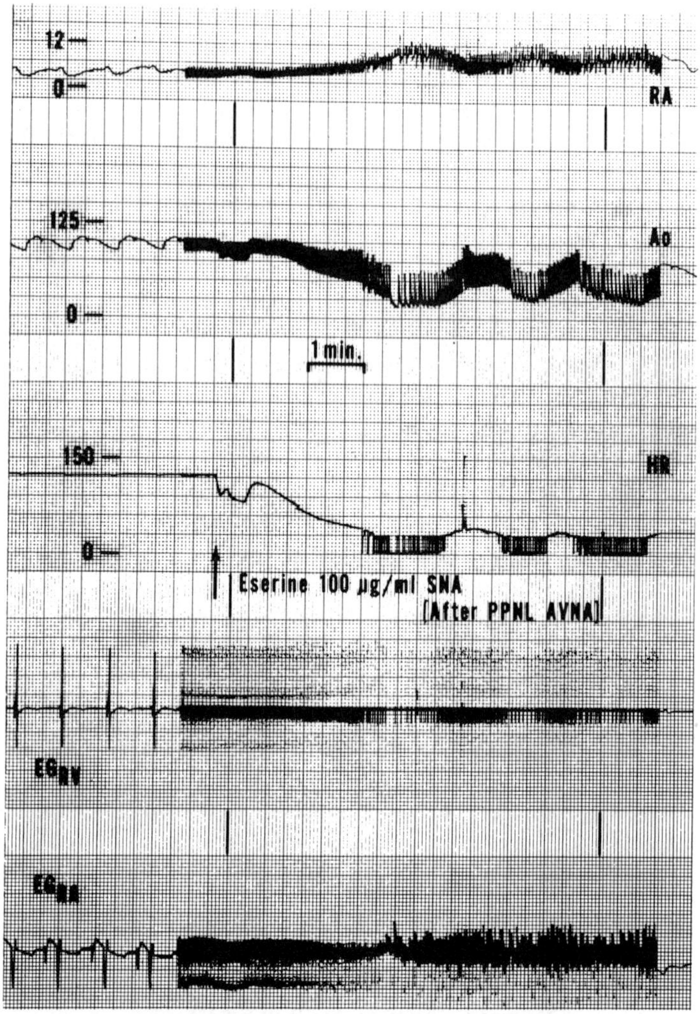

Fig. 20-1. In this anesthetized dog, local cholinesterase paralysis was produced by selective perfusion of eserine into the sinus node artery (SNA) at the arrow. Local beta-receptor blockade within the AV junction had previously been achieved with selective perfusion of propranolol (PPNL) into the AV node artery (AVNA). The steadily progressive sinus bradycardia in such experiments usually terminates with an escape AV junctional rhythm at a rate approximately two-thirds that of control sinus rate, but here the AV junction escapes very slowly and erratically. Records from top down include right atrial pressure (RA) scaled in mm Hg, aortic pressure (Ao) also in mm Hg, heart rate (HR) scaled in beats/min, and electrograms (EG) recorded from right ventricular (RV) and right atrial (RA) epicardium. (Reproduced through courtesy of *J. Pharmacol. Exp. Ther.*, ref. 50)

nergic neural influence, selective suppression of the sinus node is followed by much slower and more erratic escape AV junctional rhythm than is normally true (Figs. 20-1 to 20-3). Furthermore, in the presence of combined calcium channel blockage (verapamil) and beta receptor blockade (propranolol), selective suppression of the sinus node is followed by prolonged asystole [53]. Given the widespread and growing use of these and similar pharmacological agents, it is essential for physicians to appreciate their potential for producing serious or even catastrophic electrical instability in the heart.

In addition to whatever effect the autonomic nerves may have on stable regular rhythms, the vagus nerves facilitate both the onset and perpetuation of atrial fibrillation [38]. This vagal effect occurs by abbreviating the duration of atrial refractory periods and by doing this in a geometrically inhomogeneous pattern, and it is further facilitated by sinus slowing, which increases the dis-

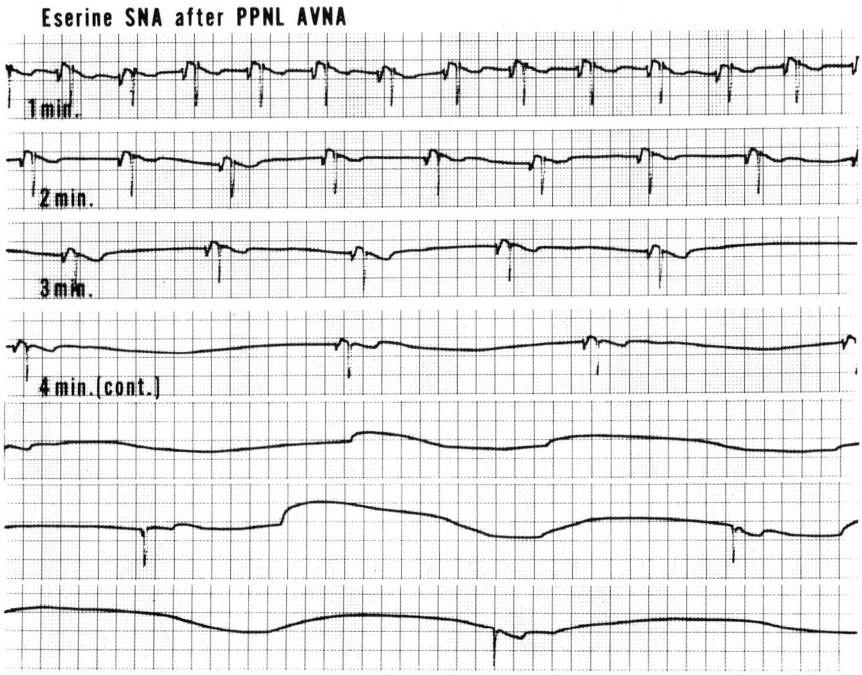

Fig. 20-2. This electrocardiogram was recorded at 25 mm/sec during the experiment illustrated in Fig. 20-1 (same dog). At this faster recording speed one can see that the rhythm continues to originate from the sinus node at very slow rates, and that when a few AV junctional escape beats occur, it is at even a slower rate. The time designations refer to the interval after administration of eserine. (Reproduced through courtesy of *J. Pharmacol. Exp. Ther.*, ref. 50)

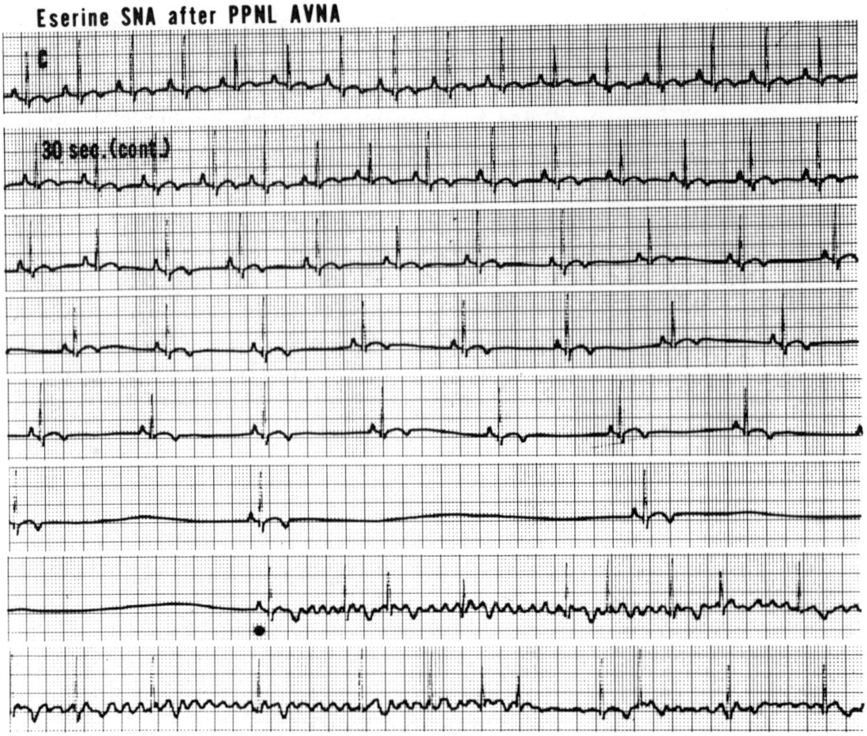

Fig. 20-3. This experiment in another anesthetized dog demonstrates a response similar to that depicted in Figs. 20-1 and 20-2, here terminating in atrial fibrillation (black dot). During the atrial fibrillation, AV conduction is nearly normal, indicating that it is not as dependent as AV junctional rhythm on local adrenergic neural effect. (Reproduced through courtesy of *J. Pharmacol. Exp. Ther.*, ref. 50)

persion of refractory periods. If the effect of acetylcholine release on the atrial myocardium is accompanied by simultaneous administration or neural release of norepinephrine, then the probability of atrial fibrillation is still further increased [12]. It is not surprising therefore that during reflexes having both vagal and sympathetic effects on atrial myocardium, transient atrial fibrillation is often observed (Fig. 20-4).

Ventricular arrhythmias are also facilitated and ventricular fibrillation threshold is lowered by sympathetic neural influence on the ventricular myocardium. In humans this may be especially important as the mediating process associated with states of anxiety, apprehension, or worry so often accompanying the acute phase of myocardial infarction or pulmonary edema. Here again, however, it is impossible to dissociate the direct effect of sympathetic nerves on putative foci of ventricular irritablity from the coexisting influence of sympathetic nerves on ventricular repolarization, cardiac rate, and the vigor of cardiac contraction which could worsen any ischemic injury already present.

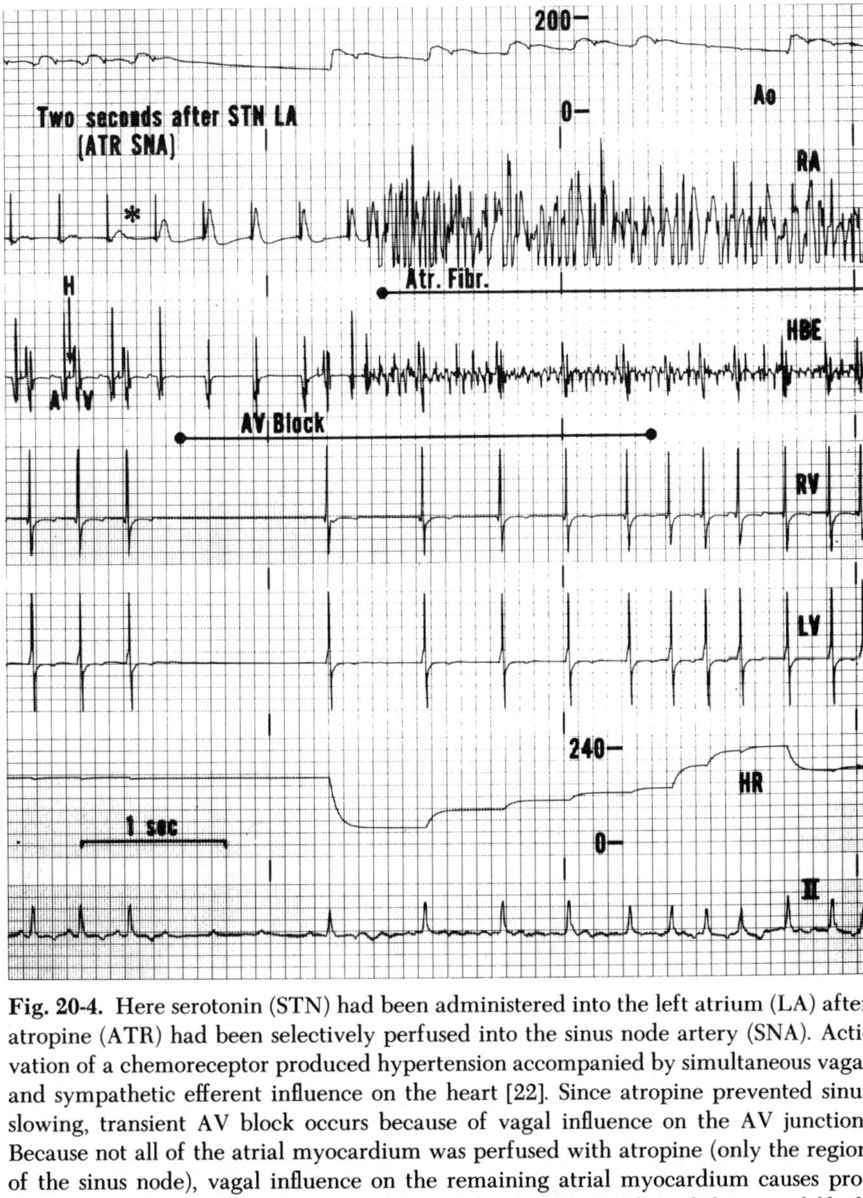

Fig. 20-4. Here serotonin (STN) had been administered into the left atrium (LA) after atropine (ATR) had been selectively perfused into the sinus node artery (SNA). Activation of a chemoreceptor produced hypertension accompanied by simultaneous vagal and sympathetic efferent influence on the heart [22]. Since atropine prevented sinus slowing, transient AV block occurs because of vagal influence on the AV junction. Because not all of the atrial myocardium was perfused with atropine (only the region of the sinus node), vagal influence on the remaining atrial myocardium causes progressive elevation of the P-Tp segment beginning at the asterisk, and then atrial fibrillation which lasted a few more seconds. During the atrial fibrillation, AV conduction was initially slow but rapidly returned to normal since the duration of the reflex vagal influence is only for a few seconds. Record labels not previously identified include bipolar electrograms from the region of the sinus node (RA), from the area of the His bundle (HBE), from right and left ventricular epicardium (RV and LV), and a surface lead II. (Reproduced through courtesy of American Heart Assoc., ref. 22)

Neural Influence on Cardiac Conduction

Easily the most important neural effect on cardiac conduction is exerted in the AV junction, particularly the AV node. Any effect of sympathetic stimulation is difficult to assess there because local automaticity is enhanced at the same time that any alteration in conduction might occur, making the reliable distinction of fusion rhythms from accelerated conduction almost impossible in humans. By contrast, the negative dromotropic effect of vagal stimulation is clearly apparent and unequivocal (19,28,51].

During most examples of vagal influence on the heart, sinus slowing is accompanied by depressed AV conduction. This permits relatively normal speed of AV conduction to be preserved when the number of stimuli arriving to the AV junction is decreased, particularly if the vagal effect is of modest intensity. However, even with less powerful vagal reflexes, a more powerful influence on the AV junction is unmasked if for some reason (e.g. the local neural disease seen with diabetes mellitus [7,35]) the sinus node is spared the slowing effect expected during vagal discharge. It is useful to realize that this form of reflex heart block can occur (Figs. 20-4 and 20-5). How often this combination (a normal AV node "overresponding" because the sinus node fails to slow) is responsible for such clinical events as cough syncope, micturition syncope, or indeed any form of so-called carotid sinus syncope, is presently unknown but merits careful study.

Neural Influence on Cardiac Repolarization

That the vagus nerves will alter repolarization of the atrial myocardium [20] can be clearly demonstrated (Fig. 20-4, 20-6, 20-7), and this has already been discussed as favoring the onset of atrial fibrillation. Whether the vagi significantly influence repolarization of the ventricular myocardium is uncertain. However, there is growing appreciation of the importance of the sympathetic nerves both for the speed and pattern of ventricular repolarization. Prolongation of ventricular repolarization may in general terms be thought of as increasing ventricular vulnerability to arrhythmias, and this effect becomes even more powerful if the normal symmetry of ventricular repolarization is distorted. Although there is little question that local disease either of ventricular myocardium or local sympathetic nerves can distort the normal symmetry of ventricular repolarization, there is both experimental [1,5] and clinical [4] evidence that asymmetry of ventricular repolarization can also be produced by extracardiac neural influence.

Much recent attention has been drawn to the role of adrenergic neural influence as an important determinant of the QT prolongation often found in victims of fainting attacks and ventricular arrhythmias, some of which end fatally [8,17,18,33]. Based on experimental observations with adrenergic neural asymmetry produced in dogs and manifest in part by prolongation of the QT interval [1,5], anesthetic blockade or surgical resection of the stellate ganglion has been shown to be successful in abbreviating a prolonged QT interval and, more

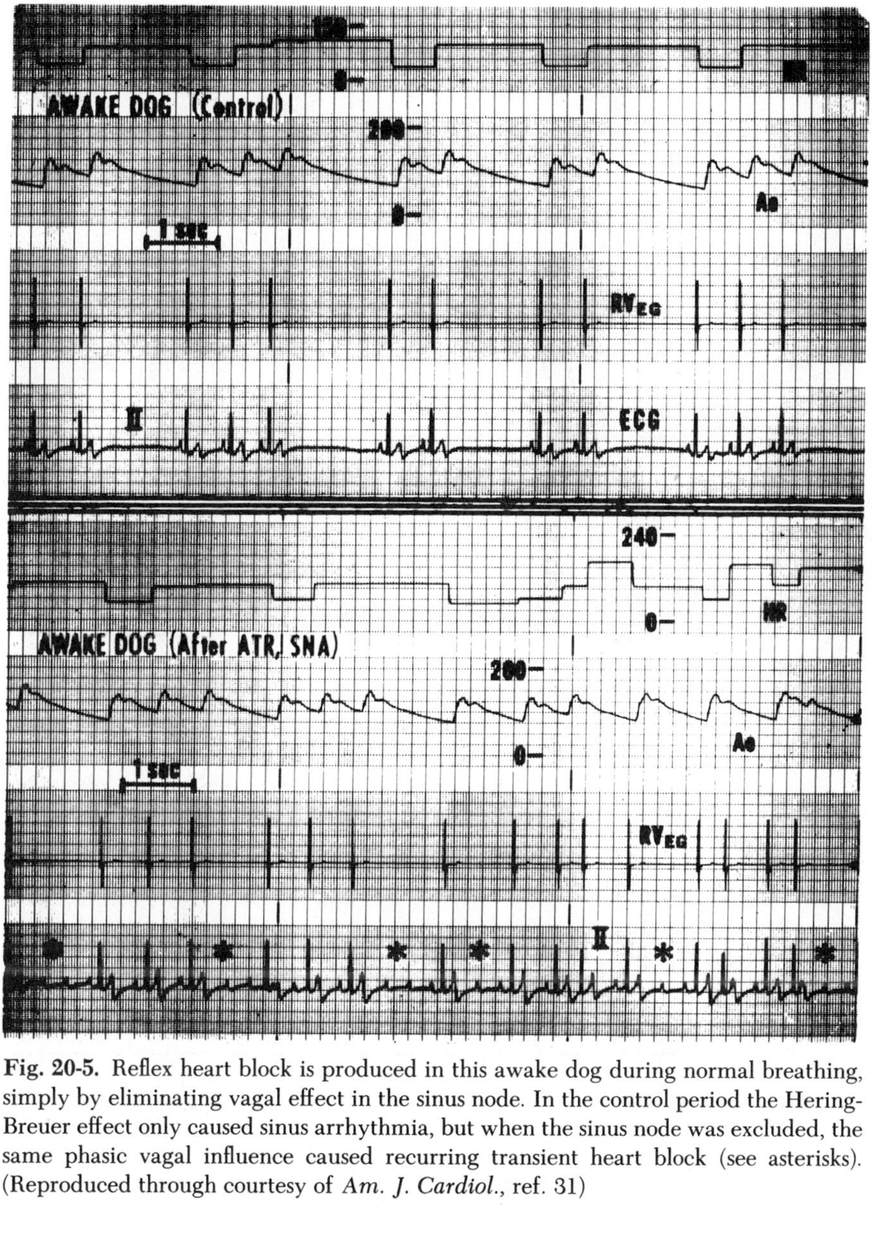

Fig. 20-5. Reflex heart block is produced in this awake dog during normal breathing, simply by eliminating vagal effect in the sinus node. In the control period the Hering-Breuer effect only caused sinus arrhythmia, but when the sinus node was excluded, the same phasic vagal influence caused recurring transient heart block (see asterisks). (Reproduced through courtesy of *Am. J. Cardiol.*, ref. 31)

importantly, in terminating or significantly reducing the episodes of documented ventricular arrhythmias in patients [39].

There is at present little question that clinical states associated with QT prolongation and manifest by paroxysms of serious ventricular arrhythmias are often caused by an asymmetry of adrenergic neural influence on the ventricular myocardium. This is equally true of such patients who are deaf and those with

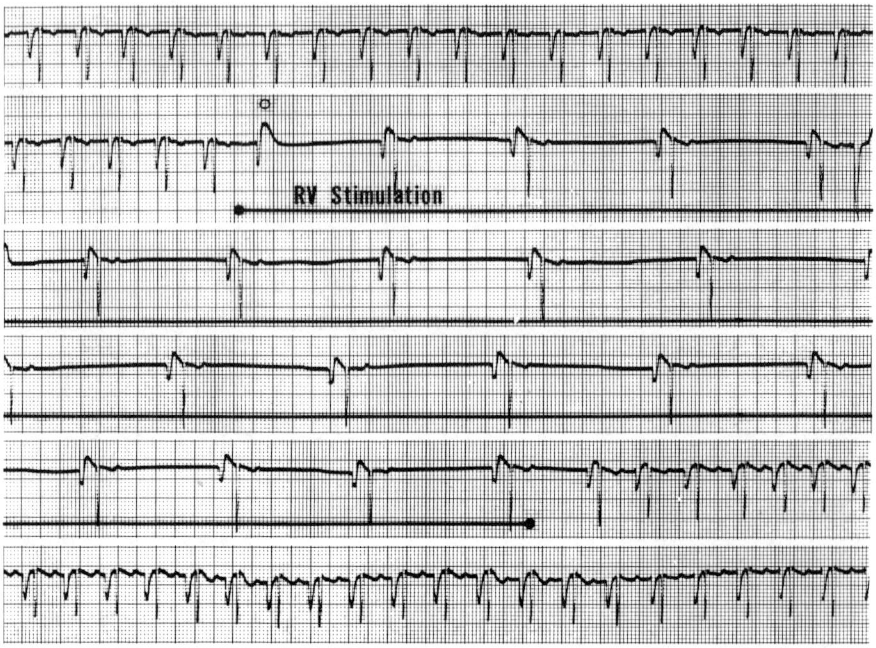

Fig. 20-6. Submaximal stimulation of the right cervical vagus nerve in this dog produced a moderate degree of sinus slowing accompanied by elevation of the P-Tp segment (unipolar wick electrogram recorded from near sinus node, 25 mm/sec). One sinus escape (marked by circle) is nonconducted and permits full appreciation of the duration of atrial repolarization, which normally extends beyond the QRS complex when the PR interval is normal. When the stimulus is terminated, both sinus rate and the P-Tp segment return to normal. (Reproduced through courtesy of *Am. J. Cardiol.*, ref. 20)

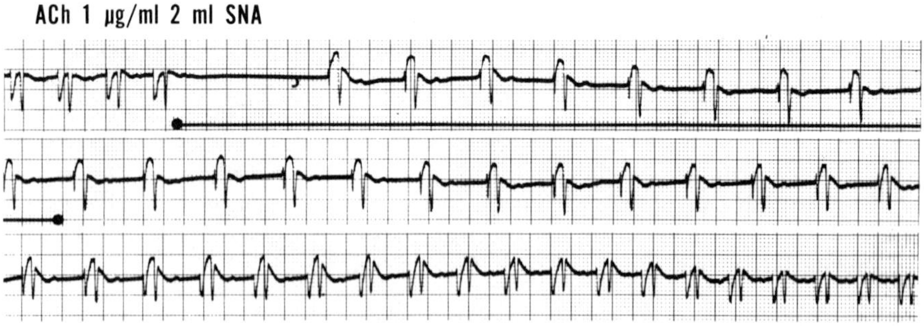

Fig. 20-7. Selective perfusion of acetylcholine (ACh) into the sinus node artery of this anesthetized dog produces an effect virtually identical to that demonstrated with vagal stimulation in Fig. 20-6 (different dog). This dog had previously received a small amount of atropine, accounting for only a minor degree of sinus slowing, since this volume of acetylcholine normally stops all sinus activity. (Reproduced through courtesy of *Am. J. Cardiol.*, ref. 20)

normal hearing. In fact, the coexistence of these problems in siblings who are deaf and others who hear normally has sometimes raised the question [17] of whether the entire process is truly an inherited defect as was originally suggested [8,33], or whether the clinical abnormalities tend to aggregate for some other reason. The more recent demonstration of ganglionitis and cardioneuropathy in the hearts of a number of such victims, some deaf and others hearing normally, has led to the suggestion [26] that the etiologic basis could be a shared familial infection, much as the varicella-zoster herpes virus is so shared [13], rather than an inherited structural or metabolic fault.

In the understandable enthusiasm for successful treatment of patients with the long QT syndromes by stellectomy, particularly since most other forms of treatment have been unpredictably successful and the outcome without treatment is often grim, there are some important caveats. The first of these is the necessary understanding that the disease, whatever its basis, is seldom stable or consistent. The hallmark of the problem, a long QT interval, is not only widely variable from day to day but even over a period of minutes in a given individual [8]. This being the case, what may be helpful by reducing the QT prolongation at one time in any patient may be responsible for worsening the situation at a different time, particularly if the neural basis for adrenergic asymmetric influence on the ventricle should change. If some viral infection of cardiac nerves is responsible, for example, it should be anticipated that the pattern of adrenergic neural asymmetry will most likely change with time and the direction of change is impossible to predict.

Somewhat similar cautions can be expressed for the use of beta-receptor blocking compounds such as propranolol or adrenergic neural blockers such as bretylium. It is attractive to think that if faulty adrenergic nerves are to blame, then blocking these nerves or their receptor sites should be clinically useful, and it sometimes is. What cannot be known beforehand is whether such drugs will be equally and completely effective for this purpose throughout the ventricular myocardium, an uneven effect perhaps resulting from uneven distribution because of local coronary disease. Furthermore, it is almost impossible to produce complete autonomic blockade safely in man, despite popular belief to the contrary by many clinicians, and the entire clinical problem could be made worse by incomplete blockade, i.e., the adrenergic neural asymmetry increased still further. In a fatal outcome of such an effect, it could too readily be misinterpreted that inadequate amounts of medication had been given rather than an inappropriate effect produced.

Neural Influence on Cardiac Contractility

It is widely appreciated that the sympathetic nervous system has an important positive inotropic influence on the ventricular myocardium. It is less widely understood that the vagi can act powerfully to depress atrial contractility [52], and even when both limbs of the autonomic nervous system are activated, the vagal efferent influence outweighs that of the sympathetic (Fig. 20-8). Under

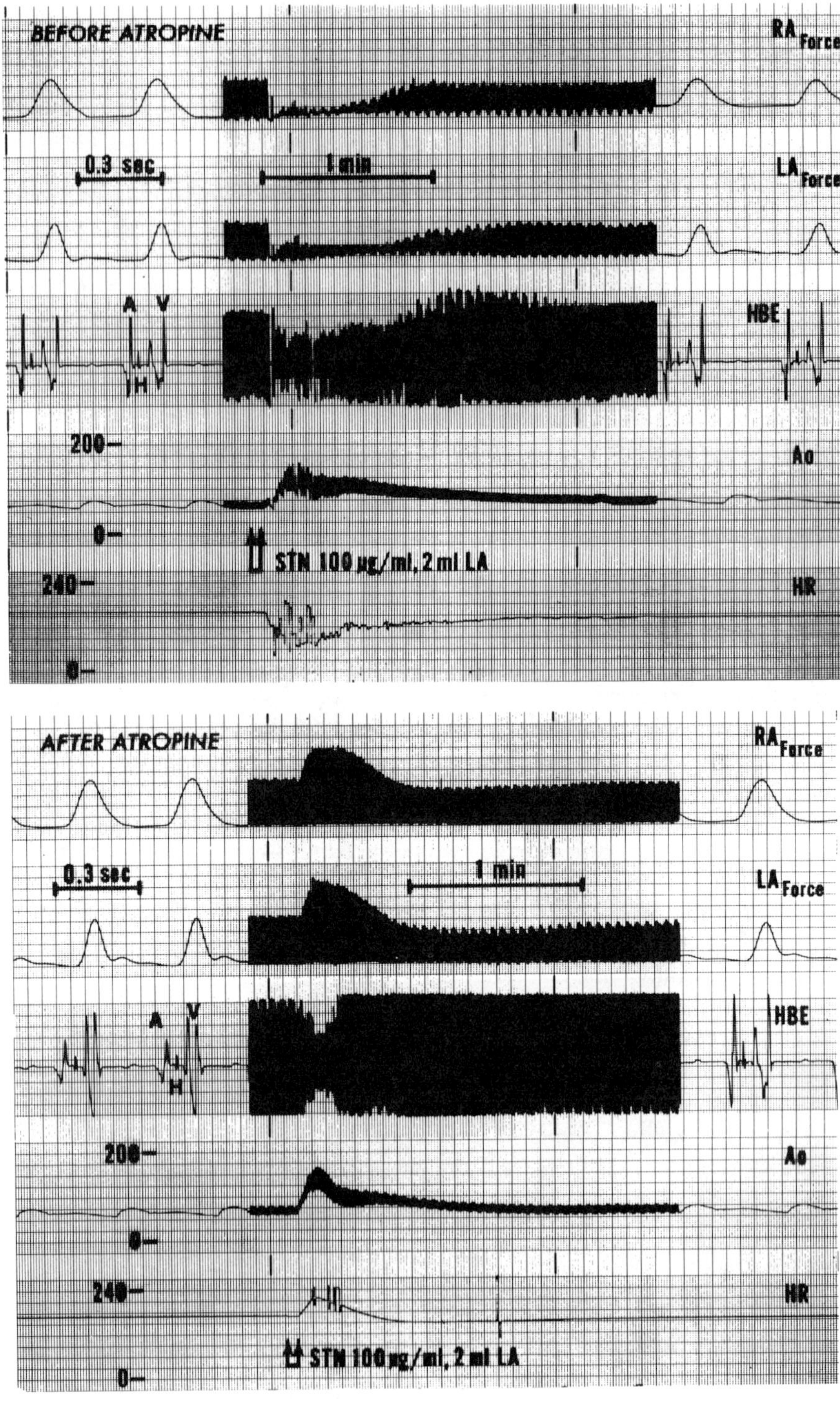
BEFORE ATROPINE
RA Force
0.3 sec
1 min
LA Force
A
V
H
HBE
200–
Ao
0–
STN 100 μg/ml, 2 ml LA
240–
HR
0–
AFTER ATROPINE
RA Force
0.3 sec
1 min
LA Force
A
V
H
HBE
200–
Ao
0–
240–
HR
STN 100 μg/ml, 2 ml LA
0–

most clinical circumstances atrial contractility has comparatively little hemodynamic effect except as it may contribute to ventricular filling. However, in certain corrective surgical procedures for congenital heart disease where the atrium is rendered a more important pumping chamber, then the potential negative inotropic effect of vagal activity becomes an essential consideration, since even the normal (i.e. unhypertrophied) atrium is capable of a significant ejecting force under appropriate circumstances [55].

In addition to the fact that sympathetic drive stimulates ventricular contractility, the local or regional neural influence in special segments of the two ventricles must also be considered. Some years ago Randall and his colleagues first demonstrated experimentally that suitably selective stimulation of small sympathetic branches near the heart was capable of producing a pressure gradient in either the left or right ventricular outflow tract of the dog [2,41,58]. Whether this is applicable to analogous human conditions, such as hypertrophic cardiomyopathy with outflow tract obstruction, is not yet determined but the possibility merits further investigation.

The general question of normal synchrony of ventricular contraction and its potential disruption by unusual or asymmetric neural influence deserves careful thought in relation to certain dysautonomic states in man. For example, patients with the mitral valve prolapse syndrome exhibit a variety of forms of dysautonomia, with inappropriate responses to challenges for cardiac rhythm or rate and for peripheral vascular control of blood pressure [6,9]. Although it is reasonable to suspect that many of their symptoms such as palpitations or labile blood pressure may logically be attributed to the dysautonomia, it is also possible (although less certain) that the mitral valve dysfunction itself may represent some form of desynchronization of normal left ventricular contraction. At the very least it is useful for clinicians to be aware of experimental and some clinical evidence that an abnormal sequence or pattern of ventricular contractions may be produced by changes in local neural control.

Neural Influence on Coronary Blood Flow

For many years it has been standard physiological dogma that the nerves might influence the terminal small coronary arteries and thereby govern coronary resistance but that the larger coronary branches were devoid of significant

Fig. 20-8. The same cardiogenic hypertensive chemoreflex illustrated in Fig. 20-4 is elicited here in another dog to demonstrate the nature of the reflex inotropic influence on the right and left atria. Before atropine there is only a negative inotropic effect, but after atropine the same reflex causes only a positive inotropic effect. Record labels not previously identified include ones for strain gauges sutured to the right (RA_{Force}) and left (LA_{Force}) atrial myocardium. Administration of atropine also converted the reflex bradycardia to tachycardia, as seen in the tachogram. (Reproduced through courtesy of American Heart Assoc., ref. 52)

neural control. With the newer clinical appreciation of the frequency and pathophysiological significance of coronary spasm in the pathogenesis of angina pectoris, acute myocardial infarction, and electrical instability of the heart, more attention has been paid to the mechanisms by which such spasm might be produced [48]. On the one hand, emotional stress and certain reflexes such as that following immersion of the hand in cold water have now been shown capable of producing coronary spasm [40]. On the other hand, coronary spasm has also been demonstrated in a transplanted human heart which is necessarily devoid of all normal neural connections and influence [3].

As a mediator of coronary spasm the other principal mechanism now suspected is platelet aggregation with the local release of thromboxane A2, a particularly powerful coronary vasoconstrictor [48]. The platelet explanation fits well with the frequent demonstration that coronary spasm tends to occur at loci where some anatomic abnormality of the artery already exists, since endothelial disease at such sites would be expected to attract platelets. But with that same logic one might suspect that local anatomical abnormalities may also represent sites of increased or deranged neural influence, either as the cause or the consequence of structural changes. While the exact comparative importance of local platelet aggregation or focal neural influence remain to be elucidated generally, one may anticipate that these roles will differ from patient to patient and perhaps from time to time even in the same patient. Thus, as the older physiological evidence indicated, coronary resistance in samll branches may prove to be constantly under neural influence but under special or abnormal circumstances the caliber of larger coronary arteries may be similarly governed by local nerves.

CLINICAL CONDITIONS RELATED TO CARDIONEUROPATHY OR OTHER FORMS OF DYSAUTONOMIA

Although there is normally some inhomogeneity in the anatomic distribution of nerves to the heart, most of the distribution is in a somewhat regular pattern with natural symmetry. It follows that efferent neural discharge during a cardiovascular reflex will have a consistently distributed and reproducible response from the heart. There are many ways in which this consistent and reproducible response can become disorganized, and most of these have been separately reviewed in the preceding section but may be summarized as follows.

One of the least studied fields in clinical cardiology, and paradoxically perhaps among the most important, is the neural control of the heart. Neural signals to the heart may originate in the brain from thoughts and emotions, from extracardiac neuroreceptors such as those in the carotid body and aortic arch, and even from within the heart itself (the cardiogenic reflexes). Put in simplest terms, many systemic diseases randomly damage some component of those elements: neuroreceptors, afferent and efferent nerves, ganglia, integrating and distributing centers in the brain, and specific target structures within the heart.

Furthermore, there may be some diseases with a special affinity for some of these structures, such as those cardioneuropathies caused by neurotropic viruses. Clinical expression of deranged neural control of the heart may range from subtle symptoms to dramatic ones, but until they are more carefully sought and defined, it is highly probable that all such derangements will be underestimated and often misunderstood.

Clinical cardiologists have long been aware of some cardioneural problems, such as vagally mediated syncope, but with a few notable exceptions such as those of Lino Rossi [43], there have rarely been any efforts to make clinicopathologic correlations in cardioneural diseases. Part of the reason for this is that an understanding of the normal neuroanatomy of the human heart, particularly its functional aspects is given low priority by most clinicians, although this book is evidence of efforts to rectify that problem. At a time when cellular receptors for neurotransmitters are being defined even to the molecular level, and when highly effective and specific pharmacological agents are already available (with more being rapidly developed) to alter or modify cardiac neural control, it seems particularly worthwhile for clinical cardiologists to consider the nerves of the heart, in the same way that its other structures have routinely been considered for understanding human cardiac disease.

A few examples of frequently encountered cardiac diseases will be presented in the next paragraph to illustrate the clinical significance of cardioneuropathy in the pathogenesis and pathophysiology of those disorders. Knowledge about the precise nature of these cardioneural mechanisms is so incomplete that for some the fragments of evidence are mainly of a physiological nature; for even fewer there is additionally anatomic evidence; and in rare cases there are both kinds of evidence which may then be correlated. Some authors may say that with pharmacological experiments in human subjects, such as those that comprise the essential basis for the increasingly popular "clinical trials," investigators can gather all the necessary and clinically useful knowledge needed about drugs influencing neural control of the heart. However, there are at least two compelling reasons to criticize those assertions: First, in the face of the present dearth of knowledge about human cardiac neural control it is probably wrong to assume that all adverse effects of such drugs can be anticipated or even recognized. Second, with fuller knowledge about nerves of the heart even better drugs, shorter and safer and cheaper clinical trials, and perhaps even the obviation of any need for such trials might be possible.

Six conditions have been selected to illustrate the importance of understanding neural control of the heart in clinical practice. These are "carotid sinus" syncope, the long QT syndromes, asymmetrical hypertrophy of the heart, mitral valve prolapse syndrome, essential hypertension (especially in its labile form), and sudden unexpected death. These are not mutually exclusive groups; for example, sudden death is one of the clinical features of several of the other groups, dysautonomia is common and clinically apparent in most of the groups, and any patient with almost any other disease may have hypertension as well. Furthermore, as indicated previously, the true mechanisms of the neural participation in the pathogenesis of any of these states is at best incompletely understood.

"Carotid Sinus" Syncope

This is a less common diagnosis than it once was, but it is a classical example among historical medical misconceptions. There is no question that the fainting spells of some elderly patients are closely mimicked by pressing on the carotid sinus. That simple clinical experiment led to a remarkable array of medical and even surgical treatments directed at the carotid sinus, which was interpreted as being hypersensitive. Cutting of the glossopharyngeal nerve, surgical denervation of the carotid sinus, and similar operations have had their vogue and some are still being practiced. And yet, the evidence that the fundamental fault was in the carotid sinus rather than in the sinus node or the AV node of the heart has never been fully persuasive. For example, there is now growing appreciation that the sinus node becomes hyperresponsive under a variety of conditions and can readily be suppressed by a vagal reflex originating anywhere, no more so from the carotid sinus than from neuroreceptors in the gall bladder, stomach, urinary bladder, aortic arch, or elsewhere. Popular use of the regrettable alliterative phrase "sick sinus syndrome" is one sign of the growing recognition by clinicians of just where the principal fault lies.

Perhaps there are a few rare circumstances in which the carotid sinus is in some way diseased or hypersensitive and can thus on its own produce cardiac reflex syncope, but the simple demonstration that carotid pressure causes marked sinus bradycardia, transient heart block, or asystole tells us nothing more than that a vagal reflex, perhaps *any* vagal reflex, can also do so. If other vagal reflexes are truly as likely to have that effect, then eliminating the carotid sinus as a source cannot be expected to be particularly effective. This is one logical explanation for the unpredictable and frequently disappointing results from such surgery in the past and its waning popularity as a suitable treatment. Lateralizing of the carotid test response cannot be accepted as much evidence for true carotid origin either, since it is well established in experimental animals and almost certainly true in humans as well that the right and left vagi differ greatly from one individual to another in their functional distribution to the heart. Although the right vagus (and as a corollary, signals coming from the right carotid sinus) usually influences predominantly the sinus node and the left vagus the AV node, there is considerable and totally unpredictable crossover innervation. But at least equally important, local disease in the target site (e.g. the sinus node) is a more plausible and logical explanation for apparent lateralization than is disease or malfunction in the carotid sinus.

Pressure on the carotid sinus is one simple and relatively reproducible clinical way to produce a vagal reflex with predictable effect on the heart, but it is equally likely that many of the commonplace events in life such as coughing, sneezing, bowel movements, voiding of urine, and laughing can have much the same result. It is inconceivable that one would consider surgical denervation of the glottis, colon, urinary bladder, nasopharynx, or bronchi; and it may be equally inappropriate to attack one carotid sinus or the other for the same purpose. The more practically important clinical point is that so-called "carotid sinus" syncope is nothing more or less than an abnormal response by either the sinus node or AV node to a vagal reflex, and that the fault may lie within any component of the reflex arc. That includes the possibility of a principal fault within the target structure in the heart, vulnerable to any vagal reflex rather than to a single particular one. Given that many such patients respond so well to demand-mode pacemakers, the question of pathophysiology may be more academic than pragmatic.

Long QT Syndromes

In 1957 Jervell and Lange-Nielsen reported sudden unexpected death occurring in several members of a Norwegian sibship in whom two of the remarkable findings were congenital deafness and a bizarre electrocardiogram, the principal feature of which was grotesque prolongation of the QT interval [33]. Despite the obvious consideration of a lethal arrhythmia as the cause, they erroneously concluded on the basis of several tenuous reasons that the fault did not lie in the heart. This remained the prevalent interpretation until 1964 when Fraser, Froggatt, and James [8] came to the different conclusion, i.e. the heart was indeed the most plausible source of the problem and that a terminal arrhythmia was the probable cause of sudden death. Since that time there have been scores of reports confirming that the mechanism both for the syncopal spells and the sudden deaths characteristic of victims of this problem is a ventricular arrhythmia.

For logical and plausible reasons it was originally suspected that the long QT syndrome was a heritable disease, interpreted as an autosomal dominant trait among those victims hearing normally [57] and an autosomal recessive trait among those born deaf [8]. However, an heritable basis began to be questioned when it was found that different members of the same family could have the long QT syndrome, whether they were deaf or heard normally [17,37]: one would be forced illogically to postulate different modes of hereditary transmission from the same two parents. More recently it has been demonstrated that both the nerves and ganglia of the heart are diseased (Figs. 20-9 and 20-10) when examined postmortem after sudden death of either deaf or normally hearing individuals who had a long QT interval and paroxysmal arrhythmias during life [26]. Although the etiology of that cardioneuropathy has not been established, viral infection must be placed high among the list of suspected etiologies [32]. As a corollary, one must now consider familial transmission of a shared infection as one possible explanation for the familial aggregation of the long QT syndrome, much in the way that the herpes zoster-varicella virus is known to behave in producing chicken pox in the children and shingles in adult members of the same family [13].

Whatever the etiology of the cardioneuropathy and the true explanation of

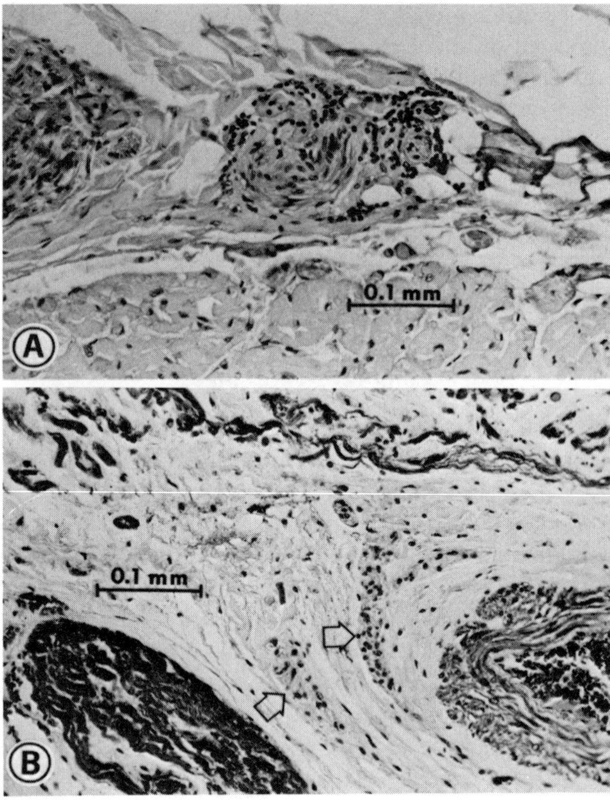

Fig. 20-9. These two photomicrographs illustrate cardioneuropathy in the heart of a patient with the long QT syndrome who died suddenly. (A) Lymphocytic infiltration of a ganglion near the sinus node. (B) Arrows mark two scarred small nerves with lymphocytes located near the sinus node artery. PAS stain in A and Goldner trichrome in B. (Reproduced through courtesy of American Heart Assoc., ref. 26)

familial aggregation may prove to be, there is now little doubt that asymmetry of adrenergic neural influence on ventricular repolarization [1,4,5,18,39,46] is the most frequent and possibly the entire explanation for the long QT interval. As discussed in a preceding section, what is *not* known is whether the adrenergic neural asymmetry is due to ventricular neuropathy or disease involving the autonomic nerves within the thorax or some problem in the reticular formation or other parts of the brain. Rossi, for example, has recently reported severe acute inflammation of the stellate ganglion removed from a patient in whom ganglionectomy was performed to treat the long QT syndrome [44].

Two other features of the long QT syndrome which have received notably little attention have been sinus bradycardia and hypochromic anemia [5]. Either of these could be attributed to some infection, causing cardioneuropathy in the vicinity of the sinus node to denervate it, in effect, but this is conjectural and neither of these two disorders has been explained. The sinus bradycardia in

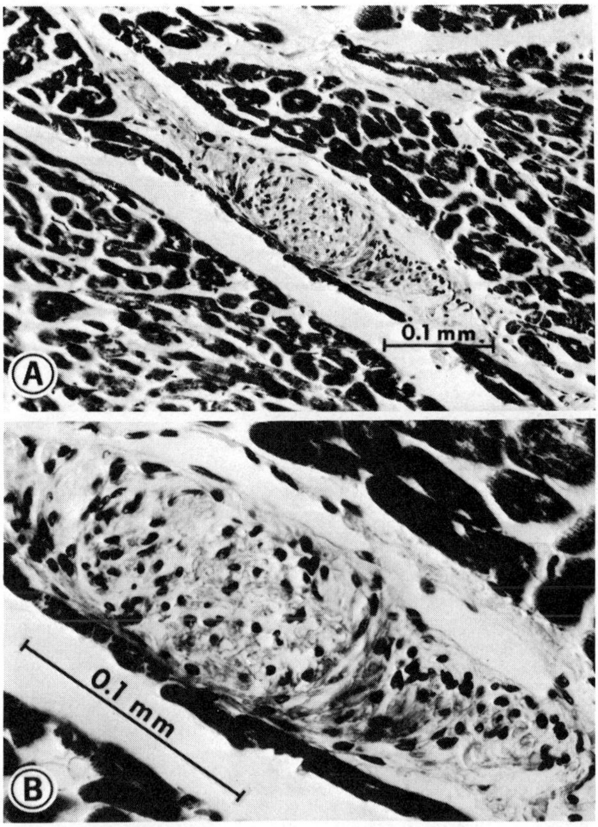

Fig. 20-10. Lymphocytic infiltration of a small nerve in the ventricular myocardium from the heart of another victim of sudden death due to the long QT syndrome, shown here at two magnifications. Goldner trichrome stain here and in all subsequent photomicrographs unless otherwise noted. (Reproduced through courtesy of American Heart Assoc., ref. 26)

particular bears some importance in the selection of treatment regimens. As cautioned in an earlier section discussing neural influence on ventricular repolarization, some forms of treatment which interfere with normal adrenergic neural transmission could be expected to worsen things as often as to improve them, and this would especially apply to the sinus bradycardia.

Asymmetrical Hypertrophy of the Heart

There are probably many ways in which a heart can grow lopsided, and much of the confusion undoubtedly stems from the fact that different etiologies produce this single common end result. Theories about etiology include abnormalities of the collagen framework, abnormal neural influence, and unexplained

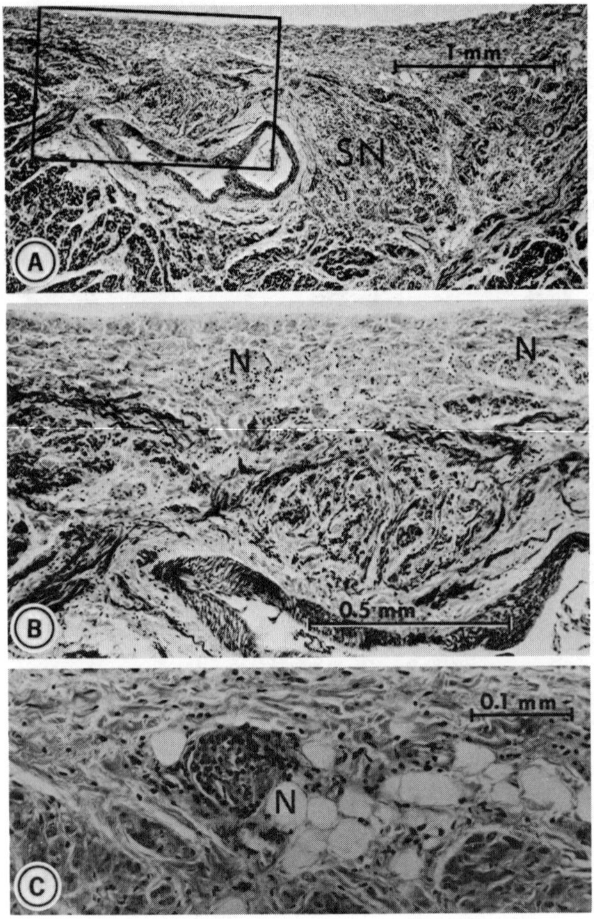

Fig. 20-11. Cardioneuropathy near the sinus node (SN) is shown here from the heart of a patient dying suddenly with asymmetrical hypertrophy of the heart. Boxed area (A) is seen at higher magnification (B), where N indicates two nerves. A different small nerve from the same heart is shown in (C), also infiltrated with lymphocytes and degenerating.

disorderly hypertrophy [36]. Much evidence favors the neural theory, including the surprising prevalence of asymmetrical hypertrophy of the heart in patients with Friedreich's ataxia, a known neuromuscular disorder [45,56]. The cardiac nerves are sometimes morphologically abnormal in both asymmetrical hypertrophy of the heart (Fig. 20-11) and in Friedreich's cardiomyopathy (Fig. 20-12). However, the small coronary arteries are also abnormal, being narrowed both in asymmetrical cardiac hypertrophy (Fig. 20-13) [23] and in Friedreich's cardiomyopathy (Fig. 20-14) [14,25]. The histological appearance of these small coronary arteries in the latter disease, at least, does not suggest that the arteriopathy is secondary to a neural fault.

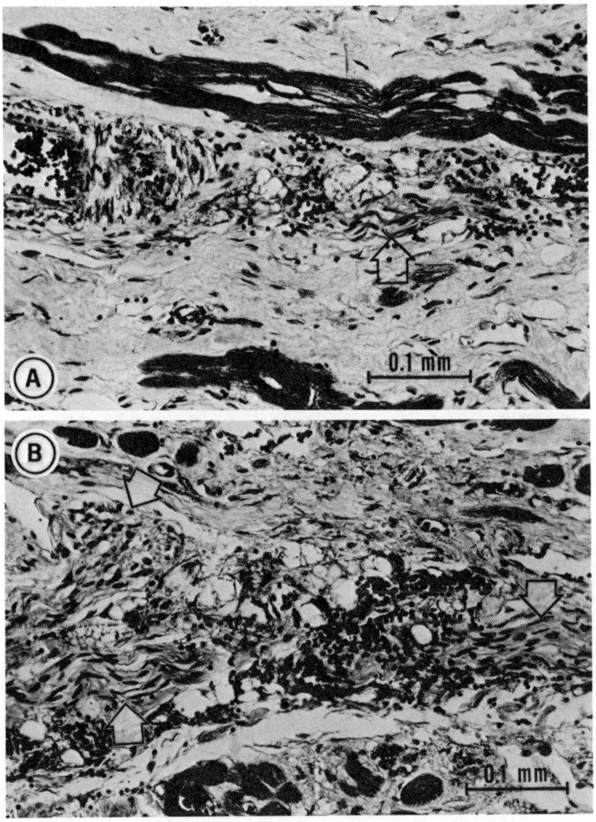

Fig. 20-12. Right atrium of the heart of a patient dying with Friedreich's cardiomyopathy, showing extensive neural degeneration. Identifiable segments of nerve are marked with arrows.

What then is the possible role of cardiac nerves in the pathogenesis or pathophysiology of asymmetrical hypertrophy of the heart? There is evidence that prolonged stimulation with norepinephrine, the normal adrenergic neurotransmitter, can cause ventricular hypertrophy [34]. As a corollary, if one had unevenly distributed focal neural disease within the heart, it would logically follow that norepinephrine effect would become uneven and any hypothetical hypertrophy become asymmetrical. Athough there is much to support such a hypothesis, the evidence is presently inconclusive. Because of the hyperdynamic behavior of these ventricles, the tendency for arrhythmias and sudden death, the presence of cardioneuropathy in some but not all examples of asymmetrical hypertrophy, and the association of the condition with certain heritable neuromuscular diseases, a neuropathic etiology remains plausible, although it seems improbable that it is the only etiology. Whether primary or secondary, however, the best presently available evidence indicates that deranged neural control of the heart deserves continued study in these patients.

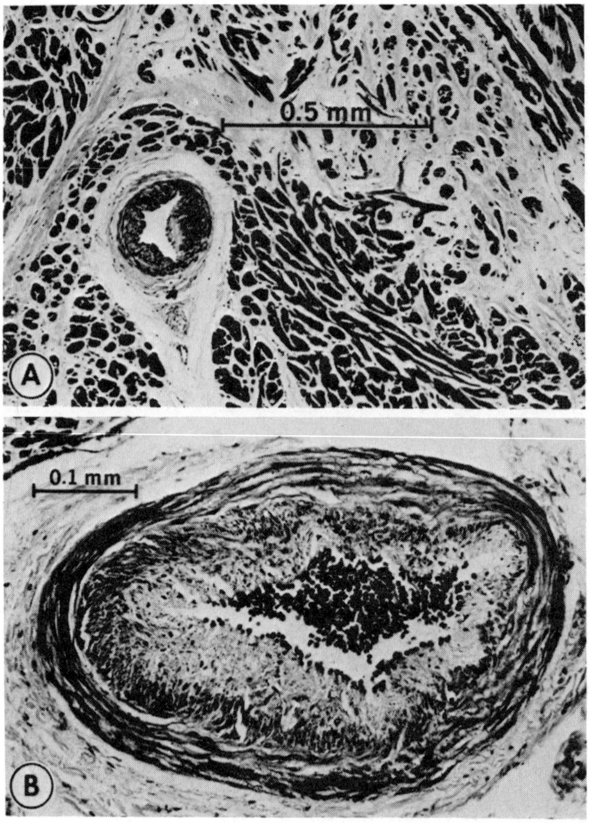

Fig. 20-13. Narrowed small coronary arteries from the heart of a patient who died suddenly with asymmetrical cardiac hypertrophy. (A) Left ventricle; (B) AV node artery. (Reproduced through courtesy of *Br. Heart J.*, ref. 56)

Mitral Valve Prolapse Syndrome

Prolapse of the mitral valve is such a frequent finding on echocardiograms that some have raised a question as to its functional significance. There is no doubt that prolapse in the absence of valvular incompetence and in the absence of any associated symptoms can be a harmless finding, and it is equally sure that extensive mitral regurgitation carries with it an important clinical significance of its own. The greatest puzzle concerns those patients with many symptoms who have a prolapsed but competent mitral valve. Can the palpitations, chest pains, lightheadedness, dyspnea, and fatigue so often encountered be attributed to the competent but prolapsed mitral valve, or is the association the other way around, namely some independent factor causes the symptoms and is also accountable for mitral prolapse?

A dysautonomic basis for this wide array of cardiovascular symptoms has been recognized for over a century, masquerading under a succession of names such as neurocirculatory asthenia, soldier's heart, and hyperventilation syn-

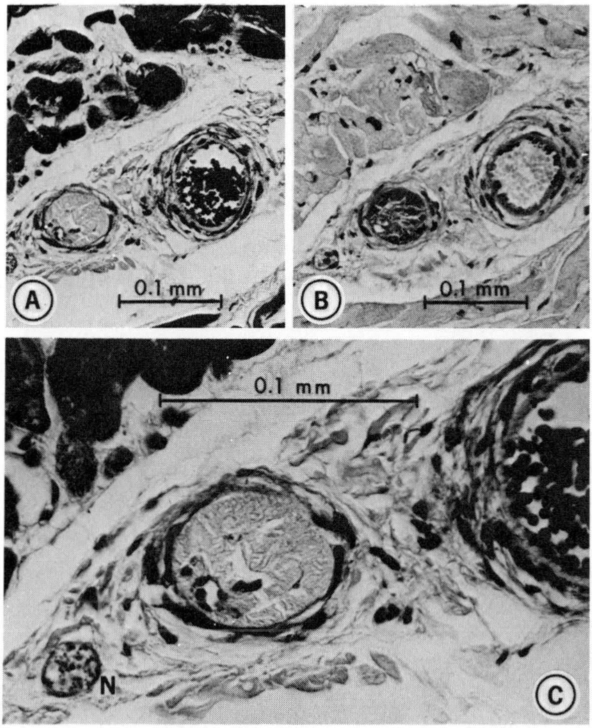

Fig. 20-14. The amorphous intramural deposit which characteristically narrows small coronary arteries in Friedreich's cardiomyopathy is illustrated here. The small artery (A) is seen at higher magnification in (C). (B) Adjacent section showing that the intramural deposit is Schiff-positive (PAS stain).

drome. Both of two recent studies conducted independently at about the same time concluded that patients with mitral valve prolapse who had all these familiar symptoms also presented evidence of abnormal autonomic neural responses by the heart and circulation [6,9]. For example, these patients responded inappropriately to simple challenges such as a Valsalva maneuver or postural tilt test, although the pattern of abnormal response varied widely from one patient to another. More pertinently, medications intended to correct the demonstrable neurocirculatory fault (e.g. diminishing the overreactive vagal or sympathetic response) produced distinct symptomatic improvement. Conversely, symptomatic improvement was accompanied by objective evidence of normalized responses to the autonomic challenges.

There is thus good reason to believe that the uncomfortable and sometimes disabling symptoms exhibited by many (but not all) patients with mitral valve prolapse have a dysautonomic basis in which the valvular deformity may or may not be a contributory factor. One must then ask if the valve is prolapsed also because of dysautonomia. Although this is easy to postulate perhaps on the basis of disorganized sympathetic neural control of the sequence or power of ventricular contraction and altered segmental wall motion), it is difficult to prove. Furthermore, there are some rare examples of biochemically abnormal collagen found in prolapsed mitral valves of symptomatic patients [11], and it is even more difficult to attribute that finding to dysautonomia. The entire subject is appropriately a current focus of active investigation, guided by what evidence has already been gathered: many patients have echocardiographically demonstrable mitral valve prolapse that is neither hemodynamically nor in any other way clinically significant; some of these patients have one or more disabling symptoms that can cause dysautonomia; and there are exceptionally rare cases of biochemically abnormal collagen in the mitral valve.

Essential Hypertension

Due to extensive public and professional educational campaigns, there is a new national awareness of the prevalence and significance of high blood pressure. Although a small percentage of such patients (probably much less than 10%) have a diagnosable cause for their hypertension (pheochromocytoma, aldosterone tumor, renal artery stenosis, chronic renal disease), the vast majority have no distinct cause and enter the diagnostic pool of "essential" hypertension. Known contributing factors to blood pressure elevation, such as smoking, obesity, alcoholism, or excessive salt intake, lend themselves to some degree of appropriate clinical management. When medications are required, most of the useful ones either directly or indirectly participate in neural control of the heart and circulation. However, it is improbable that neurally mediated processes are the sole or predominant problem, since alterations in blood volume, arterial reactivity changes independent of neural events, circulating substances such as catecholamines and those from the renin-angiotensin system, and ionic exchange processes in smooth muscle or the heart all contribute in one way or another.

Prevalent thinking today suggests that neurally mediated events act as immediate but transient factors in raising blood pressure but that more prolonged or sustained hypertension is more due to humoral perturbations [10]. On the other hand, it is a common clinical experience to find improvement even in a long-standing hypertensive patient, particularly those with labile blood pressure or accompanying tachycardia, following the use of beta-receptor blocking compounds. Although some of this improvement may be attributable to alteration of control in renin metabolism where beta-receptor mechanisms participate, it seems equally plausible that a cardiac effect was the major basis.

Early in the course of most cases of arterial hypertension, and even later in cases where blood pressure remains labile or where tachycardia and other evidence of sympathetic overdrive is present, neural events must remain high on the list of etiological considerations. Most of the neural mechanisms by which increased arterial resistance can develop are now readily amenable to pharmacological control, and this has been a recent bright chapter in treatment of such patients. But until we know more precisely how these faulty neural mechanisms come into play and what can be done to prevent this, we will continue to treat patients only after their problems have begun, and most cases of hypertension will necessarily still be classified as essential.

Sudden Unexpected Death

When one excludes readily explainable causes such as subarachnoid hemorrhage, pulmonary embolism, or rupture of the heart, most examples of sudden unexpected death are now believed to be due to a terminal lethal electrical instability of the heart. This may begin as an arrhythmia of one kind and transform into another, such as atrial fibrillation ending in ventricular fibrillation, or it can begin with prolonged asystole or heart block and either change to an arrhythmia or end as it began. The key element is the sustained abnormality of cardiac electrical activity incompatible with a survivable hemodynamic state. But for any hope of prevention it must be recognized that the terminal event observed may be only the last link in a chain of events. Thus, ventricular fibril-

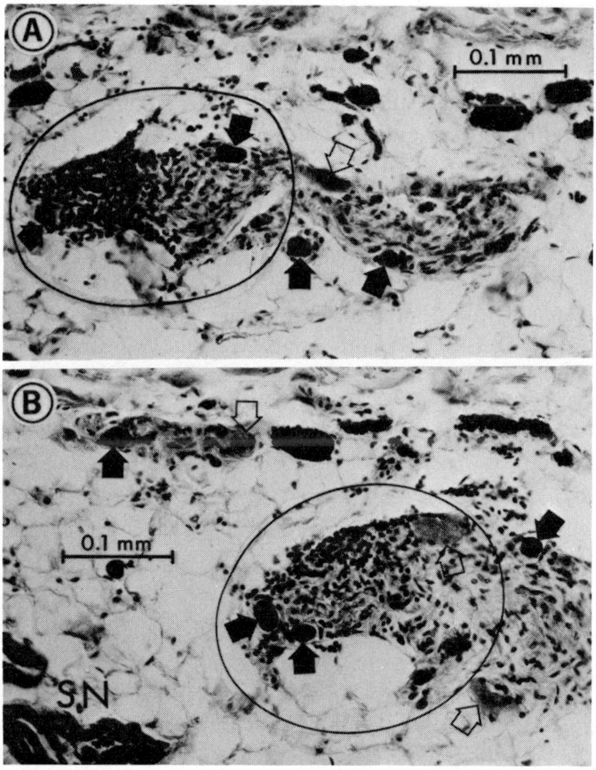

Fig. 20-15. Ganglionitis near the sinus node from the heart of a young woman who died suddenly and unexpectedly. The principal site of lymphocytic infiltration is encircled. Dark arrows mark abnormally shrunken neurons and open arrows swollen ones. (Reproduced through courtesy of *Ann. Intern. Med.*, ref. 27)

lation may have been preceded by any of several contributory and more readily treatable changes in electrical stability.

Some causes of a terminal arrhythmia can be deduced from postmortem findings such as widespread severe coronary disease, but the difficulty with that popular and frequent explanation is that the coronary disease usually had been the same or similar for a long time. Then the addition of a thrombosis or platelet aggregation with or without associated coronary spasm can be the preterminal change. There are also other structural abnormalities of the conduction system of the heart including its blood supply, which can account for lethal arrhythmias in patients without disease in the large coronary arteries [21]. However, as was discussed in a previous section, neural influence (Fig. 20-15) on cardiac rate, rhythm, conduction, and repolarization has been the long neglected factor in considering the causes of sudden unexpected death. In future studies of cardiac performance, particularly its electrical stability, we will almost certainly direct as much attention to cardiac nerves as to coronary arteries.

Mechanisms by which cardioneural control can be stabilized or disorganized, and the sites and structures where this occurs have already been reviewed. Their relevance to lethal electrical instability is in most instances self apparent. But it is fitting to close this discussion of clinical examples of the importance of the heart's nerves by a reminder that the ultimate derangement in their function may be expressed in sudden unexpected death.

REFERENCES

1. Abildskov, J. A., The prolonged QT interval. *Ann. Rev. Med. 30*: 171–179, 1979.
2. Armour, J. A. and D. A. Hopkins, Anatomy of Extrinsic Efferent Autonomic Nerves and Ganglia Innervating the Mammalian Heart, Chap. 2, this volume.
3. Buda, A. J., R. E. Fowles, J. S. Schroeder, S. A. Hunt, P. R. Cipriano, E. B. Stinson, D. C. Harrison, Coronary artery spasm in the denervated transplanted human heart. *Am. J. Med. 70*: 1144–1149, 1981.
4. Burch, G. E., R. Meyers, J. A. Abildskov, A new electrocardiographic pattern observed in cerebrovascular accidents. *Circulation 9*: 719–723, 1954.
5. Burgess, M. J. Relation of ventricular repolarization to electrocardiographic T wave-form and arrhythmia vulnerability. *Am. J. Physiol. 5*: H391-H402, 1979.
6. Coghlan, H. C., P. Phares, M. Cowley, D. Copley, T. N. James, Dysautonomia in mitral valve prolapse. *Am. J. Med. 67*: 236–244, 1979.
7. Ewing, D. J., I. W. Campbell, A. Murray, J. M. M. Neilson, B. F. Clarke, Immediate heart-rate response to standing: simple test for autonomic neuropathy in diabetes. *Br. Med. J. 1*: 145–147, 1978.
8. Fraser, G. R., P. Froggatt, T. N. James, Congenital deafness associated with electrocardiographic abnormalities, fainting attacks and sudden death. A recessive syndrome. *Q. J. Med.* 33: 361–385, 1964.
9. Gaffney, F. A., E. S. Karlsson, W. Campbell, J. E. Schutte, J. V. Nixon, J. T. Willerson, C. G. Blomqvist, Autonomic dysfunction in women with mitral valve prolapse syndrome. *Circulation 59*: 894–901, 1979.
10. Guyton, A. C., The relationship of cardiac output and arterial pressure control. The Tenth Annual George C. Griffith Lecture. *Circulation 64*: 1079–1088, 1981.

11. Hammer, D., C. V. Leier, N. Baba, J. S. Vasko, C. F. Wooley, S. R. Pinnell, Altered collagen composition in a prolapsing mitral valve with ruptured chordae tendineae. *Am. J. Med. 67*: 863–866, 1979.
12. Hashimoto, K., S. Chiba, S. Tanaka, M. Hirata, Y. Suzuki, Adrenergic mechanism participating in induction of atrial fibrillation by ACh. *Am. J. Physiol. 215*: 1183–1191, 1968.
13. Hope-Simpson, R. E., The nature of herpes zoster: a long term study and a new hypothesis. *Proc. R. Soc. Med. 58*: 9–20, 1965.
14. James, T. N. and C. Fisch, Observations on the cardiovascular involvement in Friedreich's ataxia. *Am. Heart J. 66*: 164–175, 1963.
15. James, T N. Cholinergic mechanisms in the sinus node with particular reference to the actions of hemicholinium. *Circ. Res. 19*: 347–357, 1966.
16. James, T. N. Cardiac innervation: anatomic and pharmacologic relations. *Bull. N.Y. Acad. Med. 43*: 1041–1086, 1967.
17. James, T. N. Congenital deafness and cardiac arrhythmias. *Am. J Cardiol. 19*: 627–643, 1967.
18. James. T. N. QT prolongation and sudden death. *Mod. Concepts Cardiovasc. Dis. 38*: 35–38, 1969.
19. James, T. N., E. S. Bear, R. J. Frink, K. F. Lang, J. C. Tomlinson, Selective stimulation, suppression or blockade of the AV node and His bundle. *J. Lab. Clin. Med. 76*: 240–256, 1970.
20. James, T. N., F. Urthaler, J. H. Isobe, Neurogenic influence on the P-Tp segment. *Am. J. Cardiol. 32*: 799–807, 1973.
21. James, T. N., Order and disorder in the rhythm of the heart. The Fifth Annual George C. Griffith Lecture. *Circulation 47*: 362–386, 1973.
22. James, T. N., J. H. Isobe, F. Urthaler, Analysis of components in a hypertensive cardiogenic chemoreflex. *Circulation 52*: 179–192, 1975.
23. James, T. N. and T. K. Marshall, De Subitaneis Mortibus. XII. Asymmetrical hypertrophy of the heart. *Circulation 51*: 1149–1166, 1975.
24. James, T. N. The sinus node. *Am. J. Cardiol. 40*: 965–986, 1977.
25. James, T. N. Small arteries of the heart. The 36th George E. Brown Memorial Lecture. *Circulation 56*: 2–14, 1977.
26. James, T. N., P. Froggatt, W. J. Atkinson, P. R. Lurie, D. G. McNamara, W. W. Miller, G. T. Schloss, J. F. Carroll, R. L. North, De Subitaneis Mortibus. XXX. Observations on the pathophysiology of the long QT syndromes with special reference to the neuropathology of the heart. *Circulation 57*: 1221–1231, 1978.
27. James, T. N., D. P. Zipes, R. E. Finegan, J. W. Eisele, J. E. Carter, Cardiac ganglionitis associated with sudden unexpected death. *Ann. Intern. Med. 91*: 727–730, 1979.
28. James, T. N., J. H. Isobe, F. Urthaler, Correlative electrophysiological and anatomical studies concerning the site of origin and escape rhythm during complete atrioventricular block in the dog. *Circ. Res. 45*: 108–119, 1979.
29. James, T. N., W. N. Pearce, Jr., E. G. Givhan, Jr. Sudden death while driving. *Am J. Cardiol. 45*: 1095–1102, 1980.
30. James, T. N. and W. A. H. MacLean, Paroxysmal ventricular arrhythmias and familial sudden death associated with neural lesions in the heart. *Chest 78*: 24–30, 1980.
31. James, T. N., F. Urthaler, G. R. Hageman, Reflex heart block. *Am. J. Cardiol. 45*: 1182–1188, 1980.

32. James, T. N. and K. Imamura, Virus-like particles associated with intracardiac ganglionitis in two cases of sudden unexpected death. *Jap. Heart J. 22*: 447–454, 1981.
33. Jervell, A. and F. Lange-Nielsen, Congenital deaf-mutism, functional heart disease with prolongation of the Q-T interval, and sudden death. *Am. Heart J. 54*: 59–68, 1957.
34. Laks, M. M., F. Morady, and H. J. C. Swan, Myocardial hypertrophy produced by chronic infusion of subhypertensive doses of norepinephrine in the dog. *Chest 64*: 75–78, 1973.
35. Mackay, J. D., M. McB. Page, J. Cambridge, P. J. Watkins, Diabetic autonomic neuropathy. The diagnostic value of heart rate monitoring. *Diabetologia 18*: 471–478, 1980.
36. Maron, B. J and W. C. Roberts, Hypertrophic cardiomyopathy and cardiac muscle cell disorganization revisited: relation between the two and significance. *Am. Heart J. 102*: 95–110, 1981.
37. Mathews, Jr., E. C., A. W. Blount, Jr., J. I, Townsend, Q-T prolongation and ventricular arrhythmias, with and without deafness, in the same family. *Am. J. Cardiol. 29*: 702–711, 1972.
38. Moe, G. K. and J. A. Abildskov, Atrial fibrillation as a self-sustaining arrhythmia independent of focal discharge. *Am. Heart J. 58*: 59–70, 1959.
39. Moss, A. J. and J. McDonald, Unilateral cervicothoracic sympathetic ganglionectomy for the treatment of long QT interval syndrome. *New Eng. J. Med. 285*: 903–904, 1971.
40. Raizner, A. E., R. A. Chahine, T. Ishimori, M. S. Verani, N. Zacca, N. Jamal, R. R. Miller, R. J. Luchi, Provocation of coronary artery spasm by the cold pressor test. Hemodynamic, arteriographic and quantitative angiographic observations. *Circulation 62*: 925–932, 1980.
41. Randall, W. C., Selective autonomic innervation of the heart, Chap. 3, this volume.
42. Randall, W. C. and S. B. Jones, S. L. Lipsius, G. J. Rozanski, Subsidiary atrial pacemakers and their neural control, Chap. 9, this volume.
43. Rossi, L. Histopathology of cardiac arrhythmias, 2nd ed., Milano, Casa Editrice Ambrosiana, 1978.
44. Rossi, L., International lecture of the American Heart Association, Annual Scientific Sessions, 1980.
45. Ruschhaupt, D. G., O. G. Thilenius, D. E. Cassels, Friedreich's ataxia associated with idiopathic hypertrophic subaortic stenosis. *Am. Heart J. 84*: 95–102, 1972.
46. Schwartz, P. J., Sympathetic imbalance and cardiac dysrhythmias, Chap. 10, this volume.
47. Siegel, R. J., W. R. Cabeen, Jr., W. C. Roberts, Prolonged QT interval-ventricular tachycardia syndrome from massive rapid weight loss utilizing the liquid-protein-modified-fast diet: sudden death with sinus node ganglionitis and neuritis. *Am. Heart J. 102*: 121–124, 1981.
48. Thomas, J. X., C. E. Jones, and W. C. Randall, Neural modulation of coronary blood flow, Chap. 8, this volume.
49. Urthaler, F., C. R. Katholi, J. Macy, Jr., T. N. James, Mathematical relationship between automaticity of the sinus node and the AV junction. *Am. Heart J. 86*: 189–195, 1973.
50. Urthaler, F., K. Millar, M. J. Burgess, J. A. Abildskov, T. N. James, Comparative dependence on adrenergic neural tone by automaticity in the sinus node and in the AV junction. *J. Pharmacol. Exp. Ther. 187*: 269–279, 1973.

51. Urthaler, F., C. R. Katholi, J. Macy, Jr., T. N. James, Electrophysiological and mathematical characteristics of the escape rhythm during complete AV block. *Cardiovasc. Res. 8*: 173–186, 1974.
52. Urthaler, F., G. R. Hageman, T. N. James, Hemodynamic components of a cardiogenic hypertensive chemoreflex in dogs. *Circ. Res. 42*: 135–142, 1978.
53. Urthaler, F. and T. N. James, Experimental studies on the pathogenesis of asystole after verapamil in the dog. *Am. J. Cardiol. 44*: 651–656, 1979.
54. Urthaler, F., T. N. James, G. R. Hageman, Regional flow patterns during serotonin-induced cardiogenic hypertensive chemoreflex. *Cardiovasc. Res. 14*: 169–176, 1980.
55. Urthaler, F., H. C. Coghlan, T. N. James, Effects of selectively produced changes in cardiac rhythm or conduction upon flow in the superior vena cava. *J. Thorac. Cardiovasc. Surg. 82*: 447–456, 1981.
56. Van der Hauwaert, L. G. and M. Dumoulin, Hypertrophic cardiomyopathy in Friedreich's ataxia. *Br. Heart J. 38*: 1291–1298, 1976.
57. Ward, O. C. Heritable QT prolongation without deafness. *Br. Heart J. 34*: 962, 1972.
58. Wehrmacher, W. H. and W. C. Randall, Performance of the heart in health and disease. Chap. 1, this volume.

Index

A1, A2, A5 catecholamine regions, 332, 360
Accentuated antagonism, 85–86, 147
Acetylcholine, 48
  accentuated antagonism with sympathetic system, 85, 148
  antagonism of glycogenolytic effects of beta receptor, 148
  cGMP as possible second messenger, 139, 145
  effects upon atrial refractory period, 80
  modulation of neurotransmitter release, 98ff
  reduction of K^+ conductance in SA node, 71, 137
Acetylcholinesterase, 68
  distribution within atria, 81
  in coronary arteries, 180, 182
Action potential
  as agent in information processing, 310
  atrioventricular node cells, 76
  effect of muscarinic receptor activity on, 137, 148
  sinoatrial nodal cells, 70
  sympathetic preganglion cells, 326, 331
  ventricular, effect of catecholamines on, 108
Adenosine
  modulation of neurotransmitter release, 98ff
Adenylate cyclase
  muscarinic inhibition of, 151
Adrenal gland
  compensatory responses to sympathectomy, 173
  effect of adrenalectomy on beta-receptors, 117
  importance after cardiac denervation, 284
Afferent nerves
  activity during cardiac arrhythmias, 378ff
  after surgical cardiac denervation, 286
  convergence of visceral and somatic, 376
  during acute coronary occlusion, 254
  in congestive heart failure, 13ff
  mediating cardiac pain, 369ff
  physiology of, 370ff
  reflex responses from stimulation of, 55, 369ff
Afterload
  effect on ventricular oxygen demand, 266
Ageing (aging)
  effect on alpha receptors, 107
  effect on cardiovascular system, 8
Aldosterone
  in congestive heart failure, 13
Alpha receptor, *see also* receptors
  α_1 *vs.* α_2, 418, 422
  agonists and antagonists, 97–99
  atrial *vs.* ventricular, 111
  classification, 96, 100ff, 110ff
  control of coronary circulation, 178ff, 185ff, 190, 257, 270, 407, 418
  control of inotropic state, 107
  density, 107, 110, 113ff
  distribution within coronary circulation, 190
  effect on ventricular action potential, 108
  history of research, 95
  control of neuronal norepinephrine release, 99ff
  inhibition of accelerans nerve stimulation effects, 100
  mechanism of action, 110
  modulation of acetylcholine release from vagus, 106

myocardial ischemia and, 256, 270
pharmacology, 97
presynaptic, actions of, 99ff
regulation of, 113ff, 118ff
relative potencies of agonists, 96
Amygdala
control of heart during emotion, 395ff
Angina pectoris, 369ff, 375
basis of, 189ff, 422
eliminated by beta-block, 255
surgical elimination of, 228, 293, 426, 428
Angiotensin
in congestive heart failure, 13
modulation of neurotransmitter release, 98ff
Ansa subclavia (dorsal and ventral)
cat (anatomy), 34ff
dog (anatomy), 22ff
monkey (anatomy), 37ff
Antidiuretic hormone (ADH)
in congestive heart failure, 13
Aplysia californica
control of heart in, 404
Archistriatum (pigeon)
control of the heart during emotion, 396
Arrhythmias (cardiac)
atrial fibrillation, 439
autonomic imbalance, 49, 227ff, 407, 442, 452
cardiac afferent nerve activity during, 378ff
during coronary occlusion with reversible stellectomy, 230
during emotional conditioning in monkey, 406
gluco- and mineralocorticoids and, 117
induced by cardiac nerve stimulation, 228ff, 440
intractable ventricular, treatment of, 427ff
mechanisms of, 234ff
protection by high vagal cardiac tone, 130
surgical treatment, 295, 427ff
sympathetic imbalance, 225ff, 230, 407, 442
termination (of supraventricular) by carotid massage, 130
termination by prolongation of ventricular refractory period, 81
Artery, sinoatrial nodal
distribution (dog), 205
in vitro perfusion, 215ff
selective perfusion, 204, 438
Ascending sympathetic pathways
activity in during cardiac arrhythmias, 378
locations of, 334, 366
physiology of, 371ff
referred pain and, 375
Asystole
following SA node excision
sudden cardiac death, 15
Athlete's bradycardia, 130
ATP
effect of positive inotropism upon myocardial levels, 167
Atrial activation patterns
altered by vagal stimulation, 80
Atrial contractile force
effect of muscarinic receptor activation upon, 137
effect of single vagal stimulus upon, 82, 447
frequency–force relationship for vagal stimulation, 83
response to nerve stimulation during cardiac denervation, 55
Atrial fibrillation, 439
Atrio-ventricular block
disappearance during exercise, 46
effect of autonomic blockade on, 47
induced by nerve stimulation, 59
Atrio-ventricular conduction
effect of cardiac cycle length upon, 77
in awake subject, 402ff
vagal control of, 74, 442
Atrio-ventricular node
cardiovascular disease and, 437, 442
conduction block within, 74
control in awake subject, 402ff
P-cells in, 200
relative refractory period, 76
selective parasympathetic denervation, 58
vagal effect curves, 73–75
Atrium
electrophysiological mapping, 215ff
internodal pathways in, 203
in vitro perfusion of, 215ff
subsidiary pacemakers in, 200ff
Atropine, *see* muscarinic blockade
Automaticity
ionic basis of, 219
Autonomic imbalance, *see also* dysautonomia, sympathetic imbalance
arrhythmias and, 49, 227ff, 407, 442, 452
definition, 227
Autonomic nervous system
anatomy of, 322
interaction between components of, 46
reciprocal innervation, 310
Awake subject, *see* conscious subject
Axon hillock, 309
Axonal transport
of muscarinic receptors, 102

Baboon
cardiac nerves, 39
conditioned emotional response, 393ff
coronary arteries, 182
Baroreflex, *see also* carotid sinus, 359ff
brainstem centers, 353
during acute myocardial ischemia, 253
during emotion, 400
forebrain, 361

interaction with respiratory rhythm, 315
spinal sympathetic neurons, 331, 335ff
vagal tone, 358ff
Basal autonomic tone, 321ff, 346, 351ff
Behavior
and the study of the heart, 392
Beta-blockade
deleterious effects after cardiac denervation, 284
during exercise in dog, 414
effect on A-V block, 47
effect on behaviorally induced cardiovascular responses, 401–403
effect on myocardial ATPase activity, 174
effect on myocardial metabolic efficiency, 167
reduction of myocardial infarct size, 259
Beta receptor
affinity sites (β_H, β_L), 97, 115, 116, 117
agonists and antagonists, 97
classification (β_1, β_2), 96ff, 112ff, 418
control of coronary circulation, 183ff, 418
coronary occlusion and, 118
density, 113ff
diabetes and, 117
distribution, 112
effect on ventricular action potential, 108
facilitation of neuronal norepinephrine release, 104ff
guanine nucleotides, role of, 151
heterologous regulation, 116ff
history of research, 95
homologous ("down") regulation, 114ff, 117
mechanism of action via cAMP, 109ff, 150ff
metabolic effects, 149
muscarinic receptor inhibition of, 146ff
pathological conditions, 115
pharmacology, 97, 114
physiological effects, 112ff
proteins (R_β, N_S) of, 114ff, 151
relative potencies of agonists, 96
"up regulation" of in propranolol withdrawal syndrome, 116
Bezold–Jarisch reflex
absence after cardiac denervation, 287
during cardiac reinnervation, 292
Bird, *see* pigeon
Blood pressure
after spinal transection, 337, 346
central nervous system control, 346ff
changes during cardiac denervation, 55
Blood volume
regulation after cardiac denervation, 286
"Border zone"
shift in following stellectomy, 234
Bradykinin
afferent nerve activity from intramyocardial injection, 375
Brainstem, *see* medulla oblongata
Ca^{++}, *see also* current, slow inward
cAMP modulation of current, 109
intermediary for ACh-cGMP cascade, 145
intracellular pools, 146
phospholamban and, 110
resequestration by sarcoplasmic reticulum, 173
cAMP
aberrations in spontaneously hypertensive rat, 115
antagonized by muscarinic receptor, 139, 151
changes after cardiac denervation, 285
effects antagonized by cGMP, 141
effects on protein kinase, 150, 155
mechanisms of action, 150ff
mediator of catecholamine effects on beta receptor, 109, 114, 151
role in mediating accentuated antagonism, 85
Canine, *see* dog
Cannon, W.B., 4, 17, 18
"Law of Denervation", 285
Cardiac denervation, *see also* reinnervation, 49, 278ff
afferent cardiac nerves after, 286, 427–428
cAMP changes, 285
capillary density of myocardium after, 272
clinical use, 49, 243, 295, 425ff
coronary collateral circulation after, 271ff, 429
comparison of acute and chronic effects, 268
denervation supersensitivity, 243, 285
effect on behaviorally mediated heart rate responses, 401
effect on contractile force, 262
effect on myocardial metabolism, 168ff, 429
function of heart after, 281ff, 402, 416
inadvertent, during coronary bypass, 426
increased myocardial glycogen after, 175
myocardial catecholamines after, 285
of specific regions of the heart, 49, 296
partial, 293
perfusion territory of coronary artery after, 271, 429
protective effect during coronary occlusion, 258ff, 429
reduction of myocardial blood flow after, 265
regional neural ablation, 281
selective parasympathetic denervation, 50ff, 297
surgical procedures, 50ff, 279ff
using 6-OHDA, 102
Cardiac output
during exercise, 414ff
in denervated hearts during exercise, 168
Cardiac-related sympathetic rhythm, 353ff

Cardiac transplant
  effect on cardiac performance in dog, 170
  first attempts, 278
  synchronization of donor and recipient heart rate, 74
Cardiocardiac reflex
  during acute coronary occlusion, 254, 374
  in spinal animals, 338
Cardioneuropathies, 435ff
Cardiovascular centers, 307ff, 347ff, 391
Cardiovascular disease, *see* disease
Carotid sinus
  in congestive heart failure, 13ff
  nerve, coronary vasodilation from stimulation of, 182
  syncope, 450
Cat
  cardiac nerves, 34ff
  conditional cardiovascular response, 400
  spinoreticular tract, 371
Catecholamines, *see also* norepinephrine
  actions antagonized by cGMP, 140
  denervation supersensitivity to, 284
  during exercise, 418
  effect on ventricular action potential, 108
  following acute coronary occlusion in dog, 254
  in CNS, 349
  in coronary sinus blood during cardiac nerve stimulation, 87
  influence on myocardial metabolism, 165ff, 173ff
  modulation of neurotransmitter release, 98ff
  muscarinic modulation of physiological effects, 146ff
  myocardial, during cardiac denervation and reinnervation, 285, 291
  shift of dose response curve, 111
  trophic effects, 173
Caudal medial nerve (anatomy, dog), 24
Caudal pole nerve
  cat (anatomy), 35ff
  dog (anatomy), 25ff
  evoked potentials recorded in, 33
Caudal vagal nerve (monkey, anatomy), 37ff
Central command, 391, 404
Central nervous system (CNS)
  control of the circulation, 307ff
  information processing within 310
  invertebrates, 393
cGMP
  analogues of, 139
  antagonize effects of cAMP, 141
  evidence against role in heart, 143ff
  mechanism of action, 141
  muscarinic receptors, 137, 138
  role in mediating accentuated antagonism, 86, 140
Channels (ionic)
  control by muscarinic receptors, 137
Chemoreceptors
  cardiac, 370, 375, 436, 441
  reflex coronary vasodilation, 182, 189
  sympathetic nerve discharge and, 327, 436, 441
  vagal tone and, 358
Chronotropism, *see* heart rate
Classical (Pavlovian) conditioning
Clinical considerations, *see also* disease, 453ff
Command cell, 405
Conduction velocity (sino-atrial), 70–73
Congestive heart failure, 12ff
Conscious subject, 391ff
  arrhythmias, 227, 230, 234, 239, 242
  catecholamine levels, 254
  coronary arterial diameter changes in, 184
  coronary blood flow, 168, 188, 407–408, 414ff, 418ff
  coronary occlusion, 263
  denervation of heart, 282ff
  eating, 402
  exercise, 337, 414ff
  myocardial metabolism, 168, 171
  subsidiary atrial pacemakers, 201, 206
  tonic neurogenic coronary vasoconstriction, 189, 335
Contractile force
  control in awake subject, 401, 414ff
  before and after cardiac denervation, 52
  during severe coronary stenosis, 257
  effect on alpha agonists, 107ff
  effect of chronic cardiac denervation, 262
Contractility, *see* atrial contractility, contractile force, inotropism, ventricular contractility
Convergence
  of visceral and somatic afferents in spinal cord, 376
Coronary arteries, *see also* stenosis, vasospasm
  afferent fibers from 374
  alpha receptors, 185ff
  beta receptors, 184
  histology of nervous innervation, 179
  large *vs.* small diameter, control of, 181, 182, 185
  partial stenosis, 257
  perfusion territory after cardiac denervation, 271
Coronary artery spasm, *see* vasospasm
Coronary blood flow
  autoregulation, 258
  changes in transmural distribution, 184, 192, 260
  decreases during stellate stimulation, 234
  during exercise and excitement, 168, 407–408, 414ff, 418ff
  during severe stenosis, 257
  effect of cardiac denervation, 168, 171, 265, 269, 297
  effect of stellectomy, 234
  metabolic control of, 182, 184, 258

neural control of, 171, 178ff, 185ff, 257, 407–408
parasympathetic control of, 181ff
reactive hyperemia after left stellectomy, 234
redistribution, 182
sympathetic vasocontriction during coronary occlusion, 256, 270
tonic neurogenic vasoconstriction, 185ff, 189, 420
Coronary bypass surgery
possible inadvertent cardiac denervation during, 426
Coronary collaterals
growth after cardiac denervation, 273, 429
neural vasoconstriction of, 271
resistance after cardiac denervation, 272, 429
Coronary occlusion, *see also* myocardial ischemia
afferent nerve activity during, 369ff, 373ff
epicardial electrogram mapping during, 234
infarct size, 235, 255, 258ff, 429
perfusion of ischemic myocardium in denervated heart, 269
protective effect of cardiac denervation, 258, 269
reversible stellectomy and, 230
Coronary veins, 185
Cortex (frontal)
control of the heart during emotion, 396
Cortisol
effects on beta receptors following adrenalectomy, 117
Cranial pole nerve (dog, anatomy), 22
Cranial vagal nerve
cat (anatomy), 34ff
dog (anatomy), 22ff
monkey (anatomy), 37ff
postganglionic neurons of, 30
stimulation of, 30
Creatine phosphokinase (myocardial)
changes following cardiac denervation and coronary occlusion, 260
Crista terminalis
as site of subsidiary atrial pacemaker, 215
Crosscorrelation analysis, 327, 352ff
Current, slow inward
effect of muscarinic receptor, 137, 143
in subsidiary atrial pacemaker, 219

Decompensation, 6
Defense area (hypothalamus)
coronary circulation and, 183
modulation of baroreflex, 400
Dendrites
as agents of information processing, 309, 318
Denervation supersensitivity, *see* cardiac denervation
2-Deoxyglucose
mapping techniques using, 312
Descending spinal sympathetic pathways, 332ff
locations of, 334–335
sources of, 332, 349ff
Diabetes
atrioventricular node and, 442
beta receptors, 117
Differential autonomic responses, 312
Digitalis
action via modification of cardiac vagal tone, 130
Disease (cardiovascular), *see also* specific examples
cardioneuropathies, 435ff
possible biobehavioral bases of, 405ff, 422
Dog
cardiac nerves in, 21ff, 32ff
Dorsal motor nucleus of the vagus
control of heart rate during emotion, 398
origin of cardiac vagal nerves, 26, 39
Dorsolateral funiculus (spinal cord)
site of descending sympathoexcitatory pathways, 333
Dromotropism
control in awake subject, 402ff
responses to nerve stimulation during cardiac denervation, 52ff
Dysautonomia, *see also* autonomic imbalance, sympathetic imbalance, 448ff
during stress, 16
hypertension, 5
mitral valve prolapse, 447
sudden infant death, 15

Efficiency (metabolic)
effects of catecholamines on myocardial, 165ff
Electrocardiogram
neurally induced changes during ischemia, 255
Electrograms
from atrial and ventricular plunge electrodes, 59
Electron microscopy
of coronary arterial nerves, 180
Electrophysiology of cardiac nerves, 32ff
Emotion, *see also* classical conditioning, 17ff
arrhythmias during, 239
control of heart during, 394ff
coronary blood flow during, 168, 178
Endogenous pyrogen, 8
Ergot alkaloids
and coronary vasospasm, 190, 293
Evoked potentials in cardiac nerves, 33, 328
Exercise, 414ff
after cardiac denervation, 282
arrhythmias during, 239, 242
cardiovascular response to, 3, 5ff, 394
neural control of circulation during, 337, 414ff
metabolism during, 5
stress testing, 6

Fallot, tetrology of, 14
Familial Dysautonomia (Riley Day
Syndrome), 10
Fever, 8ff
Forebrain
baroreflex and, 361ff
Frank–Starling Law, 12
during exercise after cardiac denervation, 284
in intact subject, 417
Frostbite, 9

Ganglia, *see* mediastinal, middle cervical, nodose and stellate ganglia
Glucocorticoids
effects on beta receptor, 117
Glycogenolysis
effect of beta receptor, 149
in sympathectomized heart, 174
Growth
change in myocardial beta receptors during, 116
GTP
and regulation of beta adrenergic effects on the heart, 151
Guanylate cyclase
as regulator of cGMP in heart, 144ff

H_2 receptors
and cAMP, 141
Heart
in vitro study of, 98
Heart failure, *see* congestive heart failure
Heart rate
accentuated antagonism and control of, 85ff
after cardiac denervation, 282
behaviorally induced changes in, 397
central neural control of, 350
control after left stellectomy, 237
control during disease, 436
control during emotion, 391ff, 401
control during exercise, 414ff
control of in invertebrate *(Aplysia californica)*, 404–405
increase from interganglionic nerve stimulation, 30
independent effects of right atrial pressure upon, 285
interaction with A-V conduction, 74ff, 78
neurally induced changes during selective SA *vs.* AV nodal denervation, 63ff
paradoxical response to vagal stimulation, 73
potentiation of response by alpha blockade, 104
response to nerve stimulation during cardiac denervation, 55
subsidiary atrial pacemaker, 202, 208
synchronization with vagal stimulation rate, 72
vagus nerve stimulation effects upon, 68ff, 76
Heart transplant, *see* cardiac transplant
Hemorrhage and acute hypotension, 9ff
response after cardiac denervation, 284
Heterometric autoregulation, *see* Frank–Starling Law
Homeometric autoregulation, 13
Human, *see* man
Hyperbaric conditions
Hyperpolarization
in SA node during vagal stimulation, 70
Hypertension, 10ff, 458
alpha receptors, 118
beta receptors, 115, 116
clinical course, 11, 458
DOCA, 12, 118
physiological consequences, 11
renal hypertensive rat, 118
spontaneously hypertensive rat (SHR), 12
Hypertrophy (myocardial)
asymmetrical, 453ff
beta receptors, 116
Hypobaric conditions, 6ff
Hypotension, 10
Hypothalamus
baroreflex and, 361, 400
control of coronary circulation, 183
control of heart in awake animal, 393ff
multiple "spheres of influence" of, 318
positive inotropic responses from stimulation, 179
projections from, 349
response to electrical stimulation, 393ff
spinal cord degeneration from lesions, 321
Hypothermia
total body, 9
Hypoxia
response after cardiac denervation, 284

Imbalance, *see* autonomic imbalance, dysautonomia, sympathetic imbalance
Infarct(ion) size
beta block, 255
cardiac denervation, 258ff, 429
left stellectomy, 235
Inferior cardiac nerve (cat)
oscillatory activity in, 316
Innominate nerve (cat, anatomy), 36
Inotropism
alpha receptor control, 107
central nervous system control, 351
cGMP effects on, 140
control in awake subject, 401
effect of chronic cardiac denervation, 262
effect on myocardial oxygen consumption, 166ff
gluco- and mineralocorticoid effects, 117
muscarinic receptor modulation, 155
persistent vagal effects, 76, 445
phospholamban as possible mediator of changes, 155
response to nerve stimulation during cardiac denervation, 52ff
response to hypothalamic stimulation, 179

Intact subject, *see* conscious subject
Interaction
  between sympathetic preganglionic neurons, 329
  between sinotrial and atrioventricular nodes, 74
  lack of in sympathetic and parasympathetic control of A-V conduction, 74
  sympathetic and parasympathetic control of SA node, 74
  sympathetic and parasympathetic control of ventricular refractory period, 80
  vagal–sympathetic, 84ff, 147ff, 380ff, 399
Interganglionic nerve (right and left)
  dog (anatomy), 22ff
  increase in heart rate from stimulation, 30
Intermediate medial nerve (dog, anatomy), 26
Intermediate zone (of medulla)
  as origin of cardiac vagal nerves, 27, 39
Intermediolateral nucleus, *see* spinal cord
Internal thoracic nerve (dog, anatomy), 25ff
Interneurons, spinal sympathetic, 330
Internodal pathways, 203
Invertebrates, *see Aplysia californica*
Ionophores, 141, 145
Iontophoresis
  of cGMP into sinoatrial node cells, 139

Junction, atrio-ventricular, *see* atrio-ventricular node
Junctional pacemaker
  cardiovascular disease and, 437
  induction by nerve stimulation, 65

Lactate
  myocardial production of, 171, 189, 257, 261, 430
Lateral sympathetic nerves (monkey, anatomy), 38
Life expectancy, 4
Limbic system
  control of the heart during emotion, 396

Man
  arrhythmias following unilateral stellectomy, 231
  blood pressure in paraplegic, 337
  cardiac nerves, 39
  cardiac denervation for treatment of disease, 49
  Frank–Starling Law, 417
  sympathetic imbalanced studied in, 246
Mayer waves, 315, 325
Medial cardiac nerve
  dog (anatomy), 25
  monkey (anatomy), 38
  stimulation in monkey, 40
Mediastinal ganglion
  dog (anatomy), 22ff
  monkey (anatomy), 38
Medulla oblongata, 346ff
  control of heart during emotion, 397ff
  descending projections, 332
  effect on spinal cord sympathetic neurons, 331
  history of study, 347
  origin of cardiac vagal nerves, 26
  sympathetic nerve discharge generator, 353
  sympathetic–parasympathetic interactions, 383
Metabolism (myocardial)
  after cardiac denervation or sympathectomy, 168ff, 258ff, 264ff, 283, 430
  during exercise, 418
  effect of after load, 266
  effect of catecholamines, 165ff
  mechanism of neurogenic changes, 173ff
  trophic influence of cardiac nerves, 173
Microcircuits, 310, 318, 347ff
  generator of sympathetic nerve discharge, 353
  interneurons in, 330
  rhythm generator, hypothetical model, 355
Microspheres
  loss of from ischemic myocardium, 172
Middle cervical ganglion
  evoked potentials from stimulation, 33
  cat (anatomy), 34ff
  dog (anatomy), 22ff
  monkey (anatomy), 37ff
  postganglionic sympathetic neurons in, 27ff
'Milieu interne', 3
Mineralocorticoids
  effect on beta receptor, 117
Mitral valve prolapse, 447, 456
Mollusks, *see Aplysia californica*
Monge's disease, 6ff
Monkey, *see also* baboon
  arrhythmias during emotion, 406
  cardiac nerves, 38ff
  spinothalamic tract, 371
Muscarinic blockade
  effect upon ventricular refractory period, 80
  effect on A-V block, 47
Muscarinic receptors
  agonists, 134ff
  axonal transport of, 102
  cAMP-independent antagonism of catecholamine effects, 153
  cation channels controlled by, 137
  classes of binding sites, 135
  coronary circulation, control of, 182
  density, 136
  distribution, 133
  heterotropic regulation, 136
  inhibition of norepinephrine release by, 102
  molecular mechanisms, 135, 137ff
  multiple states of, 134ff
  pharmacology, 131ff
  physiology, 131ff
  prejunctional, evidence for, 133
  radioligand binding studies, 131

regulation by guanine nucleotides, 135
thyroid hormones and, 136
Mustard procedure, 201
Myocardial contractility, *see* atrial contractility, inotropism, ventricular contractility
Myocardial hypertrophy, *see* hypertrophy, myocardial
Myocardial infarct size, *see* infarct size
Myocardial ischemia
afferent nerves activated, 374
arrhythmias during, 229ff, 406
behavior and, 407
coronary vasoconstriction during, 256, 427
effects of sympathetic nerves during, 253ff, 427
sympathetic imbalance resultant from, 242
transmural distribution of blood flow during, 184
Myocardial metabolism, *see* metabolism
Myocytes, alpha receptor location in transsynaptic hypothesis, 101

N-protein (beta receptor), *see* beta receptor
Nerves, cardiac, *see* specific nerves
Networks (neural), *see* microcircuits
Neural rhythms, *see* oscillator
Neurotransmitters, *see also* acetylcholine, norepinephrine, 360
Nitroprusside
effects on myocardial cGMP, 140, 142, 143
Nodose ganglion
cat (anatomy), 34ff
dog (anatomy), 22ff
monkey (anatomy), 37ff
Nonhuman primate, *see also* monkey, baboon, 38ff
Norepinephrine, *see also* catecholamines
effects on intermediary metabolism of myocardium, 174
inhibition of release by alpha receptor, 98ff
ischemia-induced release in heart, 254
overflow into coronary sinus, 86
(presynaptic) negative feedback regulation, 103ff
released from atrium during accentuated antagonism study, 86
Nucleus ambiguus, 27, 37, 39, 350
Nucleus tractus solitarius
baroreflex and, 359, 364
destruction of, effects on conditional cardiovascular response, 400
projections from 349

Orienting response, 392, 398
Oscillator (in CNS)
importance, 313
nature, 315, 355
sympathetic nerve discharge rhythm, 325ff
within brainstem, 346ff
Overdrive suppression, 210ff
Oxygen, utilization by myocardium, *see also* myocardial metabolism
after cardiac denervation, 168, 253ff, 283, 430
during myocardial ischemia, 255
effect of beta-blockade, 167
effect of catecholamines, 165
oxygen "wasting", 165ff, 173ff

P-cells, 200
P-wave
after surgical excision of SA node, 201, 206
shift during stellate stimulation, 62, 65
Pacemaker (cardiac)
A-V junctional, 204
beta receptors and, 113
hierarchy of, 201
history of discovery, 199
overdrive suppression, 210
P-cells, 200
selective parasympathetic denervation of, 56ff
shift from stimulation of interganglionic nerve, 30
shift from stimulation of sympathetic nerves, 210
shift from stimulation of vagus nerve, 80
subsidiary atrial, 199ff
vagal stimulation, effect on, 48, 148
"wandering", 207, 211
Pacemaker potential
effect of vagus nerve stimulation, 70
effect of sympathetic nerve stimulation and catecholamines, 109
iontophoresis of cGMP into sinoatrial node, 139
Pacing (heart rate)
A-V block, 46ff, 74ff, 211, 402
during exercise, 46
during selective SA vs AV nodal parasympathetic denervation, 61
Pain (cardiac), 369ff
"Pale region" (of right atrium), 218
referred, theory of origin, 376
Papillary muscle, 179
referred, theory of origin, 376
neural control of, 179
Paraplegic patient
blood pressure regulation in, 337
Parasympathetic cardiac nerves, *see also* vagus nerve
anatomical projection to heart, 57, 64
basal tone in, basis of, 358ff
brainstem origin, 350
during exercise, 417–418
innervating coronary arteries, 180
selective denervation of, 56ff, 297ff
Pavlov, I. P., *see also* classical conditioning, 4
study of A-V conduction, 77
Pericoronary nerves (anatomy), 180

Pharmacology (α and β receptors), 95ff
Phase response curve, *see* sinoatrial node
Phospholamban, 110, 150, 155
Pigeon
control of heart in, 394ff, 397
Plateau phase (of cardiac action potential)
effect of catecholamines, 109
Platelet aggregation, 448
Postganglionic neurons, 95, 27ff, 40ff, 323
Potassium ion
diminished conductance in SA node during vagal stimulation, 71
effect of muscarinic receptor activation on channel, 137
Preganglionic neurons (parasympathetic), 26ff, 37, 39
Preganglionic neurons (sympathetic), 322ff
Preload, 12
action potentials of, 326
anatomical organization of, 324
convergence of inputs upon, 328
inputs onto, 332ff
silent period in, 328
spontaneous discharge of, 326
Presynaptic receptors, *see* alpha receptors; receptors, presynaptic
Primate, *see* monkey, baboon, man
Principal optic nucleus (pigeon), 397
Prinzmetal angina, *see* vasospasm
Prostaglandins
heterologous regulation of beta receptors, 114
modulation of neurotransmitter release, 98ff, 103
Pulmonary artery nerves, 51
stimulation during cardiac denervation, 54ff
Purkinje system
effect of catecholamines on action potential, 109
effect of acetylcholine on action potential, 148
sympathetic innervation, 95

QT interval
effects of autonomic nerves, 227, 442
long, deafness and, 444
long, pathogenesis of, 232, 444, 451
long, surgical treatment of, 294, 445
sudden infant death, 241

Radioligand binding, 131ff
study of adrenergic receptor types, 96, 97, 101, 110, 112
study of muscarinic receptors, 131ff
Raphe nucleus (brainstem)
control of heart during emotion, 398
Reactive hyperemia (coronary circulation)
effect of left stellectomy on, 188, 234
Receptors (low pressure)
in congestive heart failure, 13
Receptors (muscarinic), *see* muscarinic receptors
Receptors (presynaptic), *see also* alpha receptors, beta receptors
influence on neurotransmitter release (α) 95; (β) 104ff
location of (α) 101
physiological role of (α) 103ff; (β) 106
Reciprocal innervation. 310
Recurrent cardiac nerve
cat (anatomy), 34ff
dog (anatomy), 25ff
monkey (anatomy), 37ff
postganglionic cells of origin, 30
Reentry
neurally induced arrhythmias from, 228ff
Reflex, *see* baroreflex, cardiocardiac reflex, spinal cord
Refractory period
atrioventricular node and A-V conduction, 76
catecholamine effects, 109
vagal effects upon atrial and ventricular, 80ff
Regeneration
of cardiac nerves following denervation, 243
Regional neural ablation, *see* cardiac denervation
Reinnervation (cardiac), 287ff
as limiting factor for clinical use, 294
Relaxation (ventricular)
effect of beta receptor activation on, 108
Renin
in congestive heart failure, 13
Repetitive extrasystole threshold
effect of unilateral stellectomy on, 232
Repolarization, ventricular, 442
Respiration
rhythmic interactions within CNS, 315, 325, 357
Reticular formation, 347ff
Rhythms, *see also* oscillators, sympathetic nerve discharge
generator within brainstem, 347, 356
junctional, 202, 210ff
vagal, 358
Right stellate cardiac nerve, *see* interganglionic nerve

Sarcolemma
locus of muscarinic receptor, 134
Segmental organization (spinal cord), 324
Selective parasympathetic denervation, 56ff
Septal artery, 272
Septum (brain)
control of the heart during emotion, 396
Serotonergic pathways, 349
Sexual intercourse
sudden death during, 18
Shock (circulatory), *see also* hemorrhage

SHR, *see* spontaneously hypertensive rats
Sick sinus syndrome, *see* syndrome, sick sinus
Signs
  Branhams bradycardia, 14
Silent period, *see* preganglionic neurons (sympathetic)
Shunts, 14ff
Sinoatrial node, *see also* artery, sinoatrial
  action potentials of, 70
  entrainment, 71
  history of discovery, 199
  interaction with atrio-ventricular node, 74
  neural control during emotion, 399
  selective parasympathetic denervation of, 58ff
  sick sinus syndrome, 450
  vagal stimulation, 70ff
Slow inward current, *see* current, slow inward
Slow waves, *see also* sympathetic nerve discharge
  cortical potentials correlated with learned HR changes, 396
Sodium ion
  in SA node during vagal stimulation, 71
Spasm, *see* vasospasm
Species differences
  alpha receptors, 101, 107
  beta receptors, 112
  coronary circulation, 182
  muscarinic receptors, 134, 138
  presynaptic inhibition, 104
Spinal cord, *see also* ascending spinal pathways, descending spinal pathways
  anatomical organization, 322
  baroreflex and, 331, 360
  cardiocardiac reflex mediated by, 254, 321ff, 371ff
  convergence of visceral and somatic afferents on, 376
  descending pathways in, 332, 349
  interneurons, sympathetic, 330
  reflexes mediated by, 321, 337, 371
Spontaneously hypertensive rats
  cAMP aberrations in, 115
Starling Law of the Heart, *see* Frank–Starling Law
Stellate cardiac nerve (cat, anatomy), 35
Stellate ganglion
  arrhythmias and, 225ff
  cat (anatomy), 34ff
  dog (anatomy), 22ff
  left stellectomy, treatment of long QT syndrome, 239, 445
  monkey (anatomy), 37ff
  postganglionic sympathetic neurons in, 28ff
  right stellectomy, arrhythmogenetic effects of, 226, 230
  right *vs.* left stellate in etiology of arrhythmias, 227ff
  right *vs.* left stellate influence on coronary blood flow, 191
  stimulation of and A-V block, 47
  stimulation of during cardiac denervation, 54
Stenosis (coronary)
  alpha vasoconstriction during, 257
Stress, *see also* specific examples, 5ff
  as cause of sudden death, 17
Stroke volume
  changes during exercise after cardiac denervation, 283
  during exercise, 414
Subsidiary atrial pacemaker(s)
  action potential recordings from, 217ff
  afterhyperpolarization in, 220
  cardiovascular disease and, 437
  catecholamine dose-response *in vitro*, 216
  hierarchy, 201
  identification, 200
  innervation, 201
  instability, 213
  in vitro study of, 215ff
  location, 202
  neural control, 209
  overdrive suppression of, 210
  "pale region" and, 217ff
  physiology in conscious dog, 206ff
Sudden cardiac death, 4ff, 15ff, 459
  animal models of, 16
  autonomic imbalance and, 49, 225ff
Sudden infant death, *see* syndrome
Sulcus terminalis
  and subsidiary atrial pacemakers, 201, 204
Sun stroke, 7
Sweating, 7ff
Sympathectomy (selective ventricular)
  changes in intermediary metabolism after, 174
  effect on coronary blood flow, 188, 265
  effect on myocardial metabolic efficiency, 169, 172, 265
  reduction in myofibrillar ATPase after, 173
  treatment of angina and vasospasm, 293; arrhythmias, 428
Sympathetic cardiac nerves, *see also* alpha receptors, beta receptors
  activity during learned heart rate changes, 398
  clinical importance of, 435ff
  distribution of coronary vasoconstrictor, 190ff
  during exercise, 414ff, 418ff
  effect on subsidiary atrial pacemaker, 210
  effect on ventricular action potential, 108
  innervating coronary arteries, 179ff, 182ff
  interaction with vagus, 84ff, 380ff
  myocardial ischemia and, 253ff
  patterns of activity in, 244, 398
  selective activation of, 178, 310
  selective distribution to SA *vs.* AV nodes, 62ff
  stimulation during vagal activation, 85
  trophic effects of, 173

Sympathetic cholinergic nerves
anatomy, 324
lacking in the coronary circulation, 183
Sympathetic imbalance, see also autonomic imbalance, dysautonomia
cardiac arrhythmias and, 225, 407, 442
clinical implications, 238
definition, 227
methodological considerations, 244
sudden infant death, 241
Sympathetic nerve discharge, 346ff
genesis of, 352
preganglionic sympathetic neurons and, 325
Sympathetic neurons
adrenergic receptor control of, 98ff
muscarinic control of norepinephrine release, 133
Sympathoexcitation
spinal interneurons and, 330
spinal pathways for, 333
Sympathoinhibition
baroreflex and, 336
spinal interneurons and, 330
Synapses, types of, 309
Synchronization of sympathetic nerve discharge, 355ff
Syndrome
Bradbury–Eggleston, 10
Horner's, 246
Long QT, pathogenesis of, 232, 238
Mitral valve prolapse, 447, 456
Parkinson's, 10
Propranolol withdrawal, 115
Raynaud's arrhythmias in, 230
Riley Day, 10
Shy–Drager, 10
Sick sinus, 200
Sudden Infant Death, 15, 241
Systole
effect of beta and alpha receptor activation on duration, 108

Telencephalon
control of the heart during emoton, 396
Thermal stress, 7ff
Thyroid
regulation of cardiac beta receptors, 116; alpha receptors, 118
hyperthyroidism, 117
Tissue culture
superior ganglion cells for study of presynaptic inhibition, 102
Tissue slice
myocardial metabolism studied using, 171
Torsades de pointe, 239
Tracts (spinal), *see* ascending, descending
Transsynaptic hypothesis, 99
Traub–Hering waves, 315
Troponin—I
influence of cAMP on, 110
Type A and B personality, 5, 16, 408

Vagal death, 4
Vagosympathetic complex (trunk)
cat (anatomy), 34ff
dog (anatomy), 22ff
Vagus nerve, *see also* muscarinic receptor, parasympathetic cardiac nerves
afferent fibers in, 380
alterations in atrial activation pattern, 80
atrial fibrillation, induction of, 439
basal activity in, origin of, 358ff
cat (anatomy), 34ff
comparison of inotropic and chronotropic effect, 83
control of atrioventricular conduction, 74ff, 404
control of coronary blood flow, 181ff
decay of stimulation effects, 84
depression of atrial and ventricular contractility, 81ff, 445
dog (anatomy), 22ff
during exercise, 417–418
effect on subsidiary atrial pacemaker, 210
effects of brief stimuli on atrial contraction, 82
effects of brief stimulation on heart rate, 69ff
interaction with sympathetic nerves, 84ff, 147ff, 380
monkey (anatomy), 37ff
origin of cardiac nerves, 26ff, 350
persistent effects of stimulation, 79
phase-response curve of stimulation effects on heart rate, 71ff
presynaptic modulation of acetylcholine release, 106
shifts in dominant pacemaker site by, 80
stimulation of during cardiac denervation, 48ff, 297
stimulation of, heart rate *vs.* A-V conduction changes, 57
stimulation of during cardiac pacing, 61
stimulation frequency *vs.* heart rate change, 69
stimulation induced hyperpolarization of SA nodal cells, 70
termination of supraventricular arrhythmia by increased activity in, 130
transection, effects of, 297
Vasoconstriction
neural basis of, 327
Vasospasm (coronary), 18, 178
cardiac denervation, effect of, 49, 427
clinical evidence for, 189
nature of, 178, 448
role of nerves in, 181, 256, 448
treatment, 243, 293
Velocity of contraction
oxygen consumption, 166
Ventral lateral cardiac nerve
arrhythmogenetic properties of, 227, 407
cat (anatomy), 36

dog (anatomy), 26, 50
monkey, *see* lateral sympathetic nerve
Ventral medial nerve (cat, anatomy), 37
Ventricular contractile force
accentuated antagonism and control of, 86
control in awake subject, 401, 414ff
effect of muscarinic receptor activation, 137
response to nerve stimulation during cardiac denervation, 55
vagal influences, 81, 440
Ventricular escape, 61
Ventricular fibrillation
after ventricular denervation, 297
as cause of sudden death, 15, 460
increased incidence following right stellectomy, 230
induced by cardiac nerves, 229, 440
Ventricular fibrillation threshold
effect of sympathetic nerves, 232, 428
Ventricular function curves
after cardiac autotransplantation in dog, 170
shift due to vagus nerve stimulation, 81
Ventricular refractoriness
sympathetic and parasympathetic influences on, 235
Ventricular tachycardia
cardiac denervation, effect of, 49
Ventrolateral cardiac nerve, *see* ventral lateral cardiac nerve
Ventrolateral nucleus ambiguus
as origin of cardiac vagal nerves, 27, 39
Veratrum alkaloids
reflex coronary vasodilation after injection of, 182
Viscerosomatic convergence, 376ff
Voltage clamp
study of slow inward current, 138

Wandering pacemaker (P-wave), *see* pacemaker
Wenckebach phenomenon, 76